# Outcome Measures and Metrics in Systemic Lupus Erythematosus

Zahi Touma
Editor

# Outcome Measures and Metrics in Systemic Lupus Erythematosus

Springer

*Editor*
Zahi Touma
Medicine
University of Toronto
Toronto, ON
Canada

ISBN 978-3-030-73302-5 ISBN 978-3-030-73303-2 (eBook)
https://doi.org/10.1007/978-3-030-73303-2



This Springer imprint is published by the registered company Springer Nature Switzerland AG
The registered company address is: Gewerbestrasse 11, 6330 Cham, Switzerland

# Preface

Systemic lupus erythematosus (SLE) is a chronic autoimmune disease that manifests with a myriad of clinical and laboratory features. The assessment of SLE is comprehensive and includes different core set domains: disease activity, damage, health-related quality of life, adverse events, and economic impact.

This book is focused on the metrics and outcome measures utilized in the assessment of SLE. It targets different audiences including physicians, scientists/researchers, and other health professionals interested in learning about the art of measurement in SLE.

The book highlights the importance of measurement in the assessment of SLE in a clinical setting, research, and clinical trials. Each of the chapters provides a systematic approach to the measures utilized in the assessment of a specific construct in SLE (e.g., disease activity and fatigue) and incorporates a comprehensive coverage of disease-specific and disease-generic measures. This book also discusses different patient-reported outcomes that are crucial to reflect patient perceptions of their health condition and cover constructs such as fatigue, pain, anxiety and depression, cognition, frailty, and many others.

Researchers will find this book very useful to understand different measures in SLE and it will help them to choose the appropriate instrument.

We hope readers will enjoy the content of this book. An immense acknowledgment to the authors who contributed to this book despite their very busy schedule during this unprecedented pandemic due to COVID-19.

Toronto, ON, Canada Zahi Touma

# Acknowledgment

Dr. Touma is supported by funding from the Arthritis Society, Young Investigator Award and the Canadian Rheumatology Association (CIORA) - Arthritis Society Clinician Investigator Award and by the Department of Medicine, University of Toronto. Dr. Touma's laboratory is supported by donations from the Kathi and Peter Kaiser family, the Lou and Marissa Rocca family and the Bozzo family.

May Y. Choi is supported by the Lupus Foundation of America Gary S. Gilkeson Career Development Award.

# Contents

# Contributors

**Janice Abbott** School of Psychology, University of Central Lancashire, Preston, UK

**Prabjit Ajrawat** University of Toronto, Division of Rheumatology, Department of Medicine, Toronto, ON, Canada

**Martin Aringer** Division of Rheumatology, Department of Medicine III, University Medical Center and Faculty of Medicine at the TU Dresden, Dresden, Germany

**Pinar Ozge Avar-Aydin** Department of Pediatric Rheumatology, Ankara University School of Medicine, Ankara, Turkey

**Megan R. W. Barber** Division of Rheumatology, Department of Medicine, Cumming School of Medicine, University of Calgary, Calgary, AB, Canada

**Dorcas E. Beaton** Institute for Work & Health, Toronto, ON, Canada

**Kathleen Bingham** Centre for Mental Health, University Health Network, Department of Psychiatry, University of Toronto, Toronto, ON, Canada

**Hermine I. Brunner** Department of Rheumatology, Cincinnati Children's Hospital Medical Center, Cincinnati, OH, USA

**Madhura Castelino** Department of Rheumatology, University College London Hospital NHS Foundation Trust, London, UK

Centre for Musculoskeletal Research, University of Manchester, Manchester, UK

**Yashaar Chaichian** Division of Immunology & Rheumatology, Department of Medicine, Stanford University School of Medicine, Stanford, CA, USA

**May Y. Choi** Cumming School of Medicine, University of Calgary, Calgary, AB, Canada

**Ann E. Clarke** Division of Rheumatology, Department of Medicine, Cumming School of Medicine, University of Calgary, Calgary, AB, Canada

**Stephanie Ensworth** Division of Rheumatology, Department of Medicine, Faculty of Medicine, University of British Columbia, Vancouver, BC, Canada

**Titilola Falasinnu** Department of Epidemiology & Population Health, and Department of Anesthesiology, Perioperative and Pain Medicine, Stanford University School of Medicine, Stanford, CA, USA

**Marvin J. Fritzler** Cumming School of Medicine, University of Calgary, Calgary, AB, Canada

**Dafna D. Gladman** Centre for Prognosis Studies in the Rheumatic Diseases, University Health Network, Toronto, ON, Canada

**Ambika Gupta** Division of Rheumatology, Department of Medicine, University of Toronto, Toronto, ON, Canada

**John G. Hanly** Division of Rheumatology, Department of Medicine, and Department of Pathology, Dalhousie University and Queen Elizabeth II Health Sciences Centre, Halifax, NS, Canada

**Sindhu R. Johnson** Division of Rheumatology, Department of Medicine, Toronto Western Hospital, Mount Sinai Hospital, Toronto, ON, Canada

Institute of Health Policy, Management and Evaluation, University of Toronto, Toronto, ON, Canada

**Mahta Kakvan** University of Toronto Lupus Clinic, Centre for Prognosis Studies in Rheumatic Diseases, Toronto Western Hospital, Toronto, ON, Canada

**Diane L. Kamen** Division of Rheumatology, Medical University of South Carolina, Charleston, SC, USA

**Patricia P. Katz** University of California San Francisco, Department of Medicine and Institute for Health Policy Studies, San Francisco, CA, USA

**Stephanie Keeling** Division of Rheumatology, Department of Medicine, University of Alberta, Edmonton, AB, Canada

**Alfred H. J. Kim** Division of Rheumatology, Department of Medicine, Washington University School of Medicine, St. Louis, MO, USA

**Andrew Kwan** University of Toronto, Department of Medicine, Toronto, ON, Canada

**Diane Lacaille** Division of Rheumatology, Department of Medicine, University of British Columbia, Vancouver, BC, Canada

**Alexandra Legge** Division of Rheumatology, Department of Medicine, Dalhousie University and Queen Elizabeth II Health Sciences Centre, Halifax, NS, Canada

**Jerik Leung** Department of Behavioral Science and Health Education, College for Public Health and Social Justice, Saint Louis University, St. Louis, MO, USA

**Deborah M. Levy** Division of Rheumatology, The Hospital for Sick Children, University of Toronto, Toronto, ON, Canada

**Lily S. H. Lim** Section of Rheumatology, Department of Paediatrics and Child Health, Children's Hospital Research Institute of Manitoba, University of Manitoba, Winnipeg, MB, Canada

**Mark Matsos** McMaster University, Division of Rheumatology, Department of Medicine, Hamilton, ON, Canada

**Kathleen McElhone** Division of Musculoskeletal and Dermatological Sciences, University of Manchester, Manchester, UK

**Taneisha K. McGhie** Department of Medicine, University of the West Indies-Mona, Kingston 7, Jamaica

**Lily McMorrow** Division of Rheumatology, Department of Medicine, Washington University School of Medicine, St. Louis, MO, USA

**Mandana Nikpour** Department of Medicine at St Vincent's Hospital, The University of Melbourne, Parkville, VIC, Australia

Department of Rheumatology, St Vincent's Hospital, Fitzroy, VIC, Australia

**Behdin Nowrouzi-Kia** Department of Occupational Science and Occupational Therapy, Temerty Faculty of Medicine, University of Toronto, Toronto, ON, Canada

**Shereen Oon** Department of Medicine at St Vincent's Hospital, The University of Melbourne, Parkville, VIC, Australia

Department of Rheumatology, St Vincent's Hospital, Fitzroy, VIC, Australia

Department of Rheumatology, The Royal Melbourne Hospital, Parkville, VIC, Australia

**Christine Peschken** University of Manitoba, Department of Medicine, Winnipeg, MB, Canada

**Janet Pope** Division of Rheumatology, Department of Medicine, University of Western Ontario, London, ON, Canada

**Nathalie Rozenbojm** University of Toronto Lupus Clinic, Centre for Prognosis Studies in Rheumatic Diseases, Toronto Western Hospital, Toronto, ON, Canada

**Jorge Sanchez-Guerrero** Division of Rheumatology, Sinai Health System/ University Health Network, University of Toronto, Toronto, ON, Canada

**Katherine Schultz** Department of Rheumatology, Cincinnati Children's Hospital Medical Center, Cincinnati, OH, USA

**Julia F. Simard** Department of Epidemiology & Population Health, and Division of Immunology & Rheumatology, Department of Medicine, Stanford University School of Medicine, Stanford, CA, USA

**Lee S. Simon** SDG, LLC, Cambridge, MA, USA

**Vibeke Strand** Division of Immunology & Rheumatology, Department of Medicine, Stanford University School of Medicine, Palo Alto, CA, USA

**Herman H. Y. Tam** Division of Rheumatology, British Columbia Children's Hospital, University of British Columbia, Vancouver, BC, Canada

**Oshrat E. Tayer-Shifman** Department of Internal Medicine and Rheumatology Service, Meir Medical Center, Kfar Saba, Israel

**Lee-Suan Teh** Department of Rheumatology, Royal Blackburn Teaching Hospital, Blackburn, UK

Faculty of Clinical and Biomedical Sciences, University of Central Lancashire (UCLan), Preston, UK

**Taraneh Tofighi** Faculty of Medicine, University of Toronto, Toronto, ON, Canada

**Zahi Touma** Centre for Prognosis in Rheumatic Disease, Toronto Lupus Clinic, Division of Rheumatology, Department of Medicine, Institute of Health Policy, Management and Evaluation, University of Toronto, Toronto, ON, Canada

University of Toronto Lupus Clinic, Centre for Prognosis Studies in Rheumatic Diseases, Toronto Western Hospital, Toronto, ON, Canada

**Konstantinos Tselios** Centre for Prognosis Studies in the Rheumatic Diseases, University Health Network, Toronto, ON, Canada

**Murray B. Urowitz** Centre for Prognosis Studies in the Rheumatic Diseases, University Health Network, Toronto, ON, Canada

University of Toronto Lupus Clinic; Centre for Prognosis Studies in the Rheumatic Diseases, Toronto Western Hospital, Toronto, ON, Canada

**Evelyne Vinet** Divisions of Rheumatology & Clinical Epidemiology, McGill University Health Centre, Montreal, QC, Canada

**Joan E. Wither** Schroeder Arthritis Institute, University Health Network, University of Toronto, Toronto, ON, Canada

**Kimberley Yuen** Queen's University School of Medicine, Kingston, ON, Canada

**Eric Zollars** Division of Rheumatology, Medical University of South Carolina, Charleston, SC, USA

# Chapter 1
# Introduction: Metrics and Domains Measured in SLE

**Taneisha K. McGhie, Dorcas E. Beaton, Diane Lacaille, Joan E. Wither, Jorge Sanchez-Guerrero, and Zahi Touma**

## Introduction

Systemic lupus erythematosus (SLE) is an autoimmune, chronic multisystem disease that is characterized by remissions and exacerbations. The SLE disease waxes and wanes, and patients often experience recurrent flares during the course of their disease. While some patients may achieve a remission of disease activity, others continue to experience persistently active disease (PAD) [1–3]. The management of

T. K. McGhie
Department of Medicine, University of the West Indies-Mona, Kingston 7, Jamaica

D. E. Beaton
Institute for Work & Health, Toronto, ON, Canada
e-mail: Dbeaton@iwh.on.ca

D. Lacaille
Division of Rheumatology, Department of Medicine, University of British Columbia, Vancouver, BC, Canada
e-mail: dlacaille@arthritisresearch.ca

J. E. Wither
Schroeder Arthritis Institute, University Health Network, University of Toronto, Toronto, ON, Canada
e-mail: Joan.Wither@uhnresearch.ca

J. Sanchez-Guerrero
Division of Rheumatology, Sinai Health System/University Health Network, University of Toronto, Toronto, ON, Canada
e-mail: Jorge.Sanchez-Guerrero@sinaihealth.ca

Z. Touma (✉)
Centre for Prognosis in Rheumatic Disease, Toronto Lupus Clinic, Division of Rheumatology, Department of Medicine, Institute of Health Policy, Management and Evaluation, University of Toronto, Toronto, ON, Canada
e-mail: zahi.touma@uhn.ca

 
Z. Touma (ed.), *Outcome Measures and Metrics in Systemic Lupus Erythematosus*, https://doi.org/10.1007/978-3-030-73303-2_1

SLE is complex, and patients often develop irreversible damage over the course of their disease, and the accrual of damage over time is proportional to the cumulative burden of disease activity [4]. In addition, patients can experience health consequences from adverse events of medications. Together, disease activity, damage, and adverse events from medications impact patient health-related quality of life. In clinical practice and research settings, it is crucial to achieve an appropriate monitoring of all these constructs, and this can be facilitated with the use of validated and reliable measures in SLE [4, 5].

In 1987, a group of 15 rheumatologists with expertise in SLE met at the University of Birmingham (Birmingham, England), supported by a research grant from the North Atlantic Treaty Organization (NATO). The object of the exercise was to determine the type of instruments that would be required to obtain a complete assessment of patients with SLE during the course of randomized clinical trials and long-term observational studies. Several members of this group had already developed disease activity instruments of their own, but it was concluded that the core domains needed were a disease activity instrument, a damage instrument, and a patient perception instrument which should be determined to be valid and reliable. This was the genesis of the concept of SLE-related domains. The NATO group enlarged subsequently into the Systemic Lupus International Collaborating Clinics (SLICC). This group led the development of the SLICC/American College of Rheumatology (ACR) Damage index (SDI).

## Core Set of Domains in SLE, Classification, and Response Criteria

In 1998, the SLE working group led the Outcome Measure in Rheumatology (OMERACT) international consensus collaboration through an evaluation of 21 different domains that were candidates for inclusion in clinical trials of SLE. At that meeting, the OMERACT community recommended five domains for an appropriate assessment of patients with SLE in randomized controlled trials (RCTs) and longitudinal observational studies (LOS): (1) disease activity, (2) chronic damage resulting from lupus activity or its treatment, (3) health-related quality of life (HRQoL), (4) adverse events, and (5) economic impact [6]. To date, there is no universal agreement as to the "gold standard" instrument to be used in any of the five domains in SLE.

One of the subcommittees of the ACR Quality of Care Committee is the ACR Subcommittee on Classification and Response Criteria which provides guidance on the methods required for the development and validation of such criteria sets [7]. This subcommittee works in conjunction with the European League Against Rheumatism (EULAR) on several projects to facilitate ACR/EULAR endorsement of newly developed classification and response criteria. An example of this rigorous process is the recently developed EULAR/ACR SLE classification criteria [8].

Response criteria (disease state and change in disease state) are very important in clinical trials and facilitate the demonstration of efficacy of new drugs [9].

**Why Is It Important to Incorporate Core Clinical Outcomes and Their Measures into Practices?**

(i) *Clinical practice*: In clinical practice, they provide dynamic data on disease status that informs clinical care in ways that can directly relate to attaining evidence-based guideline directed goals, for example, remission. As such, goal-directed care can be modified appropriately as per the treat-to-target paradigm.

(ii) *Clinical trials*: Standardized ways of measuring core domains with evidence of good performance in key psychometric properties for use in the SLE population are crucial for conducting multicenter clinical trials, particularly for investigating the effectiveness of novel therapeutic agents and for comparison of existing management strategies. A core set of outcomes reduces research waste and assures communication between trials.

(iii) *Communication*: The effective and efficient communication among practitioners for shared learning and among collaborators in research is facilitated by measures serving as a common language.

(iv) *Patient engagement*: Improved patient engagement in clinical care may be facilitated by measures, particularly when they are meaningful to them and their lived experiences. Measurement outcome instruments serve as information that may be presented to patients to enable them to make informed decisions about treatment choices.

(v) *Regulatory bodies*: Measurements may have a direct impact on the pharmacological management of SLE at the individual patient level as increasingly, measures are being linked to regulatory frameworks governing drug coverage accessibility. Focusing on certain instruments could help researchers develop a body of evidence to allow it to be considered fit for purpose in clinical trials of drug development and product labels.

(vi) *Self-appraisal for the health-care team*: On an individual practitioner level, the consistent use of measures allows for self-appraisal of quality and outcome of care delivered by stimulating mindful reflection on what is being done well and what needs to be changed. This process of self-appraisal should inspire the clinician's aspiration and development [8].

(vii) *Quality improvement*: On a system level, documented measures provide a readily available trove of historical and current data. Having access to both allows for the identification of gaps which, when filled, will enable the achievement of improvement to the existing strategies. Data generated by measurements in SLE serve as resources that instruct quality improvement initiatives.

Overall, instruments help to focus attention on what is important that may be overlooked amidst the noise of myriad disease manifestations and associated clinical challenges in the day-to-day management of SLE. Ultimately measurements in

SLE should continuously advance our understanding of a very complex disease, its patterns and processes in different patient populations.

The heterogeneity of SLE clinical phenotypes' presentations, the variability of the disease course between patients overtime (monophasic, relapsing-remitting, and persistently active), and the variability in the severity of disease activity within a patient overtime (from mild to moderate and severe disease activity) have made finding a unifying metric of disease activity very challenging. Current randomized trials [6, 10] have recognized the need to encompass a variety of measures to capture all the facets of the constructs being measured (e.g., SLE disease activity, damage, or HRQoL).

We will now review the status of each of the recommended core domains.

## Core Domain 1: Disease Activity

Disease activity in rheumatic diseases including SLE can be defined as a "reversible state, manifested by clinical, laboratory or radiographical features" [11, 12]. Disease activity primarily reflects the immunologic and inflammatory processes associated with SLE and involves a specific organ or multiple organs at a specific point in time [11, 12].

The multifaceted nature of clinical presentations in adults as well as pediatric patients makes the assessment of SLE disease activity challenging, and this requires the use of valid, reliable, and interpretable instruments. The use of disease activity instruments enables clinicians, patients, and researchers to quantify and evaluate disease activity in a standardized way [13, 14].

The application of these instruments in clinical care and research settings presents several challenges, namely, administrative and cost burden of the instrument. Other factors also play an important role when deciding on the use of a specific instrument: the preparedness and skillfulness of the assessor on a specific instrument, the mode of administration of instruments (copied forms, software programs, or both), the time required to complete the measure and whether it is self-administered or requires a facilitator to administer it, and sometimes the complexity of scoring. All of these factors need to be taken into consideration when choosing instruments applicable in a particular setting [15, 16].

Whether in clinical practice or in research settings, the ability to measure and grade SLE disease activity is fundamental to the management of patients and to the study of the disease. The most efficient way of assessing disease activity is to choose validated measures for this purpose with an appropriate glossary and scoring instructions [10]. The main two categories of disease activity measures which have been developed are global measures which describe the overall burden of SLE disease and organ-specific instruments which describe disease activity within each organ system (Chap. 6) [5].

Table 1.1 summarizes the instruments developed to assess disease activity in SLE. They are all valid, reliable, and responsive measures that have been shown to

**Table 1.1** Assessment of lupus by five domains

| Domains | Tools | Where developed | Score range | Time frame | Refs |
|---|---|---|---|---|---|
| *Disease activity* | | | | | |
| SLEDAI, its versions and modifications | SLEDAI | Toronto | 0–105 (low to high disease activity) | Last 10 days | [11] |
| | SLEDAI-2K | Toronto | 0–105 | Last 10 days | [17] |
| | SLEDAI-2K 30 days | Toronto | 0–105 | Last 30 days | [18, 19] |
| | MEX-SLEDAI | Mexico | 0–32 | Last 10 days | [20, 21] |
| | SELENA-SLEDAI[a] | Study investigators[a] | 0–105 | Last 10 days | [22] |
| SRI-50 | SRI-50 (S2K RI-50) | Toronto | 0–105 | Last 30 days | [23–25] |
| SLEDAI-2K glucocorticoid index | SLEDAI-2KG | Toronto | 0–113 | Last 30 days | [14, 26] |
| BILAG and its version | BILAG | United Kingdom | Categories A-E[b] | Previous month | [27, 28] |
| | BILAG 2004 | United Kingdom | Categories A-E[b] | Previous month | [29] |
| SLAM and its versions | SLAM | Boston | 0–86 | Previous month | [30] |
| | SLAM-R | Boston | 0–81 | Previous month | [31, 32] |
| | SLAQ | | 0–44 | Previous month | [33] |
| ECLAM | ECLAM | European Union Concerted | 0–17.5 | Previous month | [34–36] |
| LAI | LAI | UCSF, Hopkins | 0–3 | Last 2 weeks | [37] |
| SIS | SIS | NIH | 0–52 | Last week | [38] |
| RIFLE | RIFLE | | | | [39] |
| *Damage* | | | | | |
| Physician completed | SDI | SLICC/ACR | 0–49 (low to high disease activity) | Present for 6 months | [40] |
| Patients completed | LDIQ<br>LDIQ Spanish, Portuguese, and French | | | Present for 6 months | [41, 42] |

(continued)

**Table 1.1** (continued)

| Domains | Tools | Where developed | Score range | Time frame | Refs |
|---|---|---|---|---|---|
| *HRQOL* | | | | | |
| Generic | SF-36 | Boston, MA | 0–100 (8 domains – higher score = better health state) | Previous month | [43] |
| Specific | LupusQoL<br>LupusQoL-US<br>LupusQoL Spanish (Dutch, French, Greek, Italian, Hyperion, Portuguese, and Chinese) | Blackburn, UK<br>Chicago, USA<br>Spain | 0–100<br>0–100<br>0–100 | Previous month<br>Previous month<br>Previous month | [44–46] |
| | SLE Symptom Checklist (SSC) (Dutch and English) | Netherland | | Previous month | [47] |
| | SLE specific Quality of Life instrument (SLEQOL) (English, Portuguese, and Chinese) | Singapore | | Previous month | [48] |
| | L-QoL (English, Hungarian, and Turkish) | UK | | Previous month | [49] |
| *Adverse events* | | | | | |
| | As reported by patients and/or determined by physicians | | | | |
| *Economic costs and impact* | | | | | |
| | Direct/indirect costs, work productivity | | | | |

[a]The Safety of Estrogen in Lupus National Assessment – Systemic Lupus Erythematosus Disease Activity Index (SELENA-SLEDAI) flare index developed by the Study investigators in the Safety of Estrogen in Lupus Erythematosus-National Assessment Trial using a modified version of SLEDAI includes flare assessment and Physician's Global Assessment (PGA)
[b]BILAG 2004 grade: A = Active (severe), B=Beware (moderate), C=Contentment (mild), D=Discount (inactive but previously affected), E = No Evidence (inactive with no previous involvement)

correlate with each other despite there being significant differences between them [5, 8]. A key feature of all of these instruments is the attribution of the manifestations to SLE.

Disease activity measures allow for the determination of "clinically meaningful change" in the disease state representing either a flare or an improvement. Flare is considered one of the most commonly used outcome endpoints of disease activity where the goal is to hold disease in a steady state. Flare can be determined by various instruments. Although flare has been considered the most commonly used outcome endpoint to describe worsening disease activity, persistent active disease

(PAD) also is a common and clinically relevant disease state in patients with active disease and is often used in clinical and research settings [2, 5].

Recent SLE drug trials have evolved to define responders to treatment based on composite indices. Composite indices encompass different components of measurements of disease activity in SLE. A responder index in SLE integrates several relatively independent measures of disease activity into a single construct that defines a patient as either a responder or non-responder [6]. The SLE Responder Index (SRI) is a validated composite measure for disease activity which was introduced in 2009 based on data from belimumab phase II SLE trial [50]. Currently SRI is one of the most commonly used composite indices in SLE drug trials. Chapters 6, 7, 18, and 19 delve into the development of all the current disease activity instruments and variants thereof, their components including scoring, along with appraisal of psychometric properties.

## Core Domain 2: Chronic Damage Resulting from Lupus Activity or Its Treatment

Whereas disease activity is a measure of reversible manifestations of SLE, damage refers to irreversible occurrences. Damage is defined as an "irreversible change in an organ or system that has occurred since the onset of SLE," which can often be attributed to either the disease process or its sequelae [51].

Over the past decades, we have witnessed a remarkable improvement in the survival of SLE patients [52–54]. This may have been facilitated by several factors such as increased knowledge about the pathogenesis of the disease and its manifestations, improvement in the management of SLE disease activity and associated comorbidities, as well as management of chronic irreversible damage that lupus patients accrue over time. The diagnosis of lupus was linked to high mortality in the first half of the twentieth century, but recent studies have shown a drastic improvement in standardized mortality ratio (SMR) – SMR have decreased from 12.6 during the early 1970s to 3.5 in the first decade of the twenty-first century [53].

As SLE patients are living longer, they are accruing organ damage secondary to the disease process itself and to its therapy particularly glucocorticoids (GC). Studies confirmed that patients with severe disease (which is often linked to a higher doses of glucocorticoids) accrue damage faster compared to patients with mildly active disease or disease in remission [55–57] Thus, achieving remission or low disease activity is fundamental to preventing damage in SLE patients and the attendant increased morbidity and mortality [12, 51].

The need for a reliable and valid measure for damage was recognized as a priority by expert investigators in the field of SLE during the Conference of Prognosis Studies in SLE in 1985 [58]. This ultimately led to the publication of the Systemic Lupus International Collaborating Clinics/American College of Rheumatology (SLICC/ACR) damage index (SDI) in 1996 [40]. SDI items reflect irreversible damage occurring after the diagnosis of SLE, and for some items damage has to be present for at least 6 months to be included in the score. Accrued damage on SDI is permanent and the score cannot decrease. This valid and reliable index captures the fact that patients continue to accrue damage over time [59, 60]. The SDI has allowed for the standardized measurement of damage in clinical practice and in clinical trials where it has become an independent outcome measure (Chap. 7) [51, 61].

## Disease Activity and Damage in Special Circumstances: Childhood and Pregnancy

### *Childhood*

Many of the disease activity measures used in adults with SLE have been used in children with the disease, although none were developed specifically for this purpose. In light of this, the Pediatric Rheumatology International Trials Organization (PRINTO) and the ACR Provisional Criteria for the Evaluation of Response to Therapy for children with childhood SLE sought to prospectively validate proposed criteria for the evaluation of response in children with SLE [62].

The activity and damage instruments commonly used to assess disease burden in juvenile systemic lupus erythematosus (JSLE) are the SLEDAI, BILAG, and SLAM. All three tools were found to be valid and reliable and showed responsiveness in pediatric patients [63]. The European Consensus Lupus Activity Measurement (ECLAM) was also found to have construct validity in JSLE and is sensitive to clinically important change in disease activity [64]. Subsequently the modified SLEDAI-2K, a SLEDAI variant, was tested and found to have a high correlation with ECLAM indicating that both tools can be/may be useful for longitudinal estimates of JSLE activity [65]. To date, there is no gold standard for disease activity measurement in JSLE or adult SLE.

Regarding assessment of damage, the SDI has some limitations for application in the pediatric age group. One of the main concerns is the inability to capture some forms of damage that are unique to children and adolescents such as growth failure [63]. A modified version of the SDI (Ped-SDI) has been proposed for use in pediatric patients (Chap. 8).

### *Pregnancy*

SLE primarily affects women in their reproductive years and requires special management, with the aim of controlling maternal disease activity and avoiding fetomaternal complications. The disease impact on pregnancy largely relates to the extent of active inflammation at the time of conception. The effect of pregnancy on disease flares in SLE was recently estimated using data from a large cohort of pregnant and non-pregnant women with lupus [66]. In keeping with previous study results, the incidence of flare was found to be increased during pregnancy. Additionally, the rate of flare was also increased within 3 months postpartum [66].

Therefore, objective assessment of disease activity is crucial for the best management of pregnant SLE patients, and international guidelines have emphasized the need to objectively assess disease activity before and during any pregnancy using validated indices [67]. However, the physiological changes related to pregnancy may influence symptoms and laboratory parameters used in conventional disease activity measures and thus attribution to active lupus. As such, since 1999, several lupus activity instruments have been adapted for use during pregnancy, in particular, the Systemic Lupus Erythematosus Pregnancy Disease Activity Index (SLEPDAI), the modified SLAM (m-SLAM) index, and the lupus activity index in pregnancy (LAI-P). Demonstrating validity of all of these modifications is key to future use of these measures in research [68, 69]. Chapter 9 dedicated to childhood/adolescence aspects of SLE and pregnancy addresses unifying characteristics of these distinct populations while covering monitoring and disease metrics.

## Core Domain 3: Health-Related Quality of Life

Several definitions of HRQoL exist, and clinical researchers agree that HRQoL is a multidimensional construct [70]. Most definitions of HRQoL refer to "the impact that the disease and its treatment have on an individual's ability to function and his or her perceived well-being in physical, mental, and social domains of life" [44]. For example, fatigue, day-to-day functioning, sleep, general appearance, anxiety and depression, the fear of future, and the inability to plan ahead are particular concerns of SLE patients [71, 72].

Though over the last four decades the survival of patients with SLE has improved significantly and SMR also decreased, several studies have shown that SLE-related physical, psychological, emotional, and social burdens are associated with remarkable worsening of patients' HRQoL [66, 70]. In fact, HRQoL in SLE patients is lower compared with matched healthy control subjects or patients with other chronic diseases and is associated with a high prevalence of disability (25–57%) [73] and unemployment (59%) [74]. Importantly, disease effects on HRQoL are often considered of greater overall importance to patients with SLE than many other aspects of their disease [71].

Many of the components of the HRQoL domain are invisible to the clinician and dependent on patient reporting and are therefore better captured using patient-reported outcomes (PROs). This invisibility combined with the heterogeneous manifestations of SLE and its variable clinical course render the measurement of HRQoL challenging. Chapters 11 and 12 provide details on the measures of HRQoL in SLE.

The measurement of HRQOL, or its components, is accomplished using a patient-reported outcome. Patient-reported outcomes (PROs) complement the assessment of SLE and are very important to highlight patients' perceptions of their health conditions. PROs are essential in the assessment of HRQoL: pain, fatigue, anxiety, depression, physical function, cognitive function, and others [75, 76]. Current PROs can be grouped as generic questionnaires and SLE-specific questionnaires (see Table 1.1). Generic questionnaires such as the Medical Outcomes Study Short-Form 36-item Health Survey (SF-36) [44] are limited in their ability to assess issues important to SLE patients (such as sleep, sexual function, and body image) [77]. To overcome these limitations, lupus-specific HRQoL questionnaires have been developed to describe the specific impact of SLE on patients' everyday life. Some of these SLE-specific questionnaires published in the literature include the lupus quality-of-life (LupusQoL) instrument and its versions, the SLE symptom checklist (SSC) and the SLE-specific quality-of-life (SLEQoL) instrument, Lupus-specific Patient-Reported Outcomes measure (LupusPRO), and lupus impact tracker (LIT) [47–49, 78, 79]. OMERACT has recommended the inclusion of both generic and disease-specific instruments in the assessment of HRQoL in patients with SLE.

The US Food and Drug Administration (FDA) guidance for PRO measures maps the road to support labelling claims for new treatments [80]. It provides an appropriate guide on the methodology and evidence required in this process and highlights the psychometric properties of the measures in the studied population (e.g., SLE) (content validity, reliability, construct validity, and responsiveness of the measure). A recent review evaluated these measurement properties for three tools: SF-36, LupusQoL, and functional assessment of chronic illness therapy-fatigue scale (FACIT-F) [75] (Fig. 1.1). It demonstrated that the available evidence for the psychometric properties of SF-36, LupusQoL, and FACIT-F in patients with SLE supports the use of these instruments as secondary endpoints to support labelling claims in RCTs evaluating the efficacy of treatments for SLE [75].

Additionally, low correlations were identified between PRO measures (SF-36, LupusQol, and FACIT-F) and disease activity and damage measures (SLEDAI, BILAG, SDI, and others) [75]. This underscores the usefulness of PROs as tools that complement the assessment and management of patients with SLE.

Other recent explorations of PROs involved the examination of the National Institutes of Health's (NIH's) Patient-Reported Outcomes Measurement Information System (PROMIS) measures in adult SLE. PROMIS measures encompass several SLE domains (e.g., pain, fatigue, and physical functioning) as well as domains that are relevant and important to patients with SLE (e.g., social functioning and sleep) [81]. Katz et al. examined the longitudinal performance of PROMIS measures and showed adequate responsiveness to changes in related PROs and identified meaningful changes to aid in interpretation of scores [81]. The results of this study contribute additional evidence on the validity of PROMIS in SLE.

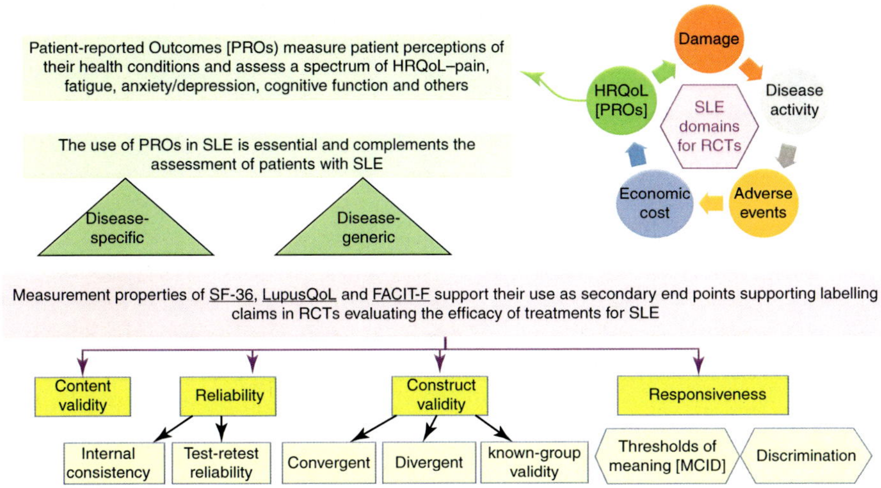


**Fig. 1.1** The measurement properties of selected patient-reported outcome measures with published data from RCTs and longitudinal observational studies. RCTs randomized controlled trials, HRQoL health-related quality of life, SF-36 Medical Outcomes Survey Short-Form 36, LupusQoL Lupus Quality of Life questionnaire, FACIT-F Functional Assessment of Chronic Illness Therapy-Fatigue Scale, MCID minimal clinically important difference

PROs in general are explored in Chap. 11. Chapter 12 covers the relevant instruments for measurement of the HRQoL domain.

## Core Domains 4: Adverse Events of Drugs

Toxicity, safety, and tolerability are essential elements to be assessed in facilitating patient risk/benefit analysis and therefore decision-making on interventions (medications, procedures, etc.). Nevertheless, the measures to quantify these constructs are underdeveloped compared to efficacy measures [82].

In clinical practice, clinicians and patients are often faced with the challenge of choosing between drugs of equivalent efficacy by taking into consideration various potential adverse effects (AEs) for a specific drug. However, mainly because of an absence of head-to-head trials and AE data, the comparative safety of drugs used in SLE is largely unknown [83].

Clinical decision-making should be supported by an objective assessment of the balance of harm compared with the apparent benefit. However, a major obstacle to that is the absence of a measurement instrument designed specifically for this purpose.

The Safety Working Group of OMERACT (previously called the Drug Safety Working Group, but now the mandate has been broadened to all types of interventions) continues to lead the drive to develop patient-derived measures for assessing safety components of interventions in rheumatology [84, 85].

## Core Domain 5: Economic Impact

SLE is associated with substantial economic burden which may vary with specific treatments or vary by disease severity and disease manifestations. The economic toll will also vary between geographic locations depending on the level of disparity in the needs of patients with SLE and the resources available. Furthermore, financial climates are ever-changing dynamic processes. In that regard, one has only to observe the financial fallout of the unprecedented COVID-19 pandemic unfolding during the writing of this book though it represents an extreme and unusual global scenario.

The measurement of the economic impact of SLE is critically important, and studies have highlighted the association of socioeconomic status with long-term survival in patients with SLE [86].

Although complex to measure, the different components of economic impact are well-defined and measurable. The "direct costs" capture "expenditures for diagnosis, treatment, continuing care and rehabilitation" [87]. "Indirect costs" are the costs resulting from "loss of productivity resulting from the illness (diminished labor market and non-labor or household activity)" [87]. Several utility measures such as the EuroQoL's EQ-5D instrument and the Health Utilities Index Mark III (HUI) have been used in the assessment of quality-adjusted life years and in evaluating cost utility of treatments to inform health policies [87].

The impact of SLE on patients' HRQoL, self-esteem, family and marital relationships, and psychosocial health refers to "intangible cost" [88]. The intangible costs associated with SLE are difficult to evaluate, and most studies focus mainly on the assessment of HRQoL as a state of health in that regard.

Several studies have examined the costs associated with SLE [4, 88–90]. Early studies have shown that SLE is associated with high health-care costs and significant productivity loss which impact patients' quality of life [88, 91]. Health-care costs have been found to be higher in patients with a long disease duration, high SLE disease activity and damage, the presence of lupus nephritis, poor physical and mental health, and high education and employment level [88, 90, 92, 93].

Recently, a multistate model was used to describe costs specifically associated with damage states across the SLE disease course. Ten-year cumulative costs (Canadian dollars) were almost ninefold higher in patients with the highest SDIs than those with the lowest SDIs [93]. The final chapter will expound on this multistate model along with the fundamental concepts of direct and indirect costs.

Analysis of economic impact will become increasingly important in clinical practice and clinical trials when comparing the outcome of different therapeutic strategies, particularly with the emergence of new biologic treatments which are significantly more expensive than the more traditional therapies (details are in Chap.

20). Incremental cost-effectiveness and cost-utility analyses will be necessary to inform health policies around coverage of expensive new treatments.

## Emerging Concepts in SLE and Deep Insights on Selected Concepts

Beyond the measurement in the five domains and their embedded constructs, the SLE field is witnessing the emergence of new concepts such as frailty. Currently, further work is being conducted on existing concepts, in particular cognition, depression, and anxiety as well as fatigue. Each of these concepts are highlighted in detail in Chaps. 13, 14, 15, 16, and 17. Some of these concepts are constituent components of the core domains discussed. All have significant prognostic implications warranting the development of valid, reliable, and responsive tools.

## Cognitive Impairment

The American College of Rheumatology (ACR) defined 19 central and peripheral nervous system syndromes as NPSLE [94] including cognitive dysfunction and mood disorders. Any of the following cognitive functions as defined by the ACR nomenclature may be involved in cognitive impairment: "memory (learning and recall), complex attention, simple attention, executive skills (planning, organizing, and sequencing), visual-spatial processing, language (e.g. verbal, fluency), reasoning/problem solving and psychomotor speed" [94].

Cognitive impairment (CI) is among the most commonly reported neuropsychiatric symptoms among patients with SLE, with a prevalence of 33–43%, and it may occur at any time in the course of disease [95, 96]. The severity ranges from mild impairment to severe dementia and is associated with significant negative effects on functioning, employment potential, and quality of life.

Cognitive impairment has been shown to be independent of disease activity [97, 98] and may be persistent. Analysis of longitudinal data from the University of California San Francisco Lupus Outcomes Study has shown that persistently low cognitive performance occurs in 28% of patients and did not significantly improve over 7 years. This highlights the importance of periodic, yearly, assessment of cognitive function in SLE [13].

Traditionally, the assessment for CI relies on tests which are time-consuming, associated with cost burden and specifically require trained psychometrists and neuropsychologists for the administration, scoring, and interpretation. For instance, the 1 to 2 h American College of Rheumatology Neuropsychological Battery (ACR-NB) of tests is considered the gold standard test recommended by the ACR to evaluate CI [96]. Recently, a new study showed evidence of validity for the computer-based, 40-minute self-administered test, the Automated Neuropsychological Assessment

Metrics (ANAM) test [99] in screening for cognitive impairment, when compared to the gold standard ACR-NB. In the future, this has potential to change the accessibility and ease of screening of this understudied and challenging clinical manifestation of lupus. Chapter 13 elaborates on cognitive function assessment in SLE.

## Depression and Anxiety

Anxiety and mood disorders such as depression are prominent conditions among the 19 syndromes defined by the ACR nomenclature "Neuropsychiatric SLE" (NPSLE) [94]. The mood state of depression includes "feelings of sadness, despair, emptiness, discouragement, or hopelessness; having no feelings; or appearing tearful" [100]. "The severity of depression can range from mild depressive symptoms to more severe clinical major depressive disorders" as defined by the *Diagnostic and Statistical Manual of Mental Disorders* [100].

Anxiety, on the other hand, has been defined as anticipation of danger or misfortune accompanied by apprehension, dysphoria, or tension, and it includes generalized anxiety, phobias, panic disorders, panic attacks, and obsessive-compulsive disorders [101].

Anxiety and depression are among the most frequent neuropsychiatric complications exhibited by SLE patients [102]. In a recent study using instruments and cutoff scores that have been studied and validated, in SLE patient cohorts, the prevalence was 27% and 34%, respectively [103], consistent with a recent systematic review and meta-analysis revealing a prevalence of 30–40% for depression [104].

Patients with anxiety and depression universally experience significant morbidity including reduced health-related quality of life [105] and have a tenfold increase in mortality rate compared with the general population [106]. Severe anxiety and depressive symptoms ultimately impair patients' ability to engage in their health-related treatment plans resulting in poor control of their SLE [44]. The causes and the contributing factors of these manifestations are multifactorial and intertwined. For example, clinical phenotypes such as skin and musculoskeletal systems involvement, as well as employment and shorter disease duration, are some factors found to be associated with anxiety or depression [103].

The more commonly used instruments in the measurement of depression and anxiety as identified by a recent systematic review were the Center for Epidemiological Studies-Depression (CES-D), Beck Depression Inventory (BDI), Beck Anxiety Inventory (BAI), Hospital Anxiety and Depression Scale (HADS-A/D), and Hamilton Rating Scale for Depression/Anxiety (HAM-D/A)] [104]. Understanding the various measures used to assess depression and anxiety is important to understanding the burden of SLE. Evidence-based metrics are vital in identifying patients with these conditions and in developing intervention plans to improve symptoms, daily living, and HRQoL. Routine patient screening with validated instruments may facilitate the timely diagnosis of depression and anxiety and thus facilitate prompt intervention strategies. Chapter 14 will explore the assessment of depression and anxiety in detail.

## Fatigue and Pain

Fatigue is a very common symptom of SLE with prevalence in SLE trials varying between 67 and 90% as measured by the Fatigue Severity Scale (FSS) [47, 73, 107]. Defined as an "overwhelming sense of tiredness, a lack of energy and recurrent feelings of exhaustion" [108], fatigue is perceived by many SLE patients to be a symptom that is more severe than pain, depression, or anxiety [109].

Pain is often one of the first symptoms of SLE [110], and chronic pain is one of the most frequently reported problems among SLE patients affecting approximately 50–90% of patients during the course of the disease [3]. Musculoskeletal disease is a common source of chronic pain [110]. However, the etiology of pain in SLE is varied including inflammatory, neuropathic, and central causes.

Both fatigue and pain are frequently rated by SLE patients as having a strong negative effect on quality of life [111, 112] and patient perception of disease burden [112]. They portend increased risk of work disability and consequential negative socioeconomic impact [112, 113]. These two potentially debilitating disease manifestations are often interlinked in patients with SLE as fatigue is a multidimensional phenomenon, which can manifest itself with physical and/or mental symptoms and pain is a contributory factor to fatigue [113].

Often pain and fatigue are not associated with the constructs measured by disease activity and damage [109, 112, 113]. As such, several measures have been developed and validated to assess fatigue and pain in SLE. Because it is a subjective symptom that is difficult to define, fatigue is challenging to measure, contributing to the development of a variety of instruments. In 2007, the Ad Hoc Committee on SLE Response Criteria for Fatigue conducted a systematic review of fatigue instruments used in SLE studies. Among the 15 instruments identified, the Krupp Fatigue Severity Scale (FSS) was recommended [114]. A recent systematic review found that the Visual Analog Scale (VAS), the FSS, and the Functional Assessment of Chronic Illness Therapy (FACIT)-Fatigue scale were the most frequently used instruments in adult SLE studies [115]. SLE-related pain measurement in clinical practice and research depends on PROs. Tools used include self-assessments: visual analogue scale of pain and the short-form McGill Pain Questionnaire [3].

Although treatment continues to advance, fatigue remains one of the most poorly understood manifestations of lupus, and the evaluation of fatigue and pain continues to be areas of unmet needs in SLE management [116, 117]. Application of core measures may facilitate greater understanding of the mechanisms of fatigue and may help guide the development of interventions to improve health outcomes. Chapter 15 elaborates on pain and fatigue assessment in SLE.

## Frailty

The concept of frailty began to emerge as a medically distinct syndrome in the 1980s in the field of geriatrics [118]. The frailty construct may be defined as a state of increased vulnerability due to degradation of homeostatic mechanisms, resulting in diminished ability to respond to physiologic stressors, and it signals susceptibility to adverse outcomes [119]. The basis of the development of frailty is the interrelation between aging and diseases through various mechanisms including neuroendocrine dysregulation, metabolic alterations, and inflammation leading to clinical manifestations such as osteoporosis, sarcopenia, weight loss, and decreased performance, to name a few [120].

The evaluation of frailty in lupus is an emerging area with data in recent years determining its prevalence to be higher in SLE patients than in similarly aged individuals in the general population [121, 122]. Poor physical and cognitive function and increased risk of functional decline and mortality were some outcomes found to be associated with frailty in SLE patients [121].

As an emerging entity, the need for metrics has been recognized. To that end, the ground-breaking Systemic Lupus International Collaborating Clinics Frailty Index (SLICC-FI) was recently developed [122]. Using data from the international SLICC inception cohort and a novel approach of deficit accumulation, this novel index identifies a full spectrum of vulnerability associated with the frailty construct. Validation of this index including its association with the risk of future adverse health outcomes is required prior to its use.

A fundamental element of the concept of frailty is the ability to predict it, so it can be modified or even prevented [119]. With the extension of life expectancy and the rising percentage of older individuals in the SLE population, the use of a validated frailty tool in SLE may enable clinicians to modify important health outcomes in this population. Chapter 16 seeks to explore the development of SLICC-FI and its potential application in clinical practice and research.

## Instrument Selection: The OMERACT Process

Having established what needs to be measured in SLE (constructs such as disease activity, damage, etc.) for research and clinical settings, investigators and rheumatologists must then identify the appropriate instruments suited to the particular research or clinical needs. This decision-making process involves identifying candidate instruments and then determining if an instrument is a match for the target construct (e.g., disease activity) and population (e.g., patients with SLE). The "Outcome Measures in Rheumatology" (OMERACT) process provides the methodology by which this can be accomplished.

Since its inception in 1992, the OMERACT process has been used to select domains and identify appropriate instruments that measure the constructs in each domain, for use in clinical trials and observational studies in each defined disease category according to three pillars: *truth*, *discrimination*, and *feasibility* [6]. These pillars guide researchers through a process providing a body of evidence to answer the question: "Is there enough evidence to support the use of this instrument in clinical research of the benefits and harms of treatments in the population and study setting described?" [123]. *Truth* reflects the evidence on the ability of the instrument to measure what is intended to be measuring. *Feasibility* refers to issues related to practicality: time, cost, and burden associated with the use of a particular instrument. *Discrimination* answers questions on the ability of the instrument to discriminate between different groups and situations (responders and nonresponders in a drug trial) and to accurately measure change when it has occurred.

OMERACT's current methodology for instrument selection is a data-driven, evidence-based approach summarized in the OMERACT Filter 2.1 Instrument Selection Algorithm (OFISA). This process is based on the concept of "3 pillars, 4 signaling questions, 7 measurement properties, 1 answer" [123].

There are two dimensions to the *truth pillar* reflected by two questions. First, "the truth pillar is reflected by practical appraisal of the instrument and its content with the signalling question – Is it a match with the target domain?" For instance, if you aim to study depression in patients with SLE, the first step is to review the literature and identify the measures on depression and carefully evaluate the evidence relayed to the use of these instruments in SLE and on the concept of interest. Each chapter in this book guides you through this process and provides you with a list of the required instruments for each construct and the evidence on its use in SLE. The second dimension of truth is "a more data-driven, hypothesis-testing assessment of the instrument's scores reflected by a second question: "Do the numeric scores make sense (i.e., are the scores relating to other measures or the testing situation in a way it should if it measures the domain well)?" In this step, you will be gathering more evidence on different aspects of validity of the instrument that you have selected for your research question. For instance, you need to determine if low SLEDAI scores are associated with mild disease and high SLEDAI scores are associated with severe disease activity. An instrument is never valid, it is more that each piece of evidence gives you a bit more confidence in how much you can trust that numeric score to capture your target domain (i.e., fatigue). We need a high degree of confidence in our scores. The question reflecting the *discrimination pillar* is "Can it discriminate between groups of interest?" [123]. In this step, you will gather the evidence to determine if a particular instrument is able to discriminate between two groups (e.g., SLEDAI is able to discriminate between patients receiving placebo and patients receiving biologic treatment in a drug trial). The signaling question for the *feasibility pillar* is "Is it practical to use?", and this covers aspects related to cost, burden on patients and assessors, and access. For instance, if you have to choose a disease activity instrument in an observational study, the cost, equipment, and time burden associated with its use are key factors in making your decision, while in a drug trial, probably there is less restrain on the time and particularly cost burden [123].

For each of these "4 signaling questions, there are 7 measurement properties that require data-oriented answers: *truth* [domain match (content validity, face validity)], *discrimination* [test-retest reliability, longitudinal construct validity (responsiveness), clinical trial discrimination, thresholds of meaning], and *feasibility* (practical assessment of burden of use)" [123].

The OMERACT Filter 2.1 Instrument Selection Algorithm (OFISA) provides a template that may be adapted for the instrument selection process in SLE (Fig. 1.2).

In OFISA, each of the four signaling questions receive traffic light ratings which will be combined into an overall rating. **Red** always means "stop, do not continue," **Amber** means "a caution is raised, but you can continue," and **Green** means "go, this question is definitely answered affirmatively." White circles indicate an absence of evidence, and in this case, the working group should create this evidence by designing new studies to fill this gap [123]. Responding to the red light "no" at the first two questions of truth (domain match) and feasibility saves time and resources. This means that a particular instrument is not the best match for the targeted population and concept, and it is recommended to invest into different instruments.

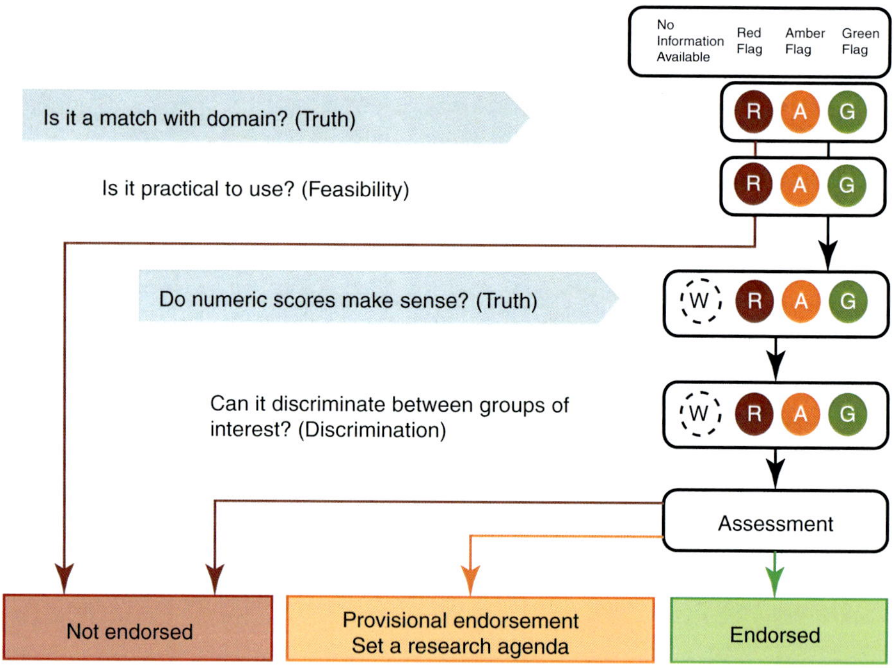


**Fig. 1.2** The OMERACT Filter 2.1 Instrument Selection Algorithm (OFISA) [123]. OMERACT Filter 2.1 Instrument Selection Algorithm (OFISA). The 4 signaling questions are linked to a results column (traffic light ratings) and a renewed emphasis on the setting aside of instruments that receive a red rating for either of the first two questions. Amber and green continue to the last two signaling questions, though the former are to be used with care and caution. OMERACT Outcome Measure in Rheumatology, W white, R red, A amber, G green

Regarding review of the evidence to support performance of an instrument at questions 3 and 4, the OMERACT Filter 2.1 recommend the techniques described by Slavin [124] which encompasses "gathering the evidence, appraisal of quality of the evidence, data extraction, and synthesis of findings" [125].

Once all four questions in the OMERACT Filter 2.1 are answered, an overall level of endorsement for a specific measure can be recommended. Instruments with **Green** color become endorsed by OMERACT, while instruments with **Amber** color receive a provisional endorsement. The amber-rated instrument requires further research by the working group which can bring the instrument again for reassessment and potential full endorsement once further evidence is gathered.

## Facilitating Development of Response Criteria and Classification Criteria: EULAR/ACR Collaborative Projects

The collaboration between the relevant standing committee from EULAR with the ACR Quality of Care Committee has led to the development of several published initiatives in rheumatology. This cooperation has led to the development and validation of classification criteria in SLE (Chap. 3). Such criteria facilitate the development of recommendations regarding conducting clinical trials [126]. In addition to classification criteria, the ACR and EULAR review proposals and provide funding for new collaborative projects in the area of response criteria [126]. With greater exploration of emerging concepts in SLE and the prospect of new pharmacological agents comes the need for developing and validating new instruments. The joint expertise of EULAR and ACR is crucial in these processes especially for initiatives of international relevance.

## Conclusion

With the use of more sensitive screening and diagnostic tests, earlier diagnosis, and a treat-to-target therapeutic strategy, the overall prognosis of patients with SLE has improved significantly. Additionally, new pharmacological agents being licensed and those in the pipeline may further improve life expectancy. As such, the therapeutic drive in SLE is to control disease activity and reduce flares and limit organ damage and drug toxicity while maintaining or improving HRQoL. The use of validated and reliable instruments is fundamental in achieving these goals.

Whether in clinical practice settings or clinical trials, clinicians and investigators should try to identify the appropriate measures suited to their needs. The choice of a specific instrument will largely depend on the setting (clinical practice vs research), the purpose of the study or clinical goal, and the psychometric properties of the instruments and may be influenced by the personal preference of the investigator.

This ground-breaking textbook outlines the development and application of various SLE measurement tools that have been in use for many years and those newly developed or enhanced for evaluation of domains and organ-specific dimensions. The psychometric properties of these measures including, validity, reliability, and sensitivity to change along with feasibility are outlined.

While often no individual measure is sufficient to measure all constructs (disease activity, damage, etc.), a combination of the most appropriate metrics needs to be selected for the purpose of assessing all clinically important constructs and endpoints. Combining instruments is especially important in clinical trial settings where composite response endpoints need to be defined.

With the promise of new therapies on the horizon, particularly biologics, instruments in SLE will become even more crucial going forward. Data provided by measures for SLE domains now will facilitate the appraisal of the effect of these new therapies in the future.

## Bibliography

1. Petri M, Buyon J, Kim M. Classification and definition of major flares in SLE clinical trials. Lupus. 1999;8(8):685–91. PubMed PMID: 10568907. Epub 1999/11/24
2. Nikpour M, Urowitz MB, Ibanez D, Gladman DD. Frequency and determinants of flare and persistently active disease in systemic lupus erythematosus. Arthritis Rheum. 2009;61(9):1152–8. PubMed PMID: 19714602. Epub 2009/08/29
3. Waldheim E, Elkan AC, Bergman S, Frostegard J, van Vollenhoven R, Henriksson EW. Extent and characteristics of self-reported pain in patients with systemic lupus erythematosus. Lupus. 2013;22(2):136–43. PubMed PMID: 23192324. Epub 2012/11/30
4. Gladman DD, Urowitz MB, Rahman P, Ibanez D, Tam LS. Accrual of organ damage over time in patients with systemic lupus erythematosus. J Rheumatol. 2003;30(9):1955–9. PubMed PMID: 12966597. Epub 2003/09/11
5. Touma Z, Gladman D, Urowitz M. Clinical measures, metrics and indices. In: Wallace DJ, Hahn BH, editors. Dubois' lupus erythematosus and related syndromes. 8th ed: Elsevier Inc; 2013. p. 532–81.
6. Strand V, Gladman D, Isenberg D, Petri M, Smolen J, Tugwell P. Endpoints: consensus recommendations from OMERACT IV. Outcome measures in rheumatology. Lupus. 2000;9(5):322–7. PubMed PMID: 10878722. Epub 2000/07/06
7. Johnson SR, Goek ON, Singh-Grewal D, Vlad SC, Feldman BM, Felson DT, et al. Classification criteria in rheumatic diseases: a review of methodologic properties. Arthritis Rheum. 2007;57(7):1119–33. PubMed PMID: 17907227. Epub 2007/10/02
8. Aringer M, Costenbader K, Daikh D, Brinks R, Mosca M, Ramsey-Goldman R, et al. 2019 European League Against Rheumatism/American College of Rheumatology classification criteria for systemic lupus erythematosus. Arthritis Rheumatol. 2019;71(9):1400–12. PubMed PMID: 31385462. PubMed Central PMCID: PMC6827566. Epub 2019/08/07
9. Singh JA, Solomon DH, Dougados M, Felson D, Hawker G, Katz P, et al. Development of classification and response criteria for rheumatic diseases. Arthritis Rheum. 2006;55(3):348–52. PubMed PMID: 16739201. Epub 2006/06/02
10. Nuttall A, Isenberg DA. Assessment of disease activity, damage and quality of life in systemic lupus erythematosus: new aspects. Best Pract Res Clin Rheumatol. 2013;27(3):309–18. PubMed PMID: 24238688. Epub 2013/11/19

11. Bombardier C, Gladman DD, Urowitz MB, Caron D, Chang CH. Derivation of the SLEDAI. A disease activity index for lupus patients. The Committee on Prognosis Studies in SLE. Arthritis Rheum. 1992;35(6):630–40. PubMed PMID: 1599520. Epub 1992/06/01
12. Gladman DD, Urowitz MB, Kagal A, Hallett D. Accurately describing changes in disease activity in Systemic Lupus Erythematosus. J Rheumatol. 2000;27(2):377–9. PubMed PMID: 10685800. Epub 2000/02/24
13. Touma Z, Moghaddam B, Su J, Katz P. Cognitive function trajectories are associated with the depressive symptoms trajectories in systemic lupus erythematosus over time. Arthritis Care Res. 2020. PubMed PMID: 32526080. Epub ahead of print.
14. Touma Z, Gladman DD, Su J, Anderson N, Urowitz MB. A novel lupus activity index accounting for glucocorticoids: SLEDAI-2K glucocorticoid index. Rheumatology. 2018;57(8):1370–6. PubMed PMID: 29688532.
15. Touma Z, Urowitz MB, Gladman DD. Systemic lupus erythematosus disease activity index 2000 responder index-50 website. J Rheumatol. 2013;40(5):733. PubMed PMID: 23637378. Epub 2013/05/03
16. Pike MC, Kelley L. Data quality challenges in systemic lupus erythematosus trials: how can this be optimized? Curr Rheumatol Rep. 2012;14(4):324–33. PubMed PMID: 22580894. PubMed Central PMCID: PMC3387490. Epub 2012/05/15
17. Gladman DD, Ibanez D, Urowitz MB. Systemic lupus erythematosus disease activity index 2000. J Rheumatol. 2002;29(2):288–91. PubMed PMID: 11838846. Epub 2002/02/13. eng
18. Touma Z, Urowitz MB, Gladman DD. SLEDAI-2K for a 30-day window. Lupus. 2010;19(1):49–51. PubMed PMID: 19910390.
19. Touma Z, Urowitz MB, Ibanez D, Gladman DD. SLEDAI-2K 10 days versus SLEDAI-2K 30 days in a longitudinal evaluation. Lupus. 2011;20(1):67–70. PubMed PMID: 21233149. Epub 2011/01/15. eng
20. Guzman J, Cardiel MH, Arce-Salinas A, Sanchez-Guerrero J, Alarcon-Segovia D. Measurement of disease activity in systemic lupus erythematosus. Prospective validation of 3 clinical indices. J Rheumatol. 1992;19(10):1551–8. PubMed PMID: 1464867. eng.
21. Uribe AG, Vila LM, McGwin G Jr, Sanchez ML, Reveille JD, Alarcon GS. The Systemic Lupus Activity Measure-revised, the Mexican Systemic Lupus Erythematosus Disease Activity Index (SLEDAI), and a modified SLEDAI-2K are adequate instruments to measure disease activity in systemic lupus erythematosus. J Rheumatol. 2004;31(10):1934–40. PubMed PMID: 15468356. eng.
22. Petri M, Kim MY, Kalunian KC, Grossman J, Hahn BH, Sammaritano LR, et al. Combined oral contraceptives in women with systemic lupus erythematosus. N Eng J Med. 2005;353(24):2550–8. PubMed PMID: 16354891. eng.
23. Touma Z, Gladman DD, Ibañez D, Urowitz MB. Systemic lupus erythematosus disease activity index 2(SLEDAI-2K) Responder Index (SRI-50): a valid index for measuring improvement in disease activity. Arthritis &Rheumatism. 2010;62(Suppl 10):1878.
24. Touma Z, Gladman DD, Ibanez D, Urowitz MB. Development and initial validation of the systemic lupus erythematosus disease activity index 2000 responder index 50. J Rheumatol. 2011;38(2):275–84. PubMed PMID: 21123323. Epub 2010/12/03. eng
25. Touma Z, Urowitz MB, Fortin PR, Landolt C, Toloza SM, Riddell C, et al. SLEDAI-2K responder index (SRI)-50:a reliable index for measuring improvement in disease activity. J Rheumatol. 2011;38(6):1171–2.
26. Touma Z, Gladman DD, Zandy M, Su J, Anderson N, Urowitz MB. Identifying a response for the systemic lupus erythematosus disease activity glucocorticoid index (SLEDAI-2KG). Arthritis Care Res. 2020. PubMed PMID: 32433815. Epub ahead of print.
27. Symmons DP, Coppock JS, Bacon PA, Bresnihan B, Isenberg DA, Maddison P, et al. Development and assessment of a computerized index of clinical disease activity in systemic lupus erythematosus. Members of the British Isles Lupus Assessment Group (BILAG). Q J Med. 1988;69(259):927–37. PubMed PMID: 3271336. eng.
28. Hay EM, Bacon PA, Gordon C, Isenberg DA, Maddison P, Snaith ML, et al. The BILAG index: a reliable and valid instrument for measuring clinical disease activity in systemic lupus erythematosus. Q J Med. 1993;86(7):447–58. PubMed PMID: 8210301. eng.

29. Isenberg DA, Rahman A, Allen E, Farewell V, Akil M, Bruce IN, et al. BILAG 2004. Development and initial validation of an updated version of the British Isles Lupus Assessment Group's disease activity index for patients with systemic lupus erythematosus. Rheumatology. 2005;44(7):902–6. PubMed PMID: 15814577. eng.
30. Liang MH, Socher SA, Larson MG, Schur PH. Reliability and validity of six systems for the clinical assessment of disease activity in systemic lupus erythematosus. Arthritis Rheum. 1989;32(9):1107–18. PubMed PMID: 2775320. eng.
31. Olesinska M, Saletra A. Quality of life in systemic lupus erythematosus and its measurement. Reumatologia. 2018;56(1):45–54. PubMed PMID: 29686443. PubMed Central PMCID: PMC5911658. Epub 2018/04/25
32. Bae SC, Koh HK, Chang DK, Kim MH, Park JK, Kim SY. Reliability and validity of systemic lupus activity measure-revised (SLAM-R) for measuring clinical disease activity in systemic lupus erythematosus. Lupus. 2001;10(6):405–9. PubMed PMID: 11434575. eng.
33. Karlson EW, Daltroy LH, Rivest C, Ramsey-Goldman R, Wright EA, Partridge AJ, et al. Validation of a Systemic Lupus Activity Questionnaire (SLAQ) for population studies. Lupus. 2003;12(4):280–6. PubMed PMID: 12729051. eng.
34. Bencivelli W, Vitali C, Isenberg DA, Smolen JS, Snaith ML, Sciuto M, et al. Disease activity in systemic lupus erythematosus: report of the Consensus Study Group of the European Workshop for Rheumatology Research. III. Development of a computerised clinical chart and its application to the comparison of different indices of disease activity. The European Consensus Study Group for Disease Activity in SLE. Clin Exp Rheumatol. 1992;10(5):549–54. PubMed PMID: 1458711. eng.
35. Vitali C, Bencivelli W, Isenberg DA, Smolen JS, Snaith ML, Sciuto M, et al. Disease activity in systemic lupus erythematosus: report of the Consensus Study Group of the European Workshop for Rheumatology Research. I. A descriptive analysis of 704 European lupus patients. European Consensus Study Group for Disease Activity in SLE. Clin Exp Rheumatol. 1992;10(5):527–39. PubMed PMID: 1458709. eng.
36. Vitali C, Bencivelli W, Isenberg DA, Smolen JS, Snaith ML, Sciuto M, et al. Disease activity in systemic lupus erythematosus: report of the Consensus Study Group of the European Workshop for Rheumatology Research. II. Identification of the variables indicative of disease activity and their use in the development of an activity score. The European Consensus Study Group for Disease Activity in SLE. Clin Exp Rheumatol. 1992;10(5):541–7. PubMed PMID: 1458710. eng.
37. Petri M, Hellmann D, Hochberg M. Validity and reliability of lupus activity measures in the routine clinic setting. J Rheumatol. 1992;19(1):53–9. PubMed PMID: 1556700. Epub 1992/01/01. eng
38. Smolen JS. Clinical and serological features: incidence and diagnostic approach. In: Smolen JS, Zielinski CC, editors. Systemic lupus erythematosus: clinical and experimental aspects. Berlin/Heidelberg: Springer-Verlag; 1987. p. 170–96.
39. Petri M, Barr SG, Buyon J, Davis J, Ginzler E, Kalunian K, et al. RIFLE: responder index for lupus erythematosus. Arthritis Rheum. 2000;43:S244.
40. Gladman D, Ginzler E, Goldsmith C, Fortin P, Liang M, Urowitz M, et al. The development and initial validation of the Systemic Lupus International Collaborating Clinics/American College of Rheumatology damage index for systemic lupus erythematosus. Arthritis Rheum. 1996;39(3):363–9. PubMed PMID: 8607884. Epub 1996/03/01. eng
41. Costenbader KH, Khamashta M, Ruiz-Garcia S, Perez-Rodriguez MT, Petri M, Elliott J, et al. Development and initial validation of a self-assessed lupus organ damage instrument. Arthritis Care Res. 2010;62(4):559–68. PubMed PMID: 20391512. eng.
42. Pons-Estel BA, Sanchez-Guerrero J, Romero-Diaz J, Iglesias-Gamarra A, Bonfa E, Borba EF, et al. Validation of the Spanish, Portuguese and French versions of the Lupus Damage Index questionnaire: data from North and South America, Spain and Portugal. Lupus. 2009;18(12):1033–52. PubMed PMID: 19762375. eng.

43. McHorney CA, Ware JE Jr, Lu JF, Sherbourne CD. The MOS 36-item Short-Form Health Survey (SF-36): III. Tests of data quality, scaling assumptions, and reliability across diverse patient groups. Med Care. 1994;32(1):40–66. PubMed PMID: 8277801.
44. McElhone K, Abbott J, Shelmerdine J, Bruce IN, Ahmad Y, Gordon C, et al. Development and validation of a disease-specific health-related quality of life measure, the LupusQol, for adults with systemic lupus erythematosus. Arthritis Rheum. 2007;57(6):972–9. PubMed PMID: 17665467.
45. Jolly M, Pickard AS, Wilke C, Mikolaitis RA, Teh LS, McElhone K, et al. Lupus-specific health outcome measure for US patients: the LupusQoL-US version. Ann Rheum Dis. 2010;69(1):29–33. PubMed PMID: 19126561. Epub 2009/01/08
46. Gonzalez-Rodriguez V, Peralta-Ramirez MI, Navarrete-Navarrete N, Callejas-Rubio JL, Santos Ruiz AM, Khamashta M. Adaptation and validation of the Spanish version of a disease-specific quality of life measure in patients with systemic lupus erythematosus: the Lupus quality of life. Med Clin. 2010;134(1):13–6. PubMed PMID: 19647276. Adaptacion y validacion de la version espanola de una medida especifica de la calidad de vida en los pacientes con lupus eritematoso sistemico: el Lupus Quality of Life. spa.
47. Grootscholten C, Ligtenberg G, Derksen RH, Schreurs KM, de Glas-Vos JW, Hagen EC, et al. Health-related quality of life in patients with systemic lupus erythematosus: development and validation of a lupus specific symptom checklist. Qual Life Res. 2003;12(6):635–44. PubMed PMID: 14516173. Epub 2003/10/01
48. Leong KP, Kong KO, Thong BY, Koh ET, Lian TY, Teh CL, et al. Development and preliminary validation of a systemic lupus erythematosus-specific quality-of-life instrument (SLEQOL). Rheumatology. 2005;44(10):1267–76. PubMed PMID: 15797980. Epub 2005/03/31
49. Doward LC, McKenna SP, Whalley D, Tennant A, Griffiths B, Emery P, et al. The development of the L-QoL: a quality-of-life instrument specific to systemic lupus erythematosus. Ann Rheum Dis. 2009;68(2):196–200. PubMed PMID: 18385276. Epub 2008/04/04
50. Furie RA, Petri MA, Wallace DJ, Ginzler EM, Merrill JT, Stohl W, et al. Novel evidence-based systemic lupus erythematosus responder index. Arthritis Rheum. 2009;61(9):1143–51. PubMed PMID: 19714615. PubMed Central PMCID: PMC2748175. Epub 2009/08/29
51. Gladman DD, Urowitz MB, Goldsmith CH, Fortin P, Ginzler E, Gordon C, et al. The reliability of the Systemic Lupus International Collaborating Clinics/American College of Rheumatology Damage Index in patients with systemic lupus erythematosus. Arthritis Rheum. 1997;40(5):809–13. PubMed PMID: 9153540. Epub 1997/05/01
52. Doria A, Iaccarino L, Ghirardello A, Zampieri S, Arienti S, Sarzi-Puttini P, et al. Long-term prognosis and causes of death in systemic lupus erythematosus. Am J Med. 2006;119(8):700–6. PubMed PMID: 16887417. Epub 2006/08/05
53. Urowitz MB, Gladman DD, Tom BD, Ibanez D, Farewell VT. Changing patterns in mortality and disease outcomes for patients with systemic lupus erythematosus. J Rheumatol. 2008;35(11):2152–8. PubMed PMID: 18793004. Epub 2008/09/17
54. Tektonidou MG, Lewandowski LB, Hu J, Dasgupta A, Ward MM. Survival in adults and children with systemic lupus erythematosus: a systematic review and Bayesian meta-analysis of studies from 1950 to 2016. Ann Rheum Dis. 2017;76(12):2009–16. PubMed PMID: 28794077. Epub 2017/08/11
55. Stoll T, Sutcliffe N, Mach J, Klaghofer R, Isenberg DA. Analysis of the relationship between disease activity and damage in patients with systemic lupus erythematosus–a 5-yr prospective study. Rheumatology. 2004;43(8):1039–44. PubMed PMID: 15161983. Epub 2004/05/27
56. Keeling SO, Vandermeer B, Medina J, Chatterley T, Nevskaya T, Pope J, et al. Measuring disease activity and damage with validated metrics: a systematic review on mortality and damage in systemic lupus erythematosus. J Rheumatol. 2018;45(10):1448–61. PubMed PMID: 30111638. Epub 2018/08/17
57. Keeling SO, Alabdurubalnabi Z, Avina-Zubieta A, Barr S, Bergeron L, Bernatsky S, et al. Canadian rheumatology association recommendations for the assessment and monitor-

ing of systemic lupus erythematosus. J Rheumatol. 2018;45(10):1426–39. PubMed PMID: 30173152.
58. Gladman D, Ginzler E, Goldsmith C, Fortin P, Liang M, Urowitz M, et al. Systemic lupus international collaborative clinics: development of a damage index in systemic lupus erythematosus. J Rheumatol. 1992;19(11):1820–1. PubMed PMID: 1362779. Epub 1992/11/01
59. Touma Z, Gladman DD, Tulloch-Reid D, Toloza SM, Ibanez D, Fortin PR, et al. Burden of autoantibodies and association with disease activity and damage in systemic lupus erythematosus. Clin Exp Rheumatol. 2010;28(4):525–31. PubMed PMID: 20659409.
60. Sutton EJ, Davidson JE, Bruce IN. The systemic lupus international collaborating clinics (SLICC) damage index: a systematic literature review. Semin Arthritis Rheum. 2013;43(3):352–61. PubMed PMID: 23786872. Epub 2013/06/22
61. Rahman P, Gladman DD, Urowitz MB, Hallett D, Tam LS. Early damage as measured by the SLICC/ACR damage index is a predictor of mortality in systemic lupus erythematosus. Lupus. 2001;10(2):93–6. PubMed PMID: 11237132. Epub 2001/03/10
62. Brunner HI, Higgins GC, Wiers K, Lapidus SK, Olson JC, Onel K, et al. Prospective validation of the provisional criteria for the evaluation of response to therapy in childhood-onset systemic lupus erythematosus. Arthritis Care Res. 2010;62(3):335–44. PubMed PMID: 20391479. PubMed Central PMCID: PMC2946212. Epub 2010/04/15
63. Lattanzi B, Consolaro A, Solari N, Ruperto N, Martini A, Ravelli A. Measures of disease activity and damage in pediatric systemic lupus erythematosus: British Isles Lupus Assessment Group (BILAG), European Consensus Lupus Activity Measurement (ECLAM), Systemic Lupus Activity Measure (SLAM), Systemic Lupus Erythematosus Disease Activity Index (SLEDAI), Physician's Global Assessment of Disease Activity (MD Global), and Systemic Lupus International Collaborating Clinics/American College of Rheumatology Damage Index (SLICC/ACR DI; SDI). Arthritis Care Res. 2011;63(Suppl 11):S112–7. PubMed PMID: 22588739. Epub 2012/05/25
64. Brunner HI, Silverman ED, Bombardier C, Feldman BM. European Consensus Lupus Activity Measurement is sensitive to change in disease activity in childhood-onset systemic lupus erythematosus. Arthritis Rheum. 2003;49(3):335–41. PubMed PMID: 12794788. Epub 2003/06/10
65. Sato JO, Corrente JE, Saad-Magalhaes C. Correlation between the Modified Systemic Lupus Erythematosus Disease Activity Index 2000 and the European Consensus Lupus Activity Measurement in juvenile systemic lupus erythematosus. Lupus. 2016;25(13):1479–84. PubMed PMID: 27230556. Epub 2016/05/28
66. Eudy AM, Siega-Riz AM, Engel SM, Franceschini N, Howard AG, Clowse MEB, et al. Effect of pregnancy on disease flares in patients with systemic lupus erythematosus. Ann Rheum Dis. 2018;77(6):855–60. PubMed PMID: 29463519. PubMed Central PMCID: PMC6037310. Epub 2018/02/22
67. Andreoli L, Bertsias GK, Agmon-Levin N, Brown S, Cervera R, Costedoat-Chalumeau N, et al. EULAR recommendations for women's health and the management of family planning, assisted reproduction, pregnancy and menopause in patients with systemic lupus erythematosus and/or antiphospholipid syndrome. Ann Rheum Dis. 2017;76(3):476–85. PubMed PMID: 27457513. PubMed Central PMCID: PMC5446003. Epub 2016/07/28
68. Buyon JP, Kalunian KC, Ramsey-Goldman R, Petri MA, Lockshin MD, Ruiz-Irastorza G, et al. Assessing disease activity in SLE patients during pregnancy. Lupus. 1999;8(8):677–84. PubMed PMID: 10568906. Epub 1999/11/24
69. Andreoli L, Gerardi MC, Fernandes M, Bortoluzzi A, Bellando-Randone S, Brucato A, et al. Disease activity assessment of rheumatic diseases during pregnancy: a comprehensive review of indices used in clinical studies. Autoimmun Rev. 2019;18(2):164–76. PubMed PMID: 30572134. Epub 2018/12/21
70. Yazdany J, Yelin E. Health-related quality of life and employment among persons with systemic lupus erythematosus. Rheum Dis Clin N Am. 2010;36(1):15–32. vii. PubMed PMID: 20202589. PubMed Central PMCID: PMC2833285. Epub 2010/03/06.

71. Panopalis P, Clarke AE. Quality of life in systemic lupus erythematosus. Clin Dev Immunol. 2006;13(2–4):321–4. PubMed PMID: 17162373. PubMed Central PMCID: PMC2270782. Epub 2006/12/13
72. Kwan A, Strand V, Touma Z. The role of patient-reported outcomes in systemic lupus erythematosus. Curr Treat Options Rheum. 2017;3:308–21.
73. Schmeding A, Schneider M. Fatigue, health-related quality of life and other patient-reported outcomes in systemic lupus erythematosus. Best Pract Res Clin Rheumatol. 2013;27(3):363–75. PubMed PMID: 24238693. Epub 2013/11/19
74. Bultink IE, Turkstra F, Dijkmans BA, Voskuyl AE. High prevalence of unemployment in patients with systemic lupus erythematosus: association with organ damage and health-related quality of life. J Rheumatol. 2008;35(6):1053–7. PubMed PMID: 18381792. Epub 2008/04/03
75. Strand V, Simon LS, Meara AS, Touma Z. Measurement properties of selected patient-reported outcome measures for use in randomised controlled trials in patients with systemic lupus erythematosus: a systematic review. Lupus Sci Med. 2020;7(1):e000373. PubMed PMID: 32591423. Epub 2020/06/28
76. Kwan A, Katz P, Touma Z. The assessment of anxiety and depression and its associated factors in SLE. Curr Rheumatol Rev. 2019;15(2):90–8. PubMed PMID: 30255761. Epub 2018/09/27
77. Yee CS, McElhone K, Teh LS, Gordon C. Assessment of disease activity and quality of life in systemic lupus erythematosus – New aspects. Best Pract Res Clin Rheumatol. 2009;23(4):457–67. PubMed PMID: 19591777. Epub 2009/07/14
78. Jolly M, Garris CP, Mikolaitis RA, Jhingran PM, Dennis G, Wallace DJ, et al. Development and validation of the Lupus Impact Tracker: a patient-completed tool for clinical practice to assess and monitor the impact of systemic lupus erythematosus. Arthritis Care Res. 2014;66(10):1542–50. PubMed PMID: 24757021. Epub 2014/04/24
79. Azizoddin DR, Weinberg S, Gandhi N, Arora S, Block JA, Sequeira W, et al. Validation of the LupusPRO version 1.8: an update to a disease-specific patient-reported outcome tool for systemic lupus erythematosus. Lupus. 2018;27(5):728–37. PubMed PMID: 29087259. Epub 2017/11/01
80. Food and Drug Administration. Patient-reported outcome measures: use in medical product development to support labeling claims. Federal Register; December 3, 2009. p. 65132–3.
81. Katz P, Pedro S, Alemao E, Yazdany J, Dall'Era M, Trupin L, et al. Estimates of responsiveness, minimally important differences, and patient acceptable symptom state in five patient-reported outcomes measurement information system short forms in systemic lupus erythematosus. ACR Open Rheumatol. 2020;2(1):53–60. PubMed PMID: 31943975. PubMed Central PMCID: PMC6957915. Epub 2020/01/17
82. Lassere MN, Johnson KR, Woodworth TG, Furst DE, Fries JF, Kirwan JR, et al. Challenges and progress in adverse event ascertainment and reporting in clinical trials. J Rheumatol. 2005;32(10):2030–2. PubMed PMID: 16206364. Epub 2005/10/06
83. Tian J, Luo Y, Wu H, Long H, Zhao M, Lu Q. Risk of adverse events from different drugs for SLE: a systematic review and network meta-analysis. Lupus Sci Med. 2018;5(1):e000253. PubMed PMID: 29644081. PubMed Central PMCID: PMC5890859. Epub 2018/04/13
84. Gazarian M, Tugwell P, Boers M, Bombardier C, Brooks P, Day R, et al. Patient based methods for assessing adverse events in clinical trials in rheumatology. Progress report for the OMERACT Drug Toxicity Working Party. Outcome Measures in Rheumatology. J Rheumatol. 1999;26(1):207–9. PubMed PMID: 9918265. Epub 1999/01/26
85. Klokker L, Tugwell P, Furst DE, Devoe D, Williamson P, Terwee CB, et al. Developing an OMERACT core outcome set for assessing safety components in rheumatology trials: the OMERACT safety working group. J Rheumatol. 2017;44(12):1916–9. PubMed PMID: 27744393. Epub 2016/10/17
86. Lau CS, Yin G, Mok MY. Ethnic and geographical differences in systemic lupus erythematosus: an overview. Lupus. 2006;15(11):715–9. PubMed PMID: 17153840. Epub 2006/12/13

87. Maetzel A, Tugwell P, Boers M, Guillemin F, Coyle D, Drummond M, et al. Economic evaluation of programs or interventions in the management of rheumatoid arthritis: defining a consensus-based reference case. J Rheumatol. 2003;30(4):891–6. PubMed PMID: 12672224. Epub 2003/04/03
88. Lau CS, Mak A. The socioeconomic burden of SLE. Nat Rev Rheumatol. 2009;5(7):400–4. PubMed PMID: 19506585. Epub 2009/06/10
89. Doria A, Briani C. Lupus: improving long-term prognosis. Lupus. 2008;17(3):166–70. PubMed PMID: 18372355. Epub 2008/03/29
90. Barber MRW, Hanly JG, Su L, Urowitz MB, St Pierre Y, Romero-Diaz J, et al. Economic evaluation of lupus nephritis in the systemic lupus international collaborating clinics inception cohort using a multistate model approach. Arthritis Care Res. 2018;70(9):1294–302. PubMed PMID: 29193883. PubMed Central PMCID: PMC6155450. Epub 2017/12/02
91. Gordon C, Clarke AE. Quality of life and economic evaluation in SLE clinical trials. Lupus. 1999;8(8):645–54. PubMed PMID: 10568902. Epub 1999/11/24
92. Katz P, Nelson WW, Daly RP, Topf L, Connolly-Strong E, Reed ML. Patient-reported lupus flare symptoms are associated with worsened patient outcomes and increased economic burden. J Manag Care Spec Pharm. 2020;26(3):275–83. PubMed PMID: 32105178. Epub 2020/02/28
93. Barber MRW, Hanly JG, Su L, Urowitz MB, St Pierre Y, Romero-Diaz J, et al. Economic evaluation of damage accrual in an international SLE inception cohort using a multistate model approach. Arthritis Care Res. 2020;72(12):1800–8. PubMed PMID: 31609532.
94. ACR Ad Hoc Committee on Neuropsychiatric Lupus Nomenclature. The American College of Rheumatology nomenclature and case definitions for neuropsychiatric lupus syndromes. Arthritis Rheum. 1999;42:599–608.
95. Hanly JG. Diagnosis and management of neuropsychiatric SLE. Nat Rev Rheumatol. 2014;10(6):338–47. PubMed PMID: 24514913.
96. Rayes HA, Tani C, Kwan A, Marzouk S, Colosimo K, Medina-Rosas J, et al. What is the prevalence of cognitive impairment in lupus and which instruments are used to measure it? A systematic review and meta-analysis. Semin Arthritis Rheum. 2018;48(2):240–55. PubMed PMID: 29571540. Epub 2018/03/25
97. Hanly JG, Fisk JD, Sherwood G, Eastwood B. Clinical course of cognitive dysfunction in systemic lupus erythematosus. J Rheumatol. 1994;21(10):1825–31. PubMed PMID: 7837145. Epub 1994/10/01. eng
98. Glanz BI, Slonim D, Urowitz MB, Gladman DD, Gough J, MacKinnon A. Pattern of neuropsychologic dysfunction in inactive systemic lupus erythematosus. Neuropsychiatry Neuropsychol Behav Neurol. 1997;10(4):232–8. PubMed PMID: 9359119. Epub 1997/11/14
99. Tayer-Shifman OE, Green R, Beaton D, Ruttan L, Wither JE, Tartaglia MC, et al. Validity evidence supports the use of automated neuropsychological assessment metrics as a screening tool for cognitive impairment in lupus. Arthritis Care Res. 2019;72(12):1809–19. PubMed PMID: 31628718. Epub 2019/10/20. eng
100. American Psychiatric Association. Diagnostic and statistical manual of mental disorders. 5th ed. Washington, DC: American Psychiatric Publishing; 2013.
101. Hanly JG, Urowitz MB, Su L. Short-term outcome of neuropsychiatric events in systemic lupus erythematosus upon enrollment into an international inception cohort study. Arthritis Rheum. 2008;59(5):721–9.
102. Hanly JG, Su L, Urowitz MB, Romero-Diaz J, Gordon C, Bae SC, et al. Mood disorders in systemic lupus erythematosus: results from an international inception cohort study. Arthritis Rheumatol. 2015;67(7):1837–47. PubMed PMID: 25778456. PubMed Central PMCID: PMC4485527. Epub 2015/03/18
103. Eldeiry D, Zandy M, Tayer-Shifman OE, Kwan A, Marzouk S, Su J, et al. Association between depression and anxiety with skin and musculoskeletal clinical phenotypes in systemic lupus erythematosus. Rheumatology. 2020;59(11):3211–20. PubMed PMID: 32221602. Epub 2020/03/30

104. Moustafa AT, Moazzami M, Engel L, Bangert E, Hassanein M, Marzouk S, et al. Prevalence and metric of depression and anxiety in systemic lupus erythematosus: a systematic review and meta-analysis. Semin Arthritis Rheum. 2020;50(1):84–94. PubMed PMID: 31303437. Epub 2019/07/16
105. Hanly JG, Omisade A, Su L, Farewell V, Fisk JD. Assessment of cognitive function in systemic lupus erythematosus, rheumatoid arthritis, and multiple sclerosis by computerized neuropsychological tests. Arthritis Rheum. 2010;62(5):1478–86. PubMed PMID: 20155829.
106. Zirkee EH, Bollen E, Buchem MA. Mortality in neuropsychiatric systemic lupus erythematosus (NPSLE). Lupus. 2014;23:31–8.
107. Shen J, Barbera J, Shapiro CM. Distinguishing sleepiness and fatigue: focus on definition and measurement. Sleep Med Rev. 2006;10(1):63–76. PubMed PMID: 16376590. Epub 2005/12/27
108. Omdal R, Mellgren SI, Koldingsnes W, Jacobsen EA, Husby G. Fatigue in patients with systemic lupus erythematosus: lack of associations to serum cytokines, antiphospholipid antibodies, or other disease characteristics. J Rheumatol. 2002;29(3):482–6. PubMed PMID: 11908560. Epub 2002/03/23
109. Jump RL, Robinson ME, Armstrong AE, Barnes EV, Kilbourn KM, Richards HB. Fatigue in systemic lupus erythematosus: contributions of disease activity, pain, depression, and perceived social support. J Rheumatol. 2005;32(9):1699–705. PubMed PMID: 16142863. Epub 2005/09/06
110. Di Franco M, Guzzo MP, Spinelli FR, Atzeni F, Sarzi-Puttini P, Conti F, et al. Pain and systemic lupus erythematosus. Reumatismo. 2014;66(1):33–8. PubMed PMID: 24938194. Epub 2014/06/19
111. Petri M, Kawata AK, Fernandes AW, Gajria K, Greth W, Hareendran A, et al. Impaired health status and the effect of pain and fatigue on functioning in clinical trial patients with systemic lupus erythematosus. J Rheumatol. 2013;40(11):1865–74. PubMed PMID: 24085548. Epub 2013/10/03
112. Elefante E, Tani C, Stagnaro C, Ferro F, Parma A, Carli L, et al. Impact of fatigue on health-related quality of life and illness perception in a monocentric cohort of patients with systemic lupus erythematosus. RMD Open. 2020;6(1):e001133. PubMed PMID: 32075876. PubMed Central PMCID: PMC7046978. Epub 2020/02/23
113. Azizoddin DR, Gandhi N, Weinberg S, Sengupta M, Nicassio PM, Jolly M. Fatigue in systemic lupus: the role of disease activity and its correlates. Lupus. 2019;28(2):163–73. PubMed PMID: 30580659. Epub 2018/12/26
114. Ad Hoc Committee on Systemic Lupus Erythematosus Response Criteria for Fatigue. Measurement of fatigue in systemic lupus erythematosus: a systematic review. Arthritis Rheum. 2007;57(8):1348–57.
115. Barbacki A, Petri M, Avina-Zubieta A, Alarcon GS, Bernatsky S. Fatigue measurements in systemic lupus erythematosus. J Rheumatol. 2019;46(11):1470–7. PubMed PMID: 30709953. Epub 2019/02/03
116. Moses N, Wiggers J, Nicholas C. Persistence of unmet need for care among people with systemic lupus erythematosus: a longitudinal study. Qual Life Res. 2008;17(6):867–76. PubMed PMID: 18553154. Epub 2008/06/17
117. Danoff-Burg S, Friedberg F. Unmet needs of patients with systemic lupus erythematosus. Behav Med. 2009;35(1):5–13. PubMed PMID: 19297299. PubMed Central PMCID: PMC2687813. Epub 2009/03/20
118. Rockwood K, Fox RA, Stolee P, Robertson D, Beattie BL. Frailty in elderly people: an evolving concept. CMAJ. 1994;150(4):489–95. PubMed PMID: 8313261. PubMed Central PMCID: PMC1486322. Epub 1994/02/15
119. Fulop T, Larbi A, Witkowski JM, McElhaney J, Loeb M, Mitnitski A, et al. Aging, frailty and age-related diseases. Biogerontology. 2010;11(5):547–63. PubMed PMID: 20559726. Epub 2010/06/19

120. Ferrucci L, Fabbri E. Inflammageing: chronic inflammation in ageing, cardiovascular disease, and frailty. Nat Rev Cardiol. 2018;15(9):505–22. PubMed PMID: 30065258. PubMed Central PMCID: PMC6146930. Epub 2018/08/02
121. Katz PP, Andrews J, Yazdany J, Schmajuk G, Trupin L, Yelin E. Is frailty a relevant concept in SLE? Lupus Sci Med. 2017;4(1):e000186. PubMed PMID: 28243456. PubMed Central PMCID: PMC5294024. Epub 2017/03/01
122. Legge A, Kirkland S, Rockwood K, Andreou P, Bae SC, Gordon C, et al. Construction of a frailty index as a novel health measure in systemic lupus erythematosus. J Rheumatol. 2020;47(1):72–81. PubMed PMID: 30988130. PubMed Central PMCID: PMC6800806. Epub 2019/04/17
123. Beaton DE, Maxwell LJ, Shea BJ, Wells GA, Boers M, Grosskleg S, et al. Instrument selection using the OMERACT filter 2.1: the OMERACT methodology. J Rheumatol. 2019;46(8):1028–35. PubMed PMID: 30709952. Epub 2019/02/03
124. Slavin RE. Best evidence synthesis: an intelligent alternative to meta-analysis. J Clin Epidemiol. 1995;48(1):9–18. PubMed PMID: 7853053.
125. Castellanos FX, Margulies DS, Kelly C, Uddin LQ, Ghaffari M, Kirsch A, et al. Cingulate-precuneus interactions: a new locus of dysfunction in adult attention-deficit/hyperactivity disorder. Biol Psychiatry. 2008;63(3):332–7. PubMed PMID: 17888409. PubMed Central PMCID: 2745053.
126. EULAR. EULAR recommendations: EULAR/ACR collaborative projects. Accessed 7 Aug 2020.

# Chapter 2
# Clinical Aspects of Systemic Lupus Erythematosus

**Diane L. Kamen and Eric Zollars**

## Introduction

Systemic lupus erythematosus (SLE) is often described as the prototypical autoimmune disease. It is a chronic, potentially severe, frequently disabling autoimmune disease with multi-organ involvement and an unpredictable, typically waxing, and waning course. As explained in Chap. 2, SLE is characterized by the production of a wide array of antibodies directed against self-antigens. It is well described that autoantibodies precede the clinical diagnosis of SLE [1, 2]. Additionally, patients report the onset of symptoms an average of 6 years prior to the diagnosis of SLE [3]. This illustrates the fact that although autoantibodies are necessary for the diagnosis of SLE, they are by no means sufficient.

Further, the clinical manifestations of SLE are much more varied than the few serologies that are commonly available for testing. SLE has the potential to affect virtually every organ, most commonly presenting with musculoskeletal, cutaneous, renal, cardiovascular, and/or central nervous system involvement.

The onset of SLE can be at any age but most often occurs in young women between puberty and menopause. The incidence and severity of SLE are also disproportionately higher among certain racial and ethnic groups, such as people of African descent who live in North America or Europe [4]. In spite of its high impact on individual lives as well as high societal cost, little is known about the etiology of SLE.

Early diagnosis can be difficult because of the insidious onset of predominantly non-specific constitutional symptoms (e.g., fatigue, joint pains, and low-grade

D. L. Kamen (✉) · E. Zollars
Division of Rheumatology, Medical University of South Carolina, Charleston, SC, USA
e-mail: kamend@musc.edu; ezollars@amgen.com



Z. Touma (ed.), *Outcome Measures and Metrics in Systemic Lupus Erythematosus*, https://doi.org/10.1007/978-3-030-73303-2_2

fever). This delay between symptom onset with inflammation and subsequent diagnosis and initiation of treatment can result in the development of organ system damage. This chapter is focused on the clinical manifestations of SLE and will, when possible, distinguish between active inflammatory features and features seen in long-standing disease due to damage.

## Classification of SLE

The clinical symptoms and laboratory manifestations of SLE are diverse, and no two patients present in the same way. To help make sense of such a wide array of manifestations, classification criteria for SLE have been developed to help identify patients, particularly for inclusion in research studies and trials. The 1982 revised American College of Rheumatology (ACR) SLE classification criteria [5] and their 1997 revision [6] are widely utilized but are missing features of SLE found to be important, such as low levels of serum complement components C3 and C4 (Table 2.1). The 2012 Systemic Lupus International Collaborating Clinics (SLICC) classification criteria included additional mucocutaneous, neuropsychiatric, and serologic criteria [7] (Table 2.2). The 2019 European League Against Rheumatism (EULAR)/ACR SLE classification criteria included hierarchical clustering and weighting of the criteria, given that certain manifestations have greater sensitivity and/or specificity for SLE compared to others [8] (Table 2.3).

## General Manifestations

Fatigue is one of the most frequent and disabling symptoms for many patients with SLE. It is the primary complaint in 50–90% of patients [9], and it is the largest negative contributor to participating with normal life in the majority of patients [3, 10].

**Table 2.1** 1997 American College of Rheumatology Classification Criteria for systemic lupus erythematosus

| |
|---|
| 1. Malar rash |
| 2. Discoid rash |
| 3. Photosensitivity – skin rash brought on by sunlight |
| 4. Oral ulcers |
| 5. Arthritis |
| 6. Serositis – pleuritic or pericarditis |
| 7. Renal disorder |
| 8. Neurologic disorder – seizures or psychosis without another explanation |
| 9. Hematologic disorder – leukopenia, hemolytic anemia, thrombocytopenia |
| 10. Immunologic disorder |
| 11. Antinuclear antibody (ANA) positive |

At least 4 out of these 11 criteria are needed for classification as definite lupus

**Table 2.2** 2012 SLICC classification criteria for systemic lupus erythematosus

| *Clinical criteria* |
|---|
| 1. Acute cutaneous lupus |
| 2. Chronic cutaneous lupus |
| 3. Oral ulcers: palate |
| 4. Non-scarring alopecia (diffuse thinning or hair fragility with visible broken hairs) |
| 5. Synovitis involving two or more joints, characterized by swelling or effusion OR tenderness in two or more joints and 30 min or more of morning stiffness |
| 6. Serositis |
| 7. Renal |
| 8. Neurologic |
| 9. Hemolytic anemia |
| 10. Leukopenia (<4000/mm3 at least once) |
| 11. Thrombocytopenia (<100,000/mm3) at least once |
| *Immunological criteria* |
| 1. ANA above laboratory reference range |
| 2. Anti-dsDNA above laboratory reference range, except ELISA: twice above laboratory |
| 3. Anti-Sm |
| 4. Antiphospholipid antibody: any of the following |
| 5. Low complement |
| 6. Direct Coombs test in the absence of hemolytic anemia |

Classification for SLE requires (1) at least 4 out of these 17 criteria, including at least 1 clinical criterion *and* 1 immunologic criterion, *or* (2) lupus nephritis as the sole clinical criterion in the presence of ANA or anti-dsDNA antibodies

Unfortunately, the number of people limited by fatigue has not changed significantly over the past 30 years. The persistence of fatigue, despite improvement overall in treatment options for SLE, is in large part attributable to its multifactorial etiology. Although treatment of active SLE with belimumab did lead to improvement in fatigue in many patients [11], fatigue is often not driven by the inflammation of SLE. In clinical cohorts of lupus patients, other features, primarily depression, correlate with fatigue [12]. Fatigue is frequently independent of serologic or other clinical manifestations of SLE. Thus, potential adverse effects of medications and manifestations of comorbid conditions including mood disorders, lack of physical activity, and sleep disorders should always be addressed.

Fever in SLE is a challenging clinical problem and can only be attributed to SLE after an extensive search for other causes. Unexplained fever >38.3 °C was newly included as one of the classification criteria for SLE in the 2019 EULAR/ACR classification criteria set, although assigned a relatively low weight at 2 points [8] (Table 2.3). A wide range (36–86%) of patients with SLE have fever reported as a manifestation of active SLE. Fever may also result from infections, medications, or malignancies. SLE as a cause of fever of unknown origin is rare, being diagnosed in less than 5% of patients. However, among hospitalized patients with known SLE, the cause of the febrile episode was often (60%) due to active SLE, with 23% due to infections.

**Table 2.3** 2019 European League Against Rheumatism and American College of Rheumatology Classification Criteria for systemic lupus erythematosus

| *Entry criterion*<br>Antinuclear antibodies (ANA) at a titer of ≥1:80 on HEp-2 cells or an equivalent positive test (ever) | |
|---|---|
| If absent, do not classify as SLE<br>If present, apply additive criteria | |
| Additive criteria<br>Do not count a criterion if there is a more likely explanation than SLE<br>Occurrence of a criterion on at least one occasion is sufficient<br>SLE classification requires at least one clinical criterion and ≥10 points<br>Criteria need not occur simultaneously<br>Within each domain, only the highest weighted criterion is counted toward the total score[b] | |
| Clinical domains and criteria | Weight |
| *Constitutional* | |
| Fever | 2 |
| *Hematologic* | |
| Leukopenia | 3 |
| Thrombocytopenia | 4 |
| Autoimmune hemolysis | 4 |
| *Neuropsychiatric* | |
| Delirium | 2 |
| Psychosis | 3 |
| Seizure | 5 |
| *Mucocutaneous* | |
| Non-scarring alopecia | 2 |
| Oral ulcers | 2 |
| Subacute cutaneous OR discoid lupus | 4 |
| Acute cutaneous lupus | 6 |
| *Serosal* | |
| Pleural or pericardial effusion | 5 |
| Acute pericarditis | 6 |
| *Musculoskeletal* | |
| Joint involvement | 6 |
| *Renal* | |
| Proteinuria >0.5 g/24 h | 4 |
| Renal biopsy Class II or V lupus nephritis | 8 |
| Renal biopsy Class III or IV lupus nephritis | 10 |
| Immunology domains and criteria | Weight |
| *Antiphospholipid antibodies* | |
| Anti-cardiolipin antibodies OR | |
| Anti-β2GP1 antibodies OR | |
| Lupus anticoagulant | 2 |
| *Complement proteins* | |
| Low C3 OR low C4 | 3 |

**Table 2.3** (continued)

| | |
|---|---|
| Low C3 AND low C4 | 4 |
| *SLE-specific antibodies* | |
| Anti-dsDNA antibody[a] *or* | |
| Anti-Smith antibody | 6 |

Classify as systemic lupus erythematosus with a score of 10 or more if entry criterion fulfilled
Note: [a]In an assay with ≥90% specificity against relevant disease controls. [b]Additional criteria items within the same domain will not be counted

Unintentional weight loss in SLE should motivate a search for active SLE. The inflammation of active SLE consumes energy, and if caloric intake is not maintained during this time, unhealthy weight loss will occur. Cachexia, defined as ≥5% weight loss, was found in close to half of patients at time of entry into the Hopkins Lupus Cohort and was strongly associated with lupus nephritis [13].

## Cutaneous Manifestations

The clinical heterogeneity that is characteristic of SLE is especially apparent among cutaneous manifestations. The SLICC classification criteria for SLE includes 13 defined and distinct lupus rashes, reflecting the broad range of rashes considered to be clinically consistent with SLE [7] (Table 2.2). Some cutaneous lesions are more specific to SLE (e.g., a photosensitive malar rash), and some are less specific (e.g., areas of alopecia). Many of the skin lesions of SLE can occur in isolation or as features of active systemic disease. Most, if not all, lesions in lupus are exacerbated by ultraviolet radiation, and protection from the sun is a necessity for patients. Broadly, the rashes can be divided into acute and chronic lesions. However, there is often overlap. The heterogeneity of clinical manifestations, severity, and potential for irrecoverable scarring lead to a great spectrum of treatment possibilities as well.

### *Acute Cutaneous Lupus*

Although there are many potential causes of an erythematous rash in the malar distribution, the "butterfly rash" is considered the classic rash of SLE, occurring in greater than 50% of patients. It is described as a raised, erythematous lesion that can be pruritic or painful and occurs over the cheeks and nose, sparing the nasolabial folds which tend to be more protected from the sun.

General photosensitivity is a feature of SLE in more than 50% of patients (Fig. 2.1). This is an exaggerated response to UV radiation than can vary in appearance from sunburn-like to a severe, raised erythematous rash. A concern for patients with SLE is that the UV exposure can trigger further systemic manifestations

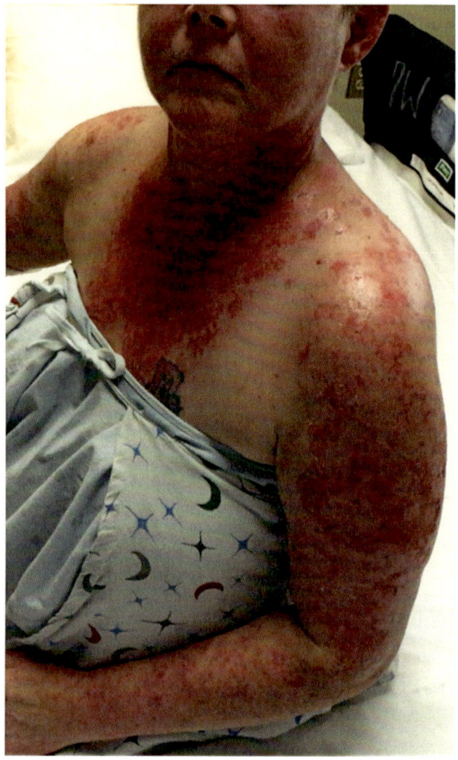

**Fig. 2.1** Photosensitive subacute cutaneous lupus erythematosus rash with a psoriasiform appearance and erythematous malar rash

as well. Photosensitivity in the form of polymorphous light eruption is common in the healthy population (10–20%), complicating the attribution of this type of rash.

Subacute Cutaneous Lupus Erythematosus (SCLE) describes a subset of non-scarring rashes which may start as erythematous papules or small plaques with scale (Fig. 2.1). These rashes can mimic psoriasis (psoriasiform) or can merge to form a polycyclic pattern or annular lesions. Although there is often central clearing, it can be differentiated from discoid lesions by the lack of scarring. As a rule, the SCLE rash is highly photosensitive. Only about 10% of people with SLE develop this rash, but about 50% of people with this rash will have SLE, with many having drug-induced SCLE. More than 90% of people will have the anti-Ro (anti-SSA) autoantibody. Of note, patients with Sjogren's syndrome can develop a similar rash.

## *Chronic Cutaneous Lupus*

Discoid lupus can be a scarring, disfiguring, and difficult-to-treat condition (Fig. 2.2). About 25% of patients with SLE will develop discoid lesions. People who present with discoid lesions are unlikely to develop SLE, with only 20% progressing to systemic involvement [14]. Discoid lesions are erythematous, initially about coin size with a raised border and prominent scale. Progression will lead to

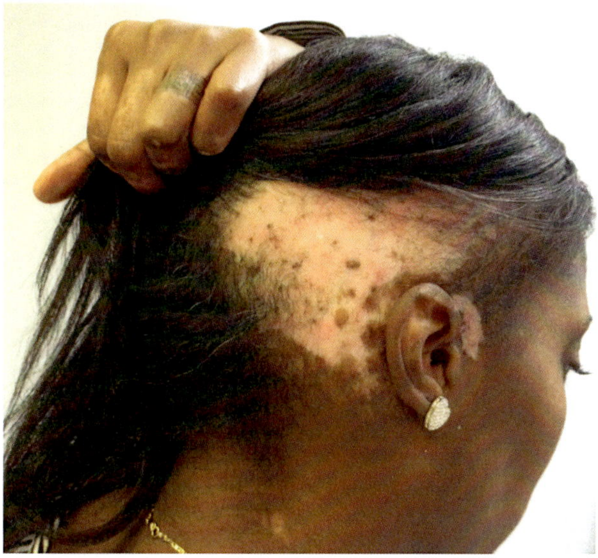

**Fig. 2.2** Patient with SLE having discoid lupus lesions (note the central scarring with hypopigmentation) and alopecia affecting the frontal and temporal regions of the scalp

the appearance of adherent scale, and there is prominent follicular plugging. Central clearing leads to atrophy and scar. When on the face, they can be quite disfiguring. When occurring on the scalp, they lead to scarring alopecia. They can occur anywhere on the body but have a predilection to the head, neck, and inside the external ear (conchal bowl).

Lupus profundus is a form of chronic cutaneous lupus which can occur independently, in association with discoid lesions or as a manifestation of SLE. Lupus profundus is a panniculitis which is inflammation of the fatty subcutaneous level. This is a rare manifestation that can lead to tender, deep nodules as well as atrophy. The atrophy of panniculitis appears as dips in the flesh. Lupus profundus unfortunately has a predisposition for the face and the upper arms.

Lupus tumidus is another rare form of chronic cutaneous lupus, which is also a photosensitive rash but does not have the same histologic features as other forms of cutaneous lupus. This rash clinically is described as erythematous, swollen plaques.

Non-scarring alopecia was added to the SLE Classification Criteria in 2012 with SLICC [7]. This is a thinning of hair, often with broken hairs and often at the temples bilaterally. This is strongly associated with increased SLE disease activity. When overall disease activity improves, the alopecia should improve as well. Notably, this is different from the scarring alopecia associated with discoid lesions in the scalp that do not improve.

## *Non-specific Cutaneous Lesions*

There are a variety of non-specific lesions that are seen in SLE and are associated with disease activity. These are often seen in other rheumatic (dermatomyositis, vasculitis) and non-rheumatic conditions (endocarditis). There is a vasculitic

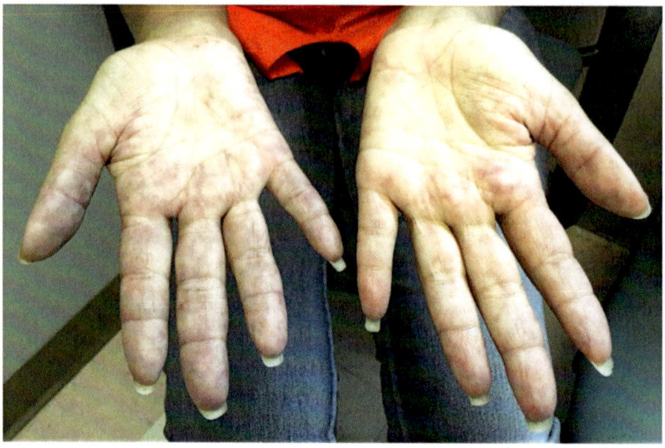

**Fig. 2.3** Patient with SLE and livedo reticularis over the palmar surface of her hands with digital angiitis

component to many of these lesions. Digital angiitis, alternatively called nodular vasculitis, consists of concerning lesions associated with elevated SLE disease activity (Fig. 2.3). These are areas of immune complex deposition or small vessel vasculitis seen on the palms and fingers as palpable purpura or raised nodules. Ischemia can result leading to gangrene. These lesions are also associated with elevated systemic disease activity and should motivate a search for other SLE manifestations.

## Musculoskeletal Features

Inflammatory lupus arthritis is experienced by the vast majority of patients at some point during the course of their disease. Arthritis is also one of the more common reasons (along with rash) for entry into lupus clinical trials. However, clinically, the arthritis is poorly described and studied. It is rarely the case that lupus has the profound proliferative synovitis of rheumatoid arthritis. Nevertheless, 10–20% of lupus patients will have an overlap rheumatoid arthritis ("rhupus"). The classic deforming arthritis of lupus is Jaccoud's that leads to reducible deformities of the fingers. The vast majority of patients have neither of these manifestations and instead have bouts of swelling of the hands, wrists, knees, and ankles. In many patients, this arthritis can be quite chronic and requires aggressive treatment for control. There is also a large component of tenosynovitis that accompanies lupus arthritis as well. The swelling of the tendons around the joints can be just as limiting as the swollen joints themselves. The arthritis and joint pain is described by the majority of lupus patients as one of the most limiting features of the disease. As the arthritis of lupus is often more subtle than that of rheumatoid arthritis, advanced imaging (e.g., ultrasound, extremity MRI) is being used more frequently to study this manifestation. Often there is subclinical (not detected by physical exam) inflammation detected by these techniques.

### *Lupus Myositis*

True muscle inflammation in SLE is rare. When it occurs, lupus myositis is different from the idiopathic inflammatory myopathies (IIMs). Pain is a larger component of lupus myositis which is rare in IIMs. Muscle biopsy is common in the evaluation of muscle inflammation, and biopsies in lupus myositis show less prominent inflammatory infiltrate than the IIMs and show a spectrum of histologic muscle damage.

### *Other Musculoskeletal Manifestations*

Patients with SLE can have many other musculoskeletal pain complaints that can complicate the attribution to lupus disease activity. Fibromyalgia, a pain processing disorder, is a comorbid condition in 20–40% of patients with SLE. As patients with SLE age, they develop degenerative arthritis similar to the rest of the population. Neither of these conditions should be treated with lupus disease-modifying drugs but unfortunately lead to over-treatment in many cases.

Lupus patients are more afflicted with avascular necrosis (AVN) of the shoulders and hips. This painful condition of bone death has no accepted medical treatment and can be very limiting. Surgical joint replacement is often required. AVN in lupus is strongly associated with steroid usage and unfortunately can occur even after relatively short amounts of time.

## Renal Manifestations

Lupus nephritis remains one of the most debilitating and potentially life-threatening manifestations of SLE, occurring in 40–60% of adults and up to 80% of children with SLE [15]. Untreated, lupus nephritis leads to chronic kidney disease (CKD), renal failure, dialysis, or death. The susceptibility and burden of SLE are substantially higher among black women compared to other groups, with blacks having 3 times the incidence rate compared to whites and females having 9–10 times the prevalence compared to males [16, 17]. Peak age of incidence for both SLE and lupus nephritis is also younger among black females. The disparities in SLE-related risk are most striking when examining renal involvement, with black patients and Hispanic patients having more frequent and more severe lupus nephritis compared to other groups [16–19].

While overall mortality in lupus has improved with the use of steroids and immune suppressants, the progression to CKD after onset of nephritis remains unacceptably high (up to 44%) [20]. Also, full remission with medical treatment is rare with the majority of patients still on immune suppression 10 years after initiation [21]. Unfortunately, lupus nephritis can be a presenting feature of SLE with significant irreversible damage occurring before diagnosis and treatment initiation. This can occur when lupus nephritis is "silent" without other features of SLE. Fortunately, lupus nephritis can be detected early with routine screening of the urine for proteinuria.

The classification of lupus nephritis is based on histological features seen on kidney biopsy, defined by the 2003 International Society of Nephrology/Renal Pathology Society criteria (Table 2.4), which were revised in 2018 [22]. Renal biopsy histology helps not only confirm the diagnosis but also guide therapy for lupus nephritis. Proliferative lupus nephritis is the most common form, often presenting as proteinuria, microscopic hematuria, urinary casts, hypertension, and potentially including renal insufficiency [23]. Membranous lupus nephritis is also frequently seen histologically either alone or in conjunction with proliferative nephritis, often presenting as nephrotic syndrome with edema, wasting, and hypercoagulability [23].

## Neuropsychiatric Manifestations

CNS lupus, also called neuropsychiatric lupus or NPSLE, is at least as common in children with SLE as in adults, with prevalence rates overall of 30–40%. CNS manifestations common in patients with SLE, such as headache, anxiety, depression and cognitive dysfunction, are also common in the general population and therefore difficult to attribute to SLE [24]. Great care must be taken with these common maladies before attributing them to increased SLE disease activity.

In a large international inception cohort of patients with SLE, 40% of patients had at least one neuropsychiatric event, and 17% had multiple events over an average of 2 years of follow-up [25]. Less than one third of the events could be attributed to SLE leaving the majority as due to non-SLE causes [25]. CNS involvement accounts for 93% of the neuropsychiatric events, with the remaining 7% involving the peripheral nervous system [25].

Although it has a lower incidence among patients with SLE compared to nephritis, CNS lupus remains a leading cause of morbidity and accounts for approximately 13–17% of deaths among patients with SLE [26]. Major events such as cerebrovascular disease, severe cognitive dysfunction, myelopathy, and optic neuritis often result in poor functional outcomes, underscoring the need for improved diagnostic tests and more effective therapeutic options [27].

Neurocognitive impairment is the most frequent of the 19 NPSLE syndromes defined by the American College of Rheumatology [28]. Up to 100% of patients with SLE have measureable abnormalities on standardized neuropsychiatric tests [29], although one study found that 70% of detectable cognitive dysfunction is mild [30]. Complicating matters is the fact that even the low doses of corticosteroids commonly taken by patients are associated with neurocognitive impairment. Impairment from corticosteroid use is most commonly manifest in declarative (verbal) memory, reflecting a hippocampus-dependent process, but severe cognitive disorders induced by corticosteroids have also been reported [28].

**Table 2.4** International Society of Nephrology/Renal Pathology Society (ISN/RPS) 2003 classification of lupus nephritis

| | |
|---|---|
| **Class I** | **Minimal mesangial lupus nephritis** |
| | Normal glomeruli by light microscopy but mesangial immune deposits by immunofluorescence |
| **Class II** | **Mesangial proliferative lupus nephritis** |
| | Purely mesangial hypercellularity of any degree or mesangial matrix expansion by light microscopy along with mesangial immune deposits |
| | May be a few isolated subepithelial or subendothelial deposits visible by immunofluorescence or electron microscopy but not by light microscopy |
| **Class III** | **Focal lupus nephritis**[a] |
| | Active or inactive focal, segmental, or global endocapillary or extracapillary glomerulonephritis involving $<50\%$ of all glomeruli, typically with focal subendothelial immune deposits, with or without mesangial alterations |
| Class III (A) | Active lesions: focal proliferative lupus nephritis |
| Class III (A/C) | Active and chronic lesions: focal proliferative and sclerosing lupus nephritis |
| Class III (C) | Chronic inactive lesions with glomerular scars: focal sclerosing lupus nephritis |
| **Class IV** | **Diffuse lupus nephritis**[b] |
| | Active or inactive diffuse, segmental, or global endocapillary or extracapillary glomerulonephritis involving $\geq 50\%$ of all glomeruli, typically with diffuse subendothelial immune deposits, with or without mesangial alterations. This class is divided into diffuse segmental (IV-S) lupus nephritis when $\geq 50\%$ of the involved glomeruli have segmental lesions and as diffuse global (IV-G) lupus nephritis when $\geq 50\%$ of the involved glomeruli have global lesions. A segmental lesion is defined as a glomerular lesion that involves less than half the glomerular tuft. This class includes cases with diffuse wire loop deposits with little or no glomerular proliferation |
| Class IV-S (A) | Active lesions: diffuse segmental proliferative lupus nephritis |
| Class IV-G (A) | Active lesions: diffuse global proliferative lupus nephritis |
| Class IV-S (A/C) | Active and chronic lesions: diffuse segmental proliferative and sclerosing lupus nephritis |
| | Active and chronic lesions: diffuse global proliferative and sclerosing lupus nephritis |
| Class IV-S (C) | Chronic inactive lesions with scars: diffuse segmental sclerosing lupus nephritis |
| Class IV-G (C) | Chronic inactive lesions with scars: diffuse global sclerosing lupus nephritis |
| **Class V** | **Membranous lupus nephritis** |
| | Global or segmental subepithelial immune deposits or their morphologic sequelae by light microscopy and by immunofluorescence or electron microscopy, with or without mesangial alterations |
| | Class V lupus nephritis may occur in combination with class III or IV, in which case both will be diagnosed |
| | Class V lupus nephritis with advanced sclerosis |
| **Class VI** | **Advanced sclerosis lupus nephritis** |
| | $\geq 90\%$ of glomeruli globally sclerosed without residual activity |

[a]Indicates the proportion of glomeruli with fibrinoid necrosis, cellular crescents, or both. Indicates the grade (mild, moderate, severe) of tubular atrophy, interstitial inflammation, and fibrosis and the severity of arteriolosclerosis or other vascular lesions

[b]Indicates the proportion of glomeruli with active and sclerotic lesions

From Weening et al. [90]

Headaches are reported by up to 57% of patients with SLE [31], but in reality, an isolated "lupus headache" that is attributable to CNS lupus is rare [32]. A headache may be a component of another NPSLE event (stroke, seizure, meningitis), but, in isolation, headache is not associated with increased disease activity. Evaluation and treatment of headache in a patient with SLE should proceed as it would in a patient without SLE. Consideration should be given to increased thrombotic risk in the presence of antiphospholipid antibodies, as well as to the possibility of SLE-related aseptic meningitis, but otherwise standard therapies for headaches apply.

Anxiety and mood disorder are also common among patients with SLE, reported in up to 37% [33], which can also be adverse effects of corticosteroid therapy and other medications [34]. Not only can depressive symptoms increase with corticosteroid use, but corticosteroid withdrawal can cause symptoms of fatigue, anorexia, and depression as well [34]. Corticosteroids therefore do not play as significant of a treatment role as compared to anxiolytics and antidepressants for anxiety and mood disorders when these are the features of CNS lupus.

Over the course of having SLE, seizures occur in 7–20% of patients, either focal or generalized, and usually in the context of increased SLE disease activity [35, 36]. Cerebrovascular disease is another common major CNS event, occurring in 5–18% of patients with SLE and comprised 80–90% of ischemic strokes, more rarely hemorrhagic [37]. Psychosis occurs in 2–3% of patients with SLE, characterized by delusions and/or both auditory and visual hallucinations, usually in the setting of active SLE [33, 38].

Acute confusional state (previously called acute organic brain syndrome) occurs in approximately 3% of patients with SLE and can present with disorganized thinking, loss of orientation, agitation, and delusions [33]. A poor prognosis is associated with progression to a reduced level of consciousness, such as stupor or coma, although symptoms may fluctuate [37]. Potential SLE-related causes include vasculitis, leukothrombosis, and autoantibodies, although non-SLE causes such as infection, medication effects, and metabolic disturbances are also common.

Lupus myelopathy occurs in approximately 1% of patients, can present with rapid onset, and involve either grey matter (lower motor neuron) or white matter (upper motor neuron) patterns. The lesions on MRI can involve any level of the spinal cord, typically appearing as cord edema and abnormalities of T2-weighted images. The cause is often multifactorial, with vasculitis documented in some cases, as well as thromboses related to antiphospholipid antibody syndrome in other cases.

## Gastrointestinal Involvement

Gastrointestinal (GI) symptoms are common among patients with SLE, although more often due to medication side effects or infections rather than due to active SLE [39]. The most prevalent GI symptoms are non-specific, such as nausea and vomiting, anorexia, and abdominal pain [40]. GI system disease activity is relatively rare among patients with SLE. But for that minority of patients, SLE activity involving the GI system can be severe and even life-threatening.

## Mucocutaneous Lesions

Ulcers in the mouth and nose are quite common among patients with SLE, with genital ulcers described much less frequently. Oral and nasal ulcers are seen in 25–50% of patients with SLE and are a component of the classification criteria sets for SLE [5–8]. Although classically described as "painless" and on the upper (hard) palate [41], they can occur anywhere in the mouth and can be painful when exposed to acidic foods or beverages.

## Lupus Enteritis

Lupus enteritis is a rare feature of SLE but has the potential for organ and life-threatening complications. Studies show a range of 0.2–5.8% of patients with SLE affected by lupus enteritis [42]. Presenting signs and symptoms of lupus enteritis are often non-specific, but seldom present without other evidence of active SLE. The three main variants of lupus enteritis are lupus mesenteric vasculitis, intestinal pseudo-obstruction, and protein losing enteropathy [43]. Lupus enteritis, as part of the British Isles Lupus Assessment Group (BILAG) disease activity index, is defined as either vasculitis or inflammation of the small bowel, with supportive image and/or biopsy findings [44].

True mesenteric vasculitis involves small vessel arteritis or venulitis [45] and can lead to the development of bowel wall infarction, ischemia, or perforation [46]. These complications hold a high rate of associated mortality. Typically, the jejunum and ileum are the most commonly GI tract locations involved. The underlying etiology for the enteric vasculitis continues to be unknown.

Intestinal pseudo-obstruction is defined as ineffective propulsion in the intestinal tract. Typical involvement implicates not only the smooth muscle but also the enteric nerves, leading to visceral autonomic nervous system dysfunction, further compromising GI motility [47]. Main areas of involvement include the lower third of the esophagus as well as the antrum and duodenum.

Protein losing enteropathy is defined as profound edema with hypoalbuminemia secondary to excessive protein loss from the GI tract. Pathophysiologic mechanisms revolve around impairment of the permeability of the gut wall [48].

## Serositis

Abdominal serositis (lupus peritonitis) is seen in 10% of SLE patients, though the 1982 Revised Criteria for Classification of SLE limits consideration of serositis to pleural and pericardial surfaces [5]. In the vast majority of cases, SLE is simultaneously active in other organ systems [49].

## *Associated Hepatobiliary Manifestations*

Elevated transaminase/transaminitis has been found among SLE patients with a frequency of between 15% and 55% [50]. Medications can be culprits, [50] and other SLE-associated conditions include viral hepatitis, hemolysis, myositis, venous congestion, and veno-occlusive disease, especially in the setting of antiphospholipid antibody syndrome. Autoimmune hepatitis and primary biliary cirrhosis should be considered if anti-mitochondrial antibodies and elevated alkaline phosphatase are present. Uncommonly, patients with SLE may develop acute cholecystitis with inflammation of the gallbladder complicated by vasculitis or serositis [43].

## Hematologic Manifestations

Hematologic abnormalities, particularly cytopenias, are common among patients with SLE and can be some of the earliest clinical manifestations detected. Over half of patients with SLE will have a form of anemia, with anemia of chronic disease and iron-deficiency anemia being the most common but autoimmune hemolytic anemia being the most specific to SLE. Autoimmune hemolytic anemia generally presents with an acute drop in hemoglobin level, anisocytosis and spherocytes on the blood smear, low serum haptoglobin, and high reticulocyte count, all reflecting active hemolysis. A positive direct antiglobulin test (Coombs test) in the context of hemolytic anemia generally confirms the diagnosis of autoimmune hemolytic anemia, although other causes such as infection and medication-induced hemolysis must still be considered.

Leukopenia, with white blood cell (WBC) counts <4000/mm$^3$, is a frequent feature of SLE, present in 22–42% of patients [51]. When due to active SLE, the WBC counts rarely go below 1500/mm$^3$, and typically the bone marrow is normal. Lymphopenia is more often due to active SLE and is one of the most common hematologic manifestations of SLE. Lymphopenia <1500/mm$^3$ is usually associated with SLE activity; however, some patients may have a genetic predisposition for lymphopenia that does not reflect active SLE. Neutropenia can also be seen with active SLE due to autoantibodies that inhibit granulocyte colony-forming units in bone marrow, but may also be the result of immunosuppressive medications and bone marrow suppression.

Thrombocytopenia is also a manifestation of SLE that can fluctuate with the level of overall disease activity. Platelet counts <100,000//mm$^3$ have been reported in 10–30% of patients with SLE. In a large multiethnic cohort of patients with SLE, early thrombocytopenia was indicative of more severe and active SLE, particularly pulmonary, neurologic, renal, and hematologic involvement. Thrombocytopenia was a predictor of mortality, and severe thrombocytopenia (with platelets <50,000/mm$^3$) predicted damage accrual [52]. Thrombocytopenia in a patient with SLE can signal other comorbidities to consider as well, such as antiphospholipid antibody syndrome and thrombotic thrombocytopenic purpura (TTP) syndrome, which can complicate SLE.

## Pulmonary Involvement

The lungs are commonly involved later in the course of SLE in the setting of other organ involvement. The most common pulmonary manifestation attributable to SLE is pleuritis, but other pleural involvement can be seen, as well as parenchymal disease, pulmonary vascular disease, diaphragmatic dysfunction, and upper airway dysfunction [53]. Finding the true prevalence of lung involvement with SLE is complicated by the high rates of pulmonary infections. An autopsy study of 90 patients with SLE found pleuropulmonary involvement in 97.8%, the most common being pleuritis (77.8%), bacterial infections (57.8%), and primary and secondary alveolar hemorrhages (25.6%), followed by distal airway alterations (21.1%), opportunistic infections (14.4%), and pulmonary thromboembolism (7.8%) [54]. In a series of 216 consecutive patients with SLE followed in the United Kingdom, 25% had evidence of lung involvement diagnosed clinically and/or by imaging [55].

The pleura is often involved in patients with SLE. Approximately 30–50% of patients with SLE will develop symptomatic pleural inflammation over the course of their disease; a larger number if asymptomatic effusions are included [56, 57]. In 5–10% of patients, pleuritis is an initial manifestation of their SLE [58]. The typical presentation of pleural involvement in SLE is sharp chest pain with a deep breath (pleurisy). Pleural effusions in SLE tend to be bilateral, but small, and may not be evident on radiographic imaging [59]. A friction rub may be present on examination; however, these can be transient. Typically, pleural disease in SLE responds well to nonsteroidal anti-inflammatory drugs (NSAIDs) or low-dose corticosteroids.

Albeit rare, occurring in 1–12% of patients, acute lupus pneumonitis is one of the most dreaded complications of SLE [60, 61]. Patients usually present with fever, cough, pleurisy, dyspnea with hypoxia, and sometimes hemoptysis. The most immediate concern for patients with suspected lupus pneumonitis is to exclude the presence of a pulmonary infection since these two diseases have similar presentations but very different treatments. It can also be difficult to distinguish acute lupus pneumonitis from diffuse alveolar hemorrhage.

Diffuse alveolar hemorrhage (DAH) is a rare and potentially fatal complication of SLE [62–64]. The exact prevalence is not known, but in one study of hospitalized patients with SLE, DAH occurred in 19 of 510 patients over 10 years [63]. Patients with DAH present acutely ill, often with dyspnea, cough, hemoptysis, and sometimes fever. It typically presents in patients with established SLE, often in the setting of active lupus nephritis or other active organ involvement. The hematocrit of a patient with active DAH will usually drop quickly. If lung function tests have been done, a significantly elevated DLCO may be suggestive of pulmonary hemorrhage. Chest radiography shows bilateral alveolar infiltrates and BAL is useful in excluding infection. The presence of persistently bloody fluid with hemosiderin-laden macrophages helps confirm DAH [63].

Chronic interstitial lung disease (ILD), also called fibrotic lupus pneumonitis, is seen in 3–13% of patients with SLE, primarily in patients with long-standing disease [65, 66]. There is an association with anti-SSA antibodies, and in one series, anti-SSA antibodies were found in 81% of patients with lupus pneumonitis, compared to 38% for all patients with SLE [67]. ILD often develops insidiously, with gradually worsening nonproductive cough, dyspnea on exertion, and pleurisy, but can also appear following acute lupus pneumonitis [68]. Similar to idiopathic pulmonary fibrosis, bibasilar inspiratory pulmonary crackles are heard on exam. Lung function tests show a restrictive pattern with reduced lung volumes and reduced diffusing capacity for carbon monoxide (DLCO).

The shrinking or "vanishing" lung syndrome (SLS) has been reported in patients with SLE who have unexplained dyspnea, elevation of the diaphragm (usually bilateral), and reduced lung volumes without evidence of ILD [69, 70]. Lung function tests show a restrictive defect and DLCO is usually normal when corrected for lung volume. A review of 77 patients with SLS reported in the literature estimates the prevalence to be 0.6–0.9% [55, 71] and finds that persistent episodes of pleuritic chest pain are common [71].

Symptomatic pulmonary hypertension (PH) is considered a rare complication of SLE, and is more often seen with SLE overlaps with other connective tissue diseases, particularly scleroderma or mixed connective tissue disease. The prevalence of PH in patients with SLE (SLE-PH) is estimated between 0.5% and 43% depending on the cohort studied and the method of diagnosis used [72–75]. Symptoms of SLE-PH most commonly include dyspnea, chest pain, nonproductive cough, and fatigue. Patients may also develop peripheral edema and other findings consistent with PH including jugular venous distension, fixed S2 splitting, murmurs of tricuspid regurgitation or pulmonic insufficiency, and hepatomegaly with ascites.

SLE can involve the upper airways in up to 30% of patients, ranging from laryngeal mucosal inflammation, mucosal ulcerations, cricoarytenoiditis, vocal cord paralysis and edema, to life-threatening necrotizing vasculitis with airway obstruction [76, 77]. Presenting symptoms can also range from hoarseness, dyspnea, and much more rarely airway obstruction from edema requiring mechanical ventilation. Corticosteroids are the first-line therapy, and symptoms typically respond well. Symptomatic bronchiolar disorders in SLE are rare, but bronchial wall thickening and/or bronchiectasis was seen in 21% of 34 patients with SLE in a prospective study using HRCT [78]. In a different series, features consistent with small airway dysfunction were found in 24% of 70 non-smoking patients with SLE [79].

## Cardiac Manifestations

SLE can involve any part of the heart, leading to pericarditis, myocarditis, endocarditis, valvular disease, and thrombosis [80].

Pericardial effusion secondary to pericarditis is the most common cardiac manifestation of SLE. Over 30% of patients have pericardial effusions on echocardiography, with 25% having symptomatic pericarditis at some point in their disease course. Classically, pericarditis presents with tachycardia and substernal or precordial positional chest pain. Some patients will have a pericardial rub detected on examination. Constrictive pericarditis and tamponade can develop, but are both rare.

Clinically apparent myocarditis is uncommon (<10% of patients with SLE) [81], but autopsy findings reveal a higher number of patients with subclinical myocarditis. Presentation of SLE myocarditis often includes symptoms of heart failure including resting tachycardia and dyspnea, as well as potential chest pain and/or fever. Imaging showing global hypokinesis without evidence of coronary artery disease would support a diagnosis of myocarditis [80]. Myocarditis should be suspected in patients with SLE presenting with otherwise unexplained arrhythmias or conduction defects, cardiomegaly with or without congestive heart failure, or tachycardia [80].

Patients with SLE can also develop myocarditis, either directly SLE induced, atherosclerosis-related, or, rarely, secondary to hydroxychloroquine [82]. Cardiomyopathy secondary to small vessel disease and thrombosis of the microcirculation have also been described [83]. Additionally, cardiac autonomic dysfunction is seen among patients with SLE. Older patients with SLE, particularly those with hypertension and peripheral neuropathy, are at a higher risk for cardiac sympathetic dysfunction, and older obese patients with a history of CVA are at a higher risk for cardiac parasympathetic dysfunction [80].

Libman-Sacks (nonbacterial thrombotic) endocarditis involves sterile, verrucous, atypical valvular lesions associated with SLE and antiphospholipid antibodies. These valvular lesions, appearing as leaflet thickening or vegetations, can affect any of the valves but most commonly mitral and aortic. A study of trans-esophageal echocardiograms found valvular thickening in 51% of patients with SLE and valvular vegetations in 43% [84]. Among patients with SLE, valvular regurgitation was found in 25% and stenosis in 4%, with both more common in patients compared to controls [84]. Initially patients with valvular lesions may be asymptomatic, but valvular insufficiency, heart failure, and consequences of embolic disease such as neurologic deficits [85].

## *Accelerated Atherosclerosis*

Patients with SLE have an increased risk of premature cardiovascular disease and atherosclerosis is the most prevalent mortality risk for older adult patients with SLE [86–88]. SLE is an independent risk factor for cardiovascular disease and is included in the American Heart Association recommendations for screening and treating for cardiovascular disease prevention. The accelerated atherosclerosis among patients with SLE may be manifested as coronary artery disease, cerebral vascular disease, and/or peripheral vascular disease. Even children with SLE have evidence of developing premature atherosclerosis and the risk of fatal myocardial infarction and other cardiovascular events increases in proportion to SLE disease duration [89].

## References


1. Arbuckle MR, McClain MT, Rubertone MV, Scofield RH, Dennis GJ, James JA, et al. Development of autoantibodies before the clinical onset of systemic lupus erythematosus. N Engl J Med. 2003;349(16):1526–33.
2. Heinlen LD, McClain MT, Merrill J, Akbarali YW, Edgerton CC, Harley JB, et al. Clinical criteria for systemic lupus erythematosus precede diagnosis, and associated autoantibodies are present before clinical symptoms. Arthritis Rheum. 2007;56(7):2344–51.
3. Morgan C, Bland AR, Maker C, Dunnage J, Bruce IN. Individuals living with lupus: findings from the LUPUS UK Members Survey 2014. Lupus. 2018;27(4):681–7.
4. Kaul A, Gordon C, Crow MK, Touma Z, Urowitz MB, van Vollenhoven R, et al. Systemic lupus erythematosus. Nat Rev Dis Primers. 2016;2:16039.
5. Tan EM, Cohen AS, Fries JF, Masi AT, McShane DJ, Rothfield NF, et al. The 1982 revised criteria for the classification of systemic lupus erythematosus. Arthritis Rheum. 1982;25(11):1271–7.
6. Hochberg MC. Updating the American College of Rheumatology revised criteria for the classification of systemic lupus erythematosus. Arthritis Rheum. 1997;40(9):1725.
7. Petri M, Orbai AM, Alarcon GS, Gordon C, Merrill JT, Fortin PR, et al. Derivation and validation of the Systemic Lupus International Collaborating Clinics classification criteria for systemic lupus erythematosus. Arthritis Rheum. 2012;64(8):2677–86.
8. Aringer M, Costenbader K, Daikh D, Brinks R, Mosca M, Ramsey-Goldman R, et al. 2019 European league against rheumatism/American college of rheumatology classification criteria for systemic lupus erythematosus. Arthritis Rheumatol. 2019;71(9):1400–12.
9. Schmeding A, Schneider M. Fatigue, health-related quality of life and other patient-reported outcomes in systemic lupus erythematosus. Best Pract Res Clin Rheumatol. 2013;27(3):363–75.
10. Krupp LB, LaRocca NG, Muir J, Steinberg AD. A study of fatigue in systemic lupus erythematosus. J Rheumatol. 1990;17(11):1450–2.
11. Strand V, Berry P, Lin X, Asukai Y, Punwaney R, Ramachandran S. Long-term impact of belimumab on health-related quality of life and fatigue in patients with systemic lupus erythematosus: six years of treatment. Arthritis Care Res (Hoboken). 2019;71(6):829–38.
12. Azizoddin DR, Gandhi N, Weinberg S, Sengupta M, Nicassio PM, Jolly M. Fatigue in systemic lupus: the role of disease activity and its correlates. Lupus. 2019;28(2):163–73.
13. Stojan G, Li J, Wittmaack A, Petri M. Cachexia in systemic lupus erythematosus: risk factors and relation to disease activity and damage. Arthritis Care Res (Hoboken). 2020. https://doi.org/10.1002/acr.24395.
14. Wieczorek IT, Propert KJ, Okawa J, Werth VP. Systemic symptoms in the progression of cutaneous to systemic lupus erythematosus. JAMA Dermatol. 2014;150(3):291–6.
15. Mina R, Abulaban K, Klein-Gitelman M, Eberhard A, Ardoin S, Singer N, et al. Validation of the lupus nephritis clinical indices in childhood-onset systemic lupus erythematosus. Arthritis Care Res. 2015;68(2):195–202.
16. Lim SS, Bayakly AR, Helmick CG, Gordon C, Easley KA, Drenkard C. The incidence and prevalence of systemic lupus erythematosus, 2002-2004: the Georgia Lupus Registry. Arthritis Rheumatol. 2014;66(2):357–68.
17. Somers EC, Marder W, Cagnoli P, Lewis EE, Deguire P, Gordon C, et al. Population-based incidence and prevalence of systemic lupus erythematosus: the Michigan lupus epidemiology and surveillance program. Arthritis Rheumatol. 2014;66(2):369–78.

18. Bastian HM, Roseman JM, McGwin G Jr, Alarcon GS, Friedman AW, Fessler BJ, et al. Systemic lupus erythematosus in three ethnic groups. XII. Risk factors for lupus nephritis after diagnosis. Lupus. 2002;11(3):152–60.
19. Korbet SM, Schwartz MM, Evans J, Lewis EJ. Severe lupus nephritis: racial differences in presentation and outcome. J Am Soc Nephrol. 2007;18(1):244–54.
20. Tektonidou MG, Dasgupta A, Ward MM. Risk of end-stage renal disease in patients with lupus nephritis, 1971–2015: a systematic review and Bayesian meta-analysis. Arthritis Rheumatol. 2016;68(6):1432–41.
21. Tamirou F, D'Cruz D, Sangle S, Remy P, Vasconcelos C, Fiehn C, et al. Long-term follow-up of the MAINTAIN Nephritis Trial, comparing azathioprine and mycophenolate mofetil as maintenance therapy of lupus nephritis. Ann Rheum Dis. 2016;75(3):526–31.
22. Bajema IM, Wilhelmus S, Alpers CE, Bruijn JA, Colvin RB, Cook HT, et al. Revision of the International Society of Nephrology/Renal Pathology Society classification for lupus nephritis: clarification of definitions, and modified National Institutes of Health activity and chronicity indices. Kidney Int. 2018;93(4):789–96.
23. Ward MM. Recent clinical trials in lupus nephritis. Rheum Dis Clin N Am. 2014;40(3):519–35. ix
24. Fanouriakis A, Boumpas DT, Bertsias GK. Pathogenesis and treatment of CNS lupus. Curr Opin Rheumatol. 2013;25(5):577–83.
25. Hanly JG, Urowitz MB, Su L, Bae SC, Gordon C, Wallace DJ, et al. Prospective analysis of neuropsychiatric events in an international disease inception cohort of patients with systemic lupus erythematosus. Ann Rheum Dis. 2010;69(3):529–35.
26. Wang Z, Wang Y, Zhu R, Tian X, Xu D, Wang Q, et al. Long-term survival and death causes of systemic lupus erythematosus in China: a systemic review of observational studies. Medicine (Baltimore). 2015;94(17):e794.
27. Bertsias GK, Ioannidis JP, Aringer M, Bollen E, Bombardieri S, Bruce IN, et al. EULAR recommendations for the management of systemic lupus erythematosus with neuropsychiatric manifestations: report of a task force of the EULAR standing committee for clinical affairs. Ann Rheum Dis. 2010;69(12):2074–82.
28. Nishimura K, Omori M, Katsumata Y, Sato E, Gono T, Kawaguchi Y, et al. Neurocognitive impairment in corticosteroid-naive patients with active systemic lupus erythematosus: a prospective study. J Rheumatol. 2015;42(3):441–8.
29. Kremer JM, Rynes RI, Bartholomew LE, Rodichok LD, Pelton EW, Block EA, et al. Non-organic non-psychotic psychopathology (NONPP) in patients with systemic lupus erythematosus. Semin Arthritis Rheum. 1981;11(1):182–9.
30. Ainiala H, Loukkola J, Peltola J, Korpela M, Hietaharju A. The prevalence of neuropsychiatric syndromes in systemic lupus erythematosus. Neurology. 2001;57(3):496–500.
31. Mitsikostas DD, Sfikakis PP, Goadsby PJ. A meta-analysis for headache in systemic lupus erythematosus: the evidence and the myth. Brain. 2004;127(Pt 5):1200–9.
32. Hanly JG, Urowitz MB, O'Keeffe AG, Gordon C, Bae SC, Sanchez-Guerrero J, et al. Headache in systemic lupus erythematosus: results from a prospective, international inception cohort study. Arthritis Rheum. 2013;65(11):2887–97.
33. Unterman A, Nolte JE, Boaz M, Abady M, Shoenfeld Y, Zandman-Goddard G. Neuropsychiatric syndromes in systemic lupus erythematosus: a meta-analysis. Semin Arthritis Rheum. 2011;41(1):1–11.
34. Bhangle SD, Kramer N, Rosenstein ED. Corticosteroid-induced neuropsychiatric disorders: review and contrast with neuropsychiatric lupus. Rheumatol Int. 2013;33(8):1923–32.
35. Andrade RM, Alarcon GS, Gonzalez LA, Fernandez M, Apte M, Vila LM, et al. Seizures in patients with systemic lupus erythematosus: data from LUMINA, a multiethnic cohort (LUMINA LIV). Ann Rheum Dis. 2008;67(6):829–34.
36. Hanly JG, Urowitz MB, Su L, Gordon C, Bae SC, Sanchez-Guerrero J, et al. Seizure disorders in systemic lupus erythematosus results from an international, prospective, inception cohort study. Ann Rheum Dis. 2012;71(9):1502–9.

37. West SG. Clinical aspects of the nervous system. In: Wallace DJ, Hahn BH, editors. Systemic glucocorticoid therapy in SLE. 8th ed. Philadelphia: Lippincott Williams & Wilkins; 2013. p. 368–81.
38. Pego-Reigosa JM, Isenberg DA. Psychosis due to systemic lupus erythematosus: characteristics and long-term outcome of this rare manifestation of the disease. Rheumatology (Oxford). 2008;47(10):1498–502.
39. Alves SC, Fasano S, Isenberg DA. Autoimmune gastrointestinal complications in patients with systemic lupus erythematosus: case series and literature review. Lupus. 2016;25(14):1509–19.
40. Ebert EC, Hagspiel KD. Gastrointestinal and hepatic manifestations of systemic lupus erythematosus. J Clin Gastroenterol. 2011;45(5):436–41.
41. Urman JD, Lowenstein MB, Abeles M, Weinstein A. Oral mucosal ulceration in systemic lupus erythematosus. Arthritis Rheum. 1978;21(1):58–61.
42. Koo BS, Hong S, Kim YJ, Kim YG, Lee CK, Yoo B. Lupus enteritis: clinical characteristics and predictive factors for recurrence. Lupus. 2015;24(6):628–32.
43. Brewer BN, Kamen DL. Gastrointestinal and hepatic disease in systemic lupus erythematosus. Rheum Dis Clin N Am. 2018;44(1):165–75.
44. Isenberg DA, Rahman A, Allen E, Farewell V, Akil M, Bruce IN, et al. BILAG 2004. Development and initial validation of an updated version of the British Isles Lupus Assessment Group's disease activity index for patients with systemic lupus erythematosus. Rheumatology. 2005;44(7):902–6.
45. Lee CK, Ahn MS, Lee EY, Shin JH, Cho YS, Ha HK, et al. Acute abdominal pain in systemic lupus erythematosus: focus on lupus enteritis (gastrointestinal vasculitis). Ann Rheum Dis. 2002;61(6):547–50.
46. Yuan S, Ye Y, Chen D, Qiu Q, Zhan Z, Lian F, et al. Lupus mesenteric vasculitis: clinical features and associated factors for the recurrence and prognosis of disease. Semin Arthritis Rheum. 2014;43(6):759–66.
47. Wang JL, Liu G, Liu T, Wei JP. Intestinal pseudo-obstruction in systemic lupus erythematosus: a case report and review of the literature. Medicine (Baltimore). 2014;93(29):e248.
48. Chen Z, Li MT, Xu D, Yang H, Li J, Zhao JL, et al. Protein-losing enteropathy in systemic lupus erythematosus: 12 years experience from a Chinese academic center. PLoS One. 2014;9(12):e114684.
49. Man BL, Mok CC. Serositis related to systemic lupus erythematosus: prevalence and outcome. Lupus. 2005;14(10):822–6.
50. Witt M, Zecher D, Anders HJ. Gastrointestinal manifestations associated with systemic lupus erythematosus. Eur J Med Res. 2006;11(6):253–60.
51. Carli L, Tani C, Vagnani S, Signorini V, Mosca M. Leukopenia, lymphopenia, and neutropenia in systemic lupus erythematosus: prevalence and clinical impact–a systematic literature review. Semin Arthritis Rheum. 2015;45(2):190–4.
52. Fernandez M, Alarcon GS, Apte M, Andrade RM, Vila LM, Reveille JD. Systemic lupus erythematosus in a multiethnic US cohort: XLIII. The significance of thrombocytopenia as a prognostic factor. Arthritis Rheum. 2007;56(2):614–21.
53. Orens JB, Martinez FJ, Lynch JP 3rd. Pleuropulmonary manifestations of systemic lupus erythematosus. Rheum Dis Clin N Am. 1994;20(1):159–93.
54. Quadrelli SA, Alvarez C, Arce SC, Paz L, Sarano J, Sobrino EM, et al. Pulmonary involvement of systemic lupus erythematosus: analysis of 90 necropsies. Lupus. 2009;18(12):1053–60.
55. Pego-Reigosa JM, Medeiros DA, Isenberg DA. Respiratory manifestations of systemic lupus erythematosus: old and new concepts. Best Pract Res Clin Rheumatol. 2009;23(4):469–80.
56. Good JT Jr, King TE, Antony VB, Sahn SA. Lupus pleuritis. Clinical features and pleural fluid characteristics with special reference to pleural fluid antinuclear antibodies. Chest. 1983;84(6):714–8.
57. Pines A, Kaplinsky N, Olchovsky D, Rozenman J, Frankl O. Pleuro-pulmonary manifestations of systemic lupus erythematosus: clinical features of its subgroups. Prognostic and therapeutic implications. Chest. 1985;88(1):129–35.

58. Winslow WA, Ploss LN, Loitman B. Pleuritis in systemic lupus erythematosus: its importance as an early manifestation in diagnosis. Ann Intern Med. 1958;49(1):70–88.
59. Bouros D, Pneumatikos I, Tzouvelekis A. Pleural involvement in systemic autoimmune disorders. Respiration. 2008;75(4):361–71.
60. Wiedemann HP, Matthay RA. Pulmonary manifestations of systemic lupus erythematosus. J Thorac Imaging. 1992;7(2):1–18.
61. Cheema GS, Quismorio FP Jr. Interstitial lung disease in systemic lupus erythematosus. Curr Opin Pulm Med. 2000;6(5):424–9.
62. Eagen JW, Memoli VA, Roberts JL, Matthew GR, Schwartz MM, Lewis EJ. Pulmonary hemorrhage in systemic lupus erythematosus. Medicine (Baltimore). 1978;57(6):545–60.
63. Zamora MR, Warner ML, Tuder R, Schwarz MI. Diffuse alveolar hemorrhage and systemic lupus erythematosus. Clinical presentation, histology, survival, and outcome. Medicine (Baltimore). 1997;76(3):192–202.
64. Badsha H, Teh CL, Kong KO, Lian TY, Chng HH. Pulmonary hemorrhage in systemic lupus erythematosus. Semin Arthritis Rheum. 2004;33(6):414–21.
65. Weinrib L, Sharma OP, Quismorio FP Jr. A long-term study of interstitial lung disease in systemic lupus erythematosus. Semin Arthritis Rheum. 1990;20(1):48–56.
66. Haupt HM, Moore GW, Hutchins GM. The lung in systemic lupus erythematosus. Analysis of the pathologic changes in 120 patients. Am J Med. 1981;71(5):791–8.
67. Boulware DW, Hedgpeth MT. Lupus pneumonitis and anti-SSA(Ro) antibodies. J Rheumatol. 1989;16(4):479–81.
68. Matthay RA, Schwarz MI, Petty TL, Stanford RE, Gupta RC, Sahn SA, et al. Pulmonary manifestations of systemic lupus erythematosus: review of twelve cases of acute lupus pneumonitis. Medicine (Baltimore). 1975;54(5):397–409.
69. Karim MY, Miranda LC, Tench CM, Gordon PA, D'Cruz DP, Khamashta MA, et al. Presentation and prognosis of the shrinking lung syndrome in systemic lupus erythematosus. Semin Arthritis Rheum. 2002;31(5):289–98.
70. Warrington KJ, Moder KG, Brutinel WM. The shrinking lungs syndrome in systemic lupus erythematosus. Mayo Clin Proc. 2000;75(5):467–72.
71. Toya SP, Tzelepis GE. Association of the shrinking lung syndrome in systemic lupus erythematosus with pleurisy: a systematic review. Semin Arthritis Rheum. 2009;39(1):30–7.
72. Winslow TM, Ossipov MA, Fazio GP, Simonson JS, Redberg RF, Schiller NB. Five-year follow-up study of the prevalence and progression of pulmonary hypertension in systemic lupus erythematosus. Am Heart J. 1995;129(3):510–5.
73. Simonson JS, Schiller NB, Petri M, Hellmann DB. Pulmonary hypertension in systemic lupus erythematosus. J Rheumatol. 1989;16(7):918–25.
74. Johnson SR, Gladman DD, Urowitz MB, Ibanez D, Granton JT. Pulmonary hypertension in systemic lupus. Lupus. 2004;13(7):506–9.
75. Quismorio FP Jr, Sharma O, Koss M, Boylen T, Edmiston AW, Thornton PJ, et al. Immunopathologic and clinical studies in pulmonary hypertension associated with systemic lupus erythematosus. Semin Arthritis Rheum. 1984;13(4):349–59.
76. Teitel AD, MacKenzie CR, Stern R, Paget SA. Laryngeal involvement in systemic lupus erythematosus. Semin Arthritis Rheum. 1992;22(3):203–14.
77. Langford CA, Van Waes C. Upper airway obstruction in the rheumatic diseases. Rheum Dis Clin N Am. 1997;23(2):345–63.
78. Fenlon HM, Doran M, Sant SM, Breatnach E. High-resolution chest CT in systemic lupus erythematosus. AJR Am J Roentgenol. 1996;166(2):301–7.
79. Keane MP, Lynch JP 3rd. Pleuropulmonary manifestations of systemic lupus erythematosus. Thorax. 2000;55(2):159–66.
80. Miner JJ, Kim AH. Cardiac manifestations of systemic lupus erythematosus. Rheum Dis Clin N Am. 2014;40(1):51–60.

81. Apte M, McGwin G Jr, Vila LM, Kaslow RA, Alarcon GS, Reveille JD, et al. Associated factors and impact of myocarditis in patients with SLE from LUMINA, a multiethnic US cohort (LV). [corrected]. Rheumatology. 2008;47(3):362–7.
82. Tselios K, Deeb M, Gladman DD, Harvey P, Urowitz MB. Antimalarial-induced cardiomyopathy: a systematic review of the literature. Lupus. 2018;27(4):591–9.
83. Vaccaro F, Caccavo D, Roumpedaki E, De Vincentis G, Di Gioia CR, Gallo P, et al. Dilated cardiomyopathy due to thrombotic microangiopathy as the only manifestation of antiphospholipid syndrome: a case report. Int J Immunopathol Pharmacol. 2008;21(1):237–41.
84. Roldan CA, Shively BK, Crawford MH. An echocardiographic study of valvular heart disease associated with systemic lupus erythematosus. N Engl J Med. 1996;335(19):1424–30.
85. Ruiz D, Oates JC, Kamen DL. Antiphospholipid antibodies and heart valve disease in systemic lupus erythematosus. Am J Med Sci. 2018;355(3):293–8.
86. Gustafsson JT, Herlitz Lindberg M, Gunnarsson I, Pettersson S, Elvin K, Ohrvik J, et al. Excess atherosclerosis in systemic lupus erythematosus,-a matter of renal involvement: case control study of 281 SLE patients and 281 individually matched population controls. PLoS One. 2017;12(4):e0174572.
87. McMahon M, Skaggs B. Pathogenesis and treatment of atherosclerosis in lupus. Rheum Dis Clin N Am. 2014;40(3):475–95.
88. Stojan G, Petri M. Atherosclerosis in systemic lupus erythematosus. J Cardiovasc Pharmacol. 2013;62(3):255–62.
89. Schanberg LE, Sandborg C, Barnhart HX, Ardoin SP, Yow E, Evans GW, et al. Premature atherosclerosis in pediatric systemic lupus erythematosus: risk factors for increased carotid intima-media thickness in the atherosclerosis prevention in pediatric lupus erythematosus cohort. Arthritis Rheum. 2009;60(5):1496–507.
90. Weening JJ, D'Agati VD, Schwartz MM, et al. on behalf of the International Society of Nephrology and Renal Pathology Society Working Group on the Classification of Lupus Nephritis.Special feature: the classification of glomerulonephritis in systemic lupus erythematosus revisited. J Am Soc Nephrol. 2004;15:241–50.

# Chapter 3
# Diagnosis and Classification of Systemic Lupus Erythematosus

**Sindhu R. Johnson and Martin Aringer**

## Introduction

The complexity of systemic lupus erythematosus (SLE) makes its diagnosis and classification challenging. Part of the challenge is that the nature of the disease is not fully understood [1]. At its most basic level, it is a systemic rheumatic disease characterized by cellular immune activation, antibody formation, immune complex deposition, and inflammation of end organ tissues [2]. Yet SLE manifests as numerous, non-identical, but overlapping constellations of organ involvement in different people [3]. The ability to recognize the correct patterns of these symptoms, signs, and laboratory findings requires years of training and practice [4]. Many healthcare professionals have been relying on the presence of any 4 of 11 American College of Rheumatology Classification criteria for SLE (1982 and revised 1997 criteria) for making a diagnosis [5, 6]. However, classification criteria are not meant to be diagnostic criteria [7, 8]. In the modern era, our understanding of SLE has expanded far beyond this limited list. Indeed, the 2012 Systemic Lupus Erythematosus International Collaborating Clinics (SLICC) criteria greatly broadened the list of manifestations to be considered [9].

The diagnosis of SLE is further challenged by the conflation of many of its manifestations with disease activity, damage, disease trajectory, severity, and prognosis. Many features, which contribute to the diagnosis, can also reflect disease activity,

S. R. Johnson (✉)
Division of Rheumatology, Department of Medicine, Toronto Western Hospital, Mount Sinai Hospital, Toronto, ON, Canada

Institute of Health Policy, Management and Evaluation, University of Toronto, Toronto, ON, Canada
e-mail: Sindhu.Johnson@uhn.ca

M. Aringer
Division of Rheumatology, Department of Medicine III, University Medical Center and Faculty of Medicine at the TU Dresden, Dresden, Germany
e-mail: martin.aringer@uniklinikum-dresden.de



Z. Touma (ed.), *Outcome Measures and Metrics in Systemic Lupus Erythematosus*, https://doi.org/10.1007/978-3-030-73303-2_3

that is, disease that is potentially reversible. Other features contributing to the diagnosis may also reflect damage, an array of cumulative insults that are irreversible [10]. Damage and disease activity are important concepts that can contribute to organ dysfunction and morbidity [10–12]. Depending on the construct being ascertained (diagnosis, classification, activity, damage), the relative importance or weight of any given disease manifestation may differ.

The 2019 European League Against Rheumatism (EULAR)/ACR classification criteria [13, 14] is the latest iteration of criteria for SLE. The development of these criteria has taught many lessons about the current thinking around the construct of SLE. In this chapter, we discuss the development of the EULAR/ACR classification criteria and highlight insights gained into the ways experts worldwide think about SLE in the modern era.

## Classification Criteria Are Not Diagnostic Criteria

A common misconception is that classification criteria are the same as diagnostic criteria. Many systemic autoimmune rheumatic diseases lack a single diagnostic test, which uniformly characterizes the disease. Rather, the diagnosis is made by recognition of certain symptoms, signs, and/or investigational (radiographic, pathologic, biochemical, or immunologic) findings. As a result, there can be significant heterogeneity in disease presentation and a resulting wide spectrum of disease. This heterogeneity in the disease spectrum is problematic in research as it can impact the validity and reliability of observations and inferences made from the study findings. Both the American College of Rheumatology (ACR) and the European League Against Rheumatism (EULAR) have therefore encouraged the development and validation of classification criteria to identify more homogeneous groups of patients for inclusion into research studies [8, 15–17].

## 2019 EULAR/ACR Classification Criteria

The 2019 EULAR/ACR classification criteria are the result of a major international collaborative effort including more than 200 investigators and patient advocates and 4000 patients. The criteria are a defined system of classification, which produces a measure of the relative probability that an individual case with a combination of clinical features has SLE [14]. This system has defined the ten most important domains in defining that probability and defines a threshold of ten, from which on experts would classify SLE for the purpose of research studies [14]. Within each domain, every criterion has been defined carefully to improve the reliability of application [14]. This novel system of classification was developed over four phases with a balanced use of data-driven and expert-based methods (Fig. 3.1).

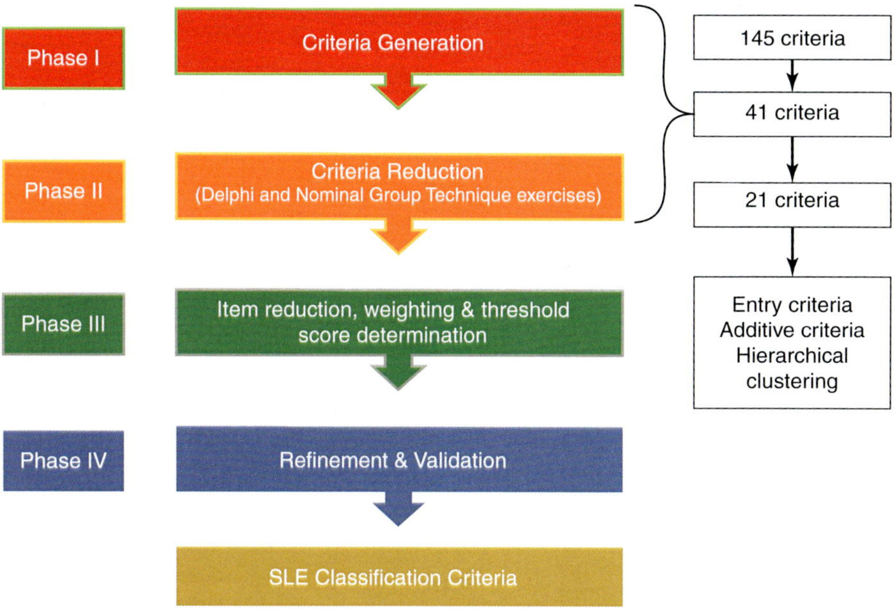


**Fig. 3.1** Methodologic overview of EULAR/ACR SLE classification criteria development

## Item Generation and New Insights About What Constitutes SLE

***ANA Is a Sensitive Screening Test and Entry Criterion*** In Phase 1, indirect immunofluorescence (IIF)-HEp-2 antinuclear antibody (ANA) was evaluated as an entry criterion for classification of SLE [18] (Fig. 3.2). In practice, ANA is used as a screening test. Thus, its use as an entry criterion reflects current practice. Using a systematic review of the literature and a meta-regression of 13,080 patient data, Leuchten et al. reported that ANA with a titer of 1:40, 1:80, 1:160, and 1:320 had a sensitivity of 98.4% (95% confidence interval (95% CI) 97.6–99.0%), 97.8% (95% CI 96.8–98.5%), 95.8% (95% CI 94.1–97.1%), and 86.0% (95% CI 77.0–91.9%), respectively [18]. The corresponding specificities were 66.9% (95% CI 57.8–74.9%), 74.7% (95% CI 66.7–81.3%), 86.2% (95% CI 80.4–90.5%), and 96.6% (95% CI 93.9–98.1%), respectively [18]. This data provided justification for ANA at a titer of at least 1:80 to be considered as an entry criterion for SLE classification.

***Novel Features of SLE*** The second, even broader objective of Phase 1 was to generate a complete, nonredundant list of candidate items that should be considered in the development of the new classification criteria. This was achieved through a cross-sectional survey of patients [19], the evaluation of an international early SLE cohort [20], and a three-step Delphi exercise of international SLE experts [21] (Fig. 3.2). Together, the studies of Phase 1 generated 145 candidate criteria to be

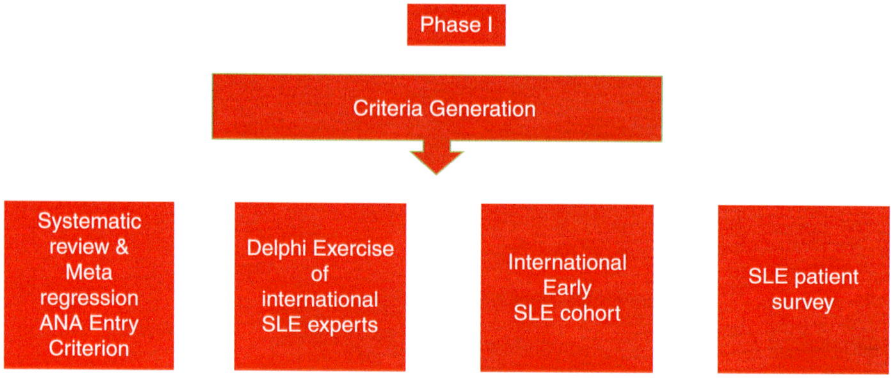


**Fig. 3.2** Methodologic components of the item generation

considered as classification criteria for SLE. In the survey of 339 German SLE patients, the majority reported fatigue (89.4%), joint pain (86.7%), photosensitivity (79.4%), and myalgia (76.1%) leading up to and in the first year after diagnosis. Of interest, more than half of the patients reported fever as an early symptom (53.7%) [19]. Using a data-driven approach, Mosca et al. evaluated an international cohort of 389 patients with early SLE and 227 patients with SLE-mimicking conditions from academic lupus centers in Asia, Europe, North America, and South America. Again, they found unexplained fever was more common in early SLE than in SLE-mimicking conditions (34.5% versus 13.7%, respectively, $p < 0.001$). In contrast, features less frequently observed in early SLE vs mimicking diseases included Raynaud's phenomenon (22.1% versus 48.5%; $p < 0.001$), sicca symptoms (4.4% versus 34.4%; $p < 0.001$), dysphagia (0.3% versus 6.2%; $p < 0.001$), and fatigue (28.3% versus 37.0%; $p = 0.024$).

The Delphi exercise surveyed 147 international SLE experts representing clinical care as well as clinical and translational lupus research (81.6% rheumatologists, 7.5% dermatologists, 6.8% nephrologists, 3.4% pediatricians, 0.7% nonclinical SLE researchers) from various geographic areas (53% from North or Central America, 46% from Europe). They suggested 145 distinct features when considering SLE [21] (Tables 3.1 and 3.2). In addition to the usual organ specific manifestations, experts suggested novel demographic features, laboratory parameters, and obstetrical and gastrointestinal manifestations to be important for classifying SLE. Interestingly, they suggested that demographic features such as age and ethnicity should be taken into consideration. They also suggested factors that should be excluded, such as systemic vasculitis, hepatitis B, hepatitis C, HIV, and parvovirus B19. Novel laboratory markers most frequently suggested included high circulating levels of IP10, MCP1, and TNF, type I interferon signature, high Th17 markers, plasma cell expansion, increased serum BLyS, hypergammaglobulinemia, lymphopenia, and anti-chromatin antibodies [21]. Due to the restricted ability to access such testing at most lupus centers, these laboratory makers were not included in the final 2019 EULAR/ACR classification criteria for SLE [13]. However, these findings reflect the ongoing shift in our understanding of what may constitute SLE (Fig. 3.3).

**Table 3.1** Body system-based features of systemic lupus erythematosus

| Cutaneous | Cardiovascular | Respiratory | Renal | Neuro-psych | Hematology | MSK | GI | OB |
|---|---|---|---|---|---|---|---|---|
| Alopecia with scalp inflammation | Early cardiovascular disease diagnosed before age 50 | Diffuse alveolar hemorrhage | Active urine sediment (without UTI) | Acute confusional state | Autoimmune hemolytic anemia | Arthritis | Hepatitis (auto-immune) | History of miscarriages |
| Bullous lupus | Libman-Sacks endocarditis | Interstitial lung disease | Elevated serum creatinine | Aseptic meningitis | Leukopenia (<4,000/mm$^3$ on 2 or more occasions) | Jaccoud's arthropathy | Peritonitis | History of pre-eclampsia |
| Chilblains lupus | Myocarditis | | Elevated urine total protein/albumin ratio | Chorea | Low reticulocyte count | Myositis | | |
| Discoid rash | Pericardial effusion | | Glomerulonephritis | Cognitive dysfunction | Lymphopenia (<1500/mm$^3$ on two or more occasions) | | | |
| Focal alopecia | Pericarditis (clinical signs) | | Lupus nephritis by renal biopsy with immune deposits | Headache | Thrombocytopenia (any) | | | |
| Focal non-scarring alopecia | Raynaud's phenomenon | | Lupus nephritis by renal biopsy with mesangial deposits | Multi-infarct dementia/ cortical atrophy | Thrombocytopenia (severe) | | | |
| Leuko-cytoclastic vasculitis | | | | Myelitis | | | | |
| Livedo reticularis | | | | Optic neuritis | | | | |
| Lupus profundus | | | | Peripheral or cranial neuropathy | | | | |
| Lupus tumidus | | | | | | | | |

(continued)

**Table 3.1** (continued)

| Cutaneous | Cardiovascular | Respiratory | Renal | Neuro-psych | Hematology | MSK | GI | OB |
|---|---|---|---|---|---|---|---|---|
| Malar rash | | | | | | | | |
| Nailfold capillary changes | | | | | | | | |
| Nasal septum perforation | | | | | | | | |
| Nasal ulcers | | | | | | | | |
| Neutrophilic urticaria | | | | | | | | |
| Non-bullous neutrophilic dermatitis | | | | | | | | |
| Oral mucosal lesions on the hard palate | | | | | | | | |
| Oral ulcers | | | | | | | | |
| Palmar erythema | | | | | | | | |
| Panniculitis | | | | | | | | |
| Photosensitivie rash | | | | | | | | |

*Neuro-psych* neuropsychiatric, *MSK* musculoskeletal, *GI* gastrointestinal, *OB* obstetrical
Adapted from Schmajuk G, Hoyer BF, Aringer M, Johnson SR, Daikh DI, Dorner T et al. Multicenter Delphi Exercise to Identify Important Key Items for Classifying Systemic Lupus Erythematosus. Arthritis Care Res (Hoboken) 2018;70(10):1488–94

**Table 3.2** Additional features of systemic lupus erythematosus

| Demographic | Antibody | Laboratory markers | Absence | Constitutional | Other |
|---|---|---|---|---|---|
| Age | ANA homogeneous pattern | Abnormal SPEP polyclonal gammopathy | Vasculitis | Constitutional symptoms (fevers, fatigue, *or* weight loss) | History of drug reaction (e.g., sulfa allergy) |
| Female gender | ANA nucleolar pattern | Complement fragments (elevated EC4d and BC4d) | Negative tests for hepatitis B and C, HIV, parvovirus B19 | Fatigue | Necrotizing lymphadenitis |
| Non-white race/ ethnicity | ANA positive any pattern aside from homogeneous | Elevated C3/C4 ratio | | Fever (≥38 °C) | Persistent adenopathy |
| | ANA positive (any pattern) >1:160 | Elevated CRP | | | |
| | ANA positive by Hep-2 | Elevated ESR | | | |
| | ANA rim pattern | Elevated ESR/CRP ratio (high ESR, low CRP) | | | |
| | ANA speckled pattern | Elevated ferritin | | | |
| | Anti c1q antibody | Hypergammaglobulinemia | | | |
| | Anti-chromatin antibody | Hypoalbuminemia | | | |
| | Anti-dsDNA antibody | Low C3 | | | |
| | Anti-erythrocyte antibodies | Low C3 AND C4 | | | |
| | Anti-factor VIII antibody | Low CH100 | | | |
| | Anti-histone antibody | Low CH50 | | | |
| | Anti-nucleosome antibody | Low total immunoglobulins | | | |
| | Antiphospholipid antibodies | Lupus band test | | | |
| | Antiplatelet antibodies | | | | |
| | Anti-ribosomal P antibody | | | | |

(continued)

**Table 3.2** (continued)

| Demographic | Antibody | Laboratory markers | Absence | Constitutional | Other |
|---|---|---|---|---|---|
| | Anti RNP antibody | | | | |
| | Anti-Smith antibody | | | | |
| | Anti-SSA antibody | | | | |
| | Anti-SSB antibody | | | | |
| | Antithyroid antibodies | | | | |
| | Anti-U1RNP | | | | |
| | APLS | | | | |
| | High titer IgA anti beta2-glycoprotein I | | | | |

Adapted from Schmajuk et al. [21]

| EULAR/ACR 2019 Classification | | For diagnosis, also consider |
|---|---|---|
| Positive ANA ever | Entry | < 3% ANA negativ |
| **Constitutional** | | Non-specific signs: Fatigue, Arthralgias, Myalgias |
| a) Fever | 2 | |
| **Hematologic** | | Non-specific signs: Lymphopenia, Anemia of chronic disease |
| a) Leukopenia < 4,000 | 3 | |
| b) Thrombocytopenia < 100,000 | 4 | |
| c) Autoimmune hemolysis | 4 | |
| **Neuropsychiatric** | | Uncommon symptoms: Neuropathy (cranial or peripheral) Chorea, Myelitis Mononeuritis multiplex |
| a) Delirium | 2 | |
| b) Psychosis | 3 | |
| c) Seizure | 5 | |
| **Mucocutaneous** | | Uncommon symptoms: Nasal ulcers, Lupus tumidus, Chilblains lupus, Lupus panniculítis Non-specific signs: Leukocytoclastic vasculitis, livedo reticularis, UV hypersensitivity |
| a) Nonscarring aplopezia | 2 | |
| b) Oral ulcers | 3 | |
| c) Discoid LE | 4 | |
| d) Subacute cutaneous LE | 4 | |
| e) Acute cutaneous LE | 6 | |
| **Serosal** | | Uncommon symptoms: Sterile peritonitis |
| a) Pleural or pericardial effusion | 5 | |
| b) Acute pericarditis | 6 | |
| **Musculoskeletal** | | Uncommon symptoms: Lupus myositis |
| a) Joint involvement | 6 | |
| **Renal** | | Additional symptoms: Hematuria, cellular casts Less specific forms of nephritis: IgA nephropathy, APS nephropathy |
| a) Proteinuria > 0.5 g/24 h | 4 | |
| b) Class II or V nephritis | 8 | |
| c) Class III or IV nephritis | 10 | |
| **Anti-phospholipid antibodies** | | |
| a) ACLA IgG, IgM, IgA | 2 | |
| b) Anti-β2 gp I IgG, IgM, IgA | 2 | |
| c) Lupus anticoagulant | 2 | |
| **Complement proteins** | | Novel tests: Cell-bound complement split products |
| a) C3 OR C4 low | 3 | |
| b) C3 AND C4 low | 4 | |
| **SLEspecific antibodies** | | Uncommon autoantibodies: Anti-ribosomal P, Anti-C1q Less specific autoantibodies: Anti-U1RNP, Anti-Ro/La, Anti-histone |
| a) Anti-dsDNA >90% specificity | 6 | |
| b) Anti-Sm | 6 | |

**Fig. 3.3** Considerations for the classification and diagnosis of SLE

***ANA Is Important for Diagnosing SLE*** The majority of experts require the presence of an ANA to make a diagnosis of SLE. 77% of experts would not feel comfortable or felt unsure classifying SLE in the absence of ANA by immunofluorescence assay (IF) [21]. Some experts noted that they would diagnose SLE in the absence of a positive ANA if historical positive values were available, that there was a subgroup of anti-Ro-positive patients that may test ANA negative, or that the variable quality of commercial ELISA testing did influence their answer [21]. Positive ANA alone was sufficient for 75% of the experts, while 25% would additionally require a specific immunofluorescence pattern [21]. 99% of experts reported anti-dsDNA and anti-Sm antibodies as the most characteristic serologic findings of SLE [21]. 61% reported that antiphospholipid antibodies would be informative in making the diagnosis, 46% for anti-Ro antibodies, 37% for anti-RNP, and 34% for anti-La, respectively [21]. Anti-C1q antibodies were also suggested as a novel laboratory finding [21].

***Similar Criteria Are Used for Classifying Childhood-Onset SLE*** Experts who care for pediatric patients rated criteria for the classification of childhood-onset SLE. Similar to adult-onset SLE, these experts reported malar rash, photosensitivity, oral ulcers, renal abnormalities, pericarditis, and pleuritis are useful for classifying pediatric SLE [21]. The difference in relative importance for pediatric lupus compared with established adult SLE was most significant for seizures (83% vs 62%) and oral ulcers (100% vs 46%) [21]. 50% of the pediatric rheumatologists in this study did not feel that there was a need for separate criteria for childhood-onset SLE [21].

## Phase 2. Reducing the Number of Criteria and Other Lessons Learned

***Manifestations Cluster Together*** The objectives of Phase 2 of EULAR/ACR classification criteria involved reducing the number of candidate criteria [22] and refining and modernizing definitions of criteria [23] (Fig. 3.1). Using the consensus methodology of nominal group technique, an international SLE expert panel was asked, "In a person with an uncertain diagnosis, which criteria most increase the likelihood that the patient has SLE? In making this judgment, you should ask yourself: If there are two patients identical in every other respect, and one has this extra feature and one doesn't, is the patient with the feature more likely to have SLE than the other?" Data for each candidate criterion were reviewed and discussed until consensus was achieved. The expert panel voted on items to be retained. Through the nominal group technique exercise, the expert panel reduced the number of candidate criteria to 21 (Fig. 3.1). The 20 remaining additive criteria included lupus nephritis by renal biopsy, autoantibodies, cytopenias, fever, arthritis, serositis, mucocutaneous, and neuropsychiatric manifestations.

In addition, novel concepts for SLE classification emerged. First was the notion of clustering criteria into "buckets," combinations of certain disease manifestations that were linked to each other. Accordingly, another step was added to evaluate the interdependence of criteria [24]. Using the early lupus cohort of Phase 1 and the Euro-lupus cohort, the inter-relationship of criteria was evaluated [24]. Associations within the mucocutaneous domain, hematologic, and the specific autoantibodies were found. Malar rash was correlated with photosensitivity (rho = 0.457 ± 0.071, $p < 0.001$), alopecia (rho = 0.360 ± 0.076, $p < 0.001$), and oral ulcers (rho = 0.270 ± 0.115, $p = 0.003$) [24]. Alopecia correlated with photosensitivity (rho = 0.227 ± 0.083, $p = 0.009$) and oral ulcers (r = 0.199 ± 0.090, $p = 0.032$). Anti-beta-2-GPI correlated with anti-cardiolipin IgG (rho = 0.828 ± 0.065, $p < 0.001$), anti-La with anti-Ro antibodies (rho = 0.840, $p < 0.001$), anti-cardiolipin IgM with IgG antibodies (rho = 0.721, $p < 0.001$), and anti-RNP and anti-Sm antibodies (rho = 0.804 ± 0.052, $p < 0.001$) [24]. Among hematologic manifestations, thrombocytopenia correlated with leukopenia (rho = 0.365 ± 0.128, $p = 0.007$) and hemolytic anemia (rho = 0.557 ± 0.132, $p = 0.001$), whereas leukopenia did not correlate with hemolytic anemia (rho = 0.108 ± 0.158, $p = 0.510$) [24]. These findings suggested multiple criteria within a domain should not be independently counted, and within a single domain only the highest ranking item should be counted to avoid overrepresentation. However, no associations were found between criteria in different domains, effectively refuting the idea of classical buckets and keeping the idea of SLE as one disease entity intact.

***Manifestations Need to Be Defined*** A second lesson from the NGT exercise was that a lack of precise definitions for the candidate criteria would result in inconsistent interpretation and application of the criteria [22]. These inconsistencies could impact the validity and reliability of the classification system. To address this challenge, an evidence-based approach was undertaken to review the literature on the sensitivity and specificity of the candidate criteria and develop hierarchical clustering of the criteria within domains [23].

## *Phase 3. Weighting and Threshold Identification*

***Manifestations Contribute to the Concept of SLE Differently*** Once a smaller, manageable list of criteria was determined, multi-criteria decision analysis [25] was used to ascertain the relative contribution of each manifestation to the classification of SLE [26] (Fig. 3.1). Using the 1982/1997 ACR criteria [5, 6], each criterion contributes to the classification of SLE equally (4 of 11 criteria are sufficient), implying that each carry the same weight. The 2012 SLICC criteria [9] similarly carry equal weight. The exception, however, is the presence of lupus nephritis. If present with an ANA or dsDNA, SLE could be classified [9]. As such, lupus nephritis carried three times more importance or weight.

Through the multi-criteria decision analysis, it became apparent that lupus nephritis continues to carry a lot of weight for classification. However, now the type of lupus nephritis matters. Compared to proteinuria >0.5 g/24 h, which carries a weight of 4 points, class II or V nephritis on renal biopsy carries 8 points [14, 26]. This conveys the importance of lupus nephritis. However, class III or IV nephritis carries a weight of 10 points, making it sufficient to classify in the presence of an ANA [14, 26]. Furthermore, other criteria such as fever, delirium, and non-scarring alopecia carry a weight of 2 each [14, 26]. Acute cutaneous lupus, acute pericarditis, and arthritis each carry a weight of 6 [14, 26]. In the modern era, disease manifestations contribute differentially to the concept of SLE.

## *Phase 4. Validation*

The SLE classification criteria were further refined in a derivation cohort of 1001 international SLE cases and control subjects with mimicking diseases [14] (Fig. 3.1). The 2019 EULAR/ACR classification criteria for SLE include positive ANA at least once as obligatory entry criterion, followed by additive weighted criteria grouped in seven clinical (constitutional, hematologic, neuropsychiatric, mucocutaneous, serosal, musculoskeletal, renal) and three immunologic (antiphospholipid antibodies, complement proteins, SLE-specific antibodies) domains, and weighted from 2 to 10 [14]. Patients accumulating ≥10 points are classified. The classification criteria were then tested in an independent international validation cohort of 1270 SLE cases and controls. The new criteria had a sensitivity of 96.1% and a specificity of 93.4%, compared with 82.8% sensitivity and 93.4% specificity of the 1997 ACR criteria and 96.7% sensitivity and 83.7% specificity of the 2012 SLICC criteria [14] (Table 3.2).

***The New Criteria Perform Well in Early Disease*** In a follow-up paper to the classification criteria paper, the same investigators demonstrated that the new criteria also perform well in early and established disease [27] (Table 3.3). In SLE patients with a disease duration of 1 to <3 years, the new criteria have a sensitivity of 97% and a specificity of 96% [27]. In SLE patients with a disease duration of 3 to <5 years, the new criteria have a sensitivity of 96% and a specificity of 99% [27]. In comparison, among SLE patients with <5 years disease duration in the Reuma.pt. and RELESSER cohorts, the ACR criteria had sensitivity of 76%, and the SLICC criteria had a sensitivity of 89% [28]. Among SLE patients with >5 years disease duration, the ACR criteria had a sensitivity of 89%, and the SLICC criteria had a sensitivity of 90% [28]. Mosca et al. reported a sensitivity of 66% and specificity 97% for the ACR criteria and a sensitivity of 84% and a specificity of 82% for the SLICC criteria [20]. Therefore, developing new classification criteria that perform well in early disease was an important objective that was met. It is hoped that by including patients with earlier disease, prevention and interventional studies may be undertaken to prevent progression of disease, prevent damage before it occurs, reduce morbidity, and improve quality of life.

**Table 3.3** Operating characteristics of the 2019 EULAR/ACR classification criteria for SLE

| | EULAR/ACR criteria | |
|---|---|---|
| | sensitivity<br>95% CI | Specificity<br>95% CI |
| *Validation cohort* | | |
| $n = 1270$ | *96.1%*<br>95–98% | *93.4%*<br>91–96% |
| *Disease duration* | | |
| *<1 year*<br>$n = 34$ | *89%*<br>52–100% | *92%*<br>74–99% |
| *1 to <3 years*<br>$n = 196$ | *97%*<br>92–99% | *96%*<br>90–99% |
| *3 to <5 years*<br>$n = 157$ | *96%*<br>88–99% | *99%*<br>94–100% |
| *≥5 years*<br>$n = 879$ | *96%*<br>94–98% | *93%*<br>89–95% |
| *Sex* | | |
| *Women*<br>$n = 1098$ | *97%*<br>95–98% | *94%*<br>91–96% |
| *Men*<br>$n = 172$ | *93%*<br>86–98% | *96%*<br>90–99% |
| *Ethnicities/race* | | |
| *Caucasian*<br>$n = 941$ | *95%*<br>93–97% | *94%*<br>91–96% |
| *Black*<br>$n = 68$ | *98%*<br>90–100% | *1.00*<br>74–100% |
| *Hispanic*<br>$n = 124$ | *100%*<br>95–100% | *96%*<br>87–100% |
| *Asian*<br>$n = 118$ | *97%*<br>91–100% | *91%*<br>79–98% |

***The New Criteria Perform Well Across Sexes and Ethnicities*** The EULAR/ACR 2019 classification criteria perform equally well in men and women [27] (Table 3.2). This is a notable finding as SLE in men may manifest differently, may be treated differently, and may be diagnosed later in life [29, 30]. Ethnic variations in SLE have been well described, particularly among African Americans, Hispanics, and Asians, compared to Caucasians [31–34]. Variations across races/ethnicities include age at diagnosis, disease manifestations, disease damage accrual, and mortality. Oku et al. reported that the ACR criteria have a sensitivity of 88% and a specificity of 85% among Asian SLE patients [35]. They also reported that among Asian SLE patients, the SLICC criteria have a sensitivity of 99% and specificity of 80% [35]. The EULAR/ACR criteria performed well among Black patients (sensitivity of 98%, specificity 100%) and have better sensitivity than the ACR criteria among Hispanic patients (100% versus 86%) and Asian patients (97% versus 77%) (Table 3.2).

## Summary

Through a rigorous methodologic approach balancing the use of data-driven and expert-based methods (cross-sectional survey, Delphi methods, nominal group technique, multi-criteria decision analysis), new classification criteria for SLE have been developed. The classification criteria reflect the paradigm shifts in our thinking about SLE: ANA is an entry criterion just as we use it as a screening test; fever assists with the classification of early SLE; the importance of disease manifestations to classification varies; and so criteria are differentially weighted and hierarchically clustered. The separation of renal biopsy findings reflects their differential impact on the probability of SLE classification. These criteria have excellent sensitivity and specificity in early and established disease, across sexes and ethnicities. The next era of SLE classification criteria will likely incorporate biologic classification based on gene expression patterns or state-of-the-art pharmacodynamic responses [3].

## References

1. Aringer M, Dorner T, Leuchten N, Johnson SR. Toward new criteria for systemic lupus erythematosus-a standpoint. Lupus. 2016;25(8):805–11. https://doi.org/10.1177/0961203316644338.
2. Tsokos GC. Systemic lupus erythematosus. N Engl J Med. 2011;365(22):2110–21. https://doi.org/10.1056/NEJMra1100359.
3. Merrill JT. Connective tissue diseases: is SLE many single-organ diseases or an overlapping spectrum? Nat Rev Rheumatol. 2015;11(7):385–6. https://doi.org/10.1038/nrrheum.2015.61.
4. Johnson SR, Tomlinson GA, Hawker GA, Granton JT, Feldman BM. Methods to elicit beliefs for Bayesian priors: a systematic review. J Clin Epidemiol. 2010;63(4):355–69.
5. Tan EM, Cohen AS, Fries JF, Masi AT, McShane DJ, Rothfield NF, et al. The 1982 revised criteria for the classification of systemic lupus erythematosus. Arthritis Rheum. 1982;25(11):1271–7.
6. Hochberg MC. Updating the American College of Rheumatology revised criteria for the classification of systemic lupus erythematosus. Arthritis Rheum. 1997;40(9):1725.
7. Aggarwal R, Ringold S, Khanna D, Neogi T, Johnson SR, Miller A, et al. Distinctions between diagnostic and classification criteria? Arthritis Care Res (Hoboken). 2015;67(7):891–7. https://doi.org/10.1002/acr.22583.
8. Johnson SR, Goek ON, Singh-Grewal D, Vlad SC, Feldman BM, Felson DT, et al. Classification criteria in rheumatic diseases: a review of methodologic properties. Arthritis Rheum. 2007;57(7):1119–33. https://doi.org/10.1002/art.23018.
9. Petri M, Orbai AM, Alarcon GS, Gordon C, Merrill JT, Fortin PR, et al. Derivation and validation of the Systemic Lupus International Collaborating Clinics classification criteria for systemic lupus erythematosus. Arthritis Rheum. 2012;64(8):2677–86. https://doi.org/10.1002/art.34473.
10. Gladman D, Ginzler E, Goldsmith C, Fortin P, Liang M, Urowitz M, et al. The development and initial validation of the Systemic Lupus International Collaborating Clinics/American College of Rheumatology damage index for systemic lupus erythematosus. Arthritis Rheum. 1996;39(3):363–9. https://doi.org/10.1002/art.1780390303.
11. van Vollenhoven RF, Mosca M, Bertsias G, Isenberg D, Kuhn A, Lerstrom K, et al. Treat-to-target in systemic lupus erythematosus: recommendations from an international task force. Ann Rheum Dis. 2014;73(6):958–67. https://doi.org/10.1136/annrheumdis-2013-205139.

12. Fanouriakis A, Kostopoulou M, Cheema K, Anders HJ, Aringer M, Bajema I, et al. 2019 update of the joint European league against rheumatism and European Renal Association-European Dialysis and Transplant Association (EULAR/ERA-EDTA) recommendations for the management of lupus nephritis. Ann Rheum Dis. 2020;79(6):713–23. https://doi.org/10.1136/annrheumdis-2020-216924.
13. Aringer M, Costenbader K, Daikh D, Brinks R, Mosca M, Ramsey-Goldman R, et al. 2019 European league against rheumatism/American college of rheumatology classification criteria for systemic lupus erythematosus. Arthritis Rheumatol. 2019;71(9):1400–12. https://doi.org/10.1002/art.40930.
14. Aringer M, Costenbader K, Daikh D, Brinks R, Mosca M, Ramsey-Goldman R, et al. 2019 European League Against Rheumatism/American College of Rheumatology classification criteria for systemic lupus erythematosus. Ann Rheum Dis. 2019;78(9):1151–9. https://doi.org/10.1136/annrheumdis-2018-214819.
15. Felson DT, Anderson JJ. Methodological and statistical approaches to criteria development in rheumatic diseases. Baillieres Clin Rheumatol. 1995;9(2):253–66. S0950-3579(05)80189-X [pii].
16. Dougados M, Betteridge N, Burmester GR, Euller-Ziegler L, Guillemin F, Hirvonen J, et al. EULAR standardised operating procedures for the elaboration, evaluation, dissemination, and implementation of recommendations endorsed by the EULAR standing committees. Ann Rheum Dis. 2004;63(9):1172–6. https://doi.org/10.1136/ard.2004.023697.
17. Dougados M, Gossec L. Classification criteria for rheumatic diseases: why and how? Arthritis Rheum. 2007;57(7):1112–5. https://doi.org/10.1002/art.23015.
18. Leuchten N, Hoyer A, Brinks R, Schoels M, Schneider M, Smolen J, et al. Performance of antinuclear antibodies for classifying systemic lupus erythematosus: a systematic literature review and meta-regression of diagnostic data. Arthritis Care Res (Hoboken). 2018;70(3):428–38. https://doi.org/10.1002/acr.23292.
19. Leuchten N, Milke B, Winkler-Rohlfing B, Daikh D, Dorner T, Johnson SR, et al. Early symptoms of systemic lupus erythematosus (SLE) recalled by 339 SLE patients. Lupus. 2018;27(9):1431–6. https://doi.org/10.1177/0961203318776093.
20. Mosca M, Costenbader KH, Johnson SR, Lorenzoni V, Sebastiani GD, Hoyer BF, et al. Brief report: how do patients with newly diagnosed systemic lupus erythematosus present? A multicenter cohort of early systemic lupus erythematosus to inform the development of new classification criteria. Arthritis Rheumatol. 2019;71(1):91–8. https://doi.org/10.1002/art.40674.
21. Schmajuk G, Hoyer BF, Aringer M, Johnson SR, Daikh DI, Dorner T, et al. Multicenter Delphi exercise to identify important key items for classifying systemic lupus erythematosus. Arthritis Care Res (Hoboken). 2018;70(10):1488–94. https://doi.org/10.1002/acr.23503.
22. Johnson SR, Khanna D, Daikh D, Cervera R, Costedoat-Chalumeau N, Gladman DD, et al. Use of consensus methodology to determine candidate items for systemic lupus erythematosus classification criteria. J Rheumatol. 2019;46(7):721–6. https://doi.org/10.3899/jrheum.180478.
23. Tedeschi SK, Johnson SR, Boumpas D, Daikh D, Dorner T, Jayne D, et al. Developing and refining new candidate criteria for systemic lupus erythematosus classification: an international collaboration. Arthritis Care Res (Hoboken). 2018;70(4):571–81. https://doi.org/10.1002/acr.23317.
24. Touma Z, Cervera R, Brinks R, Lorenzoni V, Tani C, Hoyer BF, et al. Associations among classification criteria items within systemic lupus erythematosus. Arthritis Care Res (Hoboken). 2019;72(12):1820–6. https://doi.org/10.1002/acr.24078.
25. Johnson SR, Naden RP, Fransen J, van den Hoogen F, Pope JE, Baron M, et al. Multicriteria decision analysis methods with 1000Minds for developing systemic sclerosis classification criteria. J Clin Epidemiol. 2014;67(6):706–14. https://doi.org/10.1016/j.jclinepi.2013.12.009.
26. Tedeschi SK, Johnson SR, Boumpas DT, Daikh D, Dorner T, Diamond B, et al. Multicriteria decision analysis process to develop new classification criteria for systemic lupus erythematosus. Ann Rheum Dis. 2019;78(5):634–40. https://doi.org/10.1136/annrheumdis-2018-214685.

27. Johnson SR, Costenbader K, Daikh D, Brinks R, Mosca M, Ramsey-Goldman R, et al. Performance of the 2019 EULAR/ACR classification criteria for systemic lupus erythematosus in early disease, across sexes and ethnicities. Ann Rheumatic Dis. 2020;79(10):1333–9.
28. Ines L, Silva C, Galindo M, Lopez-Longo FJ, Terroso G, Romao VC, et al. Classification of systemic lupus erythematosus: systemic lupus international collaborating clinics versus American College of Rheumatology Criteria. A comparative study of 2,055 patients from a real-life, international systemic lupus erythematosus cohort. Arthritis Care Res. 2015;67(8):1180–5. https://doi.org/10.1002/acr.22539.
29. Miller MH, Urowitz MB, Gladman DD, Killinger DW. Systemic lupus erythematosus in males. Medicine (Baltimore). 1983;62(5):327–34. https://doi.org/10.1097/00005792-198309000-00005.
30. Lu LJ, Wallace DJ, Ishimori ML, Scofield RH, Weisman MH. Review: male systemic lupus erythematosus: a review of sex disparities in this disease. Lupus. 2010;19(2):119–29. https://doi.org/10.1177/0961203309350755.
31. Johnson SR, Urowitz MB, Ibanez D, Gladman DD. Ethnic variation in disease patterns and health outcomes in systemic lupus erythematosus. J Rheumatol. 2006;33(10):1990–5.
32. Cervera R, Doria A, Amoura Z, Khamashta M, Schneider M, Guillemin F, et al. Patterns of systemic lupus erythematosus expression in Europe. Autoimmun Rev. 2014;13(6):621–9. https://doi.org/10.1016/j.autrev.2013.11.007.
33. Low ESH, Krishnaswamy G, Thumboo J. Comparing the 1997 update of the 1982 American College of Rheumatology (ACR-97) and the 2012 Systemic Lupus International Collaborating Clinics (SLICC-12) criteria for systemic lupus erythematosus (SLE) classification: which enables earlier classification of SLE in an urban Asian population? Lupus. 2019;28(1):11–8. https://doi.org/10.1177/0961203318811599.
34. Alarcon GS, McGwin G Jr, Roseman JM, Uribe A, Fessler BJ, Bastian HM, et al. Systemic lupus erythematosus in three ethnic groups. XIX. Natural history of the accrual of the American College of Rheumatology criteria prior to the occurrence of criteria diagnosis. Arthritis Rheum. 2004;51(4):609–15. https://doi.org/10.1002/art.20548.
35. Oku K, Atsumi T, Akiyama Y, Amano H, Azuma N, Bohgaki T, et al. Evaluation of the alternative classification criteria of systemic lupus erythematosus established by Systemic Lupus International Collaborating Clinics (SLICC). Mod Rheumatol. 2018;28(4):642–8. https://doi.org/10.1080/14397595.2017.1385154.

# Chapter 4
# Challenges and Advances in SLE Autoantibody Detection and Interpretation

**May Y. Choi and Marvin J. Fritzler**

## Introduction

More than a half century has lapsed since the serendipitous discovery of the lupus erythematous (LE) cell in systemic lupus erythematosus (SLE) and the development of the LE cell test by Hargraves and his colleagues at the Mayo Clinic [1]. While the description of cardiolipin and the biological false-positive venereal disease research laboratory (VDRL) test antedated the LE cell (reviewed in [2]), the LE cell discovery still serves as a historic reference point for the earliest studies of antinuclear antibodies (ANA). In the following 70 years, the spectrum of clinicians that use ANA for diagnosis and decision-making has markedly widened [3, 4]. For example, ANA testing was once regarded the exclusive domain of rheumatologists and clinical immunologists, but today, it is also used by primary care providers and virtually all other subspecialists including nephrologists, dermatologists, respirologists, and neurologists [4]. The primary driver of this change is the remarkable spectrum of autoantibodies reported in systemic autoimmune rheumatic disease (SARD) and other autoinflammatory syndromes. For example, in SLE alone, more than 180 autoantibodies have been described [5, 6]. Some might regard the continuing search for new "esoteric" or rare autoantibodies in SLE [7] unnecessary, but, for one thing, since approximately 5% of SLE patients are "seronegative" [8], at a minimum, these efforts continue to narrow that "seronegative gap" [9].

There has also been a remarkable transition in the technologies used to detect autoantibodies that has been fostered by the "Golden Age" of cell and molecular biology that emerged in the mid-1970s [3, 10, 11]. While some of the earlier immunoassays such as the LE cell test, double immunodiffusion, hemagglutination, complement fixation, radioimmunoassays, and counterimmunoelectrophoresis are

M. Y. Choi · M. J. Fritzler (✉)
Cumming School of Medicine, University of Calgary, Calgary, AB, Canada
e-mail: fritzler@ucalgary.ca



Z. Touma (ed.), *Outcome Measures and Metrics in Systemic Lupus Erythematosus*, https://doi.org/10.1007/978-3-030-73303-2_4

rarely used today [10], the contemporary ANA indirect immunofluorescence assay (IFA) on HEp-2 cell substrates is increasingly used and remains the screening test of choice for SLE [12]. One innovation that has sustained the use of ANA IFAs is automated digitized microscopy that is capable of pattern recognition and, in some devices, digital algorithms to perform single-well titers [3, 13]. In 2019, the American College of Rheumatology (ACR) and the European League Against Rheumatism (EULAR) published new classification criteria for SLE based on a scoring system including a positive ANA at a titer ≥1:80 by IFA ("or its equivalent") occurring at least once as an entry criterion [14] (and reviewed in [15, 16]).

Newer solid-phase multi-analyte arrays (SPMAA) [17] have also emerged with higher throughput, sensitivity, and specificity while detecting a broader range of autoantibodies in comparatively miniscule serum samples [18]. A technological gap, however, is that SPMAA does not employ real-time standards or calibrators for each antigen in an array, a gap that can be overcome [9]. Recent evidence also suggests that SPMAA is a more cost-effective approach than ANA IFA [19, 20]. Universally accepted, standardized, validated, and cost-effective follow-up ANA testing algorithms for SLE need to be developed. With the advent of new SLE classification criteria, improving diagnostic technologies, and novel autoantibodies, the purpose of this review is to summarize the advantages to and limitations of current ANA testing and provide a general overview of important autoantibodies in SLE (Fig. 4.1).

## Important Considerations in Interpretation of ANA Test Results and Reports

Before considering the clinical value of SLE-specific and SLE-associated autoantibodies, clinicians need to be aware of important limitations of ANA testing and interpretation of the respective test results (Table 4.1). Unfortunately, many multicenter studies and meta-analysis seemingly fail to recognize the marked variability of ANA testing across different jurisdictions and how that impacts on the conclusions of their studies [21, 22]. Autoantibodies in general and ANA in specific are extremely complex because within any individual, they can vary with time (although the precise chronological dynamics are poorly understood) and also vary between patients and even within an individual patient over the clinical course of SLE [23, 24]. This heterogeneity is likely related to the highly variable clinical course of SLE that may be "relapsing-remitting," "chronically active," or "prolonged quiescence" [25]. In addition, the impact of therapeutic interventions and coincidental comorbidities is very difficult to control for when results are obtained from cross-sectional samples. Hence, a critical factor in the interpretation of ANA test is to appreciate that results obtained from cross-sectional SLE cohorts can be markedly different from inception cohorts because single-point serological evaluations are unlikely to provide a realistic picture of the B cell response in SLE.

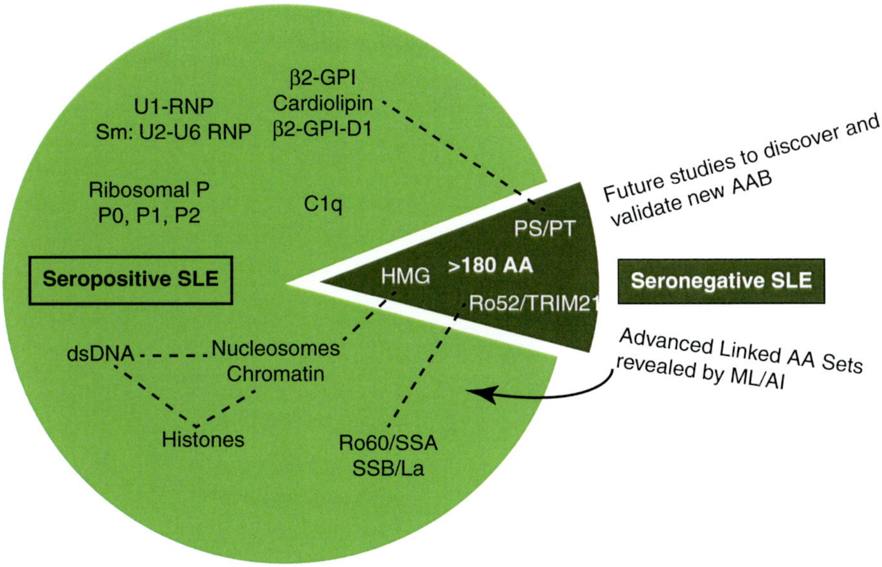


**Fig. 4.1** The prevalence of autoantibodies in seropositive SLE is approximately 95% and are represented by reactivity to a number of intracellular components and phospholipids referred to as "linked sets" (components of macromolecular complexes such as ribonucleoproteins (RNP) illustrated as dashed lines). Seronegative SLE patients do not have established SLE-related autoantibodies (AA). Future studies are needed to discover new AA and validate potentially >180 novel AA to close the "seronegative" gap. Using machine learning (ML) and artificial intelligence (AI) techniques, some AA have been shown to be linked to others. Abbreviations: β2GP1, beta 2 glycoprotein 1; dsDNA, double-stranded DNA; PS/PT, phosphatidylserine/prothrombin complex; HMG, high-mobility group proteins; RNP, ribonucleoprotein; SS-A, SS-B, Sjögren syndrome antigens A and B; SSc, systemic sclerosis; TRIM, tripartite motif

**Table 4.1** Key considerations when interpreting ANA test results

| |
|---|
| Clinicians need to be aware which ANA screening test (ANA IFA or solid-phase multi-analyte autoantigen arrays (SPMAA)) their laboratory uses. |
| Does the laboratory report all intracellular staining (i.e., cytoplasmic and mitotic patters) or only nuclear staining on the ANA IFA test? |
| What is the sensitivity, specificity, commutability, and reference range of their ANA assay? |
| In interpreting published reports on ANA, was the test performed on an inception or cross-sectional SLE cohort? |
| In SLE, autoantibodies to more than one autoantigen are typically found, and the combinations of these various antibodies can have important clinical associations. |
| An important gap in ANA testing is the need for multi-center studies that use newer SPMAA on cohorts of very early or incomplete SLE. |

Another factor impacting on ANA test results and interpretation is that the ANA IFA test lacks accuracy and commutability (traceability, harmonization) of results [23, 26]. Because achieving accuracy (closeness of a measured value to a standard or known value) of autoantibody assays is very challenging, assay precision (how close two or more assays are to each other or performance of an assay based on a predicate assay) is a common parameter used for reliable diagnostic assay design. Complete traceability [27, 28] and commutability [29] of ANA testing have yet to be achieved. As a caveat, absolute standardization of autoantibody testing is generally recognized as extremely challenging, although initiatives to improve standardization/harmonization within the wider field of *in vitro* diagnostics are underway [30].

One issue that contributes to the lack of harmonization and consensus in ANA IFA testing is whether *c*ytoplasmic and *m*itotic *p*atterns (CMP) should be considered as part of the "antinuclear antibody" (ANA) test result. In an attempt to harmonize the definition of ANA, two separate international committees recommended that CMP should be included in the definition of ANA and that the nomenclature should be more appropriately changed to anti-cellular antibodies (ACA) [31, 32]. In this chapter, the term ANA (rather than ACA) is used simply because it is most widely recognized by clinicians. Nevertheless, it is important for the clinician to know if their diagnostic laboratory reports CMP staining in their ANA IFA results.

In addition, the harmonization of ANA IFA testing is challenging because other variables such as laboratory equipment (i.e., microscope optics and light sources), serum screening dilutions, and other factors have yet to be standardized [33, 34]. There is evidence that the recent introduction of automated microscopic testing provides more harmonized ANA IFA results [35–37]. However, this technology requires a quality assurance program that addresses the total ANA IFA process. For example, the ANA IFA is semi-quantitative at best, and although immunofluorescence intensity units can be obtained, this approach has yet to be approved by regulatory agencies [23]. Next, although, in general, higher titer antibodies have better clinical correlations [38, 39], autoantibodies directed to different intracellular targets and differing IFA patterns have differing dilution curves, so that some ANA IFA systems (i.e., anti-U1RNP, anti-Sm) may be regarded as high-dilution/titer systems, whereas others (i.e., anti-SSA/Ro60, SS-B/La) are low-dilution/titer systems [39]. Last, it should be appreciated that the ANA IFA test is only useful as a screening test, and it has been recommended that specific antibodies should be confirmed through the identification of specific antibodies using SPMAA [40].

Perhaps the significant challenges to harmonization, commutability, and traceability of the ANA IFA test are inconsequential because newer diagnostic laboratories are progressively migrating to SPMAA diagnostic platforms that have higher throughput and faster turnaround times but, more importantly, utilize definable analytes/autoantigens in their test platforms [19, 41]. For the most part, SPMAAs are widely available and are currently used either as an approach to the diagnosis of specific SARDs (i.e., separate SLE, scleroderma (SSc), Sjögren's syndrome (SjS), autoimmune inflammatory myopathy (AIM) profiles) or the most common targets seen in SARDs included in a SARD screen as an alternative to the ANA IFA. However, there is some evidence that while SPMAA are a significant move forward, combining ANA IFA with SPMAA has higher clinical impact than either of the tests alone [3, 20, 36, 42, 43]. SLE serum samples that have negative SPMAA test results should ideally be tested by ANA IFA to determine if antibodies to targets not included in the SPMAA are detected.

Last, it is well-known that SLE patients commonly have more than one autoantibody, typically reflecting what has been called "linked sets" [44] or B cell responses to macromolecular complexes such as spliceosomes, nucleosomes, and/or cytoplasmic ribonucleoprotein complexes. With the advent of SPMAA, it has been increasingly appreciated that combinations and permutations of autoantibodies in SLE can be associated with unique phenotypes. For example, a combination of anti-dsDNA and anti-nucleosome antibodies is reported to differentiate lupus nephritis (LN) from SLE without LN; anti-dsDNA plus anti-histone and anti-nucleosome antibodies are associated with a higher risk of severe LN than what can be attributed to the individual autoantibodies alone [45]. When anti-Ro52/TRIM21, anti-Ro60/SS-A, and anti-SS-B/La were found together, they were associated with xerostomia and xerophthalmia ($p < 0.001$) [46]. Oral ulceration was associated with anti-Ro52/TRM21 and anti-Ro60/SS-A positivity but anti-SS-B/La negativity ($p$: 0.002), and alopecia was associated with anti-Ro60/SS-A positivity but anti-Ro52/TRIM21 and anti-SS-B/La negativity ($p$: 0.003) [46]. Further, when anti-Ro52/TRIM21 antibodies were found in isolation, there was a negative association with xerophthalmia and photosensitivity with anti-Ro60/anti-La ($p$: 0.003). These observations and others like them illustrate the limitations of interpreting the frequencies and clinical associations of any individual ANA result.

## Specific Autoantibodies

Since over 180 autoantibodies have been reported in SLE, a general context and consensus of only the key autoantibodies is discussed here. The frequency of the various autoantibodies is shown in Table 4.2. When ANA IFA patterns on HEp-2 cells are referred to, they are cross-referenced to the corresponding AC-'X' nomenclature proposed by the International Consensus on Autoantibody Patterns (ICAP: https://anapatterns.org/index.php).

### *Chromatin Components*

Autoantibodies directed against chromatin components are typically associated with a homogeneous (AC-1) or dense fine speckled (DFS) pattern (AC-2) on HEp-2 IFA. Exceptions are antibodies directed specifically to histone (H1), the inner core histones (H3, H4), and high-mobility group (HMG) proteins.

**Table 4.2** Prevalence and clinical associations of SLE autoantibodies

| Antibody target | Prevalence range[a] | Prevalence in inception SLICC cohort ($n$ = 1049)[b] | Clinical associations | Comments |
|---|---|---|---|---|
| dsDNA | 30–70% | 40.5% | **CC**, Lupus nephritis | Pathogenic: Test results can vary depending on immunoassay used |
| Nucleosomes chromatin | 20–70% | N/A | Lupus nephritis, more severe disease progressive renal failure; disease activity; DIL | Pathogenetic: Note: many drugs originally associated with anti-histone and DIL are no longer in wide use; harder to obtain validated assays because of difficulty standardizing the target macromolecular nucleocomplex |
| Histone | 10–80% | 40.1% | SLE, drug-induced SLE; NPSLE | Frequency depends on assay and which histones are included; Higher titers, especially anti-H2B, anti-H4, acetylated H4 and H2A more specific for SLE |
| High-mobility group proteins | 20–49% | N/A | SLE disease activity | Sensitivity and specificity varies depending on the HMG protein being studied |
| Dense fine speckled 70 | 1–10% | 7.1% | Monospecific antibodies rare in SLE | Reported in a variety of autoinflammatory syndromes and health individuals. Monospecific antibodies may be used to rule out diagnosis of SLE and other AARD |
| Sm (U2-U6 RNP) | 5–30% | 24.7% | **CC**, serositis, LN, NPSLE, CSF, NPSLE | Predictive: SmD3 containing a symmetrical dimethylarginine at position 112 most specific for SLE |
| U1-RNP | 15–50% | 32.4% | Leukopenia; NPSLE; ILD: IgM anti-U1RNP antibodies predominant in SLE compared to IgG anti-U1RNP without IgM more frequent in MCTD | Anti-U1RNP in CSF 64.3% sensitivity and 92.9% specificity for NPSLE |
| Ribosomal P | 10–30% | 16.1% | Renal disease; malar rash; possibly NPSLE; antibodies to C22 peptide highly specific for SLE | Associated with anti-dsDNA; although C22 of protein has the most specific SLE epitope, not all assays utilize this peptide in their assays; prevalence varies in different countries |

**Table 4.2** (continued)

| Antibody target | Prevalence range[a] | Prevalence in inception SLICC cohort ($n$ = 1049)[b] | Clinical associations | Comments |
|---|---|---|---|---|
| SS-A/Ro60 | 25–60% | 47.3% | SCLE, C4 deficiency, NLE; in pediatric SLE milder disease (cutaneous, MSK) | Predictive: Titers important in NLE |
| Ro52/ TRIM21 | 10–40% | 35.9% | Leukopenia; ~70% of patients with anti-Ro52 but not anti-Ro60-antibodies have SARD (majority have UCTD followed by SLE); ANA negative SLE | Seen in patients with malignancy with or without evidence of SARD |
| SS-B/La | 5–25% | 15.9% | SjS, SCLE; NLE, leukopenia, serositis; rare in pediatric SLE | Protective: Less renal disease |
| C1q | 15–60 | N/A | Lupus nephritis; prevalence 13% in controls (OR = 2.7, 95% CI: 1.8–4, $p < 0.001$ | Simultaneously positive anti-C1q, anti-dsDNA, and low complement were strongly associated with renal involvement (OR = 14.9, 95% CI: 5.8–38.4, $p < 0.01$); |
| Ku | 5–20% | N/A | Not specific for SLE; SSc and myositis overlap; other SARD; Raynaud's, myositis, arthritis; UCTD | Ku is a heterodimer consisting of 70 kDa (p70) and ~80 kDa (p80) protein subunits that bind blunt ends of x-ray damaged DNA |
| PCNA | 0.5–5% | 7.3% | More severe SLE; may be transiently expressed and/or decreased with therapy | PCNA is the auxiliary protein of DNA polymerase delta component of a macromolecular complex when IFA and SPMAA, specific for SLE |
| Cardiolipin | 20–60% | 12.6% | **CC**, APS; thrombosis; pulmonary hypertension | Predictive: decreased survival |
| AMA M5 | ~25% | N/A | APS | Closes serological gap in APS; thrombocytopenia, fetal loss, lupus anticoagulant; associated with anti-cardiolipin, anti-β2GP1, and biologically false-positive VDRL |

(continued)

**Table 4.2** (continued)

| Antibody target | Prevalence range[a] | Prevalence in inception SLICC cohort ($n = 1049$)[b] | Clinical associations | Comments |
|---|---|---|---|---|
| β2GP1 | 30–45% | 14.0% | **CC**, APS | Predictive of thrombosis and fetal loss: closes serological gap in APS; glycosylation of Fc domain of anti-β2GP1 may be important in pathogenesis |
| β2GP1 domain 1 | 40–56% | N/A | APS | Higher specificity than full length β2GP1; IgA antibodies important |
| PS/PT | 30–54% | N/A | APS; correlated with lupus anti-coagulant and increased risk of thrombosis | May be a surrogate biomarker for lupus anticoagulant. Commercial kit available |

*Abbreviations*: *AMA M5* anti-mitochondrial M5 type antibodies, *APS* anti-phospholipid syndrome, *β2GP1* beta 2 glycoprotein 1, *CC* classification criteria, *CI* confidence interval, *DIL* drug-induced lupus, *dsDNA* double-stranded DNA, *ILD* interstitial lung disease, *kDa* kilodalton, *LN* lupus nephritis, *SPMAA* multi-analyte antigen array, *MCTD* mixed connective tissue disease, *MSK* musculoskeletal, *NA* not assessed, *NLE* neonatal lupus erythematosus, *NPSLE* neuropsychiatric SLE, *OR* odds ratio, *PCNA* proliferating cell nuclear antigen, *PS/PT* phosphatidylserine/prothrombin complex, *RNP* ribonucleoprotein, *SARD* systemic autoimmune rheumatic disease, *SCLE* subacute cutaneous lupus erythematosus, *SjS* Sjögren's syndrome, *SS-A, SS-B* Sjögren syndrome antigens A and B, *SSc* systemic sclerosis, *TRIM* tripartite motif, *UCTD* undifferentiated connective tissue disease

[a]For interpretation, see Table 4.1 and section titled "Important Considerations in Interpretation of ANA Tests"

[b]Reference [8]

## Double-Stranded DNA

Antibodies directed to double-stranded DNA (dsDNA) were one of the first, disease-specific autoantibody targets described in SLE (reviewed in [47, 48]). Anti-dsDNA antibodies are typically associated with LN [49] and can be used to monitor disease activity [47, 50]. It is important to appreciate that the anti-dsDNA autoantibody system is highly complex, and this, in part, is reflected by the performance of different immunoassays and diagnostic platforms used to detect them. Historically, the Farr radioimmunoassay was preferred because it reputedly measured primarily high affinity antibodies and hence reflected a more "trained" B cell response in addition to antibodies that had pathogenic potential in LN. The Farr assay has become decreasingly used because of safety concerns with assays that employ radioisotopes, and there was a tendency of the kits to be in short supply. Hence, many laboratories reverted to other assays such as addressable laser bead immunoassay (ALBIA), enzyme-linked immunosorbent assay (ELISA), chemiluminescence immunoassay (CIA), and the *Crithidia luciliae* IFA [47]. One ongoing issue is whether a negative ANA IFA result is a "false negative" when the results of any of the SPMAA anti-dsDNA tests listed above are positive. To address this apparent paradox, it is important to recognize the highly complex nature of dsDNA and appreciate that in cells (i.e., HEp-2) where dsDNA is bound by histones, HMG proteins, and other DNA-binding proteins and stabilized with organic fixatives, there is no *a priori* reason to expect complete agreement of results from ANA IFA and SPMAAs when the latter use purified or synthetic dsDNA. For a more thorough discussion of limitations of anti-dsDNA testing, the reader is referred to a recent review [47].

## Histones

Histones are a class of low-molecular-weight, cationic proteins that are bound to nuclear dsDNA. Histones can be subclassified as cross-linkers of DNA in the nucleosome (H1) or components of the core nucleosome body (H2a, H2b, H3, and H4) [51]. Methylated, acetylation, and other posttranscriptional modified histones are now known to be critical in the epigenetic expression of genes [52]. In addition, they are components of apoptotic bodies [52, 53] and neutrophil extracellular traps (NETS) [54], which are considered to be important pathogenic phenomena in SLE [55]. As compared to antibodies to the core histones, antibodies directed to H1 and its variants are the least specific for SLE. Although antibodies to histones and nucleosome have been primarily linked to drug-induced lupus (DIL) [55, 56], it is important to appreciate that this association was more relevant to drugs that are no longer in wide use (e.g., hydralazine, procainamide) compared to the biological therapeutic-induced DIL that is more prevalent today. Since histones are key components of the nucleosome, antibodies to the nucleosome are considered more diagnostically relevant.

## Nucleosomes

The terms anti-nucleosome and anti-chromatin antibodies tend to be used interchangeably; however, an important distinction is that although the term "chromatin" encompasses nucleosomes, nucleosomes are more restricted in their molecular structure(s) and components, the latter largely related to dsDNA complexed to histones as described above, while chromatin contains dsDNA, HMG proteins, and other gene-regulatory elements [51]. Hence, most commercially available assays are based on purified nucleosomes that have been further processed to remove the inter-nucleosome linker DNA and less-avidly bound proteins such as HMGs and H1. In this format, anti-nucleosome antibodies are highly, but not exclusively, correlated with anti-dsDNA and are highly specific for SLE [51, 57]. In some studies, nucleosomes and anti-nucleosome antibodies are thought to be more pathogenic than anti-dsDNA. Anti-nucleosome antibodies have been reported to antedate the appearance of anti-dsDNA and predict the development of

SLE in patients who developed renal failure [58] and anti-phospholipid syndrome (APS) [59]. Despite numerous publications indicating the importance of anti-nucleosome antibodies as biomarkers for SLE [51, 60, 61], other less favorable views have been offered [62].

## High-Mobility Group Proteins

HMG proteins are a family of low-molecular-weight, chromatin-associated proteins that, except for HMG box protein-1 (HMGB1) and HMG box protein-2 (HMGB2), primarily bind to linker (i.e., non-nucleosome) DNA. Although HMGB1 is typically associated with nucleosomes, it also shuttles between the nucleus and the cytoplasm. HMGB1 consists of three separate domains: Box A, Box B, and an acidic tail of which Box A acts as a competitive antagonist for HMGB1 and has been considered as a potential treatment option for SLE [63]. Much interest has focused on HMGB1 because it is secreted by inflammatory cells and passively released from apoptotic and necrotic cells, where it has pro-inflammatory effects [64, 65]. It has been suggested that HMGB1 helps elicit anti-dsDNA antibody production in SLE [66]. The titers of anti-HMGB1 antibodies correlated with anti-dsDNA antibody levels ($r = 0.49$; $p < 0.001$), and less pronounced correlations were observed with SLE disease activity index (SLEDAI-2K) ($r = 0.15$; $p = 0.04$), low C4 ($r = -0.23$; $p$: 0.002), low C3 levels, and proteinuria [63, 67]. These observations suggested that HMGB1-anti-HMGB1 immune complexes play a role in the pathogenesis of LN. Titers of anti-Box A antibodies were also increased in 73% of patients with LN and 71% of non-LN flares. It was concluded that antibodies to the HMGB1 Box A domain of might be a novel biomarker for SLE.

Anti-HMGB1/HMGB2 antibodies were detected in SLE, rheumatoid arthritis (RA), SjS, and SSc [66]. Of interest, anti-HMGBI and HMGB2 may be target antigens of perinuclear neutrophil cytoplasmic antibodies (pANCA). However, anti-HMGB1 antibodies were not associated with ANCA-associated vasculopathies [68]. Autoantibodies to another HMG protein, the structure specific recognition protein I (SSRP1) was identified by ELISA and Western blot in 28% of SLE sera, compared to 8.3% of healthy individuals but not in other SARD [69].

## Dense Fine Speckled (DFS)

The typical DFS IIF staining pattern (AC-2) is recognized as uniformly distributed fine speckles throughout interphase nuclei and on metaphase chromatin (reviewed in [70, 71]). The priamry target antigen associated with the DFS IFA pattern was first described as dense fine speckled 70 (DFS70) based on the apparent molecular weight of 70 kDa, but the protein was later identified as the lens epithelium-derived growth factor (LEDGF) and more recently as the DNA binding transcription coactivator p75 [72]. Since the first report in interstitial cystitis, anti-DFS70 antibodies have also been reported in patients with a variety of chronic inflammatory conditions and cancer and most notably in healthy individuals [70, 71, 73]. Anti-DFS70 antibodies are now recognized as one of the key targets in high-titer-positive ANA IFA healthy and non-SARD sera [74]. Isolated (monospecific or no other detectable autoantibodies) anti-DFS70 antibodies described in healthy individuals were rarely found in SLE but were found associated with SLE-related autoantibodies in a small proportion of sera [75]. Hence, the presence of anti-DFS70 in SLE sera is currently thought to have limited clinical value. A recent report indicates geographic differences in the prevalence of anti-DFS70 antibodies and that they occur preferentially in females and young individuals [76].

## *Small Nuclear Ribonucleoproteins: Sm and U1-RNP*

Autoantibodies directed against small nuclear ribonucleoprotein (snRNP) components (Sm, U1-RNP) are typically associated with nuclear speckled (AC-4; AC-5) patterns on HEp-2 IFA. Anti-Sm antibodies are highly specific for SLE. By comparison, although anti-Sm and anti-U1RNP commonly coexist in SLE, anti-U1RNP antibodies are found in patients with a variety of other SARD (reviewed in [77]). Although anti-Sm is one of the most widely requested autoantibody tests, it lacks sensitivity because it is present in only 5–30% of SLE patients [78]. Nevertheless, largely because of its high specificity, it is one of the serologic criteria in the ACR [79], SLICC [80], and more recently the EULAR/ACR [14] classification criteria for SLE. Although anti-Sm is associated with classical SLE, it is also seen in patients with SLE-overlap syndromes [77]. Anti-Sm antibodies have been described in patients without SLE, although follow-up studies showed that some eventually developed that disease [77]. These observations highlight the importance of Sm and other SLE-specific autoantibodies as predictors of SLE [81]. The titers of anti-Sm antibodies have been reported to correlate with disease activity, milder renal and central nervous involvement, or late-onset LN, but these associations are controversial [7]. Twenty-five to forty percent (25–40%) of anti-U1RNP-positive SLE patients also have anti-Sm, although this varied in different cohorts [78]. Even though anti-U1RNP antibodies are found in a high proportion of SLE, they are also reported in SSc, AIM, SjS, and other SARD. By comparison, all (~100%) patients with mixed connective tissue disease (MCTD) are, by definition, positive for anti-U1RNP antibodies. However, anti-U1RNP antibodies are not a specific biomarker for MCTD. Regardless of the disease association, anti-U1RNP-positive patients typically have Raynaud's phenomenon, swollen digits, and leukopenia [82]. Reports of clinical association and immunologic cross-reactivity of anti-Sm with anti-ribosomal P and anti-dsDNA antibodies could be an important confounding factor.

## DNA-Dependent Protein Kinase (DNA-PK/Ku)

Ku is a heterodimer composed of 70 and ~85 kDa non-histone nuclear proteins. This antigen has gained research interest because it is a DNA-dependent protein kinase (DNA-PK) that is critical in the repair of DNA double-strand breaks induced by ionizing radiation [83]. Antibodies to various components of this macromolecular DNA-PK complex have been reported in SLE and related SARD [84]. Although initially thought to be specific for polymyositis/SSc overlap syndrome [85], subsequent studies demonstrated that anti-Ku antibodies are also found in SLE, MCTD, and SSc [86–88]. Additional studies revealed that anti-Ku antibodies were also detected in a variety of other SARD and were associated with polymyositis/SSc overlap syndrome in Japanese cohorts but with SLE and overlap syndromes in African-American cohorts [87]. In a small Japanese polymyositis/SSc overlap syndrome cohort ($n = 11$), precipitating autoantibodies to Ku were found in 55% as compared to 6% of Japanese SLE patients and <1% of other SARD [85]. In African-American individuals, these antibodies were most strongly associated with SLE (14%), whereas in Caucasian people, anti-Ku antibodies are rare regardless of the clinical diagnosis [87]. Overall, anti-Ku autoantibodies are relatively rare, being reported in 4% of patients with MCTD/overlap syndrome and in <1% of SLE, and even rarer in other SARD. More multicenter studies of inception cohorts of SLE and other SARDS using newer diagnostic platforms that include Ku proteins as analytes are needed.

## Other Nuclear Targets

### Sjögren Syndrome Antigen B/La

Autoantibodies directed against Sjögren syndrome antigen B (SS-B)/La are highly specific (~90%) and sensitive (~85%) for SjS [89, 90]. The prevalence of these antibodies is also high in mothers that gave birth to infants with neonatal lupus syndrome (NLS) [91]. In NLS, approximately 10–15% of cases of congenital heart block are not exposed to anti-Ro60/SS-A or SS-B/La [91], while the cutaneous manifestations of NLS were reported in infants exposed only to anti-U1RNP antibodies [91]. It was reported that anti-SS-B/La and Ro60/SS-A antibodies can be detected 2.8 years before the onset of the symptoms and 3.6 years before diagnosis of SLE [92], suggesting a predictive utility. SLE patients that have anti-SS-B/La antibodies usually develop secondary SjS syndrome. Anti-SS-B/La autoantibodies are rarely found alone, usually coinciding with anti-Ro60/SS-A autoantibodies [90].

## Cytoplasmic

### Ribosomal P

Autoantibodies to ribosomes were first described in the 1960s in SLE sera followed by identification of key ribosomal proteins (Rib-P) in the 1970s [93, 94] and three of the ribosomal phosphoproteins (P0, P1, P2) in the 1980s [95, 96]. The

Rib-P are largely localized to the cytoplasm and are components of the 60S ribosomal subunit [93]. Over the years, anti-Rib-P antibodies have been the subject of extensive study and have been shown to be a highly specific biomarker for the diagnosis of SLE [97–99]. They are associated with LN, autoimmune hepatitis, and, although controversial, neuropsychiatric SLE (NPSLE) [100, 101]. Experimental evidence indicates that anti-Rib-P have a pathogenic role in LN and NPSLE. Despite remarkable evidence for their high disease specificity, anti-Rib-P have not been included in classification or diagnostic criteria for SLE. A significant challenge in interpreting the published literature is the variability of diagnostic platforms and the target antigens used in anti-Rib-P immunoassays. Evidence indicates that the major epitope is localized in the C-terminal 22 amino acids [98, 102], and some diagnostic assays use this analyte in their assays, but other assays use various combinations of the other Rib-P's [103, 104]. This likely accounts for the marked discrepancies in frequencies (10–47%) and association with clinical and demographic features reported in SLE cohorts. Although Rib-P proteins are localized in the cytoplasm, ANA IFA is not a reliable screening method to detect them [104, 105], but when it is positive, it is typically associated with a cytoplasmic AC-19 pattern. Anti-Rib-P antibodies commonly co-exist with anti-dsDNA and anti-cardiolipin (aCL) antibodies [106, 107], and this may account with the observed association with LN and NPSLE.

## Ro60/SSA

In general, anti-Ro60/SS-A antibodies are not reliably detected by most ANA IFA screening assays. An exception is a specialized HEp-2 substrate (HEp-2000, Immuno Concepts) that has been transfected with the Ro60/SS-A gene where it is overexpressed in some cells and more reliably detected by IFA [108]. Depending upon the method of detection and the cohort being studied, anti-Ro60/SS-A is found in up to 50% of patients with SLE. By comparison, the prevalence of anti-Ro60/SS-A is up to 85% in SjS. The prevalence of anti-Ro60/SS-A is similarly high in mothers of infants with NLS and subacute cutaneous lupus. A much lower prevalence (<25%) of anti-Ro60/SS-A is seen in SSc, AIM, RA, and autoimmune liver diseases. In SLE, anti-Ro60/SS-A is associated with photosensitive skin rash, elevated serum immunoglobulins, lower complement levels, lymphopenia, and leukopenia. In SLE, the combination of anti-Ro60/SS-A and anti-SS-B/La may be protective against the development of neurologic and kidney disease among patients [109]. Antibodies to anti-Ro60/SS-A have been reported to appear years before a diagnosis of SLE is made [92].

## Ro52/TRIM21

Ro52/TRIM21 is a 52-kDa member of the tripartite motif-containing (TRIM) super family of proteins, is a factor in innate and acquired immunity, and is an interferon (IFN)-inducible protein in some cells [110]. Its role in pathological autoimmune processes includes the aberrant ubiquitylation of the interferon-regulatory factor

(IRF) family of proteins, regulation of type I interferon and proinflammatory cytokines [110, 111], and a key effector in the toll-like receptor 3 pathway [112] and is linked to IL-23 and BAFF expression [111]. Hence, Ro52/TRIM21 has been purported as an attractive therapeutic target for SLE [110]. Anti-Ro52/TRIM21 antibodies are not detected by conventional HEp-2 ANA IFA.

Unfortunately, Ro52/TRIM21 was initially reported to be part of the same antigenic macromolecule as Ro60/SS-A and the B cell response to these two targets were strongly linked (reviewed in [113]). Subsequently, both of these claims were shown to be incorrect, but the medical literature is confounded because many commercially available diagnostics assays included both Ro52/TRIM21 and Ro60/SS-A in a single test and many reports of clinical associations have linked both targets together. As a result, detailed studies using anti-Ro52/TRM21 as a separate analyte are now needed. When this has been done, anti-Ro52/TIRM21 was found to be not specific for any SARD [114] but in SSc and MCTD was reported to be associated with polyautoimmunity (i.e., patients that have more than one autoimmune condition), interstitial lung disease, and rheumatoid factor [114, 115] and in SjS with more aggressive disease [116]. In SLE using LIA and ELISA, monospecific anti-Ro52/TRIM21 was observed in 6/67 (5.9%) and was most commonly associated with anti-Ro60/SS-A (22/67, 32.8%) [114]. In other studies, this autoantibody was associated with leukopenia, and ~70% of patients with anti-Ro52/TRIM21, but no anti-Ro60/SS-A antibodies, had undifferentiated connective tissue disease (UCTD) or SLE [46, 117, 118].

## Cell Cycle

### Proliferating Cell Nuclear Antigen

Antibodies directed to the 35 kDa proliferating cell nuclear antigen (PCNA) were first described in a Japanese female with SLE (reviewed in [119]). The identification of anti-PCNA and its purported high specificity for SLE was based on a unique cell-cycle IFA pattern on HEp-2 cells (AC-13) and a specific immunoprecipitation line in double immunodiffusion. However, subsequent studies that used other assays such as LIA, ELISA, and ALBIA [119] indicated that anti-PCNA antibodies were not specific for SLE [120]. Further studies (unpublished) indicate that the high specificity of anti-PCNA is consistent with earlier reports of specficity for SLE if both the typical IFA AC-13 pattern and high titer anti-PCNA antibodies are detected by SPMAA [121]. The disadvantage of anti-PCNA is that it has low sensitivity (<5%) for SLE and it may be undetectable after immunosuppression treatment [119].

## *Extracellular*

### C1q

Anti-C1q antibodies are predictive of and associated with LN, especially membranoproliferative disease [122–124]. In SLE with active LN, anti-C1q antibodies are found in up to 20–90% of patients [124, 125]. The combined detection of C1q and dsDNA antibodies predicted flares of LN and have a combined sensitivity of 91% and specificity of 90% for LN [126]. Anti-C1q antibodies are as specific as high avidity dsDNA antibodies for LN and close a diagnostic and serological gap in some cases [122, 127].

## *Phospholipids and Related Antigens [128]*

Autoantibodies directed to phospholipids (aCL, beta2 glycoprotein I (β2-GPI) and phospholipid-related targets (phosphatidylserine/prothrombin complex or PS/PT) are a heterogeneous family of autoantibodies that are an important serological criteria in the classification of SLE [79, 80] and APS [128, 129]. Historically, aPL antibodies are traced to the identification of a biologically false-positive test for syphilis and the eventual link to cardiolipin, other anionic (negatively charged) phospholipids, and phospholipid-binding proteins [2, 128]. Some studies indicate that they also have predictive value [130].

### Cardiolipin

The importance of aCL antibodies in SLE and APS has had a rather tumultuous history. However, aCL remains a key criterion for APS and has a prominent place in the laboratory diagnosis of both diseases. The primary use of the aCL assay is as an adjunct to anti-β2-GPI and lupus anticoagulant (LA) tests [128]. Its importance was underscored by a study reporting that >25% of APS patients were negative for anti-β2-GPI and LA but positive for aCL [131]. Hence, it remains an important assay to close the serological gap and classification of APS. IgG and IgM aCL test results should be reported as GPL and MPL units derived from calibrators composed of a pool of polyclonal aPLs. A positive aCL result is defined as a medium or high titer of greater than 40 GPL or MPL units. As an alternative, assay cutoffs established at greater than the 99th percentile of results obtained from a control group of at least 50 individuals are considered acceptable [79]. A significant limitation of the aCL test is its lack of specificity as it can be positive in other diseases, particularly those of infectious origin.

## β2-glycoprotein 1

β2-GPI is a 326 amino acid protein, and approximately 20% of the molecule is comprised of carbohydrates. β2-GPI antibodies are reported to have a higher specificity but lower sensitivity for APS than aCL antibodies. High titer IgG and IgM isotypes are diagnostic biomarkers and classification criteria of APS [128, 129] where they are associated with vascular thrombosis and recurrent spontaneous abortion. The value of anti-β2-GPI antibodies has highest clinical value when they are detected on two or more occasions at least 12 weeks apart. The prevalence and levels of anti-β2-GPI antibodies are significantly higher in SLE with arterial or venous thrombosis than in SLE patients without these complications and represent a significant risk factor for arterial thrombosis in SLE [132]. IgA anti-β2-GPI antibodies are reported to be more prevalent than IgG or IgM isotypes. The presence of both β2-GPI and aCL antibodies is strongly associated with clinical symptoms of APS [133, 134]. Unlike aCL antibodies, anti-β2-GPI antibodies are seldom detectable in infectious diseases. β2-GPI is composed of five molecular domains, of which the exposed residues spanning the region from arginine (Arg)39 to Arg43 of domain 1 represent the primary epitope bound by APS autoantibodies. The pathogenic subsets of anti-β2-GPI associated with thrombosis are reported to also bind domain 1. An approach to increasing the specificity of anti-β2-GPI testing was the development of a commercial immunoassay that included only DI of β2-GPI [134–136]. Recent reports indicate the value of this assay in risk management [135] and predicting thrombosis and late pregnancy morbidity [137]. However, as a word of caution, there is variation of results in different commercially available assays [138].

## Non-criteria Autoantibodies: Phosphatidylserine/Prothrombin Complex

Despite over 40 years of study and research, numerous difficulties are attributed to the APS criteria assays. In particular, no single or combination of APS criteria antibodies is present in up to 25% of patients who are strongly suspected of having APS, resulting in a "seronegative gap" [128, 139]. A number of non-criteria autoantibodies, such as anti-phosphatidylethanolamine, antibodies to proteins of the coagulation cascade, and antibodies to the PS/PT complex, have been associated with APS [128, 140, 141]. Some interest has focused on the mitochondrial membrane antigen M5 which is associated with thrombocytopenia and fetal loss and co-exists with LA, aCL, anti-β2GP1, and biologically false-positive VDRL [142, 143]. With the availability of a commercial anti-PS/PT assay [144], a number of reports have focused on its value [145], particularly its use in closing the seronegative gap in APS [141, 146]. Although the presence of anti-PS/PT antibodies appears to be independent of the LA, they may be a potential substitute for the troubled LA assay [146, 147]. The clinical utility of these assays, however, is limited by a paucity of prospective clinical data and lack of standardization [138]. Therefore, additional studies are required before any "non-criteria" immunoassays are included in standard APS classification criteria.

## *Orphan Autoantibodies*

As noted above, more than 180 autoantibodies have been described in SLE, and the list continues to grow. These "orphan" autoantibodies [81, 130] were not discussed here, but the reader is referred to published studies of selected "orphan" autoantibodies [7, 148]. The reason that many of these antibodies are not commonly used is that they have yet to meet SMAARTT (specificity-sensitivity, measurable, actionable, added value, realistic, titers, timely) criteria for development by laboratory diagnostics or and neither has there been a demand for them from clinical practitioners [149]. As SPMAAs become increasingly available, it is possible that some of these "orphan" biomarkers will find new uses in the prediction, diagnosis, and prognosis of SLE.

## Summary

In summary, there is a need for evidence-based and unbiased approaches to ANA testing. In parallel, a compelling case can be made for attenuation of significant morbidity and healthcare expenditures in SLE by using ANA testing for "case finding" and making a much earlier diagnosis and prevention of high morbidity [150]. Given the shortcomings of ANA IFA testing [151], it appears that a move to SPMAAs as the screening tests of choice for SLE may be warranted.

## References

1. Hargraves MM, Richmond H, Morton R. Presentation of two bone marrow elements: the "tart" cells and the "L.E." cell. Mayo Clin Proc. 1948;23:25–8.
2. Benedek TC. History of lupus. In: Wallace DJ, Hahn BH, editors. Dubois' lupus erythematosus and related conditions. Philadelphia: Elsevier; 2019. p. 1–14.
3. Mahler M, Meroni PL, Bossuyt X, Fritzler MJ. Current concepts and future directions for the assessment of autoantibodies to cellular antigens referred to as anti-nuclear antibodies. J Immunol Res. 2014;2014:315179.
4. Fritzler MJ. Widening spectrum and gaps in autoantibody testing for systemic autoimmune diseases. J Rheum Res. 2018;1:10–8.
5. Sherer Y, Gorstein A, Fritzler MJ, Shoenfeld Y. Autoantibody explosion in systemic lupus erythematosus. Semin Arthritis Rheum. 2004;34:501–37.
6. Yaniv G, Twig G, Shor DB, Furer A, Sherer Y, Mozes O, et al. A volcanic explosion of autoantibodies in systemic lupus erythematosus: a diversity of 180 different antibodies found in SLE patients. Autoimmun Rev. 2014;14:75–9.
7. Fredi M, Cavazzana I, Quinzanini M, Taraborelli M, Cartella S, Tincani A, et al. Rare autoantibodies to cellular antigens in systemic lupus erythematosus. Lupus. 2014;23:672–7.
8. Choi MY, Clarke AE, St Pierre Y, Hanly JG, Urowitz MB, Romero-Diaz J, et al. Antinuclear antibody-negative systemic lupus erythematosus in an international inception cohort. Arthritis Care Res (Hoboken). 2018;71:893–902.

9. Fritzler MJ, Martinez-Prat L, Choi MY, Mahler M. The utilization of autoantibodies in approaches to precision health. Front Immunol. 2018;9:2682.
10. Fritzler MJ, Fritzler ML. Microbead-based technologies in diagnostic autoantibody detection. Expert Opin Med Diag. 2009;3:81–9.
11. Olsen NJ, Choi MY, Fritzler MJ. Emerging technologies in autoantibody testing for rheumatic diseases. Arthritis Res Ther. 2017;19:172.
12. Meroni PL, Schur PH. ANA screening: an old test with new recommendations. Ann Rheum Dis. 2010;69:1420–2.
13. Hammonds T. Academic-pharma drug discovery alliances: seeking ways to eliminate the valley of death. Future Med Chem. 2015;7:1891–9.
14. Aringer M, Costenbader K, Daikh D, Brinks R, Mosca M, Ramsey-Goldman R, et al. 2019 European League Against Rheumatism/American College of Rheumatology classification criteria for systemic lupus erythematosus. Ann Rheum Dis. 2019;78:1151–9.
15. Shepherd M, Shields B, Hammersley S, Hudson M, McDonald TJ, Colclough K, et al. Systematic population screening, using biomarkers and genetic testing, identifies 2.5% of the U.K. pediatric diabetes population with monogenic diabetes. Diabetes Care. 2016;39(11):1879–88.
16. Willems P, De LE, Westhovens R, Vanderschueren S, Blockmans D, Bossuyt X. Antinuclear antibody as entry criterion for classification of systemic lupus erythematosus: pitfalls and opportunities. Ann Rheum Dis. 2018;78(8):e76.
17. Colon-Franco JM, Bossuyt PMM, Algeciras-Schimnich A, Bird C, Engstrom-Melnyk J, Fleisher M, et al. Current and emerging multianalyte assays with algorithmic analyses-are laboratories ready for clinical adoption? Clin Chem. 2018;64:885–91.
18. Meroni PL, Chan EK, Damoiseaux J, Andrade LEC, Bossuyt X, Conrad K, et al. Unending story of the indirect immunofluorescence assay on HEp-2 cells: old problems and new solutions? Ann Rheum Dis. 2018;78:e46.
19. Perez D, Gilburd B, Azoulay D, Shovman O, Bizzaro N, Shoenfeld Y. Antinuclear antibodies: is the indirect immunofluorescence still the gold standard or should be replaced by solid phase assays? Autoimmun Rev. 2018;17:548–52.
20. Bizzaro N, Brusca I, Previtali G, Alessio MG, Daves M, Platzgummer S, et al. The association of solid-phase assays to immunofluorescence increases the diagnostic accuracy for ANA screening in patients with autoimmune rheumatic diseases. Autoimmun Rev. 2018;17:541–7.
21. Pisetsky DS. Antinuclear antibody testing - misunderstood or misbegotten? Nat Rev Rheumatol. 2017;13:495–502.
22. Pisetsky DS, Lipsky PE. The role of ANA determinations in classification criteria for SLE. Arthritis Care Res (Hoboken). 2018;71(5):696.
23. Jacobs JFM, Bossuyt X. Standardization and harmonization of autoimmune diagnostics. Clin Chem Lab Med. 2018;56:1563–7.
24. Perez D, Gilburd B, Cabrera-Marante O, Martinez-Flores JA, Serrano M, Naranjo L, et al. Predictive autoimmunity using autoantibodies: screening for anti-nuclear antibodies. Clin Chem Lab Med. 2018;56:1771–7.
25. Barr SG, Zonana-Nacach A, Magder LS, Petri M. Patterns of disease activity in systemic lupus erythematosus. Arthritis Rheum. 1999;42:2682–8.
26. Wiik AS. Anti-nuclear autoantibodies: clinical utility for diagnosis, prognosis, monitoring, and planning of treatment strategy in systemic immunoinflammatory diseases. Scand J Rheumatol. 2005;34:260–8.
27. Sjowall C, Bentow C, Aure MA, Mahler M. Two-parametric immunological score development for assessing renal involvement and disease activity in systemic lupus erythematosus. J Immunol Res. 2018;2018:1294680.
28. Beastall GH, Brouwer N, Quiroga S, Myers GL. Traceability in laboratory medicine: a global driver for accurate results for patient care. Clin Chem Lab Med. 2017;55:1100–8.
29. Young IS. The enduring importance and challenge of commutability. Clin Chem. 2018;64:421–3.

30. Paxton A. New momentum in harmonizing lab results. CAP Today. 2018;32:1–34.
31. Agmon-Levin N, Damoiseaux J, Kallenberg C, Sack U, Witte T, Herold M, et al. International recommendations for the assessment of autoantibodies to cellular antigens referred to as antinuclear antibodies. Ann Rheum Dis. 2014;73:17–23.
32. Damoiseaux J, von Muhlen CA, Garcia-de la Torre I, Carballo OG, de Melo CW, Francescantonio PL, et al. International consensus on ANA patterns (ICAP): the bumpy road towards a consensus on reporting ANA results. Auto Immun Highlights. 2016;7:1.
33. Fritzler MJ, Wiik A, Fritzler ML, Barr SG. The use and abuse of commercial kits used to detect autoantibodies. Arthritis Res Ther. 2003;5:192–201.
34. Bossuyt X, Louche C, Wiik A. Standardisation in clinical laboratory medicine: an ethical reflection. Ann Rheum Dis. 2008;67:1061–3.
35. Van den Bremt S, Schouwers S, Van BM, Van HL. ANA IIF automation: moving towards harmonization? Results of a multicenter study. J Immunol Res. 2017;2017:6038137.
36. Claessens J, Belmondo T, De LE, Westhovens R, Poesen K, Hue S, et al. Solid phase assays versus automated indirect immunofluorescence for detection of antinuclear antibodies. Autoimmun Rev. 2018;17:533–40.
37. Kim J, Lee W, Kim GT, Kim HS, Ock S, Kim IS, et al. Diagnostic utility of automated indirect immunofluorescence compared to manual indirect immunofluorescence for antinuclear antibodies in patients with systemic rheumatic diseases: a systematic review and meta-analysis. Semin Arthritis Rheum. 2018;48(4):728–35.
38. Bossuyt X, Hendrickx A, Frans J. Antinuclear antibody titer and antibodies to extractable nuclear antigens. Arthritis Rheum. 2005;53:987–8.
39. Oyaert M, Bossuyt X, Ravelingien I, Van HL. Added value of indirect immunofluorescence intensity of automated antinuclear antibody testing in a secondary hospital setting. Clin Chem Lab Med. 2016;54:e63–6.
40. Chan EK, Damoiseaux J, de Melo CW, Carballo OG, Conrad K, Francescantonio PL, et al. Report on the Second International Consensus on ANA Pattern (ICAP) workshop in Dresden 2015. Lupus. 2016;25:797–804.
41. Meroni PL, Borghi MO. Diagnostic laboratory tests for systemic autoimmune rheumatic diseases: unmet needs towards harmonization. Clin Chem Lab Med. 2018;56:1743–8.
42. Bossuyt X, Fieuws S. Detection of antinuclear antibodies: added value of solid phase assay? Ann Rheum Dis. 2014;73:e10.
43. Jeong S, Hwang H, Roh J, Shim JE, Kim J, Kim GT, et al. Evaluation of an automated screening assay, compared to indirect immunofluorescence, an extractable nuclear antigen assay, and a line immunoassay in a large cohort of Asian patients with antinuclear antibody-associated rheumatoid diseases: a multicenter retrospective study. J Immunol Res. 2018;2018:9094217.
44. Craft J, Hardin JA. Linked sets of antinuclear antibodies: what do they mean? J Rheumatol. 1987;14(Suppl):106–9.
45. Yang J, Xu Z, Sui M, Han J, Sun L, Jia X, et al. Co-positivity for anti-dsDNA, -nucleosome and -histone antibodies in lupus nephritis is indicative of high serum levels and severe nephropathy. PLoS One. 2015;10:e0140441.
46. Menor AR, Jurado RA, Rodriguez Gutierrez FJ, Solis DR, Cardiel MH, Salaberri Maestrojuan JJ. Association of anti-Ro52, anti-Ro60 and anti-La antibodies with diagnostic, clinical and laboratory features in a referral hospital in Jerez, Spain. Reumatol Clin. 2015;12(5):256–62.
47. Mummert E, Fritzler MJ, Sjowall C, Bentow C, Mahler M. The clinical utility of anti-double-stranded DNA antibodies and the challenges of their determination. J Immunol Methods. 2018;459:11–9.
48. Pisetsky DS. Anti-DNA antibodies - quintessential biomarkers of SLE. Nat Rev Rheumatol. 2016;12:102–10.
49. Yung S, Chan TM. Mechanisms of kidney injury in lupus nephritis – the role of anti-dsDNA antibodies. Front Immunol. 2015;6:475.
50. Andrejevic S, Jeremic I, Sefik-Bukilica M, Nikolic M, Stojimirovic B, Bonaci-Nikolic B. Immunoserological parameters in SLE: high-avidity anti-dsDNA detected by ELISA are the most closely associated with the disease activity. Clin Rheumatol. 2013;32:1619–26.

51. Gomez-Puerta JA, Burlingame RW, Cervera R. Anti-chromatin (anti-nucleosome) antibodies: Diagnostic and clinical value. Autoimmun Rev. 2008;7:606–11.
52. Van Bavel CC, Dieker JW, Kroeze Y, Tamboer WP, Voll R, Muller S, et al. Apoptosis-induced histone H3 methylation is targeted by autoantibodies in systemic lupus erythematosus. Ann Rheum Dis. 2010;70:201–7.
53. Van Bavel CC, Dieker J, Muller S, Briand JP, Monestier M, Berden JH, et al. Apoptosis-associated acetylation on histone H2B is an epitope for lupus autoantibodies. Mol Immunol. 2009;47:511–6.
54. Dwivedi N, Neeli I, Schall N, Wan H, Desiderio DM, Csernok E, et al. Deimination of linker histones links neutrophil extracellular trap release with autoantibodies in systemic autoimmunity. FASEB J. 2014;28:2840–51.
55. Vaglio A, Grayson PC, Fenaroli P, Gianfreda D, Boccaletti V, Ghiggeri GM, et al. Drug-induced lupus: traditional and new concepts. Autoimmun Rev. 2018;17:912–8.
56. Fritzler MJ, Tan EM. Antibodies to histones in drug-induced and idiopathic lupus erythematosus. J Clin Invest. 1978;62:560–7.
57. Mehra S, Fritzler MJ. The spectrum of anti-chromatin/nucleosome autoantibodies: independent and interdependent biomarkers of disease. J Immunol Res. 2014;2014:368274.
58. Stinton LM, Barr SG, Tibbles LA, Yilmaz S, Sar A, Benedikttson H, et al. Autoantibodies in lupus nephritis patients requiring renal transplantation. Lupus. 2007;16:394–400.
59. Abraham SJ, Rojas-Serrano J, Cabiedes J, Alcocer-Varela J. Antinucleosome antibodies may help predict development of systemic lupus erythematosus in patients with primary antiphospholipid syndrome. Lupus. 2004;13:177–81.
60. Cervera R, Vinas O, Ramos-Casals M, Font J, Garcia-Carrasco M, Siso A, et al. Anti-chromatin antibodies in systemic lupus erythematosus: a useful marker for lupus nephropathy. Ann Rheum Dis. 2003;62:431–4.
61. Kiss E, Lakos G, Szegedi G, Poor G, Szodoray P. Anti-nucleosome antibody, a reliable indicator for lupus nephritis. Autoimmunity. 2009;42:393–8.
62. Rekvig OP, van der Vlag J, Seredkina N. Anti-nucleosome antibodies – a critical reflection on their specificities and diagnostic impact. Arthritis Rheumatol. 2014;65:1061–9.
63. Schaper F, De Leeuw K, Horst GT, Maas F, Bootsma H, Heeringa P, Limburg PC, Westra J. Autoantibodies to Box A of high mobility group box-1 in Systemic Lupus Erythematosus. Clin Exp Immunol. 2017;188:412–9.
64. Scaffidi P, Misteli T, Bianchi ME. Release of chromatin protein HMGB1 by necrotic cells triggers inflammation. Nature. 2002;418:191–5.
65. Magna M, Pisetsky DS. The role of cell death in the pathogenesis of SLE: is pyroptosis the missing link? Scand J Immunol. 2015;82:218–24.
66. Cully M. Connective tissue diseases: HMGB1 helps elicit anti-dsDNA antibody production in SLE. Nat Rev Rheumatol. 2013;9:321.
67. Abdulahad DA, Westra J, Bijzet J, Limburg PC, Kallenberg CG, Bijl M. High mobility group box 1 (HMGB1) and anti-HMGB1 antibodies and their relation to disease characteristics in systemic lupus erythematosus. Arthritis Res Ther. 2011;13:R71.
68. de Souza AW, Westra J, Bijzet J, Limburg PC, Stegeman CA, Bijl M, Kallenberg CG. Is serum HMGB1 a biomarker in ANCA-associated vasculitis? Arthritis Res Ther. 2013;15:R104.
69. Santoro P, De Andrea M, Migliaretti G, Trapani C, Landolfo S, Gariglio M. High prevalence of autoantibodies against the nuclear high mobility group (HMG) protein SSRP1 in sera from patients with SLE, but not other rheumatic diseases. J Rheumatol. 2002;29:90–3.
70. Conrad K, Rober N, Andrade LE, Mahler M. The clinical relevance of anti-DFS70 autoantibodies. Clin Rev Allergy Immunol. 2017;52:202–16.
71. Mahler M, Meroni PL, Andrade LE, Khamashta M, Bizzaro N, Casiano CA, et al. Towards a better understanding of the clinical association of anti-DFS70 autoantibodies. Autoimmun Rev. 2016;15:198–201.
72. Ganapathy V, Casiano CA. Autoimmunity to the nuclear autoantigen DFS70 (LEDGF): what exactly are the autoantibodies trying to tell us? Arthritis Rheum. 2004;50:684–8.

73. Ochs RL, Mahler M, Basu A, Rios-Colon L, Sanchez TW, Andrade LE, et al. The significance of autoantibodies to DFS70/LEDGFp75 in health and disease: integrating basic science with clinical understanding. Clin Exp Med. 2016;16:273–93.
74. Mariz HA, Sato EI, Barbosa SH, Rodrigues SH, Dellavance A, Andrade LE. Pattern on the antinuclear antibody-HEp-2 test is a critical parameter for discriminating antinuclear antibody-positive healthy individuals and patients with autoimmune rheumatic diseases. Arthritis Rheum. 2011;63:191–200.
75. Choi MY, Clarke AE, St PY, Hanly JG, Urowitz MB, Romero-Diaz J, et al. The prevalence and determinants of anti-DFS70 autoantibodies in an international inception cohort of systemic lupus erythematosus patients. Lupus. 2017;26:1051–9.
76. Albesa R, Sachs UJ, Infantino M, Manfredi M, Benucci M, Baus Y, et al. Increased prevalence of anti-DFS70 antibodies in young females: experience from large international multicenter study on blood donors. Clin Chem Lab Med. 2018;57(7):999–1005.
77. Riemekasten G, Humrich JY, Hiepe F. Antibodies against the extractable nulcear antigens RNP, Sm, R0/SSA, and La/SSB. In: Wallace DJ, Hahn BH, editors. Dubois' systemic lupus erythematosus and related syndromes. Philadelphia: Elsevier Inc.; 2019. p. 366–71.
78. Craft J. Antibodies to snRNPs in systemic lupus erythematosus. Rheum Dis Clin N A. 1992;18:311–35.
79. Hochberg MC. Updating the American College of Rheumatology revised criteria for the classification of systemic lupus erythematosus. Arthritis Rheum. 1997;40:1725.
80. Petri M, Orbai AM, Alarcon GS, Gordon C, Merrill JT, Fortin PR, et al. Derivation and validation of systemic lupus international collaborating clinics classification criteria for systemic lupus erythematosus. Arthritis Rheum. 2012;64:2677–86.
81. Fritzler MJ. Challenges to the use of autoantibodies as predictors of disease onset, diagnosis and outcomes. Autoimmun Rev. 2008;7:616–20.
82. Sharp GC, Irvin W, Tan EM, Gould G, Holman HR. Mixed connective tissue disease - an apparently distinct rheumatic disease syndrome associated with a specific antibody to an extractable nuclear antigen (ENA). Am J Med. 1972;52:148–59.
83. Sakata K, Matsumoto Y, Satoh M, Oouchi A, Nagakura H, Koito K, et al. Clinical studies of immunohistochemical staining of DNA-dependent protein kinase in oropharyngeal and hypopharyngeal carcinomas. Radiat Med. 2001;19:93–7.
84. Belizna C, Henrion D, Beucher A, Lavigne C, Ghaali A, Levesque H. Anti-Ku antibodies: clinical, genetic and diagnostic insights. Autoimmun Rev. 2010;9:691–4.
85. Mimori T, Akizuki M, Yamagata H, Inada S, Yoshida S, Homma M. Characterization of a high molecular weight acidic nuclear protein recognized by autoantibodies in sera from patients with polymyositis-scleroderma overlap. J Clin Invest. 1981;68:611–20.
86. Reeves WH. Use of monoclonal antibodies for the characterization of novel DNA-binding proteins recognized by human autoimmune sera. J Exp Med. 1985;161:18–39.
87. Wang J, Satoh M, Kabir F, Shaw M, Domingo MA, Mansoor R, et al. Increased prevalence of autoantibodies to ku antigen in African American versus white patients with systemic lupus erythematosus. Arthritis Rheum. 2001;44:2367–70.
88. Hoa S, Hudson M, Troyanov Y, Proudman S, Walker J, Stevens W, et al. Single-specificity anti-Ku antibodies in an international cohort of 2140 systemic sclerosis subjects: clinical associations. Medicine (Baltimore). 2016;95:e4713.
89. Vitali C, Bombardieri S, Jonsson R, Moutsopoulos HM, Alexander EL, Carsons SE, et al. Classification criteria for Sjogren's syndrome: a revised version of the European criteria proposed by the American-European Consensus Group. Ann Rheum Dis. 2002;61:554–8.
90. Routsias JG, Tzioufas AG. Autoimmune response and target autoantigens in Sjogren's syndrome. Eur J Clin Investig. 2010;40:1026–36.
91. Izmirly PM, Halushka MK, Rosenberg AZ, Whelton S, Rais-Bahrami K, Nath DS, et al. Clinical and pathologic implications of extending the spectrum of maternal autoantibodies reactive with ribonucleoproteins associated with cutaneous and now cardiac neonatal lupus from SSA/Ro and SSB/La to U1RNP. Autoimmun Rev. 2017;16:980–3.

92. Arbuckle MR, McClain MT, Rubertone MV, Scofield RH, Dennis GJ, James JA, et al. Development of autoantibodies before the clinical onset of systemic lupus erythematosus. N Engl J Med. 2003;349:1526–33.
93. Grela P, Sawa-Makarska J, Gordiyenko Y, Robinson CV, Grankowski N, Tchorzewski M. Structural properties of the human acidic ribosomal P proteins forming the P1-P2 heterocomplex. J Biochem. 2008;143:169–77.
94. Lin A, Wittmann-Liebold B, McNally J, Wool IG. The primary structure of the acidic phosphoprotein P2 from rat liver 60 S ribosomal subunits. Comparison with ribosomal 'A' proteins from other species. J Biol Chem. 1982;257:9189–97.
95. Francoeur AM, Peebles CL, Heckman KJ, Lee JC, Tan EM. Identification of ribosomal protein autoantigens. J Immunol. 1985;135:2378–84.
96. Pasoto SG, Viana VS, Bonfa E. The clinical utility of anti-ribosomal P autoantibodies in systemic lupus erythematosus. Expert Rev Clin Immunol. 2014;10:1493–503.
97. Toubi E, Shoenfeld Y. Clinical and biological aspects of anti-P-ribosomal protein autoantibodies. Autoimmun Rev. 2007;6:119–25.
98. Mahler M, Agmon-Levin N, van Liempt M, Shoenfeld Y, Waka A, Hiepe F, Swart A, Gürtler I, Fritzler MJ. Multi-center evaluation of autoantibodies to the major ribosomal P C22 epitope. Rheumatol Int. 2012;32:691–8.
99. Zandman-Goddard G, Shoenfeld Y. Antiribsomal P antibodies. In: Shoenfeld Y, Meroni PL, Gershwin ME, editors. Autoantibodies. Amsterdam: Elsevier BV; 2014. p. 225–31.
100. Karassa FB, Afeltra A, Ambrozic A, Chang DM, De KF, Doria A, et al. Accuracy of anti-ribosomal P protein antibody testing for the diagnosis of neuropsychiatric systemic lupus erythematosus: an international meta-analysis. Arthritis Rheum. 2006;54:312–24.
101. Hanly JG, Urowitz MB, Siannis F, Farewell V, Gordon C, Bae SC, et al. Autoantibodies and neuropsychiatric events at the time of systemic lupus erythematosus diagnosis: results from an international inception cohort study. Arthritis Rheum. 2008;58:843–53.
102. Mahler M, Kessenbrock K, Raats J, Williams RCJr, Fritzler MJ. Characterization of the human autoimmune response to the major C-terminal epitope of the ribosomal P proteins. J Mol Med. 2003;81:194–204.
103. Lin JL, Dubljevic V, Fritzler MJ, Toh BH. Major immunoreactive domains of human ribosomal P proteins lie N-terminal to a homologous C-22 sequence: application to a novel ELISA for systemic lupus erythematosus. Clin Exp Immunol. 2005;141:155–64.
104. Mahler M, Kessenbrock K, Raats J, Fritzler MJ. Technical and clinical evaluation of anti-ribosomal P protein immunoassays. J Clin Lab Anal. 2004;18:215–23.
105. Mahler M, Ngo J, Schulte-Pelkum J, Luettich T, Fritzler MJ. Limited reliability of the indirect immunofluorescence technique for the detection of anti-Rib-P antibodies. Arthritis Res Ther. 2008;10:R131.
106. Reichlin M. Serological correlations with nephritis in systemic lupus erythematosus. Clin Immunol. 2005;117:12–4.
107. Gerli R, Caponi L. Anti-ribosomal P protein antibodies. Autoimmunity. 2005;38:85–92.
108. Fritzler MJ, Hanson C, Miller J, Eystathioy T. Specificity of autoantibodies to SS-A/Ro on a transfected and overexpressed human 60 kDa Ro autoantigen substrate. J Clin Lab Anal. 2002;16:103–8.
109. Malik S, Bruner GR, Williams-Weese C, Feo L, Scofield RH, Reichlin M, et al. Presence of anti-La autoantibody is associated with a lower risk of nephritis and seizures in lupus patients. Lupus. 2007;16:863–6.
110. Yoshimi R, Ishigatsubo Y, Ozato K. Autoantigen TRIM21/Ro52 as a possible target for treatment of systemic lupus erythematosus. Int J Rheumatol. 2012;2012:718237.
111. Bolland S, Garcia-Sastre A. Vicious circle: systemic autoreactivity in Ro52/TRIM21-deficient mice. J Exp Med. 2009;206:1647–51.
112. Kyriakidis NC, Kapsogeorgou EK, Gourzi VC, Konsta OD, Baltatzis GE, Tzioufas AG. Toll-like receptor 3 stimulation promotes Ro52/TRIM21 synthesis and nuclear redistribution in

salivary gland epithelial cells, partially via type I interferon pathway. Clin Exp Immunol. 2014;178:548–60.
113. Schulte-Pelkum J, Fritzler M, Mahler M. Latest update on the Ro/SS-A autoantibody system. Autoimmun Rev. 2009;8:632–7.
114. Dugar M, Cox S, Limaye V, Gordon TP, Roberts-Thomson PJ. Diagnostic utility of anti-Ro52 detection in systemic autoimmunity. Postgrad Med J. 2010;86:79–82.
115. Hudson M, Pope J, Mahler M, Tatibouet S, Steele R, Baron M, et al. Clinical significance of antibodies to Ro52/TRIM21 in systemic sclerosis. Arthritis Res Ther. 2012;14:R50.
116. Retamozo S, Akasbi M, Brito-Zeron P, Bosch X, Bove A, Perez-De-Lis M, et al. Anti-Ro52 antibody testing influences the classification and clinical characterisation of primary Sjogren's syndrome. Clin Exp Rheumatol. 2012;30:686–92.
117. Lu R, Robertson JM, Bruner BF, Guthridge JM, Neas BR, Nath SK, et al. Multiple autoantibodies display association with lymphopenia, proteinuria, and cellular casts in a large, ethnically diverse SLE patient cohort. Autoimmune Dis. 2012;2012:819634.
118. Go EJL, O'Neil KM. The catastrophic antiphospholipid syndrome in children. Curr Opin Rheumatol. 2017;29(5):516–22.
119. Mahler M, Miyachi K, Peebles C, Fritzler MJ. The clinical significance of autoantibodies to the proliferating cell nuclear antigen (PCNA). Autoimmun Rev. 2012;11:771–5.
120. Vermeersch P, De Beeck KO, Lauwerys BR, Van den Bergh K, Develter M, Marien G, et al. Antinuclear antibodies directed against proliferating cell nuclear antigen are not specifically associated with systemic lupus erythematosus. Ann Rheum Dis. 2009;68:1791–3.
121. Mahler M, Silverman ED, Fritzler M. Novel diagnostic and clinical aspects of anti-PCNA antibodies detected by novel detection methods. Lupus. 2010;19:1527–33.
122. Beurskens FJ, van Schaarenburg RA, Trouw LA. C1q, antibodies and anti-C1q autoantibodies. Mol Immunol. 2015;68:6–13.
123. Trouw LA, Daha MR. Role of anti-C1q autoantibodies in the pathogenesis of lupus nephritis. Expert Opin Biol Ther. 2005;5:243–51.
124. de Leeuw K, Kallenberg CGM. Antibodies against C1q antibodies. In: Wallace DJ, Hahn BH, editors. Dubois' lupus erythematosus and related syndromes. Philadelpha: Elsevier Inc.; 2019. p. 372–3.
125. Vitre B, Gudimchuk N, Borda R, Kim Y, Heuser JE, Cleveland DW, et al. Kinetochore-microtubule attachment throughout mitosis potentiated by the elongated stalk of the kinetochore kinesin CENP-E. Mol Biol Cell. 2014;25:2272–81.
126. Matrat A, Veysseyre-Balter C, Trolliet P, Villar E, Dijoud F, Bienvenu J, et al. Simultaneous detection of anti-C1q and anti-double stranded DNA autoantibodies in lupus nephritis: predictive value for renal flares. Lupus. 2011;20:28–34.
127. Eggleton P, Ukoumunne OC, Cottrell I, Khan A, Maqsood S, Thornes J, et al. Autoantibodies against C1q as a diagnostic measure of lupus nephritis: systematic review and meta-analysis. J Clin Cell Immunol. 2014;5:210.
128. Giles I, Cohen H, Ioannou Y. Pathogenesis of antiphospholipid antibody syndrome. In: Wallace DJ, Hahn BH, editors. Dubois' lupus erythematosus and related syndromes. Philadelphia: Elsevier Inc.; 2019. p. 324–37.
129. Miyakis S, Lockshin MD, Atsumi T, Branch DW, Brey RL, Cervera R, et al. International consensus statement on an update of the classification criteria for definite antiphospholipid syndrome (APS). J Thromb Haemost. 2006;4:295–306.
130. Meroni PL, Shoenfeld Y. Predictive, protective, orphan autoantibodies: the example of the anti-phospholipid antibodies. Autoimmun Rev. 2008;7:585–7.
131. Nash MJ, Camilleri RS, Kunka S, Mackie IJ, Machin SJ, Cohen H. The anticardiolipin assay is required for sensitive screening for antiphospholipid antibodies. J Thromb Haemost. 2004;2:1077–81.
132. Nojima J, Kuratsune H, Suehisa E, Futsukaichi Y, Yamanishi H, Machii T, et al. Association between the prevalence of antibodies to $\beta_2$-glycoprotein I, prothrombin, protein C, protein S,

and annexin V in patients with systemic lupus erythematosus and thrombotic and thrombocytopenic complications. Clin Chem. 2001;47:1008–15.
133. Obermoser G, Bitterlich W, Kunz F, Sepp NT. Clinical significance of anticardiolipin and anti-beta2-glycoprotein I antibodies. Int Arch Allergy Immunol. 2004;135:148–53.
134. Andreoli L, Chighizola CB, Nalli C, Gerosa M, Borghi MO, Pregnolato F, et al. Clinical characterization of antiphospholipid syndrome by detection of IgG antibodies against beta2-glycoprotein i domain 1 and domain 4/5: ratio of anti-domain 1 to anti-domain 4/5 as a useful new biomarker for antiphospholipid syndrome. Arthritis Rheumatol. 2015;67:2196–204.
135. Mahler M, Norman GL, Meroni PL, Khamashta M. Autoantibodies to domain 1 of beta 2 glycoprotein 1: a promising candidate biomarker for risk management in antiphospholipid syndrome. Autoimmun Rev. 2012;12:313–7.
136. Cousins L, Pericleous C, Khamashta M, Bertolaccini ML, Ioannou Y, Giles I, et al. Antibodies to domain I of beta-2-glycoprotein I and IgA antiphospholipid antibodies in patients with 'seronegative' antiphospholipid syndrome. Ann Rheum Dis. 2015;74:317–9.
137. Chighizola CB, Pregnolato F, Andreoli L, Bodio C, Cesana L, Comerio C, et al. Beyond thrombosis: anti-beta2GPI domain 1 antibodies identify late pregnancy morbidity in anti-phospholipid syndrome. J Autoimmun. 2018;90:76–83.
138. Chayoua W, Kelchtermans H, Moore GW, Musial J, Wahl D, et al. Identification of high thrombotic risk triple-positive antiphospholipid syndrome patients is dependent on anti-cardiolipin and anti-beta2glycoprotein I antibody detection assays. J Thromb Haemost. 2018;16:2016–23.
139. Zohoury N, Bertolaccini ML, Rodriguez-Garcia JL, Shums Z, Ateka-Barrutia O, Sorice M, et al. Closing the serological gap in the antiphospholipid syndrome: the value of "non-criteria" antiphospholipid antibodies. J Rheumatol. 2017;44:1597–602.
140. Sciascia S, Khamashta MA, Bertolaccini ML. New tests to detect antiphospholipid antibodies: antiprothrombin (aPT) and anti-phosphatidylserine/prothrombin (aPS/PT) antibodies. Curr Rheumatol Rep. 2014;16:415.
141. Zhang S, Wu Z, Zhang W, Zhao J, Norman GL, Zeng X, et al. Antibodies to phosphatidylserine/prothrombin (aPS/PT) enhanced the diagnostic performance in Chinese patients with antiphospholipid syndrome. Clin Chem Lab Med. 2018;56:939–46.
142. La Rosa L, Covini G, Galperin C, Catelli L, Del Papa N, Reina G, et al. Anti-mitochondrial M5 type antibody represents one of the serological markers for anti-phospholipid syndrome distinct from anti-cardiolipin and anti-beta2-glycoprotein I antibodies. Clin Exp Immunol. 1998;112:144–51.
143. Meroni PL, Harris EN, Brucato A, Tincani A, Barcellini W, Vismara A, et al. Anti-mitochondrial type M5 and anti-cardiolipin antibodies in autoimmune disorders: studies on their association and cross-reactivity. Clin Exp Immunol. 1987;67:484–91.
144. Sciascia S, Sanna G, Murru V, Khamashta MA, Bertolaccini ML. Validation of a commercially available kit to detect anti-phosphatidylserine/prothrombin antibodies in a cohort of systemic lupus erythematosus patients. Thromb Res. 2014;133:451–4.
145. Amengual O, Forastiero R, Sugiura-Ogasawara M, Otomo K, Oku K, Favas C, et al. Evaluation of phosphatidylserine-dependent antiprothrombin antibody testing for the diagnosis of antiphospholipid syndrome: results of an international multicentre study. Lupus. 2017;26:266–76.
146. Shi H, Zheng H, Yin YF, Hu QY, Teng JL, Sun Y, et al. Antiphosphatidylserine/prothrombin antibodies (aPS/PT) as potential diagnostic markers and risk predictors of venous thrombosis and obstetric complications in antiphospholipid syndrome. Clin Chem Lab Med. 2018;56:614–24.
147. Bertolaccini ML, Sciascia S, Murru V, Garcia-Fernandez C, Sanna G, Khamashta MA. Prevalence of antibodies to prothrombin in solid phase (aPT) and to phosphatidylserine-prothrombin complex (aPS/PT) in patients with and without lupus anticoagulant. Thromb Haemost. 2013;109:207–13.

148. Stinton LM, Eystathioy T, Selak S, Chan EKL, Fritzler MJ. Autoantibodies to protein transport and messenger RNA processing pathways: endosomes, lysosomes, Golgi complex, proteasomes, assemblyosomes, exosomes and GW Bodies. Clin Immunol. 2004;110:30–44.
149. Fritzler MJ, Mahler M. Redefining systemic lupus erythematosus — SMAARTT proteomics. Nat Rev Rheumatol. 2018;14:451–2.
150. Choi MY, Barber MR, Barber CE, Clarke AE, Fritzler MJ. Preventing the development of SLE: identifying risk factors and proposing pathways for clinical care. Lupus. 2016;25:838–49.
151. Fritzler MJ. The antinuclear antibody (ANA) test: last or lasting gasp? Arthritis Rheum. 2011;63:19–22.

# Chapter 5
# Childhood-Onset Systemic Lupus Erythematosus (cSLE): Is It Really Different Than Adult-Onset SLE?

**Herman H. Y. Tam, Deborah M. Levy, and Lily S. H. Lim**

## Introduction

In this review, we ask the provocative question of whether childhood-onset systemic lupus erythematosus (cSLE) and adult-onset SLE (aSLE) are substantively different. To do this, we review and evaluate how cSLE and aSLE differ (or not) in epidemiology, genetic predispositions, classification, racial predispositions, disease manifestations, activity and outcomes, medication use, and mental health. We highlight the unique aspects of cSLE compared to aSLE in terms of impact on growth and development and social outcomes. We present data from cSLE and aSLE cohorts that are derived from the same population (geographic locales) where available and preferentially review studies with direct cSLE and aSLE comparisons.

## What Is cSLE?

cSLE is a dynamic concept. Approximately 15–20% of patients with SLE develop their illness before adulthood [1]. The upper age cutoff is mostly based on the age

H. H. Y. Tam
Division of Rheumatology, British Columbia Children's Hospital, University of British Columbia, Vancouver, BC, Canada
e-mail: herman.tam@phsa.ca

D. M. Levy
Division of Rheumatology, The Hospital for Sick Children, University of Toronto, Toronto, ON, Canada
e-mail: deborah.levy@sickkids.ca

L. S. H. Lim (✉)
Section of Rheumatology, Department of Paediatrics and Child Health, Children's Hospital Research Institute of Manitoba, University of Manitoba, Winnipeg, MB, Canada
e-mail: llim@chrim.ca



Z. Touma (ed.), *Outcome Measures and Metrics in Systemic Lupus Erythematosus*, https://doi.org/10.1007/978-3-030-73303-2_5

limits of pediatric care in a region or country and not based on distinct cSLE pathophysiologic mechanisms. In the current literature, there are large variations in who are included in studies of cSLE. The maximum age of inclusion ranges from 14 to 20 years in existing studies [2–7], while some have focused only on those with prepubertal onset [8, 9]. Within the pediatric population, the median age of onset of cSLE is 12 years [10], and there is an age-dependent increase in cSLE incidence [11–13]. In the current review, we include studies of cSLE cohorts, as defined by their authors.

## *Epidemiology*

### Incidence and Prevalence

Worldwide incidence and prevalence rates of cSLE from epidemiological studies (regional surveys, national questionnaires, health administrative data) range from 0.3 to 10 per 100,000 children and 1.9 to 25.7 per 100,000 children, respectively [3, 13–18]. The widely varying numbers are due to differences in age stratifications, methods of case ascertainment, setting of study (e.g., clinic based or national data), ethnic backgrounds, and varying time periods. Rates are grossly higher in aSLE, with incidence and prevalence rates ranging from 0.3 to 23.2 per 100,000 persons and from 20 to 241 per 100,000 persons, respectively [13, 19, 20], influenced by similar factors.

We highlight here two large national American studies using the 2000–2004 national claims data from Medicaid, a US federal-state health program for Americans living in poverty (according to the federal annual income threshold). The studies included an eligible population of 30 million children aged 3 to less than 17 years and 23 million adults. The incidence of cSLE (2.2/100,000 person-years) was 1/10 that of aSLE (23.2/100,000 person-years), while the prevalence of cSLE (9.7/100,000 children) was 1/15 that of aSLE (143.7/100,000 adults) [11, 19]. Some caveats need to be considered in interpreting these results. The Medicaid population has higher proportions of ethnic minorities (especially African Americans and Hispanics) compared to the US population. These populations are known to have increased predilection for SLE and more severe disease manifestations; therefore, the results from these studies are likely biased toward a higher number and more severe cases. Conversely, some of the most severe cases with end-stage renal disease could have been covered under other programs and not captured in the Medicaid databases. Furthermore, the cases in this study were ascertained by administrative billing data, and not all the algorithms used were validated. Overall, there are clear epidemiologic data demonstrating lower incidence and prevalence of cSLE than aSLE, but the magnitude may differ depending on the population studied.

### Sex Predominance

Similar to aSLE, cSLE affects more females than males. The prevalence of female cSLE rises from the first to second decade of life, with the greatest prevalence among girls in the ages 15 to <18 years age group [11]. The most commonly cited ratios are from North America and western European countries where the female to male ratio of cSLE increases from 4:3 in the first decade of life to 4:1 in adolescence [21, 22]. In aSLE, the female to male ratio is 9:1 during the reproductive years which then decreases to 5:1 after 50 years old [23, 24].

This extent of female predominance has been observed in populations across the globe. In a Taiwanese population-based survey ($n$ = 1208), the overall incidence rates were 8.7 and 1.2 per 100,000 population in females and males, respectively [16]. The female to male incidence rate ratio was about 6:1 in the first two decades of life and increased to peak at about 9:1 from 30 to 49 years. Similarly, a large single-center Chinese study ($n$ = 1970) demonstrated a female to male ratio of 4.7:1 in less than 15 years old, 11:1 in ages between 15 and 50, and 5:1 in ages equal or greater than 50 years old [25].

However, this trend was not observed in a large international Latin American inception cohort (Grupo Latino Americano de Estudio del Lupus – GLADEL) with 1214 patients (18.9% cSLE and 81.1% aSLE). The female to male ratios were similar in cSLE (9:1) and aSLE (8.8:1) [4]. One possible reason for this difference compared to studies from Asia and North America is the lower observed incidence of cSLE patients less than 10 years old (7.8% of all cSLE) in this cohort, thereby lowering the numbers of affected males.

Although there is no definitive evidence, the influence of the changing female hormonal milieu likely contributes to the changing female predominance through the lifespan. This is supported by the consistent median age of cSLE diagnosis between 11 and 12 years old coinciding with common times of pubertal change [10]. In animal models of lupus-prone mice, estrogen promotes disease development, and progesterone protects against disease activity [26]. A UK health database case-control study found the use of combined oral contraceptive increased the SLE incidence in a dose-dependent manner [27]. A US prospective study also identified early age at menarche, oral contraceptive use, and use of postmenopausal hormones with increased risk of developing SLE [28].

## *Genetics*

Genetics play an important role in SLE evidenced by an estimated heritability of more than 66% [29], a tenfold increase in concordance rate between monozygotic twins compared to dizygotic twins [30], and familial aggregation [31]. Previous genome-wide association studies have identified approximately 90 SLE risk loci [29]. Human leukocyte antigen (HLA) alleles have also been shown to contribute to genetic risk such as the association of HLA-DRB1*0301 with autoantibody production [32]. A large transancestral genotyping study (European, African, and Hispanic Amerindian ancestry) identified multiple non-HLA regions and the concept of a nonlinear relationship between genetic load (risk allele count) and development of SLE [33].

As most known SLE risk loci to date are derived from European ancestry, association studies will likely exclude loci non-specific to Europeans. One study using data from the Lupus Family Registry and Repository (LFRR) analyzed 19 commonly implicated European-derived SLE risk loci [34]. For each additional risk allele carried, the odds of developing cSLE was 1.5 times in Gullah and 1.25 times in African-American children, but not significantly different in Hispanic or Caucasian children. These data suggest that more risk alleles, i.e., a higher genetic load, have an effect on earlier development and increased disease severity in cSLE.

A Toronto-based study of large multi-racial cohorts of cSLE (36% European, 26% East Asian, 10% African, 9% South Asian, 19% Amerindian/admixed, $n = 572$) and aSLE (59% European, 14% East Asian, 10% African, 5% South Asian, 12% Amerindian/admixed, $n = 665$) assessed the association of genetic risk score and lupus nephritis (LN) risk. They studied genetic risk scores (GRS) weighted by 39 non-HLA and 7 HLA European-based SLE-risk alleles separately [35]. There was a significant association of non-HLA GRS and LN only in European cSLE. In addition, the odds of cSLE patients having LN was 3.5 times greater among those in the highest quartile compared to those in the lowest for GRS [35]. This effect was not seen in European aSLE, but the difference in associations was not significant. Similar findings were found in the HLA GRS.

A rare subset of cSLE, termed "monogenic SLE," occurs when a single gene variant results in SLE disease onset early in life, typically prior to age 5 years. Moreover, an extreme phenotype is frequently observed, and genetic exploration should be considered in these children. Not surprisingly, consanguinity is a significant risk factor for developing monogenic lupus [36]. Whether the same genetic variants seen in monogenic lupus account for a proportion of patients with aSLE remains unknown. Studying the genes of monogenic SLE can provide further insight into the pathogenesis of SLE and also provide potential treatment targets, with more than 30 genes reported to date causing monogenic lupus or lupus-like disease. The main functional categories described include defects in the complement system (e.g., *C1q*), type 1 interferonopathies (e.g., *TREX1* linked to Aicardi-Goutières syndrome, *DNAases* linked to hypocomplemententemic urticarial vasculitis), immune regulatory pathways (e.g., *PRKCD*), and other pathways (e.g., *PTPN11*, *RAG1*) [37].

We have highlighted some studies exploring the link between genetic load and the age of onset of SLE. A higher genetic load and more extreme mutations (monogenic lupus) are associated with earlier disease onset [34, 35, 37]. As our understanding of genetic load expands with more SLE susceptibility loci and genes identified, further genetic studies in SLE patients are needed to examine for their differences in cSLE compared to aSLE.

## *Classification Criteria*

Several classification criteria for SLE currently exist [38–40]. The original American College of Rheumatology (ACR) SLE classification criteria have undergone three revisions in 1982, 1997, and a complete overhaul in conjunction with the European

League Against Rheumatism (EULAR) in 2019 [38, 40, 41]. In 2012, the SLE International Collaboration Clinics (SLICC) developed a classification criterion [39] with increased sensitivity, including a wider array of clinical features especially dermatological manifestations compared to the 1997 ACR criteria. The most significant change for the 2019 EULAR/ACR criteria [40] is the requirement of a positive ANA as an entry criterion, with other SLE manifestations counted using a weighted score.

Although these criteria were developed in aSLE cohorts, they are commonly applied in cSLE studies to identify study cohorts. Only a few small cSLE studies (total $n = 79$) have validated the use of ACR 1997 and SLICC 2012 criteria [42–45]. A single-center cSLE study [45] showed that the sensitivity for ACR 1997 and SLICC 2012 was only 82.5% and 91.3%, respectively, at less than 1 year from diagnosis but increased over time to 100% for both at over 10 years. A recent study compared EULAR/ACR 2019, SLICC 2012, and ACR 1997 in 122 cSLE patients. EULAR/ACR 2019 was found to have comparable sensitivity but less specificity than SLICC 2012 at both diagnosis and 1 year follow-up [46].

A systematic review and meta-analysis compared the performance of SLICC 2012 and ACR 1997 in both cSLE (four studies – Brazil, Argentina, UK, Italy, Turkey) and aSLE (nine studies) [47]. SLICC 2012 has higher sensitivity but lower specificity in cSLE compared to aSLE, and SLICC 2012 classifies cSLE earlier than ACR 1997 in most studies. Overall, it appears that SLICC 2012 is more sensitive, and ACR 1997 is more specific for both aSLE and cSLE. As these classification criteria were developed in aSLE patients and used adults with autoimmune disease as controls, they may not perform as well in cSLE. Further studies in children are needed to compare the performance of EULAR/ACR 2019 criteria against existing criteria. We also stress that using classification criteria as diagnostic criteria has not been adequately validated and is discouraged; cSLE remains a clinical diagnosis.

## *Race*

SLE is more common in patients of non-Caucasian ancestry, including Africans, Hispanics, Asians, and Native Americans [22, 48, 49]. In cSLE, the magnitude of this effect is more evident in certain races when compared to aSLE [11, 19, 50]. Two American studies of the cSLE and aSLE population insured by Medicaid (between 2000 and 2004) demonstrated SLE prevalence rates (compared to Caucasians) of approximately twofold greater in African Americans, 1.5-fold greater in Hispanics, and between 1.2- and 1.5-fold greater in Native Americans. One notable difference between cSLE and aSLE was in the Asian American population, where the prevalence rate was more than threefold greater than Caucasians in cSLE, but closer to 1.5-fold greater in aSLE [11, 19]. Similarly, two other North American cohorts, the LUpus in MInorities: NAture versus nurture (LUMINA) [6] and the 1000 Canadian Faces of Lupus [2, 51] cohorts have demonstrated proportions of up to 88% non-Caucasians, greater than the proportion of non-Caucasians in these geographic locales which ranges from 20% to 65%.

## Race and Disease Manifestations Overall

Do patterns of SLE disease manifestations differ by race? Two studies from The 1000 Faces of Canadian Lupus (a national cohort of both cSLE and aSLE) examined the difference in disease manifestations in the different races [2, 51]. The pediatric cohort (32% Caucasian) [2] analysis demonstrated three clinically distinct clusters: severe (multiorgan involvement, especially renal) in 34%, moderate (predominant hematologic involvement and arthritis) in 41%, and mild (predominant mucocutaneous involvement and arthritis) in 25%. Only 20% of Caucasian patients were in the severe group, while only 16% of Asian and 9% of Black (predominantly Afro-Caribbean) patients had mild disease. The aSLE cohort (62% Caucasian) [51] demonstrated greater renal involvement in Asians and Blacks, compared to Caucasian and Indigenous Canadians. Caucasians had more mucocutaneous features except for discoid rash, while Asians had less arthritis and serositis.

The California Lupus Surveillance Project used multiple sources of health data and included both cSLE ($n$ = 134) and aSLE ($n$ = 590) patients, with 70% non-Caucasian patients [52]. Similar to the Canadian studies, the prevalence of severe organ involvement including renal disease was up to 1.75-fold greater in patients of African, Asian, and Hispanic ethnicities compared to Caucasians [52]. Adjusted analyses showed that non-Caucasian groups (African, Asian/Pacific Islander, Hispanic) had a 2.2- to 4.3-fold increased risks of developing lupus nephritis and thrombocytopenia, and the Asian/Pacific Islander and Hispanic groups (compared to Caucasians) had a 2.5-fold increased risk of developing antiphospholipid syndrome.

## Race, Disease Manifestations, and Age of Onset

The racial distribution of cSLE and aSLE cohorts is often different, even in cohorts derived from similar geographic regions [53], which could introduce significant biases if these cohorts are compared naïvely. These differences may be due to referral biases or to inherent differences in the age of onset in populations of specific ethnicities. Here, we first describe studies comparing cSLE and aSLE manifestations starting with more racially homogeneous populations followed by appropriately adjusted studies in more racially heterogeneous SLE populations.

Three studies of Chinese patients reported rates of renal involvement in 51–58% of cSLE patients [3, 25, 54], which were similar to the rates of 45–65% in aSLE patients [3, 25]. When examined over time and adjusted for multiple comparisons, there were no differences in the prevalence of major organ involvement in cSLE compared to aSLE [3, 25].

In the Latin American GLADEL cohort [4], comprised of 1214 patients (230 cSLE, 984 aSLE) of Mestizo (44%), White (40–42%), and African-Latin American (10–15%) ethnicity, cSLE patients were significantly more likely (OR > 1 or significantly different frequency) to have malar rash, fever, oral ulcers, thrombocytopenia, hemolytic anemia, cerebrovascular accident, and IgM anti-cardiolipin and less likely to experience myalgia, sicca symptoms, cranial nerve involvement, and impaired renal function compared to aSLE. Overall, the frequency of central nervous system manifestations but not of other major organ involvement differed between cSLE and aSLE. Though the racial proportions were similar in the two groups, these results were not from race-adjusted analyses.

Turning to more heterogeneous populations, there are studies from the Canadian national cohort, the International/US-based LFRR, and the California Lupus surveillance study. When adjusted for racial differences, all of the studies suggested increased rates of some manifestations in the cSLE patients, although results were diverse. In the recent Canadian study of 552 aSLE and 276 cSLE race and ethnically diverse patients [55], the only differences in disease features were increased neurologic manifestations (OR 2.04, $p < 0.05$) and a lower rate of lupus anticoagulant positivity (OR 0.54, $p < 0.05$) in cSLE following adjustment for race/ethnicity, disease duration, and geographic location differences between the cohorts.

Another racially heterogeneous study, the LFRR included 111 cSLE and 1206 aSLE patients [34]. Their analyses, adjusted for race, sex, and disease duration, demonstrated greater odds of proteinuria, hemolytic anemia, leucopenia, hemolytic anemia, anti-dsDNA, and malar rash in cSLE compared to aSLE. However, this recruited population was enriched for multiplex SLE pedigrees and had severe disease.

In contrast, the California Lupus Surveillance study ($n$ = 724) [52], which assessed the effect of race/ethnicity while adjusting for age of onset, demonstrated no difference in the risk of developing lupus nephritis, thrombocytopenia, neuropsychiatric disease, or antiphospholipid syndrome between cSLE and aSLE (19–29 years as reference group, no other comparisons to other age groups reported).

In summary, racially homogeneous populations have not demonstrated consistent differences in at least major organ involvement between cSLE and aSLE [3, 25]; however, in racially heterogeneous populations, some studies have found differences in clinical manifestations between cSLE and aSLE, even after adjusting for race/ethnicity [34, 52, 55]. Consideration for methodological issues might explain these differences [34, 55, 56], suggesting that race/ethnicity could be more important than the age of onset as demonstrated in the most recent California Lupus Surveillance study [52].

## Race, SLE Outcomes, and Age of Onset

Is there a difference in SLE outcomes in patients of different races? Is there a difference in cSLE compared to aSLE outcomes, after adjusting for race? Using the same approach as above, we examine the data from racially homogeneous and heterogeneous populations.

Race plays an important role in mortality, a commonly studied outcome. In the USA, SLE is one of the top 10 causes of death (#7) in all females 15–24 years, but one of top 5 in African and Hispanic females in this age group. SLE continues to be one of the top 10 causes of death in young adult African and Hispanic females 25–44 years [57].

Outcomes of three subgroups of SLE [cSLE (<16 years), aSLE (16–50 years), and late-onset SLE (>50 years)] were compared in a single-center study from Hong Kong [3]. Comparing cSLE and aSLE, there were no significant differences in survival and in damage scores as measured by the ACR/SLICC SLE damage index (SDI) at ≥2 years. The GLADEL cohort [4] similarly demonstrated no difference in mortality but found a statistically significant difference in maximum SDI, apparently greater in cSLE, but the medians and interquartile ranges of cSLE and aSLE were no different for maximum SDI.

In the racially heterogeneous Canadian cohort, there was no difference in SDI between cSLE and aSLE, adjusted for race, disease duration, and center [55]. In the USA, the racially heterogeneous Lupus Outcome Study (LOS) cohort analyzed mortality and other SLE disease outcomes in two studies [58, 59]. Of note, the racial composition of cSLE ($n = 90$) and aSLE ($n = 795$) cohorts was different (~50% in cSLE, 30% in aSLE were non-Caucasians), and mean disease duration was significantly longer in cSLE (16.5 years) compared to aSLE (13.4 years). Examining outcomes, more cSLE patients were on dialysis (19% vs 6%) and required renal transplant (12% vs 4%) [58]. cSLE predicted 1.6-fold greater odds of renal involvement in race-adjusted analyses. There was no difference in the proportion with myocardial infarction (MI), but the mean age of cSLE patients at event was younger (32 versus 48 years), and cSLE patients had a 6.8 greater odds of MI. Although adjusted for sex, ethnicity, recruitment source, and age, one must consider that the number of events was very small (7 MI events). Examining mortality [59], there was no difference in the proportion of deaths in the two populations (cSLE 9%, aSLE 7%), though as expected, cSLE patients were younger at time of death. In an adjusted Cox proportional hazards model, cSLE was a predictor for mortality (compared to aSLE); this model was not adjusted for race.

In summary, in racially homogeneous or comparable racial admixture studies, outcomes of damage accrual and mortality between cSLE and aSLE are not different; however, in racially heterogeneous populations, unadjusted for the effects of race and other confounders, some studies suggest worse outcomes in cSLE compared to aSLE. Future studies seeking to answer questions about differences in manifestations or outcomes between cSLE and aSLE in racially heterogeneous populations should employ a statistical modelling approach that allows adjustment and evaluation of the effects of race/ethnicity and other confounders such as disease duration.

## *Medication Use*

The principles of treatment in cSLE and aSLE are similar with the aim to control disease activity while minimizing the impact of therapy. We compare here the use of immunosuppressants in both groups.

Several cohort studies suggest that cSLE patients receive more corticosteroids and more high-dose intravenous pulse methylprednisolone than aSLE patients overall [3, 53, 58]. The study populations have an overrepresentation of racial minorities, who may have more severe disease manifestations in cSLE requiring more corticosteroid use. Pediatric rheumatologists may perceive the disease as being more severe due to the relatively young (pediatric age) patients thus prompting greater use of corticosteroids.

Among non-biologic disease-modifying antirheumatic drugs, no significant difference in hydroxychloroquine use has been found between cSLE and aSLE [6, 18, 53, 58]. There are reports of increased intravenous cyclophosphamide use in cSLE [3, 18, 58]. This reduced use in aSLE could be due to greater and more relevant concerns of cyclophosphamide-induced fertility implications in women of reproductive age. Reported use of mycophenolate mofetil has had a proportionally greater increase in cSLE than in aSLE in recent years [18, 58].

Non-disease factors also affect the choice of medications. Pediatric use of newer drugs often lags behind the adult practice. Drug approvals, access, and financial coverage for medications may depend on jurisdictions or health insurance, thereby influencing prescribing practices. There are often institutional and individual practice differences as well.

Non-adherence is common in SLE [60], but there may be age group-specific reasons. Qualitative studies in cSLE have identified both patient and caregiver non-adherence barriers including disease knowledge deficits, pill burden, forgetfulness, refusal, perceived absence of immediate results, developmentally appropriate decision-making, disruption of family, and caregiver burnout [61, 62]. In aSLE, risk factors for non-adherence include being single, low educational level, presence of other comorbidities, limited comprehension, and pill burden [63].

In summary, although there are some differences between medication use between cSLE and aSLE, these might not all be due to the underlying disease. Instead, the differences are likely a result of non-disease factors such as physician practice patterns, age-appropriate considerations for growth and development and/or fertility, adherence, or financial or psychosocial factors.

## *Growth and Development*

cSLE often occurs during a critical time of growth and development. aSLE patients are expected to have reached final height prior to their diagnosis; therefore, their heights should not be affected by disease activity. The LOS cohort analyzed final height outcomes for 72 cSLE and 494 aSLE patients, age range 18 to 63 years [64]. The mean age of diagnosis for cSLE was 14 ± 3 years and for aSLE was 33 ± 10 years. There was no difference in medication use of corticosteroids and cyclophosphamide between the two groups. cSLE patients were 2.8 cm shorter than their target height (based on mid-parental height), while aSLE patients were 0.6 cm taller than expected

($p < 0.001$). In multivariable linear regression modelling of cSLE, females, sex, race/ethnicity, year of SLE diagnosis, cyclophosphamide, and end-stage renal failure were adjusted for. Substantially reduced height (>2 standard deviations below target height) was more likely in cSLE patients (3.9-fold), those diagnosed between 11 and 13 years (11.2-fold), and patients who received cyclophosphamide (9-fold). These results suggest that greater disease activity as suggested by need for cyclophosphamide, occurring during critical ages of rapid pubertal growth (11–13 years), adversely affects growth and development in cSLE [64].

## Mental Health

Mental health disorders in SLE can be related to SLE itself, taking many forms such as cognitive dysfunction, organic brain syndrome, psychosis, or mood disorders. More commonly, mental health disorders are comorbidities, either extant from before the diagnosis of SLE, developed as an acute reaction to a new devastating diagnosis, or develop later independent of SLE. We found only one small study comparing depression in cSLE and aSLE, but all were young adults (18–45 years) [65]. We review the data in cSLE and aSLE separately first and then examine the risk of depression in the comparative study [65].

Patients with cSLE are known to have higher prevalence of depressive (20–30%) and anxiety symptoms (36%) compared to the general US adolescent population [66, 67]. In a US Medicaid claims study, there was a high prevalence of depression (19%), anxiety (7%), and other psychiatric diagnoses (18%) in cSLE patients. These symptoms may be the consequence of living with a chronic condition, as the prevalence of major depressive disorder is 20–27% for youths with type 1 diabetes, compared to 5–8% in non-diabetic youths [68].

The prevalence of depression in aSLE is greater than in the general adult population (7% in the USA). A systematic review of 17 studies focused on the relationship between SLE and depression found widely varying definitions of the term depression, likely resulting in different estimates. "Depression" was found in 2–60%, "major depression" in 20–47%, and "mood disorders" in 17–27% [69].

The LOS included adults aged 18–45 with both cSLE and aSLE and used the Center for Epidemiological Studies-Depression (CES-D) scale to define patients with depression [65, 70]. Among 546 participants, 47% met criteria for major depression at least once during follow-up, 32% of cSLE, 29% of aSLE. While there was no difference in baseline prevalence of major depression, cSLE (compared to aSLE) participants were 1.7 times more likely to develop major depression over time and 2.2 times more likely to have recurrent depressive episodes [65]. However, the two SLE populations were substantively different; cSLE participants had longer disease duration, were more likely to be recruited from rheumatology offices (in contrast to community practices), and had more severe disease (needed dialysis and transplant). In multivariable longitudinal modelling, cSLE patients were 1.7 times more likely to develop depression over time, independent of sociodemographic factors, education attainment, disease activity, disease duration, and general health statistics (lower physical function, higher BMI, comorbid conditions, or past myocardial infarction or stroke).

In summary, mental health disorders are more frequent in SLE patients compared to the general population and are common in both cSLE and aSLE. There is a suggestion that cSLE (compared to aSLE) may be an independent predictor of depression over time, but the evidence is limited being only available from one study. Screening for and management of mental health disorders are important aspects in caring for patients with SLE. These may be especially challenging in children when screening assessments can be more difficult.

## *Social Outcomes*

Living with a chronic disease may limit one's educational and vocational attainment. It is important to consider these factors together as they are often very much intertwined, and both contribute to an individual's quality of life. cSLE patients are sick during their school years, and this can affect their performance for obvious reasons, while aSLE patients are likely to stop working and less likely to re-enter the workforce if they stopped working [71]. It is not hard to imagine that the nature of the disease with flares in symptoms, involvement of the brain, fatigue, the need for multiple medical care visits, and associated morbidities like fibromyalgia would make sustaining work challenging. However, in cSLE, patients have a longer time to adapt to their disease and have the possibility of choosing their future vocation knowing their health and limitations imposed by SLE. Would cSLE patients then have better work outcomes?

cSLE patients do not perform as well academically compared to their non-diseased peers. One study reported lower parent-rated school competence compared to demographically matched peers with similar neurocognitive function. Poor school competence was also correlated with higher disease activity [72]. A Canadian provincial study from Manitoba showed that children with chronic rheumatic disease, including cSLE, had lower educational performance compared to matched controls, even after adjusting for socioeconomic status and psychiatric comorbidities [73].

The LOS compared longitudinal education and work outcomes of 115 cSLE and 929 aSLE adults. The average age of cSLE patients was younger (29 ± 10 years) compared to aSLE patients (44 ± 9 years). They found no significant difference in completing a bachelor's degree between those with cSLE compared to aSLE, adjusted for sex, age, non-Caucasian ethnicity, rural residence, and geographic regions of residence [74]. In bivariate analysis, the proportion of the two populations that completed at least bachelor's degree was comparable (cSLE 31%, aSLE 41%, $p > 0.05$). However, given that there has been a secular trend of increasing tertiary education in the USA, this might actually be suggesting an underperformance of cSLE adults [75]. This consideration could be mitigated by the fact that

20% of the cSLE patients were still in school at the time of study; however, when these patients were dropped from analysis, there continued to be no difference in educational attainment between cSLE and aSLE. The authors hypothesized that educational programs and accommodations in place to support students with cSLE may have facilitated academic endeavors [74]. Longitudinally, cSLE patients were 38% less likely to be employed than those with aSLE, adjusted for age, sex, non-Caucasian ethnicity, education, interview year, presence of severe disease (dialysis, transplant, disease activity), and physical function [74].

We conclude that SLE affects educational and vocational outcomes, seemingly more in cSLE patients; however, this evidence is limited. Study populations are small and might be biased, such that the true magnitude of effects is unclear and awaits further robust studies.

## Summary

We examined whether cSLE and aSLE are truly different by exploring various aspects of disease including epidemiology, genetics, classification criteria, race, medication use, growth and development, mental health, and social outcomes. A unique aspect of this review is the consideration of the confounding impact of race/ethnicity in influencing observed differences in racially heterogeneous cSLE and aSLE populations.

Lupus is a continuum of disease. There are some non-substantive differences in various aspects of disease and management among cSLE and aSLE patients. On the one hand are those patients with very-early-onset cSLE due to monogenic lupus. Racially homogeneous studies have demonstrated that cSLE and aSLE have few clinical differences. In race-adjusted analyses of racially heterogeneous populations, there are differences in neurological disease but less consistent differences in the frequency of other disease manifestations. The existing classification criteria have comparable utility in both populations. There are some differences in treatment given in cSLE and aSLE, but this could be due to non-disease factors such as practice differences. There is no difference in mortality rates and SDI in properly adjusted analyses, but cSLE patients are more likely to develop depression over time. As cSLE patients are affected during their childhood/adolescence, this can have age-specific impact on their final height and social outcomes.

It has been challenging to address this question of whether cSLE and aSLE are different diseases due to the relative lack of studies that include both populations in the same study for direct comparisons. As we have shown, race is an especially important consideration. We suggest future studies seeking to compare cSLE and aSLE should adjust for the effects of race and other confounders in multivariable models to allow for better understanding (Table 5.1).

**Table 5.1** Summary of comparisons between cSLE and aSLE

| Comparison | | Conclusions |
|---|---|---|
| Incidence | | 10-fold lower in cSLE than aSLE |
| Prevalence | | 15-fold lower in cSLE than aSLE |
| Sex | | Higher male incidence proportionally in cSLE (especially <10 years old) compared to aSLE<br>Female cSLE incidence increases starting in adolescence matching aSLE |
| Genetics | | Monogenic lupus with extreme phenotypes in children less than 5 years old<br>Higher genetic load may be associated with earlier disease onset |
| Classification criteria | | SLICC 2012 has lower specificity for cSLE compared to aSLE<br>EULAR/ACR 2019 remains to be validated in cSLE |
| Race | Homogeneous populations | No significant differences in major organ involvement<br>No significant differences in damage accrual and mortality |
| | Heterogeneous populations | Neurological manifestations and some minor manifestations or serologies may be more frequent in cSLE<br>cSLE patients have worst outcomes in some studies<br>*(Inconsistent findings across studies)* |
| Medication use | | Greater corticosteroid use in cSLE<br>Similar antimalarial use in cSLE and aSLE<br>Different choices of non-steroidal immunosuppressants use may be due to non-disease factors (e.g., practice patterns, fertility, adherence, finance) |
| Mental health | | Higher risk of developing depression and mental health disorders in cSLE compared to aSLE[a] |
| *Unique aspects of cSLE* | | |
| Growth and development | | cSLE patients have reduced final height[a] |
| Social outcomes | | Potentially poorer education attainment and employment in cSLE[a] |

Abbreviations: *ACR* American College of Rheumatology, *EULAR* European League Against Rheumatism, *SLICC* SLE International Collaboration Clinics
[a]Limited data, derived from single studies

# References


1. Levy DM, Peschken CA, Tucker LB, Chedeville G, Huber AM, Pope JE, et al. Influence of ethnicity on childhood-onset systemic lupus erythematosus: results from a multiethnic multi-center Canadian cohort. Arthritis Care Res (Hoboken). 2013;65(1):152–60.
2. Hochberg MC. The incidence of systemic lupus erythematosus in Baltimore, Maryland, 1970-1977. Arthritis Rheum. 1985;28(1):80–6.
3. Mok CC, Mak A, Chu WP, To CH, Wong SN. Long-term survival of southern Chinese patients with systemic lupus erythematosus: a prospective study of all age-groups. Medicine (Baltimore). 2005;84(4):218–24.
4. Ramirez Gomez LA, Uribe Uribe O, Osio Uribe O, Grisales Romero H, Cardiel MH, Wojdyla D, et al. Childhood systemic lupus erythematosus in Latin America. The GLADEL experience in 230 children. Lupus. 2008;17(6):596–604.
5. Font J, Cervera R, Espinosa G, Pallares L, Ramos-Casals M, Jimenez S, et al. Systemic lupus erythematosus (SLE) in childhood: analysis of clinical and immunological findings in 34 patients and comparison with SLE characteristics in adults. Ann Rheum Dis. 1998;57(8):456–9.

6. Tucker LB, Uribe AG, Fernandez M, Vila LM, McGwin G, Apte M, et al. Adolescent onset of lupus results in more aggressive disease and worse outcomes: results of a nested matched case-control study within LUMINA, a multiethnic US cohort (LUMINA LVII). Lupus. 2008;17(4):314–22.
7. Rood MJ, ten Cate R, van Suijlekom-Smit LW, den Ouden EJ, Ouwerkerk FE, Breedveld FC, et al. Childhood-onset systemic lupus erythematosus: clinical presentation and prognosis in 31 patients. Scand J Rheumatol. 1999;28(4):222–6.
8. Pluchinotta FR, Schiavo B, Vittadello F, Martini G, Perilongo G, Zulian F. Distinctive clinical features of pediatric systemic lupus erythematosus in three different age classes. Lupus. 2007;16(8):550–5.
9. Chiang LL, Lin YT, Chan HY, Chiang BL. Differential manifestations of prepubescent, pubescent and postpubescent pediatric patients with systemic lupus erythematosus: a retrospective study of 96 Chinese children and adolescents. Pediatr Rheumatol Online J. 2012;10(1):12.
10. Kamphuis S, Silverman ED. Prevalence and burden of pediatric-onset systemic lupus erythematosus. Nat Rev Rheumatol. 2010;6(9):538–46.
11. Hiraki LT, Feldman CH, Liu J, Alarcon GS, Fischer MA, Winkelmayer WC, et al. Prevalence, incidence, and demographics of systemic lupus erythematosus and lupus nephritis from 2000 to 2004 among children in the US Medicaid beneficiary population. Arthritis Rheum. 2012;64(8):2669–76.
12. Chiu YM, Lai CH. Nationwide population-based epidemiologic study of systemic lupus erythematosus in Taiwan. Lupus. 2010;19(10):1250–5.
13. Rees F, Doherty M, Grainge MJ, Lanyon P, Zhang W. The worldwide incidence and prevalence of systemic lupus erythematosus: a systematic review of epidemiological studies. Rheumatology (Oxford). 2017;56(11):1945–61.
14. Pineles D, Valente A, Warren B, Peterson MG, Lehman TJ, Moorthy LN. Worldwide incidence and prevalence of pediatric onset systemic lupus erythematosus. Lupus. 2011;20(11):1187–92.
15. Al-Arfaj AS, Al-Balla SR, Al-Dalaan AN, Al-Saleh SS, Bahabri SA, Mousa MM, et al. Prevalence of systemic lupus erythematosus in central Saudi Arabia. Saudi Med J. 2002;23(1):87–9.
16. Yeh KW, Yu CH, Chan PC, Horng JT, Huang JL. Burden of systemic lupus erythematosus in Taiwan: a population-based survey. Rheumatol Int. 2013;33(7):1805–11.
17. Dave M, Rankin J, Pearce M, Foster HE. Global prevalence estimates of three chronic musculoskeletal conditions: club foot, juvenile idiopathic arthritis and juvenile systemic lupus erythematosus. Pediatr Rheumatol Online J. 2020;18(1):49.
18. das Chagas Medeiros MM, Bezerra MC, Braga FN, da Justa Feijao MR, Gois AC, Reboucas VC, et al. Clinical and immunological aspects and outcome of a Brazilian cohort of 414 patients with systemic lupus erythematosus (SLE): comparison between childhood-onset, adult-onset, and late-onset SLE. Lupus. 2016;25(4):355–63.
19. Feldman CH, Hiraki LT, Liu J, Fischer MA, Solomon DH, Alarcon GS, et al. Epidemiology and sociodemographics of systemic lupus erythematosus and lupus nephritis among US adults with Medicaid coverage, 2000-2004. Arthritis Rheum. 2013;65(3):753–63.
20. Stojan G, Petri M. Epidemiology of systemic lupus erythematosus: an update. Curr Opin Rheumatol. 2018;30(2):144–50.
21. Hiraki LT, Benseler SM, Tyrrell PN, Hebert D, Harvey E, Silverman ED. Clinical and laboratory characteristics and long-term outcome of pediatric systemic lupus erythematosus: a longitudinal study. J Pediatr. 2008;152(4):550–6.
22. McCarty DJ, Manzi S, Medsger TA Jr, Ramsey-Goldman R, LaPorte RE, Kwoh CK. Incidence of systemic lupus erythematosus. Race and gender differences. Arthritis Rheum. 1995;38(9):1260–70.
23. Mina R, Brunner HI. Update on differences between childhood-onset and adult-onset systemic lupus erythematosus. Arthritis Res Ther. 2013;15(4):218.
24. Tedeschi SK, Bermas B, Costenbader KH. Sexual disparities in the incidence and course of SLE and RA. Clin Immunol. 2013;149(2):211–8.

25. Feng JB, Ni JD, Yao X, Pan HF, Li XP, Xu JH, et al. Gender and age influence on clinical and laboratory features in Chinese patients with systemic lupus erythematosus: 1,790 cases. Rheumatol Int. 2010;30(8):1017–23.
26. Hughes GC, Choubey D. Modulation of autoimmune rheumatic diseases by oestrogen and progesterone. Nat Rev Rheumatol. 2014;10(12):740–51.
27. Bernier MO, Mikaeloff Y, Hudson M, Suissa S. Combined oral contraceptive use and the risk of systemic lupus erythematosus. Arthritis Rheum. 2009;61(4):476–81.
28. Costenbader KH, Feskanich D, Stampfer MJ, Karlson EW. Reproductive and menopausal factors and risk of systemic lupus erythematosus in women. Arthritis Rheum. 2007;56(4):1251–62.
29. Moser KL, Kelly JA, Lessard CJ, Harley JB. Recent insights into the genetic basis of systemic lupus erythematosus. Genes Immun. 2009;10(5):373–9.
30. Deapen D, Escalante A, Weinrib L, Horwitz D, Bachman B, Roy-Burman P, et al. A revised estimate of twin concordance in systemic lupus erythematosus. Arthritis Rheum. 1992;35(3):311–8.
31. Alarcon-Segovia D, Alarcon-Riquelme ME, Cardiel MH, Caeiro F, Massardo L, Villa AR, et al. Familial aggregation of systemic lupus erythematosus, rheumatoid arthritis, and other autoimmune diseases in 1,177 lupus patients from the GLADEL cohort. Arthritis Rheum. 2005;52(4):1138–47.
32. Morris DL, Fernando MM, Taylor KE, Chung SA, Nititham J, Alarcon-Riquelme ME, et al. MHC associations with clinical and autoantibody manifestations in European SLE. Genes Immun. 2014;15(4):210–7.
33. Langefeld CD, Ainsworth HC, Cunninghame Graham DS, Kelly JA, Comeau ME, Marion MC, et al. Transancestral mapping and genetic load in systemic lupus erythematosus. Nat Commun. 2017;8:16021.
34. Webb R, Kelly JA, Somers EC, Hughes T, Kaufman KM, Sanchez E, et al. Early disease onset is predicted by a higher genetic risk for lupus and is associated with a more severe phenotype in lupus patients. Ann Rheum Dis. 2011;70(1):151–6.
35. Webber D, Cao J, Dominguez D, Gladman DD, Levy DM, Ng L, et al. Association of systemic lupus erythematosus (SLE) genetic susceptibility loci with lupus nephritis in childhood-onset and adult-onset SLE. Rheumatology (Oxford). 2020;59(1):90–8.
36. Hiraki LT, Silverman ED. Genomics of systemic lupus erythematosus: insights gained by studying monogenic young-onset systemic lupus erythematosus. Rheum Dis Clin N Am. 2017;43(3):415–34.
37. Demirkaya E, Sahin S, Romano M, Zhou Q, Aksentijevich I. New horizons in the genetic etiology of systemic lupus erythematosus and lupus-like disease: monogenic lupus and beyond. J Clin Med. 2020;9(3):712.
38. Hochberg MC. Updating the American College of Rheumatology revised criteria for the classification of systemic lupus erythematosus. Arthritis Rheum. 1997;40(9):1725.
39. Petri M, Orbai AM, Alarcon GS, Gordon C, Merrill JT, Fortin PR, et al. Derivation and validation of the Systemic Lupus International Collaborating Clinics classification criteria for systemic lupus erythematosus. Arthritis Rheum. 2012;64(8):2677–86.
40. Aringer M, Costenbader K, Daikh D, Brinks R, Mosca M, Ramsey-Goldman R, et al. 2019 European League Against Rheumatism/American College of Rheumatology classification criteria for systemic lupus erythematosus. Arthritis Rheumatol. 2019;71(9):1400–12.
41. Tan EM, Cohen AS, Fries JF, Masi AT, McShane DJ, Rothfield NF, et al. The 1982 revised criteria for the classification of systemic lupus erythematosus. Arthritis Rheum. 1982;25(11):1271–7.
42. Sag E, Tartaglione A, Batu ED, Ravelli A, Khalil SM, Marks SD, et al. Performance of the new SLICC classification criteria in childhood systemic lupus erythematosus: a multicentre study. Clin Exp Rheumatol. 2014;32(3):440–4.
43. Fonseca AR, Gaspar-Elsas MI, Land MG, de Oliveira SK. Comparison between three systems of classification criteria in juvenile systemic lupus erythematous. Rheumatology (Oxford). 2015;54(2):241–7.

44. Lythgoe H, Morgan T, Heaf E, Lloyd O, Al-Abadi E, Armon K, et al. Evaluation of the ACR and SLICC classification criteria in juvenile-onset systemic lupus erythematosus: a longitudinal analysis. Lupus. 2017;26(12):1285–90.
45. Tao JJ, Hiraki LT, Levy DM, Silverman ED. Comparison of sensitivities of American College of Rheumatology and Systemic Lupus International Collaborating Clinics Classification Criteria in childhood-onset systemic lupus erythematosus. J Rheumatol. 2019;46(7):731–8.
46. Rodrigues Fonseca A, Felix Rodrigues MC, Sztajnbok FR, Gerardin Poirot Land M, Knupp Feitosa de Oliveira S. Comparison among ACR1997, SLICC and the new EULAR/ACR classification criteria in childhood-onset systemic lupus erythematosus. Adv Rheumatol. 2019;59(1):20.
47. Hartman EAR, van Royen-Kerkhof A, Jacobs JWG, Welsing PMJ, Fritsch-Stork RDE. Performance of the 2012 Systemic Lupus International Collaborating Clinics classification criteria versus the 1997 American College of Rheumatology classification criteria in adult and juvenile systemic lupus erythematosus. A systematic review and meta-analysis. Autoimmun Rev. 2018;17(3):316–22.
48. Hiraki LT, Benseler SM, Tyrrell PN, Harvey E, Hebert D, Silverman ED. Ethnic differences in pediatric systemic lupus erythematosus. J Rheumatol. 2009;36(11):2539–46.
49. Siegel M, Lee SL. The epidemiology of systemic lupus erythematosus. Semin Arthritis Rheum. 1973;3(1):1–54.
50. Lau CS, Yin G, Mok MY. Ethnic and geographical differences in systemic lupus erythematosus: an overview. Lupus. 2006;15(11):715–9.
51. Peschken CA, Katz SJ, Silverman E, Pope JE, Fortin PR, Pineau C, et al. The 1000 Canadian faces of lupus: determinants of disease outcome in a large multiethnic cohort. J Rheumatol. 2009;36(6):1200–8.
52. Maningding E, Dall'Era M, Trupin L, Murphy LB, Yazdany J. Racial and ethnic differences in the prevalence and time to onset of manifestations of systemic lupus erythematosus: the California Lupus Surveillance Project. Arthritis Care Res (Hoboken). 2020;72(5):622–9.
53. Brunner HI, Gladman DD, Ibanez D, Urowitz MD, Silverman ED. Difference in disease features between childhood-onset and adult-onset systemic lupus erythematosus. Arthritis Rheum. 2008;58(2):556–62.
54. Lee PY, Yeh KW, Yao TC, Lee WI, Lin YJ, Huang JL. The outcome of patients with renal involvement in pediatric-onset systemic lupus erythematosus--a 20-year experience in Asia. Lupus. 2013;22(14):1534–40.
55. Kim H, Levy DM, Silverman ED, Hitchon C, Bernatsky S, Pineau C, et al. A comparison between childhood and adult onset systemic lupus erythematosus adjusted for ethnicity from the 1000 Canadian Faces of Lupus Cohort. Rheumatology (Oxford). 2019:kez006.
56. Rasmussen A, Sevier S, Kelly JA, Glenn SB, Aberle T, Cooney CM, et al. The lupus family registry and repository. Rheumatology (Oxford). 2011;50(1):47–59.
57. Yen EY, Singh RR. Brief report: lupus-an unrecognized leading cause of death in young females: a population-based study using nationwide death certificates, 2000-2015. Arthritis Rheumatol. 2018;70(8):1251–5.
58. Hersh AO, von Scheven E, Yazdany J, Panopalis P, Trupin L, Julian L, et al. Differences in long-term disease activity and treatment of adult patients with childhood- and adult-onset systemic lupus erythematosus. Arthritis Rheum. 2009;61(1):13–20.
59. Hersh AO, Trupin L, Yazdany J, Panopalis P, Julian L, Katz P, et al. Childhood-onset disease as a predictor of mortality in an adult cohort of patients with systemic lupus erythematosus. Arthritis Care Res (Hoboken). 2010;62(8):1152–9.
60. Mehat P, Atiquzzaman M, Esdaile JM, AviNa-Zubieta A, De Vera MA. Medication nonadherence in systemic lupus erythematosus: a systematic review. Arthritis Care Res (Hoboken). 2017;69(11):1706–13.
61. Harry O, Crosby LE, Smith AW, Favier L, Aljaberi N, Ting TV, et al. Self-management and adherence in childhood-onset systemic lupus erythematosus: what are we missing? Lupus. 2019;28(5):642–50.

62. Bugni VM, Ozaki LS, Okamoto KY, Barbosa CM, Hilario MO, Len CA, et al. Factors associated with adherence to treatment in children and adolescents with chronic rheumatic diseases. J Pediatr. 2012;88(6):483–8.
63. Koneru S, Kocharla L, Higgins GC, Ware A, Passo MH, Farhey YD, et al. Adherence to medications in systemic lupus erythematosus. J Clin Rheumatol. 2008;14(4):195–201.
64. Heshin-Bekenstein M, Perl L, Hersh AO, von Scheven E, Yelin E, Trupin L, et al. Final adult height of patients with childhood-onset systemic lupus erythematosus: a cross sectional analysis. Pediatr Rheumatol Online J. 2018;16(1):30.
65. Knight AM, Trupin L, Katz P, Yelin E, Lawson EF. Depression risk in young adults with Juvenile- and adult-onset lupus: twelve years of followup. Arthritis Care Res (Hoboken). 2018;70(3):475–80.
66. Neufeld KSF, Ng L, Danguecan A, Dominguez D, Schachter R, Quilter M, Couture J, Korczak D, Levy D, Hiraki L, Silverman E, Knight A. Depression and anxiety symptoms in childhood-onset systemic lupus erythematosus [abstract]. Arthritis Rheumatol. 2019:71.
67. Knight A, Weiss P, Morales K, Gerdes M, Gutstein A, Vickery M, et al. Depression and anxiety and their association with healthcare utilization in pediatric lupus and mixed connective tissue disease patients: a cross-sectional study. Pediatr Rheumatol Online J. 2014;12:42.
68. Kovacs M, Goldston D, Obrosky DS, Bonar LK. Psychiatric disorders in youths with IDDM: rates and risk factors. Diabetes Care. 1997;20(1):36–44.
69. Palagini L, Mosca M, Tani C, Gemignani A, Mauri M, Bombardieri S. Depression and systemic lupus erythematosus: a systematic review. Lupus. 2013;22(5):409–16.
70. Julian LJ, Gregorich SE, Tonner C, Yazdany J, Trupin L, Criswell LA, et al. Using the Center for Epidemiologic Studies Depression Scale to screen for depression in systemic lupus erythematosus. Arthritis Care Res (Hoboken). 2011;63(6):884–90.
71. Yelin E, Tonner C, Trupin L, Panopalis P, Yazdany J, Julian L, et al. Work loss and work entry among persons with systemic lupus erythematosus: comparisons with a national matched sample. Arthritis Rheum. 2009;61(2):247–58.
72. Zelko F, Beebe D, Baker A, Nelson SM, Ali A, Cedeno A, et al. Academic outcomes in childhood-onset systemic lupus erythematosus. Arthritis Care Res (Hoboken). 2012;64(8):1167–74.
73. Lim SHLM, R.A, Ekuma O, Brownell M, Peschken CA, Hitchon CA, Gerhold K, Lix L. A population based study of high school academic outcomes in individuals with childhood-onset chronic rheumatic diseases in Manitoba, Canada [abstract]. Arthritis Rheumatol. 2018:70.
74. Lawson EF, Hersh AO, Trupin L, von Scheven E, Okumura MJ, Yazdany J, et al. Educational and vocational outcomes of adults with childhood- and adult-onset systemic lupus erythematosus: nine years of followup. Arthritis Care Res (Hoboken). 2014;66(5):717–24.
75. Roser M, Ortiz-Ospina E. Tertiary education 2013 [Available from: https://ourworldindata.org/tertiary-education.

# Chapter 6
# Metrics in Disease Activity Measures in Systemic Lupus Erythematosus

**Konstantinos Tselios, Dafna D. Gladman, and Murray B. Urowitz**

## Introduction

Systemic lupus erythematosus (SLE) is a multisystem autoimmune disease characterized by unpredictable remissions and exacerbations. Disease course varies from prolonged quiescence (after the initial diagnosis) to relapsing-remitting and persistently active disease [1, 2]. Patients with SLE may experience events that are related to disease activity, chronic irreversible damage, as well as drug-related adverse events, all of which impact their quality of life and overall prognosis. Close monitoring of all these aspects and appropriate attribution to the occasional pathogenetic process (disease activity or irreversible damage) is essential for the optimal management of the patients. Therefore, the use of validated and reliable tools is fundamental not only for the daily management but also for standardization purposes in order to promote a common language between investigators and improve the quality of research in the field.

K. Tselios · D. D. Gladman
Centre for Prognosis Studies in the Rheumatic Diseases, University Health Network, Toronto, ON, Canada

M. B. Urowitz (✉)
Centre for Prognosis Studies in the Rheumatic Diseases, University Health Network, Toronto, ON, Canada

University of Toronto Lupus Clinic; Centre for Prognosis Studies in the Rheumatic Diseases, Toronto Western Hospital, Toronto, ON, Canada
e-mail: m.urowitz@utoronto.ca



Z. Touma (ed.), *Outcome Measures and Metrics in Systemic Lupus Erythematosus*, https://doi.org/10.1007/978-3-030-73303-2_6

## Principles for the Assessment of SLE Patients

The assessment of patients with lupus includes the determination of the following domains [3]:

1. Disease activity
2. Chronic damage, resulting either from the disease itself or other factors
3. Adverse events of drugs
4. Health-related quality of life (HRQoL)

To date, there has been no universal agreement regarding the optimal tools to be used for the assessment of these domains. Whether in research or in the clinical care setting, investigators and physicians must identify and choose the most appropriate tools suited to the particular research question or clinical needs. This chapter focuses on describing the available measures to assess disease activity in SLE patients.

## Disease Activity Indices

Disease activity can be defined as the constellation of reversible clinical and/or laboratory features that reflect the immune-mediated and inflammatory manifestations of organ involvement in the context of SLE at a specific point in time [4]. Several measures have been developed and validated to assess disease activity. Appropriate measures must be proven to be reliable and valid as well as sensitive to change. In addition, the practical applicability of the measure includes the ease of administration and method of scoring, an uncomplicated interpretation, as well as the low cost of data collection [5]. Two types of disease activity measures have been developed. Global indices describe the overall burden of active disease, whereas organ-specific indices relate to disease activity within each organ system, either individually or incorporated into one summary score.

### *Global Indices*

#### Systemic Lupus Erythematosus Disease Activity Index and Its Versions

The Systemic Lupus Erythematosus Disease Activity Index (SLEDAI) was introduced in Toronto, Canada, in 1985 [4]. The index was modeled on the clinicians' judgment of global disease activity and developed by a group of rheumatologists and methodologists with expertise in lupus. A consensus-based nominal group process was used to ensure the wide acceptance of the resulting index. An initial literature review identified 37 items (descriptors) that had been used to describe disease activity in lupus, out of which 24 (the most prevalent) were retained. The elimination of the 13 descriptors occurred in the first phase of the development and was based on their low prevalence in SLE. Multiple regression models were used to derive the relative weighted scores for each of the 24 descriptors of 9 organ systems, based on the experts' evaluation of 1400 case scenarios. The definitions of the descriptors were based on the

American College of Rheumatology (ACR) glossary of rheumatic disease terms, and they were further refined throughout the development process [6, 7]. The values obtained from the regression models were used to generate the relative score of each descriptor (ranging from 1 to 8), and the maximum possible score was 105.

The initial validation of the resulting SLEDAI was conducted throughout the primary development phase, and the descriptors were used to evaluate disease activity in the University of Toronto Lupus Clinic cohort. The SLEDAI descriptors were precisely defined in the 10-day period before the patient's assessment. As such, the manifestation must be documented if present (and attributed to SLE) within that period [4]. The remarkable intra- and inter-rater reliability of the index was proven on a set of case scenarios of lupus patients [4]. Its reliability was also shown in a multicenter study in real patients with rheumatologists from four different countries successfully using and interpreting SLEDAI [8]. The index is highly reproducible in routine clinical and research settings and has been demonstrated to be reliable even when used by less experienced physicians (e.g., rheumatology trainees) [9, 10]. SLEDAI has been shown to correlate with other validated measures of disease activity, such as the British Isles Lupus Assessment Group (BILAG) index, the Lupus Activity Index (LAI), and the Systemic Lupus Activity Measure (SLAM) [8, 10, 11]. Moreover, it has been used in both research and clinical settings and as a predictive variable and outcome measure in prognostic studies of SLE [10, 12, 13]. It has also shown high sensitivity to change over time and validity in the assessment of childhood lupus [14–16]. Lupus disease activity, as determined by the SLEDAI, has been associated with mortality and survival in SLE and has been the major determinant of damage accrual [17, 18]. Regarding short-term mortality (within the next six months) in particular, a SLEDAI between 1 and 5 carries a relative risk of 1.28 that increases to 2.34 for a score between 6 and 10, 4.74 for a score between 11 and 19, and 14.1 for a SLEDAI greater or equal to 20 [19].

### Mexican Version of the SLEDAI (Mex-SLEDAI)

The Mex-SLEDAI was developed in Mexico in 1992 in an attempt to reduce the inherent cost in the SLEDAI calculation by eliminating the included laboratory tests [20]. Hence, it excludes the immunologic descriptors (anti-dsDNA antibodies and complements C3/C4). Moreover, certain clinical and laboratory manifestations were added. Fatigue, mononeuritis, and myelitis were clustered in the neurologic disorders, while peritonitis was grouped with serositis. An increase in serum creatinine was added to the renal disorders, whereas hemolysis and lymphopenia were added to the hematologic disorders. Other descriptors were eliminated, mainly lupus headache, visual disturbances, and pyuria. The total number of descriptors in the Mex-SLEDAI was reduced to 10 (from the initial 24 of the SLEDAI). The investigators also modified the definitions for some descriptors. Different weighted scores were assigned to the descriptors of Mex-SLEDAI with a maximum possible score of 32. The Mex-SLEDAI was originally validated during the development process in Spanish-speaking countries [20]. In 2004, the modifications of SLEDAI 2000 (SLEDAI-2K) were incorporated for the first time into the Mex-SLEDAI version and applied to patients of non-Hispanic descent (Mex-SLEDAI-2K) [21]. The Mex-SLEDAI-2K was shown to have convergent validity with the SLEDAI-2K and the revised Systemic Lupus Activity Measure (SLAM-R) as well as moderate correlation ($r = 0.54$) with the Physician's Global Assessment (PGA) [21]. Nevertheless, the sensitivity to change of the Mex-SLEDAI needs to be studied further [20, 21]. The index has not been used extensively in clinical trials and is limited to lupus centers in South America.

### Safety of Estrogens in Lupus Erythematosus National Assessment Trial (SELENA)-SLEDAI

The Safety of Estrogens in Lupus Erythematosus National Assessment Trial (SELENA) proposed a new modification of the SLEDAI to which a composite flare outcome, the SELENA-SLEDAI Flare Index (SFI), was added [22]. Several descriptors were modified in this version. The definition of *seizures* was modified to exclude events that were attributed to previous irreversible central nervous system damage, and the *cerebrovascular accident* was modified to exclude hypertensive causes. These modifications were redundant since both descriptors are scored as present only if the features are attributed to current lupus activity in the original SLEDAI [4]. The descriptor *visual disturbance* was modified to include scleritis and episcleritis. This modification has not been validated since both features do not reflect similar changes included under the *visual disturbances* in the original SLEDAI. In addition, they are usually not severe enough to deserve a score of 8. In the descriptor *cranial nerve disorder*, vertigo due to lupus was added. Vertigo is one of the manifestations of vestibulocochlear cranial nerve involvement and was reflected in the original SLEDAI as one of the manifestations of the *cranial nerve disturbance*. The definitions of *pleurisy* and *pericarditis* were modified by adding the phrase "classic and severe" to ensure the attribution of the descriptors to lupus disease activity. Of note, both SLEDAI and SLEDAI-2K mandate the presence of subjective (e.g., pleuritic or pericardial pain) and objective (e.g., rub, effusion, electrocardiographic or echocardiographic confirmation, or pleural thickening) findings for pleurisy and pericarditis to be scored as present [4, 23]. In the SELENA-SLEDAI, the researchers accepted the presence of either the objective or the subjective findings to score the descriptor as present [22]. Concerning *arthritis*, the SELENA-SLEDAI mandates more than two (three or more) joints to be affected, whereas the SLEDAI-2K defined arthritis as two or more actively inflamed joints as in the definition of lupus arthritis in the ACR glossary of terms [6, 7]. The SELENA-SLEDAI defines *proteinuria* as new onset or recent increase of more than 0.5 grams/24 h as in the original SLEDAI. However, SLEDAI-2K modified proteinuria to be >0.5 grams/24 h [23]. As in the original SLEDAI, the score of the SELENA-SLEDAI may range from 0 to 105 [22, 23].

Despite the modifications in the aforementioned descriptors, the SELENA-SLEDAI appears similar to the SLEDAI-2K. Most importantly, the modifications introduced in the SELENA-SLEDAI have not been validated yet. Thus, the SELENA-SLEDAI version lacks the stringent validation that is essential before the application of a measure in clinical trials or research settings. In general, the SLEDAI-2K can serve as well as the SLEDAI component of the SELENA instrument, which also includes a flare measure. The SELENA-SLEDAI Flare Index is presented in detail in Table 6.1.

**Table 6.1** SELENA-SLEDAI Flare Index

| **Physician's Global Assessment (0 none, 1 mild, 2 moderate, 3 severe) on a visual analogue scale** | | | | |
|---|---|---|---|---|
| (Enter weight in SLEDAI-2K Score column if descriptor is present at the time of the visit or in the preceding 30 days) | | | | |
| **Weight** | **Score** | **Descriptor** | **Definition** | **Flare Index** |
| 8 | | Seizure | Recent onset (last 10 days). Exclude metabolic, infectious, or drug causes *or seizure due to past irreversible CNS damage* | **Mild/moderate flare** |
| 8 | | Psychosis | Altered ability to function in normal activity due to severe disturbance in the perception of reality. Include hallucinations, incoherence, marked loose associations, impoverished thought content, marked illogical thinking, and bizarre, disorganized, or catatonic behavior. Exclude uremia and drug causes | **SLEDAI change 3 or more points**<br>**New/worse**<br>Discoid<br>Photosensitive<br>Profundus<br>Cutaneous vasculitis<br>Bullous lupus<br>Nasopharyngeal ulcers<br>Pleuritis<br>Arthritis<br>Fever (SLE)<br>Increase in prednisone (but not >0.5 mg/kg/day)<br>Added NSAID or Plaquenil (for disease activity)<br>≥1 increase in PGA (but not >2.5) |
| 8 | | Organic brain syndrome | Altered mental function with impaired orientation, memory, or other intellectual function, with rapid-onset and fluctuating clinical features, inability to sustain attention to environment, plus at least 2 of the following: perceptual disturbance, incoherent speech, insomnia or daytime drowsiness, or increased or decreased psychomotor activity. Exclude metabolic, infectious, or drug causes | |
| 8 | | Visual disturbance | Retinal *and eye* changes of SLE. Include cytoid bodies, retinal hemorrhages, serous exudate or hemorrhages in the choroid, or optic neuritis, *scleritis, or episcleritis.* Exclude hypertension, infection, or drug causes | |
| 8 | | Cranial nerve disorder | New onset of sensory or motor neuropathy involving cranial nerves. *Include vertigo due to lupus* | |
| 8 | | Lupus headache | Severe, persistent headache; may be migrainous, but must be nonresponsive to narcotic analgesia | |
| 8 | | CVA | New onset of cerebrovascular accident(s). Exclude arteriosclerosis *or hypertensive causes* | |

(continued)

**Table 6.1** (continued)

| | | | | |
|---|---|---|---|---|
| 8 | | Vasculitis | Ulceration, gangrene, tender finger nodules, periungual infarction, splinter hemorrhages, or biopsy or angiogram proof of vasculitis | |
| 4 | | Arthritis | *>2 joints* with pain and signs of inflammation (i.e., tenderness, swelling, or effusion) | |
| 4 | | Myositis | Proximal muscle aching/ weakness associated with elevated creatine phosphokinase or electromyogram changes or a biopsy showing myositis | **Severe flare** |
| 4 | | Urinary casts | Heme-granular or red blood cell casts | **Change in SLE-DAI > 12 points**<br>**New/worse**<br>CNS-SLE<br>Vasculitis<br>Myositis<br>PLT < 60,000<br>Anemia Hb < 7 g/l or decrease >3 g/l<br>**Requiring:**<br>Double prednisone<br>Hospitalization<br>Prednisone >0.5 mg/kg/day<br>New cytoxan, azathioprine, or methotrexate<br>Hospitalization (SLE)<br>Increase in PGA to >2.5 |
| 4 | | Hematuria | >5 red blood cells/high power field. Exclude stone, infection, or other causes | |
| 4 | | Proteinuria | *New onset or recent increase of more than* 0.5 gram/24 hours | |
| 4 | | Pyuria | >5 white blood cells/high power field. Exclude infection | |
| 2 | | Rash | *Ongoing* inflammatory *lupus* rash | |
| 2 | | Alopecia | *Ongoing* abnormal, patchy, or diffuse loss of hair *due to active lupus* | |
| 2 | | Mucosal ulcers | Oral or nasal ulcerations *due to active lupus* | |
| 2 | | Pleurisy | *Classic and severe* pleuritic chest pain *or* pleural rub or effusion or pleural thickening *due to lupus* | |
| 2 | | Pericarditis | *Classic and severe* pericardial pain, rub, effusion, or electrocardiogram confirmation | |
| 2 | | Low complement | Decrease in CH50, C3, or C4 below the lower limit of normal for testing laboratory | |
| 2 | | Increased DNA binding | *≥25% binding* by Farr assay *or* above normal range for testing laboratory | |
| 1 | | Fever | >38 °C. Exclude infectious cause | |
| 1 | | Thrombocytopenia | <100,000 platelets/× $10^9$/L | |
| 1 | | Leukopenia | <3000 white blood cells/× $10^9$/L, exclude drug causes | |
| Total score | | | | |

The Safety of Estrogens in Lupus Erythematosus–National Assessment Trial and Systemic Lupus Erythematosus Disease Activity Index (SELENA-SLEDAI) Flare Index. From: Petri et al. [22]

## SLEDAI-2000 (SLEDAI-2K)

The SLEDAI-2K was introduced and validated in 2002 [23]. In the glossary of the original SLEDAI, certain descriptors were scored as active only if they were new; thus, persistently active disease would not be captured. This would lead to an apparent improvement that, in fact, was not truly observed. Among the SLEDAI descriptors, *rash*, *alopecia*, and *mucosal ulcers* were scored only if they were new or recurrent and, in the case of proteinuria, if new onset or a recent increase of more than 0.5 grams in 24 hours was present. The SLEDAI-2K was modified to allow the documentation of ongoing disease activity in the descriptors *rash*, *alopecia*, *mucosal ulcers*, and *proteinuria* [23]. Hence, the SLEDAI-2K includes the presence of any inflammatory rash, alopecia, or mucosal ulcers and new, recurrent, or persistent proteinuria greater than 0.5 grams/24 h. As in the original SLEDAI, all the descriptors of the SLEDAI-2K must be attributed to lupus activity [23]. In the validation phase of SLEDAI-2K against SLEDAI, the entire cohort of the University of Toronto Lupus Clinic was used. Of 18,636 visits, 78% of the scores were concordant in SLEDAI-2K and SLEDAI. In the remaining 22% of the visits, the differences were the result of proteinuria, rash, alopecia, and mucosal ulcers. The initial SLEDAI-2K was equivalent to SLEDAI at presentation as a predictor of mortality. Moreover, the SLEDAI-2K described disease activity at different levels comparably to the original SLEDAI. The indices were equivalent in describing changes in disease activity from one visit to the next [23].

## SLEDAI-2K: 30-Day Version

In the original SLEDAI and its 2000 modification, the time frame for the individual components was a 10-day period before the patient assessment [4, 23]. Other major disease activity indices for SLE measure disease activity in the preceding 30 days [24–26]. Moreover, the usual time frame of observations within a clinical trial is 30 days; thus, validating SLEDAI-2K 30 days against SLEDAI-2K 10 days was relevant. The first validation study was conducted on 149 patients who were seen over 9 weeks at the University of Toronto Lupus Clinic. The results showed that SLEDAI-2K 30 days is similar to SLEDAI-2K 10 days in both patients who were in remission and patients with a spectrum of disease activity levels [27]. The second study validated SLEDAI-2K 30 days against SLEDAI-2K 10 days in a group of 41 patients who were followed at monthly intervals for 12 months. These studies confirmed that having a manifestation of active lupus present at 11 to 30 days before a visit and a complete resolution in the 10 days before the visit is unusual. Therefore, the 30-day time frame for SLEDAI-2K was reliable for use in observational studies and clinical trials to describe disease activity in SLE [27, 28].

The SLEDAI-2K can detect only complete resolution of the active descriptors and, thus, cannot reflect a partial improvement in a given disease manifestation. Another pitfall is that the index cannot detect worsening of a previously active descriptor; nevertheless, this particular descriptor will continue to be scored as active (present). Despite the fact that SLEDAI-2K is a global index and generates a total score reflecting overall disease activity, disease activity in each of the nine organ systems can be derived if required for clinical trials. The practical applicability of SLEDAI-2K in clinical settings, its ease of administration, and its simplicity in scoring are fundamental properties. These benefits have enabled SLEDAI-2K to be one of the most widely used global disease activity measures in longitudinal observational studies and clinical trials. The SLEDAI-2K 30 days is shown in detail in Table 6.2.

**Table 6.2** SLEDAI-2K (30 days) data collection sheet

| **Patient Name:** | | | **Visit date:** |
|---|---|---|---|
| (Enter weight in SLEDAI-2K Score column if descriptor is present at the time of the visit or in the preceding 30 days) | | | |
| **Weight** | **Score** | **Descriptor** | **Definition** |
| 8 | | Seizure | Recent onset. Exclude metabolic, infectious or drug causes |
| 8 | | Psychosis | Altered ability to function in normal activity due to severe disturbance in the perception of reality. Include hallucinations, incoherence, marked loose associations, impoverished thought content, marked illogical thinking, or bizarre, disorganized, or catatonic behavior. Exclude uremia and drug causes |
| 8 | | Organic brain syndrome | Altered mental function with impaired orientation, memory, or other intellectual function, with rapid onset and fluctuating clinical features and inability to sustain attention to environment, plus at least two of the following: perceptual disturbance, incoherent speech, insomnia or daytime drowsiness, or increased or decreased psychomotor activity. Exclude metabolic, infectious, or drug causes |
| 8 | | Visual disturbance | Retinal changes of SLE. Include cytoid bodies, retinal hemorrhages, serous exudate or hemorrhages in the choroid, or optic neuritis. Exclude hypertension, infection, or drug causes |
| 8 | | Cranial nerve disorder | New onset of sensory or motor neuropathy involving cranial nerves |
| 8 | | Lupus headache | Severe, persistent headache; may be migrainous, but must be nonresponsive to narcotic analgesia |
| 8 | | CVA | New onset of cerebrovascular accident(s). Exclude arteriosclerosis |
| 8 | | Vasculitis | Ulceration, gangrene, tender finger nodules, periungual infarction, splinter hemorrhages, or biopsy or angiogram proof of vasculitis |
| 4 | | Arthritis | $\geq$2 joints with pain and signs of inflammation (i.e., tenderness, swelling, or effusion) |
| 4 | | Myositis | Proximal muscle aching/weakness associated with elevated creatine phosphokinase/aldolase or electromyogram changes or a biopsy showing myositis |

**Table 6.2** (continued)

| | | | |
|---|---|---|---|
| 4 | | Urinary casts | Heme-granular or red blood cell casts |
| 4 | | Hematuria | >5 red blood cells/high power field. Exclude stone, infection, or other cause |
| 4 | | Proteinuria | >0.5 gram/24 hours |
| 4 | | Pyuria | >5 white blood cells/high power field. Exclude infection |
| 2 | | Rash | Inflammatory type rash |
| 2 | | Alopecia | Abnormal, patchy, or diffuse loss of hair |
| 2 | | Mucosal ulcers | Oral or nasal ulcerations |
| 2 | | Pleurisy | Pleuritic chest pain with pleural rub or effusion or pleural thickening |
| 2 | | Pericarditis | Pericardial pain with at least one of the following: rub, effusion, or electrocardiogram or echocardiogram confirmation |
| 2 | | Low complement | Decrease in CH50, C3, or C4 below the lower limit of normal for testing laboratory |
| 2 | | Increased DNA binding | Increased DNA binding by Farr assay above normal range for testing laboratory |
| 1 | | Fever | >38 °C. Exclude infectious cause |
| 1 | | Thrombocytopenia | <100,000 platelets/× $10^9$/L, exclude drug causes |
| 1 | | Leukopenia | <3000 white blood cells/× $10^9$/L, exclude drug causes |

The Systemic Lupus Erythematosus Disease Activity Index 2000 (SLEDAI-2K). From Gladman et al. [23]

## SLEDAI-2K Glucocorticoid Index (SLEDAI-2KG)

The SLEDAI-2KG is the latest suggested revision of the SLEDAI-2K and incorporates the variable of glucocorticoid dose (prednisone or equivalent) in the traditional SLEDAI-2K [29]. It was developed by the Toronto Lupus Clinic on 150 real patients and based on a quadratic linear regression model to derive the relative weight of the different glucocorticoid doses. Briefly, the daily prednisone dose is weighted and added to the regular SLEDAI-2K score as follows: 0 for prednisone <5 mg/day, 2 for 5–7.5 mg/day, 3 for 10 mg/day, 4 for 12.5–15 mg/day, 5 for 17.5–20 mg/day, 6 for 22.5–27.5 mg/day, 7 for 30–35 mg/day, and 8 for ≥37.5 mg/day. The index was validated in a separate cohort and found to capture 10–16% more responders than the traditional SLEDAI-2K at 6 and 12 months. The advantage of the SLEDAI-2KG is the potential ability to differentiate evolving disease activity within a certain organ/system or the disease as a whole. For example, a patient with thrombocytopenia (and a SLEDAI-2K of 1) may be considered active by the attending physician and treated with 60 mg of prednisone (for a SLEDAI-2KG of 9). On the contrary, a patient with chronic mild thrombocytopenia and no need for glucocorticoid treatment would have had the same SLEDAI-2K (again 1) and a similar score of 1 on SLEDAI-2KG.

## Systemic Lupus Activity Measure (SLAM)

The Systemic Lupus Activity Measure (SLAM) index was introduced in Boston in 1989 to measure global disease activity. It uses disease manifestations derived from the American Rheumatology Association Council on SLE and includes 30 items (23 clinical and 7 laboratory) in 11 organ/systems with a total possible score of 86. The SLAM index assesses global disease activity in the previous month [6, 11, 26]. Most clinical and laboratory items are categorized as present or absent and scored from 0 to 3, based on the severity of the manifestation regardless of the significance of the organ involved [11, 30]. For instance, mild fatigue or oral ulcers are considered to be of the same importance as lupus headache or seizures. A few items can score only 1 or 2, in particular, fatigue, oral ulcers, headache, alopecia, Raynaud's phenomenon, lymphadenopathy, and hepatomegaly or splenomegaly. The revised index (SLAM-R) includes 23 clinical manifestations and the same seven laboratory parameters and has a possible range of 0 to 81 with a score of 7 being considered clinically significant [30]. The definitions of several items were modified. In particular, pleurisy, pericarditis, and pneumonitis were abandoned because of the difficulty in scoring. The definitions and weighting of fatigue, stroke, seizure, and headache were modified. The SLAM-R index does not include immunologic tests as in the SLEDAI-2K. Both SLAM and SLAM-R are reliable and valid in measuring disease activity across patients from different ethnic backgrounds and when compared to other global disease activity measures [8, 11]. Moreover, they capture the patient's global assessment better than the other indices since they include several subjective items that reflect the patients' perception of the disease [31, 32]. The SLAM-R index is also valid for assessing disease activity in childhood [15, 16]. A potential drawback in the SLAM-R index is that it includes subjective items, such as fatigue, shortness of breath, chest pain, abdominal pain, myalgia, and arthralgia, which are then scored based on severity. All these features may as well be attributed to fibromyalgia and not active disease. The assessment of these items has been associated with ambiguity in research settings and clinical trials, and a score of 7 on the SLAM-R index is not unusual for subjective complaints that can be misinterpreted as disease activity. The SLAM-R index is presented in detail in Table 6.3.

## European Consensus Lupus Activity Measurement (ECLAM)

The European Consensus Lupus Activity Measurement (ECLAM) index was developed by the Consensus Study Group of the European Workshop for Rheumatology Research in 1992 [33, 34]. It was based on the analysis of 704 lupus patients from 29 centers in 14 countries. The 15 items of the ECLAM index were derived through univariate logistic regression to reflect the most prevalent clinical and laboratory features of SLE and weighted according to their respective coefficient as

**Table 6.3** SLE Activity Measure R (SLAM-R) (present during last month)

| | | |
|---|---|---|
| **Constitutional**<br>**1. Weight Loss**<br>0 Absent<br>1 ≤ 10% body weight<br>3 > 10% body weight<br>Unknown | **Reticuloendothelial**<br>**11. Lymphadenopathy**<br>0 Absent<br>1 Shotty<br>2 Diffuse or nodes >1 cm × 1.5 cm<br>Unknown | **21. Headache (including migraine equivalents and aseptic meningitis)**<br>0 Absent<br>1 Symptoms only<br>2 Interferes with normal activities/aseptic meningitis<br>Unknown |
| **2. Fatigue**<br>0 Absent<br>1 Little or no limit on normal activity<br>2 Limits normal activity<br>Unknown | **12. Hepato- or splenomegaly**<br>0 Absent<br>1 Palpable only with inspiration<br>2 Palpable without inspiration<br>Unknown | **22. Myalgia/myositis**<br>0 Absent<br>1 Symptoms only<br>2 Limits some activity<br>3 Incapacitating<br>Unknown |
| **3. Fever**<br>0 Absent<br>1 37.5–38.5 °C or 99.5–101.3 °F<br>3 > 38.5 °C or >101.3 °F<br>Unknown | **Pulmonary**<br>**13. Pleurisy/pleural effusion**<br>0 Absent<br>1 Shortness of breath or pleuritic pain<br>2 Shortness of breath or pleuritic pain<br>with exercise<br>3 Shortness of breath or pleuritic pain at rest<br>Unknown | **Joints**<br>**23. Joint pain**<br>0 Absent<br>1 Arthralgia only<br>2 Objective synovitis<br>3 Limits function<br>Not recorded |
| **Integumentary system**<br>**4. Oral/nasal ulcers, periungual erythema, malar rash, photosensitive rash, or nail fold infarct**<br>0 Absent<br>1 Present<br>Unknown | **Cardiovascular**<br>**14. Raynaud's**<br>0 Absent<br>1 Present<br>Unknown | **Laboratory**<br>**24. Hematocrit (mL/dL)**<br>0 > 0.35<br>1 0.30–0.35<br>2 0.25–0.29<br>3 < 0.25<br>Not recorded |
| **5. Alopecia**<br>0 Absent<br>1 Hair loss with trauma<br>2 Alopecia observed<br>Unknown | **15. Hypertension (diastolic pressure, mm Hg)**<br>0 < 90<br>1 90–104<br>2 105–114<br>3 ≥ 115<br>Unknown | **25. White blood cell count (per mm$^3$)**<br>0 > 3.5<br>1 2.0–3.5<br>2 1.0–1.9<br>3 < 1.0<br>Not recorded |
| **6. Erythematous, macular, or papular rash, discoid lupus, lupus profundus, or bullous lesions**<br>0 Absent<br>1 < 20% Total body surface area (TBA)<br>2 20–50% TBA<br>3 > 50% TBA | **16. Pericarditis/carditis**<br>0 Absent<br>2 Positional chest pain or arrhythmia<br>3 Myocarditis with hemodynamic compromise and/or arrhythmia<br>Unknown | **26. Lymphocyte count (per mm$^3$)**<br>0 1.5–4.0<br>1 1.0–1.49<br>2 0.5–0.99<br>3 < 0.5<br>Not recorded |

(continued)

**Table 6.3** (continued)

| | | |
|---|---|---|
| **7. Vasculitis (leucocytoclastic vasculitis, urticaria, palpable purpura, livedo reticularis, ulcer, or panniculitis)**<br>0 Absent<br>1 < 20% TBA<br>2 20–50% TBA<br>3 > 50% TBA<br>Unknown | **Gastrointestinal**<br>**17. Abdominal pain (serositis, pancreatitis, or ischemic bowel, etc.)**<br>0 Absent<br>1 Complaint<br>2 Limiting pain<br>3 Peritoneal signs/ascites<br>Unknown | **27. Platelet count (×1000 per mm$^3$)**<br>0 > 150<br>1 100–150<br>2 50–99<br>3 < 50<br>Not recorded |
| **Eye**<br>**8. Cytoid bodies**<br>0 Absent<br>1 Present<br>3 Visual acuity <20/200<br>Unknown | **Neuromotor**<br>**18. Stroke syndrome (includes mononeuritis multiplex, reversible neurologic deficit (RND), cerebrovascular accident (CVA), or retinal vascular thrombosis)**<br>0 Absent<br>1 RND, mononeuritis multiplex, cranial neuropathy or chorea<br>2 CVA, myelopathy, or retinal vascular occlusion<br>Unknown | **28. ESR (Westergren, mm/hr)**<br>0 < 25<br>1 25–50<br>2 51–75<br>3 > 75<br>Not recorded |
| **9. Hemorrhages (retinal or choroidal) or episcleritis**<br>0 Absent<br>1 Present<br>3 Visual acuity <20/200<br>Unknown | **19. Seizure**<br>0 Absent<br>2 1 or more/month<br>3 Status epilepticus<br>Unknown | **29. Serum creatinine (μmol/L) or creatinine clearance (% normal)**<br>0 44–123 or80–100%<br>1 124–185 or 60–79%<br>2 186–354 or 30–59%<br>3 > 354 or <30%<br>Not recorded |
| **10. Papillitis or pseudotumor cerebri**<br>0 Absent<br>1 Present<br>3 Visual acuity <20/200 or field cut<br>Unknown | **20. Cortical dysfunction**<br>0 Absent<br>1 Mild depression/personality disorder or cognitive deficit<br>2 Change in sensorium, severe depression, or limiting cognitive impairment<br>3 Psychosis, dementia, or coma<br>Unknown | **30. Urine sediment (per hpf)**<br>0 Normal<br>1 6–10 RBC or 6–10 WBC; *or* 0–3 granular or 0–3 non RBC casts; *or* trace to 1+ (on dipstick) (<500 mg/L 24 urine protein)<br>2 11–25 RBC or 11–25 WBC; *or* >3 granular or >3 non RBC casts; *or* 2 to 3+ (on dipstick) (500 mg–3.5 g/L 24 urine protein)<br>3 > 25 RBC or >25 WBC; *or* any RBC casts; *or* 4+ (on dipstick) (>3.5 g/L urine protein)<br>Not recorded |
| | **Total SLAM-R score** | |

The Revised Systemic Lupus Activity Measure (SLAM-R). Bae et al. [30]

determined by multivariate regression analyses. The Physician's Global Assessment was considered the "gold standard" for lupus disease activity for the development of the index. The ECLAM evaluates disease activity over the previous month, and the maximum possible score is 10. It is reliable, valid, and sensitive to change when compared to other indices including the SLEDAI and the British Isles Lupus Assessment Group (BILAG) index [31]. It can also be used to evaluate disease activity retrospectively from the data provided in clinical charts [35]. It has also been validated for the assessment of disease activity in childhood-onset lupus [15]; however, it has not been extensively used in clinical trials. The ECLAM index is presented in detail in Table 6.4.

## *Lupus Activity Index*

The Lupus Activity Index (LAI) was proposed in 1989 to assess the global disease activity over the previous 2 weeks [10]. The LAI includes five sections, eight organ systems, and three laboratory measures. It incorporates the Physician's Global Assessment (PGA) as well as treatment with glucocorticoids and immunosuppressive drugs. The severity of the disease is based on the physician's judgment. The

**Table 6.4** European Consensus Lupus Activity Measurement (ECLAM)

| | | |
|---|---|---|
| **Generalized manifestations** | Fever, fatigue | 0.5 |
| **Articular manifestations** | Arthritis, evolving arthralgia | 1 |
| **Active mucocutaneous manifestations** | Malar rash, generalized rash, discoid rash, skin vasculitis, oral ulcers | 0.5 |
| **Evolving mucocutaneous** | | 1 |
| **Myositis*** | | 2 |
| **Pericarditis** | | 1 |
| **Intestinal manifestations** | Intestinal vasculitis, sterile peritonitis | 2 |
| **Pulmonary manifestations** | Pleurisy, pneumonitis, ingravescent dyspnea | 1 |
| **Evolving neuropsychiatric manifestations*** | Headache/migraine, seizures, stroke, organic brain disease, psychosis | 2 |
| **Renal manifestations*** | Proteinuria, urinary casts, hematuria, raised serum creatinine, or reduced creatinine clearance* | 0.5 |
| **Evolving renal manifestations** | | |
| **Hematologic features** | Non-hemolytic anemia, hemolytic anemia*, leukopenia (or lymphopenia), thrombocytopenia | 1 |
| **Erythrocyte sedimentation rate** | Raised ESR | 1 |
| **Hypocomplementemia** | C3, CH50 | 1 |
| **Evolving hypocomplementemia** | | 1 |

**The European Consensus Lupus Activity Measurement (ECLAM) index.** From: Vitali C, Bencivelli W, Isenberg DA, et al.: Disease activity in systemic lupus erythematosus: report of the Consensus Study Group of the European Workshop for Rheumatology Research. II. Identification of the variables indicative of disease activity and their use in the development of an activity score. The European Consensus Study Group for Disease Activity in SLE. Clin Exp Rheumatol 1992; 10(5): 541–7

(continued)

**Table 6.4** (continued)

| |
|---|
| **Final score** |
| If any of the above mucocutaneous manifestations are new or have worsened since the last observation, add 1 point |
| If this system (or manifestation) is the only involvement present from among items 1–10, add 2 more points |
| Excluding patients with end-stage chronic renal disease |
| If the final total score is not an integer number, round off to the lower integer for values <6 and to the higher integer for values >6 |
| If the final score is >10, round off to 10 |
| **1. Generalized manifestations** |
| Fever = Documented basal morning temperatures of 37.5 °C not due to an infective process |
| Fatigue = A subjective feeling of extraordinary tiredness |
| **2. Articular manifestations** |
| Arthritis = non-erosive arthritis involving at least two peripheral joints (wrist, metacarpophalangeal or proximal, interphalangeal joints) |
| Evolving arthralgia = new onset or worsening of specific localized pain without objective symptoms in at least two peripheral joints |
| **3a. Active mucocutaneous manifestations** |
| Malar rash = fixed erythema, flat or raised over the malar eminences, and tending to spare the nasolabial folds |
| Generalized rash = a maculo-papular rash not induced by drugs, that may be located anywhere on the body, and that is not strictly dependent on sun exposure |
| Discoid rash = erythematosus, raised patches with adherent keratotic scaling and follicular plugging |
| Skin vasculitis = including digital ulcers, purpura, urticaria, and bullous lesions |
| Oral ulcers = oral or nasopharyngeal ulcers, usually painless, observed by a physician |
| **3b. Evolving mucocutaneous** |
| If any of the above mucocutaneous manifestations are new or have worsened since the last observation, add 1 point |
| **4. Myositis*** |
| Confirmed by raised muscle enzymes and/or EMG examination and/or histology |
| **5. Pericarditis** |
| Documented by ECG or rub or evidence of pericardial effusion on ultrasound |
| **6. Intestinal manifestations** |
| Intestinal vasculitis = evidence of acute intestinal vasculitis |
| Sterile peritonitis = evidence of abdominal effusion in the absence of infective processes |
| **7. Pulmonary manifestations** |
| Pleurisy = clinical or radiological evidence of pleural effusion in the absence of infective processes |
| Pneumonitis = single or multiple lung opacities on chest X-ray thought to reflect active disease not due to an infective process |
| Ingravescent dyspnea = due to an evolving interstitial involvement |
| **8. Evolving neuropsychiatric manifestations** |
| New appearance or worsening of any of the following: |
| Headache/migraine = recently developed, persistent or recurrent. Poorly responsive to the most commonly used drugs, but partially or totally responsive to corticosteroids |
| Seizures = grand mal or petit mal seizures, Jacksonian fits, temporal lobe seizures, or choreic syndrome, in the absence of offending drugs or known metabolic derangements (e.g., uremia, ketoacidosis or electrolyte imbalance) |
| Stroke = cerebral infarction or hemorrhage, instrumentally confirmed |
| Organic brain disease = impairment of memory, orientation, perception, and ability to calculate |
| Psychosis = dissociative features in the absence of offending drugs or known metabolic derangements, e.g., uremia, ketoacidosis, or electrolyte imbalance |
| **9a. Renal manifestations** |
| Proteinuria = at least 500 mg/day |
| Urinary casts = red cells, hemoglobin, granular, tubular or mixed casts |
| Hematuria = microscopic or macroscopic |
| Raised serum creatinine or reduced creatinine clearance |
| **10. Hematologic features** |
| Non-hemolytic anemia = Coombs-negative normocytic hypochromic or normochromic anemia without reticulocytosis |
| Hemolytic anemia* = Coombs-positive hemolytic anemia, with reticulocytosis and elevated LDH, in the absence of offending drugs |
| Leukopenia (or lymphopenia) = less than 3500/mm3 WBC (or 1500/mm3 lymphocytes) in the absence of offending drugs Thrombocytopenia = less than 100,000/mm3 in the absence of offending drugs |
| **11. Erythrocyte sedimentation rate** |
| Raised ESR >25 mm/h by Westergren or comparable methods, not due to other concomitant pathological process |
| **12a. Hypocomplementemia** |
| Reduced plasma level of any of the following: |
| C3 by radial immunodiffusion or laser nephelometer |
| CH50 by standardized hemolytic methods |
| **12b. Evolving hypocomplementemia** |
| Significantly reduced level of any of the items mentioned above (plus C4) with respect to the last |

overall score reflects the mean of the PGA, physician's judgment of the severity of each clinical manifestation, degree of laboratory abnormalities, and treatment. Its total score can range from 0 to 3 [10]. Its validity was demonstrated in a study of 150 patients in which the correlation of the LAI was modified (M-LAI) so as not to contain the PGA and was scored at 0.64. The index has performed relatively well in assessing disease activity when compared to other disease activity measures and has been sensitive to change; nonetheless, its use has been limited [31].

## *SLE Activity Index Score*

The SLE activity Index Score (SIS) is a global index developed by clinicians at the National Institutes of Health (NIH). It includes 17 items that comprise both clinical manifestations and subjective features reflecting the perception of the patients (fatigue, arthralgia, myalgia) as well as laboratory items. Its score may range from 0 to 52. The SIS evaluates disease activity over the previous week into inactive, mildly active, moderately active, active, and very active disease. It has been used in both clinical trials and research settings [34, 36]. The validity of the SIS has been demonstrated against other disease activity indices, in particular, the SLEDAI, SLAM, and BILAG. In this study, all four indices were closely correlated with each other ($r = 0.86$ between SIS and SLAM); nevertheless, it has not been used as extensively as the SLEDAI or the BILAG [34, 37]. The index is presented in detail in Table 6.5.

**Table 6.5** SLE Activity Index Score (SIS)

| Clinical variables | | Laboratory variables | |
|---|---|---|---|
| Fatigue | 1 | ESR 25–50 mm/h | 1 |
| Temperature >38 °C | 1 | ESR >50 mm/h | 2 |
| Arthralgia | 1 | DNA binding <50% | 1 |
| Arthritis (joint effusion) | 1 | DNA binding ≥50% | 2 |
| Myalgia | 1 | Mild hypocomplementemia (CH50 80–150 U/ml) | 1 |
| Muscle weakness | 2 | Severe hypocomplementemia (CH50 < 80 U/ml) | 2 |
| Serositis (pain) | 1 | CPK >100, aldolase >10 U/ml | 2 |
| Serositis (friction rub/X-ray/sonography) | 2 | Lupus Anticoagulant | 1 |
| Vasculitis (minor*) | 1 | Proteinuria <1.5 g/24 h | 1 |
| Vasculitis (major*) | 3 | Proteinuria >1.5 g/24 h | 2 |
| Bullous skin lesions | 3 | 5–15 RBC or 1–3 casts/HPF | 1 |
| Active SLE rash | 1 | >15 RBC or >3 casts/HPF | 2 |
| Active alopecia | 1 | Hemolytic anemia (>8 g Hb) | 1 |
| Mucosal ulcers | 1 | Hemolytic anemia (<8 g Hb) | 2 |
| CNS (minor*) | 2 | Thrombocytopenia (40–100,000/mm$^3$) | 1 |
| CNS (major*) | 3 | Thrombocytopenia (<40,000/mm$^3$) | 2 |

(continued)

**Table 6.5** (continued)

| Clinical variables | | Laboratory variables | |
|---|---|---|---|
| Cranial nerve palsy | 2 | Neutropenia (<3000/mm$^3$) | 1 |
| Blood pressure >150/90 mmHg | 1 | Lymphopenia (<1000/mm$^3$) | 1 |
| Lymphadenopathy | 1 | | |
| Non-infectious lung infiltrates | 3 | | |
| Active thromboembolic event | 1 | | |
| Maximum score | 33 | Maximum score | 19 |
| Total SIS (maximum: 52) | | | |

**The SLE activity index score (SIS).** From: Smolen JS. Clinical and serological features: incidence and diagnostic approach. In: Smolen JS, Zielinski CC (Eds): Systemic Lupus Erythematosus: clinical and experimental aspects. Germany 1987, Springer-Verlag: Berlin/Heidelberg, pp. 170–196

**Physician's assessment of disease activity (0–100 mm scale from none to most severe activity)**

**Categories of SIS**

SIS 0–4: Inactive disease
SIS 5–8: Mildly active disease (+)
SIS 9–12: Moderate activity (++)
SIS 13–15: Active disease (+++)
SIS >15: Very active disease (++++)

**Minor vasculitis:** Raynaud's phenomenon, periungual infarcts, purpura
**Major vasculitis:** ulcerations, cystoid bodies, mononeuritis
**CNS minor:** confusion, depression, organic brain syndrome
**CNS major:** stupor, coma, seizures, CVA
**Hypocomplementemia:** consider possibility of inborn C4 deficiency
Usually there will be no very active manifestations in vital organs without concomitant involvement of other organ systems and/or abnormal laboratory findings

## *British Isles Lupus Assessment Group (BILAG) Index*

The BILAG index was developed in the United Kingdom and Ireland in 1988 using a nominal consensus approach [38]. It is based on the principle of the physician's intention to treat. BILAG comprises 86 items including clinical signs, symptoms, and laboratory variables in eight organ/systems. The items recorded must have been attributed to active lupus and present during the 4 weeks before the assessment [38]. Based on the presence of certain features, each system is categorized into one of four levels as follows: A for action, B for beware, C for content, and D for discount [24]. The BILAG was shown to have good inter-rater reliability and be valid when compared to the "gold standard" criterion (i.e., starting or increasing disease-modifying therapy) [24]. Further validation of the BILAG showed that disease activity in different systems does not follow a common pattern in SLE [39]. This study recommended the use of the individual BILAG components rather than the total score as a primary endpoint in clinical and epidemiologic studies [39]. Its sensitivity to change over time was proven in a study of 23 patients who were prospectively followed every 2 weeks for up to 40 weeks, with a standardized response means of 0.57 [31]. The index was reliable and valid in several studies conducted by the BILAG group and other investigators and has correlated well with other disease activity measures, in particular, the SLEDAI and the SLAM indices [11, 14, 15, 24, 31, 39, 40]. It was also adapted and validated in the assessment of SLE in children [15]. It has been successfully used in clinical trials and research settings and has been particularly effective for demonstrating new organ flares [8, 15, 40–44].

The classic BILAG index has undergone a series of revisions to the current BILAG-2004 [11, 24, 38]. The BILAG-2004 index included further changes in some organs/systems, refinements in the definitions of certain descriptors such as the central nervous system manifestations, the removal of items attributed to damage rather than activity such as avascular necrosis and tendon contracture, as well as modifications in the glossary and scoring [44]. As in the classic index, the BILAG-2004 is based on the physician's intention to treat. The index contains 97 items, whereas the classic BILAG index had only 86. The descriptor *vasculitis* was removed, and its items were included in other systems. The *gastrointestinal* and *ophthalmic* systems were added [44]. In the classic BILAG index, all items that are improving can only contribute to a C score, which does not reflect the appropriate level of disease activity for more severe manifestations. In the BILAG-2004 index, features that contribute to an A score when recorded as being the same, worse, or new will contribute to a B score when improving [44].

A complete history and physical examination are required to determine disease activity and attribution of each clinical or laboratory manifestation by the BILAG-2004. The index generates a score for each of the nine systems assessed. The scoring of lupus activity in each system is graded with A through E (for organ/systems that were never affected during disease course), based on the assessment of the clinical features and/or the laboratory findings for the occasional organ/system. Like the classic BILAG index, the BILAG-2004 is a transitional index that is able to capture changing severity of clinical manifestations. The items in each system are rated using a scale from 0 to 4 (0 = not present, 1 = improving, 2 = same, 3 = worse, and 4 = new), and some items are scored as present or absent, reflecting disease activity over the last four weeks. The classic BILAG index and its versions, including the BILAG-2004 index, are ordinal scale indices, and an additive numerical scoring scheme for the BILAG-2004 index is available (A grade = 12 points, B = 8, C = 1, D = 0, and E = 0) [45]. This scoring system is mainly adopted in studies in which the BILAG-2004 index needs to be compared with other numerical indices or to facilitate the statistical analysis, if required; however, the BILAG-2004 index was not designed to be used in this way [44, 45]. The British Lupus Integrated Prospective System (BLIPS) is a computerized program that calculates the BILAG scores with the option to derive the SLEDAI, the SLAM-R index, the Systemic Lupus International Collaborating Clinics (SLICC)/ACR Damage Index, and the Medical Outcomes Study (MOS) Short-Form 36 (SF-36) [46]. BLIPS has also undergone refinement to reflect the BILAG-2004 index, and several amendments were made to the other activity indices [44, 46].

The BILAG-2004 index has shown a good reliability and high levels of physician agreement in almost all systems [44]. Its reliability was evaluated in a large study involving 11 centers across the United Kingdom with the participation of 14 raters and 97 patients. This study showed that the BILAG-2004 is a reliable index to assess SLE activity and recommended the training of raters to ensure its optimal performance [47]. More recently, the construct validity of the BILAG-2004 index was confirmed by its association with the erythrocyte sedimentation rate (ESR), C3/C4 levels, anti-double-stranded DNA (anti-dsDNA) titers, and the SLEDAI-2K index [48]. The criterion validity of BILAG-2004, defined as change in therapy, was confirmed by the association between the BILAG-2004 index and the increase in therapy [48]. In this study, higher SLEDAI-2K scores were significantly associated with overall BILAG-2004 scores reflecting higher disease activity. Although the BILAG index has been extensively used in clinical trials, its routine use in long-term studies has some drawbacks, in particular, the practical applicability, the complicated glossary of the clinical features, and the scoring analysis. The BILAG-2004 is presented in detail in Table 6.6. The numerical scoring for the BILAG-2004 index is shown in Table 6.7.

**Table 6.6** BILAG-2004

Only record manifestations/items due to SLE disease activity
Assessment refers to manifestations occurring in the last 4 weeks (compared with the previous 4 weeks)
To be used with the glossary

Record: N/A not available, 0 not present, 1 improving, 2 same, 3 worse, 4 new

| | Yes/no | | Yes/no |
|---|---|---|---|
| **Constitutional** | | 49. Pleural effusion with dyspnea | |
| 1. Pyrexia – documented >37.5 °C | | 50. Pulmonary hemorrhage/ vasculitis | |
| 2. Weight loss – unintentional >5% | | 51. Interstitial alveolitis/pneumonitis | |
| 3. Lymphadenopathy/splenomegaly | | 52. Shrinking lung syndrome | |
| **Mucocutaneous** | | 53. Aortitis | |
| 4. Skin eruption – severe | | 54. Coronary vasculitis | |
| 5. Skin eruption – mild | | **GASTROINTESTINAL** | |
| 6. Angio-oedema – severe | | 55. Lupus peritonitis | |
| 7. Angio-oedema – mild | | 56. Abdominal serositis or ascites | |
| 8. Mucosal ulceration – severe | | 57. Lupus enteritis/colitis | |
| 9. Mucosal ulceration – mild | | 58. Malabsorption | |
| 10. Panniculitis/bullous lupus – severe | | 59. Protein-losing enteropathy | |
| 11. Panniculitis/bullous lupus – mild | | 60. Intestinal pseudo-obstruction | |
| 12. Major cutaneous vasculitis/ thrombosis | | 61. Lupus hepatitis | |
| 13. Digital infarcts or nodular vasculitis | | 62. Acute lupus cholecystitis | |
| 14. Alopecia – severe | | 63. Acute lupus pancreatitis | |
| 15. Alopecia – mild | | **Ophthalmic** | |
| 16. Periungual erythema/chilblains | | 64. Orbital inflammation/myositis/ proptosis | |
| 17. Splinter hemorrhages | | 65. Keratitis – severe | |
| **Neuropsychiatric** | | 66. Keratitis – mild | |
| 18. Aseptic meningitis | | 67. Anterior uveitis | |

**Table 6.6** (continued)

| | | | |
|---|---|---|---|
| 19. Cerebral vasculitis | | 68. Posterior uveitis/retinal vasculitis – severe | |
| 20. Demyelinating syndrome | | 69. Posterior uveitis/retinal vasculitis – mild | |
| 21. Myelopathy | | 70. Episcleritis | |
| 22. Acute confusional state | | 71. Scleritis – severe | |
| 23. Psychosis | | 72. Scleritis – mild | |
| 24. Acute inflammatory demyelinating polyradiculoneuropathy | | 73. Retinal/choroidal vaso-occlusive disease | |
| 25. Mononeuropathy (single/multiplex) | | 74. Isolated cotton-wool spots (cytoid bodies) | |
| 26. Cranial neuropathy | | 75. Optic neuritis | |
| 27. Plexopathy | | 76. Anterior ischemic optic neuropathy | |
| 28. Polyneuropathy | | **Renal** | |
| 29. Seizure disorder | | 77. Systolic blood pressure (mmHg) | |
| 30. Status epilepticus | | 78. Diastolic blood pressure (mmHg) | |
| 31. Cerebrovascular disease (not due to vasculitis) | | 79. Accelerated hypertension | Value |
| 32. Cognitive dysfunction | | 80. Urine dipstick protein (+ = 1, ++ = 2, +++ = 3) | Value |
| 33. Movement disorder | | 81. Urine albumin-creatinine ratio (mg/mg) | |
| 34. Autonomic disorder | | 82. Urine protein-creatinine ratio (mg/mg) | Value |
| 35. Cerebellar ataxia (isolated) | | 83. 24-hour urine protein (g) | Value |
| 36. Lupus headache – severe unremitting | | 84. Nephrotic syndrome | Value |
| 37. Headache from intracranial hypertension | | 85. Creatinine (plasma/serum) | Value |
| **Musculoskeletal** | | 86. GFR (calculated, in mL/min/1.73 m$^2$) | |
| 38. Myositis – severe | | 87. Active urinary sediment | Value |
| 39. Myositis – mild | | **Hematological** | **Value** |
| 40. Arthritis (severe) | | 88. Hemoglobin (g/dL) | |
| 41. Arthritis (moderate)/tendonitis/tenosynovitis | | 89. Total white cell count (×10$^9$/L) | |
| 42. Arthritis (mild)/arthralgia/myalgia | | 90. Neutrophils (×10$^9$/L) | |
| **Cardiorespiratory** | | 91. Lymphocytes (×10$^9$/L) | |
| 43. Myocarditis – mild | | 92. Platelets (×10$^9$/L) | |
| 44. Myocarditis/endocarditis + cardiac failure | | 93. TTP | |
| 45. Arrhythmia | | 94. Evidence of active hemolysis | |
| 46. New valvular dysfunction | | 95. Coombs test positive (isolated) | |
| 47. Pleurisy/pericarditis | | | |
| 48. Cardiac tamponade | | | |

The British Isles Lupus Assessment Group (BILAG) 2004 index. From Isenberg et al. [44]

**Table 6.7** Scoring of disease activity of the BILAG-2004 based on the principle of physician's intention to treat

| Scoring by grade | Disease severity | Numerical scores | Assumption about the treatment for each grade |
|---|---|---|---|
| **A = Active** | Severe | 12 | Severe disease activity requiring any of the following treatment:<br>1. Systemic high-dose oral glucocorticoids (equivalent to prednisolone >20 mg/day)<br>2. Intravenous pulse glucocorticoids (equivalent to pulse methylprednisolone 500 mg)<br>3. Systemic immunomodulators (include biologicals, immunoglobulins, and plasmapheresis)<br>4. Therapeutic high-dose anticoagulation in the presence of high-dose steroids or immunomodulators, e.g., warfarin with target INR 3-4 |
| **B = Beware** | Moderate | 8 | Moderate disease activity requiring any of the following treatment:<br>1. Systemic low-dose oral glucocorticoids (equivalent to prednisolone 20 mg/day)<br>2. Intramuscular or intra-articular or soft tissue glucocorticoids injection (equivalent to methylprednisolone <500 mg)<br>3. Topical glucocorticoids<br>4. Topical immunomodulators<br>5. Antimalarials or thalidomide or prasterone or acitretin<br>6. Symptomatic therapy, e.g., NSAIDs for inflammatory arthritis |
| **C = Contentment** | Mild | 1 | Patient requires symptomatic treatment (e.g., analgesics or NSAIDs) |
| **D = Discount** | Inactive but previously affected | 0 | Not applicable |
| **E = No Evidence** | Inactive with no previous involvement | 0 | Not applicable |

Scoring of the British Isles Lupus Assessment Group (BILAG) index. From: Yee et al. [45]

All the aforementioned indices have been extensively used for both clinical trials and observational studies. A literature search of the PubMed database (dated 09 December 2019) with the indices mandated to appear in the title and/or abstract of the paper revealed the following: SLEDAI has been mentioned in 2238 articles, BILAG in 265, SLAM in 247, ECLAM in 152, SELENA-SLEDAI in 133, Mex-SLEDAI in 55, LAI in 28, and SIS in 13.

# Organ-Specific Indices

## *Renal Outcome Measures*

Several renal composite outcome measures have been proposed and adopted in the assessment of lupus nephritis for both clinical trials and observational studies. These measures mostly include the quantitative changes in the urinary sediment (e.g., hematuria, pyuria, cellular casts), proteinuria (e.g., 24-hour urine protein, 24-hour urine protein/creatinine ratio, spot urine protein/creatinine ratio, spot urine albumin/creatinine ratio), and renal function (e.g., serum creatinine and estimated glomerular filtration rate, eGFR). The patient's response is usually defined as improvement (complete or partial response) or no response [49, 50]. The incidence of renal flares and the time to the next flare have also been used as outcome measures in clinical trials. Moreover, histologic features have been considered to assess renal response in lupus nephritis trials whenever feasible [50]. The most widely accepted definition of complete renal response is the reduction of proteinuria to a level of <0.5 g/24 h along with no significant change in serum creatinine (<10–20% of the baseline value). Partial response is defined as a 50% reduction in proteinuria (based on the initial protein excretion) with no significant change in serum creatinine (<10–20% of the baseline value) [50].

In an effort to standardize the assessment of lupus nephritis and achieve optimal detection of the renal response in clinical trials, the members of the SLICC group in collaboration with nephrologists developed a measure of renal activity in SLE [51]. The measure was then used to develop an SLE renal response index [51]. The renal activity score was computed as follows: proteinuria 0.5 to 1 g/day (3 points), proteinuria >1 to 3 g/day (5 points), proteinuria >3 g/day (11 points), urine red blood cell count >10/high-power field (HPF) (3 points), and urine white blood cell count >10/HPF (1 point). A reasonable agreement was reached among physician ratings in a pilot study. Nevertheless, the developers of the index suggested further refinement, testing, and validation [51].

## *Cutaneous Lupus Erythematosus Disease Area and Severity Index*

The Cutaneous Lupus Erythematosus Disease Area and Severity Index (CLASI) was developed to facilitate the quantification of disease activity and damage of cutaneous lupus erythematosus in 2005 [52]. The index has separate scores for damage and activity of skin manifestations. Activity is graded as a summary score of erythema, scaling, and hypertrophy of the skin, mucous membrane lesions, and non-scarring recent alopecia. Damage is scored in terms of dyspigmentation or scarring that also includes scarring alopecia. Patients' subjective symptoms (pruritus, pain, fatigue) are recorded separately on 0–100 mm visual analog scales. The total possible score for activity and damage is 70 and 56, respectively. The CLASI has good content validity as well as inter- and intra-rater reliability when used by dermatologists. A study conducted on patients with cutaneous lupus assessed by academic rheumatologists and dermatologists showed superior results with dermatologists in the use of the CLASI. It was recommended that rheumatologists may benefit from incorporating input from dermatologists for the use of the index [53]. The revised CLASI (R-CLASI) was proposed to describe accurately all types of cutaneous lupus [54]. This is an expanded version of the original index, in which the accuracy of the description of the existing parameters was increased (scaling, hypertrophy, dyspigmentation). In parallel, new parameters were added such as edema, infiltration, subcutaneous nodules, and plaque [54]. Its validity and reliability were proven only among dermatologists [54]. Hence, the CLASI and its revision require further validation and assessment among rheumatologists before being adopted in clinical trials for SLE.

## Measures of Disease Activity over Time

### *Adjusted Mean SLEDAI-2K*

SLEDAI-2K assesses disease activity at a single point in time [23]. To summarize disease activity over time, the Adjusted Mean SLEDAI-2K (AMS) was developed. The AMS calculates the area under the curve of SLEDAI-2K divided by the length of the time interval [55]. It has been used as a predictor of major outcomes in lupus, including mortality, damage, and atherosclerotic vascular events (AVEs) [55–57]. An increase of AMS by one point was associated with increased risk of mortality by 16%, damage by 6%, and AVEs by 12% [57]. The frequency of visits within 1 year (quarterly, semi-annually, or annually) does not have a significant impact on the AMS [58]. However, in individual patients, only visits up to 3 months apart provided an accurate estimation of disease activity over time, while visits beyond 3 months compromised this measure [58]. The AMS plays an important role in measuring disease activity over time in addition to its prognostic value, especially in patients with prolonged follow-up in longitudinal studies.

## Responder Measures

### *Flares*

The SELENA-SLEDAI Flare Index (SFI) was proposed by the SELENA trial investigators to define flares [59]. The original SFI proposed mild/moderate and severe flares, and this separation was applied in a number of randomized controlled trials (RCTs) [22]. SFI is a composite outcome that incorporates the SELENA-SLEDAI index, the classification of flares in mild/moderate/severe, and the PGA (0 = none, 1 = mild, 2 = moderate, 3 = severe) [22]. In a study conducted on patient scenarios, the reliability of the SFI was substantial for severe flares and fair for mild/moderate flares [59]. Previous training of the examiners on SFI improves its performance, in particular for mild/moderate flares [59]. Interestingly, a different group evaluated the reliability and validity of the SELENA-SLEDAI, PGA, and SFI retrospectively on patients' charts. The findings of that study were that the PGA and SELENA-SLEDAI components of the SFI are more reliable and valid than the SFI as a whole. Both the intra- and inter-rater reliability of the PGA and the SELENA-SLEDAI were better than the SFI [60]. Moreover, the PGA and the SELENA-SLEDAI demonstrated adequate agreement with each other. However, the SFI displayed poor agreement with PGA- and SELENA-SLEDAI-defined flares. This study raised questions regarding the validity of the SFI; nevertheless, the authors attributed the inadequate performance of the SFI to the methods of the retrospective chart abstraction and study design [60]. The SFI was revised later to accurately detect mild and moderate flares that were observed in clinical trials [61]. The revised SFI suggested specific clinical manifestations for each organ system and categorizes flares (mild, moderate, severe) based on the treatment decision. In this new version of the SFI, two of the major components of the original SFI (PGA and SELENA-SLEDAI) have been excluded [61].

## *Improvement*

### Responder Index for Lupus Erythematosus

The Responder Index for Lupus Erythematosus (RIFLE) was developed to measure partial and complete response to therapy, particularly in clinical trials [62]. The RIFLE is able to detect considerable variation in disease activity and is sensitive to change over time. It classified patients as worsening, present or no change, partial response, resolution, and not present on the basis of their SLE manifestations. The RIFLE has been used in a limited number of clinical trials and research studies and needs further validation [51, 63]. One study evaluated the minimal clinically important differences of validated measures of lupus activity in childhood-onset SLE. This study showed that the RIFLE appears to be less useful for the assessment of childhood-onset SLE than it is for adult SLE, as compared to the SLEDAI-2K, SLAM-R, ECLAM, and BILAG indices [64].

### SLE Responder Index

The SLE Responder Index (SRI) was developed in the context of a phase II clinical trial with belimumab, a B lymphocyte-stimulator antagonist, to define a clinically meaningful change in disease activity [42]. This is a composite outcome that incorporates the modification of the SLEDAI, SELENA-SLEDAI, BILAG, and PGA [4, 22, 24, 39]. The SELENA-SLEDAI score was used to determine global improvement. The BILAG domain scores were used to ensure that no significant worsening in previously unaffected organ systems had occurred. The PGA ensured that improvement in disease activity was not achieved at the expense of the patient's overall condition [42]. In that trial, patients with serologically active disease treated with belimumab plus standard of care therapy showed a statistically significant response [46% vs. 29% of the patients receiving placebo] at week 52 [42]. The subsequent phase III trial used the same outcome measure and demonstrated a statistically significant difference in responders between belimumab and placebo [43]. In the EMBODY trials (testing epratuzumab versus placebo), the researchers proposed a modification of the SRI, in which the BILAG index was used to define primary improvement, whereas the SLEDAI and PGA were used to ensure no deterioration in disease activity [65]. The most widely used versions of the SRI are the SRI-4 and the SRI-5. Both measures require no new BILAG A score or just one B score and no deterioration >0.3 (or 10%) in the PGA. The decrease in the SLEDAI-2K score should reach 4 or 5 points, respectively. More stringent endpoints (SRI-6 to SRI-10) were also used as secondary endpoints.

### BILAG-Based Composite Lupus Assessment (BICLA)

The BICLA was initially described and used as a primary endpoint in certain randomized, controlled trials [65]. The BICLA response is defined as (1) at least one gradation of improvement in baseline BILAG scores in all body systems with moderate or severe disease activity at entry (e.g., all A (severe disease) scores falling to B (moderate), C (mild), or D (no activity) and all B scores falling to C or D); (2) no new BILAG A or more than one new BILAG B scores; (3) no worsening of total SLEDAI-2K score from baseline; (4) ≤10% deterioration in Physicians Global Assessment; and (5) no initiation of non-protocol treatment.

### SLEDAI-2K Responder Index 50

The SLEDAI and its versions record descriptors of disease activity as present or absent [4, 20, 22, 23, 27, 28]. Any manifestation has to be resolved completely for the index to demonstrate improvement. This is a major limitation of the index since it does not allow the detection of a partial response or a signal toward improvement such as an ACR20 response, which has been the most commonly used endpoint in studies on rheumatoid arthritis. This disadvantage led to modifications aiming to capture partial improvement in disease activity. A minimum of 50% was considered by the investigators to reflect a clinically important improvement and gave rise to the concept of the SLEDAI-2K Responder Index 50 (S2K RI-50) [66]. The SLEDAI-2K 30 days was used to build the S2K RI-50. The index comprises the same 24 descriptors as the SLEDAI-2K and covers 9 organ systems. The new definitions of the S2K RI-50 were generated to identify a 50% improvement in each of the 24 descriptors of the SLEDAI-2K. Content and face validity of each definition were confirmed according to the adopted methodology. As in the SLEDAI-2K 30 days, each descriptor in the S2K RI-50 refers to the preceding 30 days [27, 28]. The assigned scores for the descriptors of the S2K RI-50 were derived by dividing the score of the corresponding SLEDAI-2K descriptor by 2. As in the SLEDAI-2K, the score of the S2K RI-50 can range from 0 to 105 (if there is no improvement in any clinical or laboratory manifestation) or less, of course, if there is complete or 50% improvement in any of the activity variables. The scoring method is simple, cumulative, and intuitive as in the original SLEDAI-2K [23, 66]. To familiarize physicians with both the definitions of the S2K RI-50 and the S2K RI-50 data retrieval form, a dedicated web site was developed for training purposes (www.s2k-ri-50.com/).

In the initial validation, the concurrent construct validity of the S2K RI-50 and the physician-response assessment were evaluated in 141 patients. The S2K RI-50 scores decreased more than the SLEDAI-2K scores in patients who improved, and more patients were classified as responders using the S2K RI-50. A moderate correlation was found between the S2K RI-50 and the physician-response assessment. More importantly, the decrease in the S2K RI-50 scores was clinically more important than the decrease in the SLEDAI-2K scores in patients who improved and met the definition of improvement by decreasing by 4 points or more [2, 66]. In a multicenter study, the S2K RI-50 was evaluated on patient profiles and demonstrated both intra- and inter-rater reliability with average intraclass correlation coefficients of 0.99 and 1.00, respectively [67]. More recently, it was shown to enhance the ability of the SLE Responder Index to identify patients with clinically important improvement in disease activity [68]. The definitions of the S2K RI-50 descriptors are shown in detail in Table 6.8.

## Measures of Clinically Meaningful Change in Disease Activity

### *Improvement*

Improvement has been accepted as a relevant outcome measure in clinical trials. At present, improvement is defined on the basis of disease activity measures, in particular, the SLEDAI-2K and BILAG index: improvement is a reduction in SLEDAI-2K of 4 or higher or a reduction in the BILAG scores. A major clinical response by the BILAG index is a BILAG C score or better at 6 months with no new BILAG A or B scores and the maintenance of response with no new BILAG A or B scores between 6 and 12 months [50]. Although the BILAG-2004 index was significantly associated with a decrease in therapy with a major improvement from Grade A or B to C or D, it was not definitively responsive to the improvement in disease activity from very active to moderately active (Grade A to B). In fact, a reduction

**Table 6.8** Definitions of improvement for the S2K-RI-50 index

| Descriptor | SLEDAI-2K defintion | Definition of S2K-RI-50 improvement |
|---|---|---|
| **Seizure** | Recent onset. Exclude metabolic, infectious, or drug causes | ≥50% reduction in frequency of baseline seizure days/month |
| **Psychosis**[a] | Altered ability to function in normal activity due to severe disturbance in the perception of reality. Include hallucinations, incoherence, marked loose associations, impoverished thought content, marked illogical thinking, or bizarre, disorganized, or catatonic behavior. Exclude uremia and drug causes | ≥50% improvement of the psychotic manifestations judged by physician |
| **Organic brain syndrome**[a] | Altered mental function with impaired orientation, memory, or other intellectual function, with rapid onset and fluctuating clinical features. Include clouding of consciousness with reduced capacity to focus and inability to sustain attention to environment, plus at least two of the following: perceptual disturbance, incoherent speech, insomnia or daytime drowsiness, or increased or decreased psychomotor activity. Exclude metabolic, infectious, or drug causes | ≥50% improvement of the organic brain manifestations judged by physician |
| **Visual disturbance** | Retinal changes of SLE. Include cytoid bodies, retinal hemorrhages, serous exudate or hemorrhages in the choroid, or optic neuritis. Exclude hypertension, infection, or drug causes | ≥50% improvement of the retinal exam assessed by physician |
| **Cranial nerve disorder**[c] | New onset of sensory or motor neuropathy involving cranial nerves | ≥50% recovery of motor or sensory function in affected nerve within 1 month from the event on the basis of decrease in lupus disease activity or ≥50% decrease of the severity of pain within 1 month from the event on the basis of decrease in lupus disease activity as determined by patient on numerical scale of 1–10 if applicable with no worsening in either |
| **Lupus headache**[b] | Severe, persistent headache; may be migrainous, but must be nonresponsive to narcotic analgesia | ≥50% decrease of the severity of pain as determined by patient on numerical scale of 1–10 |

**Table 6.8** (continued)

| Descriptor | SLEDAI-2K defintion | Definition of S2K-RI-50 improvement |
|---|---|---|
| **CVA**[c] | New onset of cerebrovascular accident(s). Exclude arteriosclerosis | ≥50% recovery of motor or sensory function related to CVA within 1 month from the event on the basis of decrease in lupus disease activity as determined by physician without worsening in either |
| **Vasculitis**[d] | Ulceration, gangrene, tender finger nodules, periungual infarction, splinter hemorrhages, or biopsy or angiogram proof of vasculitis | ≥50% improvement of the vasculitis lesions present with no new lesion or worsening in either<br>A ≥50% improvement for ulceration or gangrene is defined as ≥50% decrease in the body surface area; for periungual infarction, splinter hemorrhages, or tender finger nodules a ≥50% improvement is defined as ≥50% decrease in the total number of involved digits with periungual infarction, splinter hemorrhages, and tender finger nodules<br>Multiple lesions in a single digit, count only one |
| **Arthritis** | ≥2 joints with pain and signs of inflammation (i.e., tenderness, swelling, or effusion) | ≥50% reduction in the number of joints with pain and signs of inflammation (i.e., tenderness, swelling or effusion) |
| **Myositis** | Proximal muscle aching/weakness, associated with elevated creatinine phosphokinase/aldolase or electromyogram changes or a biopsy showing myositis<br>*Motor strength by MRC scale:*<br>0 No contraction<br>1 A flicker or trace of contraction<br>2 Active movement with gravity eliminated<br>3 Active movement against gravity<br>4 – Active movement against gravity/slight resistance<br>4 Active movement against gravity/moderate resistance<br>4 + Active movement against gravity/strong resistance<br>5 Normal power | ≥50% increase in muscles power judged by physician or increase by<br>or 1 grade upon a scale of zero to five<br>or<br>≥50% decrease in the level of creatinine phosphokinase/aldolase level comparing to previous visit with no worsening in either |
| **Urinary casts** | Heme-granular or red blood cell casts | Decrease by ≥50% in the total number of casts (heme-granular and red blood cell casts) |
| **Hematuria** | >5 red blood cells/high power field. Exclude stone, infection, or other cause | Decrease by ≥50% in the number of red blood cell/high power field at this visit |

(continued)

**Table 6.8** (continued)

| Descriptor | SLEDAI-2K defintion | Definition of S2K-RI-50 improvement |
|---|---|---|
| **Proteinuria** | New onset, recurrent, or persistent proteinuria of more than >0.5 gram/24 hours | Decrease by ≥50% in the range of proteinuria |
| **Pyuria** | >5 white blood cells/ high power field. Exclude infection | Decrease by ≥50% in the number of white blood cells/ high power field |
| **Rash**[d] | New onset, recurrent, or persistent inflammatory lupus rash<br>Activity of skin lesions should be based on the evaluation of the most active lesion | Decrease by ≥50% of involved body surface area and/or activity of most active lesion with no worsening in either<br>Activity of the lesion should be determined by the color of the lesions:<br>0 – absent<br>1 – pink, faint erythema<br>2 – red<br>3 – dark red/purple/violaceous/crusted/ hemorrhagic<br>A ≥50% decrease in the activity of the lesion is defined by decreasing by 2 grades<br>Dyspigmentation, scarring, and atrophy are not active lesions |
| **Alopecia**[d] | New onset, recurrent, or persistent abnormal, patchy, or diffuse loss of hair<br>Size of patchy alopecic lesion should be determined based on involved total scalp surface. Total scalp surface is 4.5%<br>Diffuse alopecia is determined by patient on numerical scale of 1–10<br>Activity of alopecia should be based on the evaluation of the most active lesion | Decrease by ≥50% of total scalp involved area for patchy alopecic lesion or ≥50% reduction in the diffuse alopecia as determined by patient on numerical scale of 1–10, and/or activity of the most active alopecic lesions with no worsening in either<br>Activity of the alopecic lesion should be determined by the color of the most active lesion:<br>0 – absent<br>1 – pink, faint erythema<br>2 – red<br>3 – dark red/purple/violaceous/crusted/ hemorrhagic<br>A ≥50% decrease in the activity of the lesion is defined by decreasing by 2 grades |
| **Mucosal Ulcers** | New onset, recurrent, or persistent oral or nasal ulcerations | Decrease by ≥50% in the number of ulcers at this visit |
| **Pleurisy** | Pleuritic chest pain with pleural rub or effusion, or pleural thickening | ≥50% reduction in the pain severity as determined by patient on numerical scale of 1–10 and/or ≥50% reduction in the amount of fluid (on imaging) with no worsening in either |
| **Pericarditis** | Pericardial pain with at least one of the following: rub, effusion, electrocardiogram or echocardiogram confirmation | ≥50% reduction in the pain severity as determined by patient on numerical scale of 1–10 and/or ≥50% reduction in the amount of fluid (on imaging) with no worsening in either |

**Table 6.8** (continued)

| Descriptor | SLEDAI-2K defintion | Definition of S2K-RI-50 improvement |
|---|---|---|
| **Low complement** | Decrease in CH50, C3, or C4 below the lower limit of normal for testing laboratory | ≥50% increase in the level of any complement or normalization of one of them without a drop in either |
| **Increased anti-DNA antibodies** | Increase in the level of anti-DNA antibodies above normal range for testing laboratory | ≥50% reduction in the level of anti-DNA antibodies |
| **Fever** | >38 °C. Exclude infectious causes | ≥50% reduction in the degree of fever above normal |
| **Thrombocyto-penia** | <100,000 platelets/ × $10^9$/L. Exclude drug causes | ≥50% increase in platelets but <100,000 platelets/$mm^3$ |
| **Leukopenia** | <3000 white blood cells/x $10^9$/L. Exclude drug causes | ≥50% increase in white blood cells but <3000/$mm^3$ |

**Numerical scale: 1 is mild and 10 is most severe**

To determine body surface area, use rule of nines for skin scoring: head 9%, chest 9%, abdomen 9%, back 18%, legs 36%, arms/hands 18%, genitalia/perineum 1%, and patient's palm for 1%.

[a]Overlap of symptoms will count for only one descriptor either psychosis or organic brain syndrome

[b]Lupus headache improvement will count regardless of whether patient is using narcotic analgesia or not though it has to be part of the baseline lupus headache

[c]CVA and cranial nerve improvement will count if it occurs within 1 month from the event on the basis of decrease in lupus disease activity as this is more likely on the basis of decrease disease activity

[d]Vasculitis, rash, and alopecia; if the total BSA is ≤1%, a ≥50% improvement is defined by ≥50% decrease in the activity of the most active lesion by a decrease of 2 grades or ≥50% decrease in the size of the biggest lesion with no worsening in either

from Grade A to B is not always reflected by a reduction in therapy. Hence, it is recommended that the efficacy criterion of improvement to low-level activity (Grade C or D) instead of improvement from Grade A to B should be used as the main outcome in clinical trials using the BILAG-2004 [69].

Until recently, few responder indices have been developed that measure response to treatment in multiple systems. Of the available indices, the BILAG has been the most commonly used in clinical trials. In 2010, the US Food and Drug Administration (FDA) referred to the BILAG as being the best available index to study the reduction in disease activity for clinical trials [70]. Nevertheless, the American College of Rheumatology expressed the need for the development and validation of new reliable indices to measure improvement in clinical trials for the development of new drugs for SLE.

Although the SLEDAI-2K has been used to define improvement in disease activity, it is important to highlight that the captured improvement is actually a complete resolution of any given clinical or laboratory manifestation. The S2K RI-50 was developed to detect an improvement of 50% or greater, which was considered to be clinically meaningful [66]. The performance of the S2K RI-50 was evaluated prospectively and retrospectively in longitudinal studies and was shown to identify patients with 50% or greater improvement [71]. More importantly, the S2K RI-50 enhances the ability of the composite outcome SRI to identify patients with clinically important improvement in disease activity [41, 68].

## Flare and Persistently Active Disease

Flare is defined as an increase in the SLEDAI-2K of 4 points or more, an increase in the SELENA-SLEDAI score of 3 points or more, or one new category A or two new category B grades on the BILAG index [13, 22, 40]. In terms of specific flare indices, the SELENA researchers initially proposed the SFI and, more recently, the revised SFI version in an effort to differentiate mild and moderate flares [59, 61]. The revised SFI suggested specific clinical manifestations for each organ system and categorized flares (mild, moderate, severe) on the basis of the treatment decision [61]. One study individually evaluated mild, moderate, and severe flares and showed that the intraclass correlation coefficients were 0.54, 0.21, and 0.18 for a BILAG-2004 flare, SELENA flare, and PGA flare, respectively. The results of this study highlight the difficulty in the distinction between mild and moderate flares, and the results among the examiners were much less consistent, despite the use of the new SFI version [61]. Similarly, the separation between mild and moderate flares remains problematic even with the use of the BILAG-2004 [69]. More importantly, the BILAG-2004 index appears to perform better at detecting increases in disease activity, as compared to improvement, leading to the recommendation that the BILAG-2004 index should be used in longitudinal studies that aim to determine worsening in disease activity. Moreover, the renal scoring in the BILAG-2004 index is powered to detect new-onset lupus nephritis or significant improvement (Grade C or D), and using more specific criteria is advisable to define response in longitudinal studies on lupus nephritis and, ultimately, in clinical trials [69].

Besides flares, SLEDAI-2K scores are used to define persistently active disease (PAD) with a SLEDAI-2K score change of 4 or less between visits and a remission as a SLEDAI-2K score of 0. A recent study from the Toronto Lupus Clinic showed that among inception patients, about 10% will follow a persistently active disease course over the first 10 years of disease [1]. At least 25% of these patients never achieved the definition of flare since the fluctuation of their SLEDAI-2K scores was minimal (1 or 2 points) for the entire decade. As expected, these patients had higher cumulative damage and mortality over time compared to patients who achieved even a short-lived remission [1]. Although flare has been the most commonly used outcome measure to describe worsening disease activity, PAD is also relevant and should be used in clinical and research settings [2].

## Assessment of Disease Activity in Special Patient Groups

### *Childhood*

The Pediatric Rheumatology International Trial Organization (PRINTO) and the ACR Provisional Criteria for the Evaluation of Response to Therapy for children with SLE attempted to prospectively validate the provisional criteria for the evaluation of response. The PRINTO could not firmly select a specific index for the assessment of global disease activity. The differences in sensitivity and specificity among the evaluated indices (SLEDAI-2K, ECLAM, SLAM-R, and BILAG) were small, and all of them performed equally in evaluating disease activity [16]. Although the BILAG index showed a slightly higher sensitivity than the others, the PRINTO emphasized the complexity of its scoring system, which could result in considerable measuring error with less experienced raters.

### *Pregnancy*

The assessment of lupus during pregnancy is affected by the physiologic changes that influence the clinical and laboratory features of lupus. Since 1999, several lupus activity scales have been adapted for use during pregnancy, in particular, the Systemic Lupus Erythematosus Pregnancy Disease Activity Index (SLEPDAI), the modified SLAM (m-SLAM) index, and the lupus activity index in pregnancy (LAI-P) [72]. None of these indices demonstrated an acceptable reliability and validity to date.

## Low Disease Activity in SLE

Complete remission is rare in SLE and has not been strictly defined yet [73]. Therefore, a more realistic target, such as low disease activity, may be of value in daily clinical practice as well as in clinical trials. In order to be meaningful, low disease activity should capture a disease state that will lead to favorable long-term outcomes, preferably as close to complete remission as possible. In this context, different definitions of low disease activity emerged during the last few years [74–76].

Zen et al. first introduced the concept of minimal disease activity (MDA) based on a clinical SLE Disease Activity Index-2000 (SLEDAI-2K) ≤1 (excluding serology) that is maintained on antimalarials, standard doses of immunosuppressives, and low doses of prednisone (≤5 mg/day) [74]. The damage accrual of those patients (all Caucasians) was comparable to that of patients who achieved clinical remission after 7 years of follow-up [74]. Moreover, sustained MDA was associated with improved survival in the long term [77]. Practically, MDA allows only for the presence of hematological manifestations, such as isolated leukopenia or thrombocytopenia, which must be attributable to lupus and exclude secondary causes, since these are the only (along with fever) SLEDAI-2K components with a weighted score of 1 [23].

Polachek et al. expanded the concept of MDA to that of low disease activity (LDA), allowing for a clinical SLEDAI-2K ≤ 2 on antimalarials only (active serology was permitted) [75]. In that context, only the SLEDAI-2K components with a weighted score of 1 (hematologic manifestations) or 2 (mucocutaneous manifestations, pleuritis, pericarditis) could be accepted in the definition of low disease activity. Although a validated instrument for the assessment of the severity of skin involvement, such as the CLASI (Cutaneous Lupus Erythematosus Area and Severity Index) was not included in the definition, mucocutaneous manifestations (rash, alopecia, oral/nasal ulcerations) must have been minor enough to be treated with topical medications and antimalarials only. Concerning pleuritis and pericarditis, the other manifestations with a weighted score of 2 in the SLEDAI-2K [23], those patients requiring glucocorticosteroids and/or immunosuppressives are excluded by definition. Only those treated with nonsteroidal anti-inflammatories and/or antimalarials meet this definition of low disease activity. Sustained LDA for 1 year occurred in 13% of the 620 patients and led to outcomes (damage accrual and mortality) comparable to the patients who had achieved clinical remission after 2 years of follow-up [75]. Moreover, patients who sustained LDA or clinical remission for ≥10 years had comparable damage accrual and mortality, regardless of the administered therapy [78].

Franklyn et al. from the Asia Pacific Lupus Collaboration further expanded the concept of low disease activity with the Lupus Low Disease Activity State (LLDAS), a definition that was based on expert consensus [76]. This definition consisted of five criteria, namely, a SLEDAI-2K ≤ 4 with no major organ (renal, central nervous system, cardiopulmonary, vasculitis, fever, gastrointestinal system, and hemolytic anemia) involvement, no new clinical activity compared to the previous assessment, PGA ≤1, current prednisone dose ≤7.5 mg/day, and standard (not exceeding the maximum recommended) maintenance doses of immunosuppressive drugs or biologics. Any given patient can be classified as LLDAS if he/she fulfils all five criteria, while serology counts toward disease activity. From a clinical perspective, LLDAS allows for the presence (and persistence) of all minor clinical manifestations (mucocutaneous, hematological) either alone or in combinations (e.g., a skin rash and leukopenia). Potentially, it may even include arthritis or myositis, as long as there are no other clinical manifestations or active serology. Severe cases of musculoskeletal involvement (arthritis or myositis) will expectedly not be included in LLDAS due to higher PGA and/or a possible increase in the prednisone dose. During the initial validation process, the authors showed that patients who spent more than 50% of the time in LLDAS accrued significantly less irreversible damage as compared to the rest of the patients after an average follow-up of 3.9 years. LLDAS is protective against new damage as well as all-cause mortality as long as it has been sustained for 2 years [79–82].

## References


1. Tselios K, Gladman DD, Touma Z, et al. Disease course patterns in systemic lupus erythematosus. Lupus. 2019;28(1):114–22.
2. Nikpour M, Urowitz MB, Ibañez D, et al. Frequency and determinants of flare and persistently active disease in systemic lupus erythematosus. Arthritis Rheum. 2009;61(9):1152–8.
3. Smolen JS, Strand V, Cardiel M, et al. Randomized clinical trials and longitudinal observational studies in systemic lupus erythematosus: consensus on a preliminary core set of outcome domains. J Rheumatol. 1999;26(2):504–7.
4. Bombardier C, Gladman DD, Urowitz MB, et al. Derivation of the SLEDAI. A disease activity index for lupus patients. The Committee on Prognosis Studies in SLE. Arthritis Rheum. 1992;35(6):630–40.
5. Boers M, Brooks P, Strand CV, et al. The OMERACT filter for outcome measures in rheumatology. J Rheumatol. 1998;25(2):198–9.
6. American Rheumatism Association Glossary Committee. Dictionary of the rheumatic diseases. Vol. I: signs and symptoms. New York: Contact Associates International; 1982.
7. American Rheumatism Association Glossary Committee. Dictionary of the rheumatic diseases. Vol. II: diagnostic testing. New York: Contact Associates International; 1985.
8. Gladman DD, Goldsmith CH, Urowitz MB, et al. Cross-cultural validation and reliability of 3 disease activity indices in systemic lupus erythematosus. J Rheumatol. 1992;19(4):608–11.
9. Hawker G, Gabriel S, Bombardier C, et al. A reliability study of SLEDAI: a disease activity index for systemic lupus erythematosus. J Rheumatol. 1993;20(4):657–60.
10. Petri M, Hellmann D, Hochberg M. Validity and reliability of lupus activity measures in the routine clinic setting. J Rheumatol. 1992;19(1):53–9.
11. Liang MH, Socher SA, Larson MG, et al. Reliability and validity of six systems for the clinical assessment of disease activity in systemic lupus erythematosus. Arthritis Rheum. 1989;32(9):1107–18.
12. McLaughlin JR, Bombardier C, Farewell VT, et al. Kidney biopsy in systemic lupus erythematosus. III. Survival analysis controlling for clinical and laboratory variables. Arthritis Rheum. 1994;37(4):559–67.
13. Gladman DD, Urowitz MB, Kagal A, et al. Accurately describing changes in disease activity in systemic lupus erythematosus. J Rheumatol. 2000;27(2):377–9.
14. Gladman DD, Goldsmith CH, Urowitz MB, et al. Sensitivity to change of 3 systemic lupus erythematosus disease activity indices: international validation. J Rheumatol. 1994;21(8):1468–71.
15. Brunner HI, Feldman BM, Bombardier C, et al. Sensitivity of the systemic lupus erythematosus disease activity index, British Isles lupus assessment group index, and systemic lupus activity measure in the evaluation of clinical change in childhood-onset systemic lupus erythematosus. Arthritis Rheum. 1999;42(7):1354–60.
16. Brunner HI, Higgins GC, Wiers K, et al. Prospective validation of the provisional criteria for the evaluation of response to therapy in childhood-onset systemic lupus erythematosus. Arthritis Care Res (Hoboken). 2010;62(3):335–44.
17. Zonana-Nacach A, Yañez P, Jimènez-Balderas FJ, et al. Disease activity, damage and survival in Mexican patients with acute severe systemic lupus erythematosus. Lupus. 2007;16(12):997–1000.
18. Becker-Merok A, Nossent HC. Damage accumulation in systemic lupus erythematosus and its relation to disease activity and mortality. J Rheumatol. 2006;33(8):1570–7.
19. Cook RJ, Gladman DD, Pericak D, et al. Prediction of short term mortality in systemic lupus erythematosus with time dependent measures of disease activity. J Rheumatol. 2000;27(8):1892–5.
20. Guzman J, Cardiel MH, Arce-Salinas A, et al. Measurement of disease activity in systemic lupus erythematosus. Prospective validation of 3 clinical indices. J Rheumatol. 1992;19(10):1551–8.
21. Uribe AG, Vila LM, McGwin G Jr, et al. The systemic lupus activity measure–revised, the Mexican Systemic Lupus Erythematosus Disease Activity Index (SLEDAI), and a modified

SLEDAI-2K are adequate instruments to measure disease activity in systemic lupus erythematosus. J Rheumatol. 2004;31(10):1934–40.
22. Petri M, Kim MY, Kalunian KC, et al. Combined oral contraceptives in women with systemic lupus erythematosus. N Engl J Med. 2005;353(24):2550–8.
23. Gladman DD, Ibañez D, Urowitz MB. Systemic lupus erythematosus disease activity index 2000. J Rheumatol. 2002;29(2):288–91.
24. Hay EM, Bacon PA, Gordon C, et al. The BILAG index: a reliable and valid instrument for measuring clinical disease activity in systemic lupus erythematosus. Q J Med. 1993;86(7):447–58.
25. Vitali C, Bencivelli W, Isenberg DA, et al. Disease activity in systemic lupus erythematosus: report of the Consensus Study Group of the European Workshop for Rheumatology Research. II. Identification of the variables indicative of disease activity and their use in the development of an activity score. The European Consensus Study Group for Disease Activity in SLE. Clin Exp Rheumatol. 1992;10(5):541–7.
26. Fellows of Harvard College: SLE Activity Measure-Revised (SLAM-R). Revised 1998.
27. Touma Z, Urowitz MB, Gladman DD. SLEDAI-2K for a 30-day window. Lupus. 2010;19(1):49–51.
28. Touma Z, Urowitz MB, Ibañez D, et al. SLEDAI-2K 10 days versus SLEDAI-2K 30 days in a longitudinal evaluation. Lupus. 2011;20(1):67–70.
29. Touma Z, Gladman DD, Su J, Anderson N, Urowitz MB. A novel lupus activity index accounting for glucocorticoids: SLEDAI-2K glucocorticoid index. Rheumatology (Oxford). 2018;57:1370–6.
30. Bae SC, Koh HK, Chang DK, et al. Reliability and validity of systemic lupus activity measure-revised (SLAM-R) for measuring clinical disease activity in systemic lupus erythematosus. Lupus. 2001;10(6):405–9.
31. Ward MM, Marx AS, Barry NN. Comparison of the validity and sensitivity to change of 5 activity indices in systemic lupus erythematosus. J Rheumatol. 2000;27(3):664–70.
32. Fortin PR, Abrahamowicz M, Neville C, et al. Impact of disease activity and cumulative damage on the health of lupus patients. Lupus. 1998;7(2):101–7.
33. Vitali C, Bencivelli W, Isenberg DA, et al. Disease activity in systemic lupus erythematosus: report of the Consensus Study Group of the European Workshop for Rheumatology Research. I. A descriptive analysis of 704 European lupus patients. European Consensus Study Group for Disease Activity in SLE. Clin Exp Rheumatol. 1992;10(5):527–39.
34. Bencivelli W, Vitali C, Isenberg DA, et al. Disease activity in systemic lupus erythematosus: report of the Consensus Study Group of the European Workshop for Rheumatology Research. III. Development of a computerized clinical chart and its application to the comparison of different indices of disease activity. The European Consensus Study Group for Disease Activity in SLE. Clin Exp Rheumatol. 1992;10(5):549–54.
35. Mosca M, Bencivelli W, Vitali C, et al. The validity of the ECLAM index for the retrospective evaluation of disease activity in systemic lupus erythematosus. Lupus. 2000;9(6):445–50.
36. Aringer M, Graninger WB, Steiner G, et al. Safety and efficacy of tumor necrosis factor alpha blockade in systemic lupus erythematosus: an open-label study. Arthritis Rheum. 2004;50(10):3161–9.
37. Vitali C, Bencivelli W, Mosca M, et al. Development of a clinical chart to compute different disease activity indices for systemic lupus erythematosus. J Rheumatol. 1999;26(2):498–501.
38. Symmons DP, Coppock JS, Bacon PA, et al. Development and assessment of a computerized index of clinical disease activity in systemic lupus erythematosus. Members of the British Isles Lupus Assessment Group (BILAG). Q J Med. 1988;69(259):927–37.
39. Stoll T, Stucki G, Malik J, et al. Further validation of the BILAG disease activity index in patients with systemic lupus erythematosus. Ann Rheum Dis. 1996;55(10):756–60.
40. Gordon C, Sutcliffe N, Skan J, et al. Definition and treatment of lupus flares measured by the BILAG index. Rheumatology (Oxford). 2003;42(11):1372–9.
41. Touma Z, Gladman DD, Ibañez D, et al. SLEDAI-2K Responder Index (SRI-50) enhances the ability to identify responders in clinical trials. J Rheumatol. 2011;38(11):2395–9.

42. Furie RA, Petri MA, Wallace DJ, et al. Novel evidence-based systemic lupus erythematosus responder index. Arthritis Rheum. 2009;61(9):1143–51.
43. Navarra SV, Guzmán RM, Gallacher AE, et al. Efficacy and safety of belimumab in patients with active systemic lupus erythematosus: a randomized, placebo-controlled, phase 3 trial. Lancet. 2011;377(9767):721–31.
44. Isenberg DA, Rahman A, Allen E, et al. BILAG 2004. Development and initial validation of an updated version of the British Isles Lupus Assessment Group's disease activity index for patients with systemic lupus erythematosus. Rheumatology (Oxford). 2005;44(7):902–6.
45. Yee CS, Cresswell L, Farewell V, et al. Numerical scoring for the BILAG- 2004 index. Rheumatology (Oxford). 2010;49(9):1665–9.
46. Isenberg DA, Gordon C. From BILAG to BLIPS—disease activity assessment in lupus past, present and future. Lupus. 2000;9(9):651–4.
47. Yee CS, Farewell V, Isenberg DA, et al. Revised British Isles Lupus Assessment Group 2004 index: a reliable tool for assessment of systemic lupus erythematosus activity. Arthritis Rheum. 2006;54(10):3300–5.
48. Yee CS, Farewell V, Isenberg DA, et al. British Isles Lupus Assessment Group 2004 index is valid for assessment of disease activity in systemic lupus erythematosus. Arthritis Rheum. 2007;56(12):4113–9.
49. Touma Z, Gladman DD, Urowitz MB, et al. Mycophenolate mofetil for induction treatment of lupus nephritis: a systematic review and meta-analysis. J Rheumatol. 2011;38(1):69–78.
50. Guidance for Industry: Lupus nephritis caused by systemic lupus erythematosus—developing medical products for treatment. http://www.fda.gov/downloads/Drugs/GuidanceComplianceRegulatoryInformation/Guidances/UCM216280.pdf.
51. Petri M, Kasitanon N, Lee SS, et al. Systemic lupus international collaborating clinics renal activity/response exercise: development of a renal activity score and renal response index. Arthritis Rheum. 2010;58(6):1784–8.
52. Albrecht J, Taylor L, Berlin JA, et al. The CLASI (Cutaneous Lupus Erythematosus Disease Area and Severity Index): an outcome instrument for cutaneous lupus erythematosus. J Invest Dermatol. 2010;125(5):889–94.
53. Krathen M, Albrecht J, Werth VP. The cutaneous lupus disease activity and severity index as a validated outcome measure for cutaneous lupus erythematosus: comment on the article by Stamm et al. Arthritis Rheum. 2010;59(4):601–2.
54. Kuhn A, Meuth AM, Bein D, et al. Revised Cutaneous Lupus Erythematosus Disease Area and Severity Index (RCLASI): a modified outcome instrument for cutaneous lupus erythematosus. Br J Dermatol. 2010;163(1):83–92.
55. Ibañez D, Urowitz MB, Gladman DD. Summarizing disease features over time: I. Adjusted mean SLEDAI derivation and application to an index of disease activity in lupus. J Rheumatol. 2010;30(9):1977–82.
56. Ibañez D, Gladman DD, Urowitz MB. Adjusted mean systemic lupus erythematosus disease activity index-2K is a predictor of outcome in SLE. J Rheumatol. 2010;32(5):824–7.
57. Ibañez D, Gladman D, Urowitz M. Summarizing disease features over time: II. Variability measures of SLEDAI-2K. J Rheumatol. 2010;34(2):336–40.
58. Ibañez D, Gladman DD, Touma Z, et al. Optimal frequency of visits for patients with systemic lupus erythematosus to measure disease activity over time. J Rheumatol. 2010;38(1):60–3.
59. Petri M, Buyon J, Skovron ML, et al. Reliability of SELENA SLEDAI and flare as clinical trial outcome measures [abstract]. Arthritis Rheum. 1998;41:S218.
60. FitzGerald JD, Grossman JM. Validity and reliability of retrospective assessment of disease activity and flare in observational cohorts of lupus patients. Lupus. 2010;8(8):638–44.
61. Petri M, Buyon J, Kalunian KC, et al. Revision of the SELENA Flare Index [abstract]. Arthritis Rheum. 2009;60:S902.
62. Petri M, Barr SG, Buyon J, et al. RIFLE: responder index for lupus erythematosus [abstract]. Arthritis Rheum. 2000;43:S244.

63. Burt RK, Traynor A, Statkute L, et al. Nonmyeloablative hematopoietic stem cell transplantation for systemic lupus erythematosus. JAMA. 2010;295(5):527–35.
64. Brunner HI, Higgins GC, Klein-Gitelman MS, et al. Minimal clinically important differences of disease activity indices in childhood-onset systemic lupus erythematosus. Arthritis Care Res (Hoboken). 2010;62(7):950–9.
65. Wallace DJ, Kalunian K, Petri MA, et al. Efficacy and safety of epratuzumab in patients with moderate/severe active systemic lupus erythematosus: results from EMBLEM, a phase IIb, randomized, double-blind, placebo-controlled, multicentre study. Ann Rheum Dis. 2014;73:183–90.
66. Touma Z, Gladman DD, Ibañez D, et al. Development and initial validation of the systemic lupus erythematosus disease activity index 2000 responder index 50. J Rheumatol. 2011;38(2):275–84.
67. Touma Z, Urowitz MB, Fortin P, et al. Systemic Lupus Erythematosus Disease Activity Index (SLEDAI-2K) Responder Index (SRI)-50: a reliable index for measuring improvement in disease activity. J Rheumatol. 2011;38(5):868–73.
68. Touma Z, Gladman DD, Rose S, Fei K, Gregan Y, Gordon R, et al. Early improvement in SLEDAI-2K Responder Index-50 predicts SRI-4 response in a randomized placebo-controlled trial of ustekinumab in systemic lupus erythematosus. Arthritis Rheumatol. 2019;71(Suppl 10):2571 (Abstract).
69. Yee CS, Farewell V, Isenberg DA, et al. The BILAG-2004 index is sensitive to change for assessment of SLE disease activity. Rheumatology (Oxford). 2010;48(6):691–5.
70. Guidance for Industry: Systemic lupus erythematosus—Developing medical products for treatment. http://www.fda.gov/downloads/Drugs/GuidanceComplianceRegulatoryInformation/Guidances/ucm072063.pdf.
71. Touma Z, Gladman DD, Ibanez D, et al. SLEDAI-2K Responder Index-50 captures 50% improvement in disease activity over 10 years. Lupus. 2012;21(12):1305–11.
72. Buyon JP, Kalunian KC, Ramsey-Goldman R, et al. Assessing disease activity in SLE patients during pregnancy. Lupus. 2010;8(8):677–84.
73. van Vollenhoven R, Voskuyl A, Bertsias G, et al. A framework for remission in SLE: consensus findings from a large international task force on definitions of remission in SLE (DORIS). Ann Rheum Dis. 2017;76:554–61.
74. Zen M, Bassi N, Nalotto L, et al. Disease activity patterns in a monocentric cohort of SLE patients: a seven-year follow up study. Clin Exp Rheumatol. 2012;30:856–63.
75. Polachek A, Gladman DD, Su J, et al. Defining low disease activity in systemic lupus erythematosus. Arthritis Care Res (Hoboken). 2017;69:997–1003.
76. Franklyn K, Lau CS, Navarra SV, et al. Definition and initial validation of a Lupus Low Disease Activity State (LLDAS). Ann Rheum Dis. 2016;75:1615–21.
77. Lopez R, Davidson JE, Beeby MD, et al. Lupus disease activity and the risk of subsequent organ damage and mortality in a large lupus cohort. Rheumatology (Oxford). 2012;51:491–8.
78. Tselios K, Gladman DD, Touma Z, et al. Clinical remission and low disease activity have comparable outcomes over 10 years in systemic lupus erythematosus. Arthritis Care Res. 2019;71(6):822–8.
79. Tsang-A-Sjoe MW, Bultink IE, Heslinga M, et al. Both prolonged remission and Lupus Low Disease Activity State are associated with reduced damage accrual in systemic lupus erythematosus. Rheumatology (Oxford). 2017;56:121–8.
80. Tani C, Vagelli R, Stagnano C, et al. Remission and low disease activity in systemic lupus erythematosus: an achievable goal even with fewer steroids? Real-life data from a monocentric cohort. Lupus Sci Med. 2018;5:e000234.
81. Zen M, Iaccarino L, Gatto MA, et al. Lupus low disease activity state is associated with a decrease in damage progression in Caucasian patients with SLE, but overlaps with remission. Ann Rheum Dis. 2018;77:104–10.
82. Sharma C, Raymond W, Eilertsen G, Nossent J. FRI 0350 Lupus low disease activity state (LLDAS-50) is a significant predictor for damage accrual and mortality: a Norwegian cohort analysis. (abstract). Ann Rheum Dis. 2018;77:711.

# Chapter 7
# Metrics of Damage in SLE

**Taraneh Tofighi, Sindhu R. Johnson, and Zahi Touma**

## The Concept of Damage in SLE

With the reduction in mortality amongst patients with SLE over the past several decades, estimating the accrued impact of adverse events attributable to SLE and its treatments has become an important aspect of care. Mortality in SLE follows a bimodal pattern whereby early mortality is often related to severe SLE disease activity and associated infectious events, while mortality late in the course of disease is often a reflection of accrued damage from lupus, its treatment, or co-morbidities, particularly cardiovascular diseases [1, 2]. The Outcome Measures in Rheumatology (OMERACT) group has recognized damage as a key domain in the prognostication and management of disease, alongside disease activity, adverse events of drugs, health-related quality of life, and economic impact [3].

Damage is defined as irreversible organ dysfunction present from the time of SLE disease onset. In 1991, the Systemic Lupus International Collaborating Clinics (SLICC) group pioneered the field by conceptualizing the framework of damage in SLE and standardizing its definition and metric in the form of the SLICC/ACR

T. Tofighi
Faculty of Medicine, University of Toronto, Toronto, ON, Canada
e-mail: tara.tofighi@mail.utoronto.ca

S. R. Johnson
Division of Rheumatology, Department of Medicine, Toronto Western Hospital, Mount Sinai Hospital, Toronto, ON, Canada

Institute of Health Policy, Management and Evaluation, University of Toronto, Toronto, ON, Canada

Z. Touma (✉)
Centre for Prognosis in Rheumatic Disease, Toronto Lupus Clinic, Division of Rheumatology, Department of Medicine, Institute of Health Policy, Management and Evaluation, University of Toronto, Toronto, ON, Canada
e-mail: Zahi.Touma@uhn.ca



Z. Touma (ed.), *Outcome Measures and Metrics in Systemic Lupus Erythematosus*, https://doi.org/10.1007/978-3-030-73303-2_7

damage index (SDI) [4]. Damage as a construct reflects a clinical feature (a combination of subjective and/or objective [laboratory, pathological, or imaging]) that must be continuously present for a minimum of 6 months to score, with the intention of separating damage from active inflammation. SLE disease activity is thought to lessen or remit with treatment and is reversible by definition [4]. On this principle, nephrotic range proteinuria or elevated serum creatinine may initially reflect disease activity, but persistence for at least 6 months would qualify as renal damage as per the SDI. Several exceptions exist—for example, irreversible events such as myocardial infarction and cerebrovascular accident qualify for scoring immediately at occurrence. Thus, while persistence is fundamental for some features of damage according to SDI (e.g. renal damage), other features qualify the construct of damage upon occurrence (e.g. stroke). Additionally, events such as cataracts that occur after diagnosis and require surgical intervention are scored as damage given their contribution to disease burden.

As SLE is a multisystem, complex illness that varies with time, accurate assessment of damage lies in the development of standardized instruments that have demonstrable psychometric properties. With this in mind, the development of a damage index began.

## Conceptualization and Development of a Damage Index

The importance of measuring damage was highlighted during the 1985 Conference of Prognosis Studies in SLE, with initial development of what is now known as the Systemic Lupus International Collaborating Clinics (SLICC)/American College of Rheumatology (ACR) damage index (SDI) underway in 1991 [4, 5]. The working group tasked with the development of the SDI included members of the North Atlantic Treaty Organization (NATO) as well as rheumatologists with expertise in the assessment of damage [5]. The group sought to reduce discordance amongst raters by first establishing the definition of damage—irreversible change sustained for 6 months since the onset of disease—agreeing the index would not quantify pathologically abnormal tissue.

The group developed the index on the basis of variables present in 20 SLE real patient profiles with documented damage, which could then be tested for validity, reproducibility, and sensitivity for change. In a nominal group process, items were included in the SDI only if they could be differentiated from disease activity, and there was agreement amongst members of the working group [6]. In 1996, 5 years following its initial conceptualization, the SDI was endorsed by the American College of Rheumatology (ACR) and recommended as the damage index for SLE (Fig. 7.1).

a

Visite Date:__________________

**SLICC/ACR DAMAGE INDEX and GLOSSARY OF TERMS**

Damage occurring since diagnosis of lupus, ascertained by clinical assessment and present for at least 6 months unless otherwise stated. Repeat episodes mean at least 6 months apart to score 2. The same lesion cannot be scored twice.

| ITEM | SCORE (circle) |
|---|---|
| **OCULAR** (Either eye, by clinical assessment) | |
| Any cataract ever | 1 |
| Retinal change OR optic atrophy | 1 |
| **NEUROPSYCHIATRIC** | |
| Cognitive impairment (e.g., memory deficit, difficulty with calculation, poor concentration , difficulty in spoken or written language, impaired performance level) OR major psychosis | 1 |
| Seizures requiring therapy for 6 months | 1 |
| Cerebral vascular accident ever (Score 2 if> 1) OR resection not for malignancy | 1 2 |
| Cranial or peripheral neuropathy (excluding optic) | 1 |
| Transverse myelitis | 1 |
| **RENAL** | |
| Estimated or measured GFR <50% | 1 |
| Proteinuria 24 h, ≥3.5 g | 1 |
| OR | |
| End-stage renal disease (regardless of dialysis or transplantation) | 3 |
| **PULMONARY** | |
| Pulmonary hypertension (right ventricular prominence, or loud P2) | 1 |
| Pulmonary fibrosis (physical and X-ray) | 1 |
| Shrinking lung (X-ray) | 1 |
| Pleural fibrosis (X-ray) | 1 |
| Pulmonary infarction (X-ray) OR resection not for malignancy | 1 |
| **CARDIOVASCULAR** | |
| Angina OR coronary artery bypass | 1 |
| Myocardial infarction ever (Score 2 if > 1) | 1 2 |
| Cardiomyopathy (ventricular dysfunction) | 1 |
| Valvular disease (diastolic murmur, or a systolic murmur >3/6) | 1 |
| Pericarditis x 6 months or pericardiectomy | 1 |

**SLICC/ACR DAMAGE INDEX - Page 2**

| ITEM | SCORE |
|---|---|
| **PERIPHERAL VASCULAR** | |
| Claudication x 6 months | 1 |
| Minor tissue loss (pulp space) | 1 |
| Significant tissue loss ever (e.g., loss of digit or limb, resection) (Score 2 if >1) 1 2 | 1 2 |
| Venous thrombosis with swelling , ulceration, OR venous stasis | 1 |
| **GASTROINTESTINAL** | |
| Infarction or resection of bowel (below duodenum), spleen, liver or gallbladder ever (Score 2 if> 1) | 1 2 |
| Mesenteric insufficiency | 1 |
| Chronic peritonitis | 1 |
| Stricture OR upper gastrointestinal tract surgery ever | 1 |
| Pancreatic insufficiency requiring enzyme replacement or with pseudocys | 1 |
| **MUSCULOSKELETAL** | |
| Atrophy or weakness | 1 |
| Deforming or erosive arthritis (including reducible deformities, excluding avascular necrosis) | 1 |
| Osteoporosis with fracture or vertebral collapse (excluding avascular necrosis) | 1 |
| Avascular necrosis (Score 2 if >1) | 1 2 |
| Osteomyelitis | 1 |
| Ruptured tendons | |
| **SKIN** | |
| Alopecia | 1 |
| Extensive scarring or panniculum other than scalp and pulp space | 1 |
| Skin ulceration (excluding thrombosis) for more than 6 months | 1 |
| **PREMATURE GONADAL FAILURE** | 1 |
| **DIABETES** (regardless of treatment) | 1 |
| **MALIGNANCY** (Exclude dysplasia) | 1 2 |
| **TOTAL SCORE** | |

**Fig. 7.1** (**a**) SLICC/ACR damage index with weighted damage score in 12 systems. (**b**) SLICC/ACR damage index glossary of terms

**b**

Visit Date: ________________

**SLICC/ACR DAMAGE INDEX**
**GLOSSARY OF TERMS**

**Damage:** Non-reversible change, not related to active inflammation, occurring since diagnosis of lupus, ascertained by clinical assessment and present for at least 6 months unless otherwise stated. Repeat episodes mean at least 6 months apart to score 2. The same lesion cannot be scored twice.

**Cataract:** A lens opacity (cataract) in either eye, ever, whether primary or secondary to steroid therapy, documented by ophthalmoscopy.

**Retinal change:** Documented by ophthalmoscopic examination, may result in field defect, legal blindness.

**Optic atrophy:** Documented by ophthalmoscopic examination.

**Cognitive impairment:** Memory deficit, difficulty with calculation, poor concentration, difficulty in spoken or written language, impaired performed level, documented on clinical examination, or by formal neurocognitive testing.

**Major psychosis:** Altered ability to function in normal activity due to psychiatric reasons. Severe disturbance in the perception of reality characterized by the following features: delusions, hallucinations (auditory, visual), incoherence, marked loose associations, impoverished thought content, marked illogical thinking, bizarre, disorganized or catatonic behavior.

**Seizures:** Paroxysmal electrical discharge occurring in the brain and producing characteristic physical changes including tonic and clonic movements and certain behavioral disorders. Only seizures requiring therapy for 6 months are counted as damage.

**CVA:** Cerebral vascular accident resulting in focal findings such as paresis, weakness, etc, OR surgical resection for causes other than malignancy.

**Neuropathy:** Damage to either a cranial or peripheral nerve, excluding optic nerve, resulting in either motor or sensory dysfunction.

**Transverse myelitis:** Lower extremity weakness or sensory loss with loss of rectal and urinary bladder sphincter control.

**Renal:** Estimated or measured GFR <50%, proteinuria 2::3.5 gin 24 hours, or end-stage renal disease (regardless of dialysis or transplantation).

**Pulmonary:** Pulmonary hypertension (right ventricular prominence, or loud P2), pulmonary fibrosis (physical and X-ray), shrinking lung (X-ray), pleural fibrosis (X-ray), pulmonary infarction (X-ray), a resection for cause other than malignancy.

**Cardiovascular:** Angina or coronary artery bypass, myocardial infarction (documented by EKG and enzymes) ever, cardiomyopathy (ventricular dysfunction documented clinically), valvular disease (diastolic murmur, or a systolic murmur >316), pericarditis x 6 months pericardiectomy.

**Peripheral vascular:**
Claudication, persistent for 6 months, by history.
Minor tissue loss, such as pulp space, ever.
Significant tissue loss, such as loss of digit or limb, or resection, ever.
Venous thrombosis with swelling, ulceration, or clinical evidence of venous stasis.

**Gastrointestinal:**
Infarction or resection of bowel below duodenum, by history.
Resection of spleen, liver or gallbladder ever, for whatever cause.
Mesenteric insufficiency, with diffuse abdominal pain on clinical examination.
Chronic peritonitis, with persistent abdominal pain and peritoneal irritations, on clinical examination.
Oesophageal stricture, shown on endoscopy.
Upper gastrointestinal tract surgery, such as correction of stricture, ulcer surgery, etc., ever, by history.
Pancreatic insufficiency requiring enzyme replacement or with a pseudocyst.

**Musculoskeletal:**
Muscle atrophy or weakness, demonstrated on clinical examination.
Deforming or erosive arthritis, including reducible deformities (excluding avascular necrosis), on clinical examination.
Osteoporosis with fracture or vertebral collapse (excluding avascular necrosis) demonstrated on X-ray.
Avascular necrosis, demonstrated on any imaging technique.
Osteomyelitis, documented clinically, and supported by culture evidence.
Tendon ruptures.

**Skin:**
Scarring, chronic alopecia, documented clinically.
Extensive scarring or panniculum other than scalp and pulp space, documented clinically.
Skin ulceration (excluding thrombosis) for more than 6 months.

**Premature gonadal failure:** Secondary amenorrhea, prior to age 40.

**Diabetes:** Diabetes requiring therapy, but regardless of treatment.

**Malignancy:** Documented by pathology, excluding dysplasias.

**Fig. 7.1** (continued)

## SLICC/ACR Damage Index (SDI) and Adaptations

The SDI remains largely unchanged from the time of its inception and is the gold standard for assessing damage in SLE clinical and research settings. The index applies a weighted damage score to 12 systems: ocular (range 0–2), neuropsychiatric (0–6), renal (0–3), pulmonary (0–5), cardiovascular (0–6), peripheral vascular (0–5), gastrointestinal (0–6), musculoskeletal (0–7), skin (0–3), diabetes (0–1), gonadal (0–1), and malignancies (0–2). Unlike measures of disease activity, items do not require direct attribution to SLE to score. Of note, the haematological system was historically excluded from the SDI as the initial working group believed it would be difficult to distinguish transient drug-related cytopenia (e.g. thrombocytopenia, leukopenia) from true irreversible damage [6].

The index is clinician administered and can take up to 15 minutes to complete for a complex patient unknown to the clinician. The index was designed for accessibility amongst various centres, with scoring based on easily accessible tests and clinical judgement. Serious events such as end-stage renal disease (ESRD) and malignancies score higher on the index, with additional points for recurrent events that occur a minimum of 6 months apart. By definition, the SDI at diagnosis is 0, with damage stable or increasing over time up to a theoretical maximum of 47 points. Patients rarely score above 10 on the SDI, with a study of 146 Toronto Lupus Clinic patients initially scoring 1.3 and subsequently 2.3 over an 8.2-year interval, representing an increase of 1.08 in 54.8% of patients over this time [7]. A separate study of 2054 patients at Johns Hopkins followed for 6.4 years corroborated these findings, showing a yearly 0.13 increase in the SDI score following SLE diagnosis [8].

The original SDI has only been validated in the English language and, as intended during its original design, does not quantify pathologically abnormal tissue or assess the impact of damage on patients' lives. A modified, patient-administered adaptation of the SDI, the Lupus Damage Index Questionnaire (LDIQ) was developed in 2010 and is available in Spanish, French, and Portuguese. The LDIQ was originally developed for use where physician assessment is unavailable, although its reliability and validity in longitudinal studies have not yet been demonstrated to the same degree as the SDI [9].

## Psychometric Properties: Putting SDI to the Test

### *Validity Measures*

Content and face validity were obtained by members of the working group during initial development of the SDI, as items were only retained if there was agreement amongst members. In 1996, the instrument was distributed to 18 individuals who were not members of the SLICC group—16 of 17 individuals agreed with index scores from physicians at the original conference [6]. It should be noted that although reviewers agreed with the content of the index, there were several points of discussion, including whether cytopenia should be included as it may reflect drug toxicity, and whether hypertension should be included as it may reflect renal damage or glucocorticoid therapy. In the final index, neither were included as features of damage as both items were considered difficult to distinguish from disease activity.

Discriminant validity of the index was established in a study where 19 SLICC members completed the index based on 42 case scenarios comprised of two assessments each 5 years apart. The index was shown to identify changes in damage in patients with both active and inactive disease. The damage score did not change significantly in patients who were identified as stable, and there was a larger change in damage score amongst patients with active disease at both time points, compared with patients thought to have inactive disease at both time points. With the aim of confirming construct validity, Stoll et al. compared the SDI with the British Isles Lupus Assessment Group (BILAG) index and patients' medication scores, noting a low correlation with both (0.19 with BILAG and 0.33 for the medication index) [10].

## Reliability and Sensitivity to Change

Analyses of variance revealed the SDI score did not differ by physician rater (observer effect $p = 0.93$) or order in which the physician saw patients (order effect $p = 0.26$). As such, the index has been shown to detect differences amongst patients without rater differences, with physicians from different centres and healthcare systems (five countries, ten lupus centres) able to record accumulated damage for a particular patient in the same way among different raters. There was concordance in damage index scores amongst raters despite a wide variation in disease activity amongst included patients as detected by the Systemic Lupus Erythematosus Disease Activity Index (SLEDAI) [11]. This study further corroborated previous studies that noted no correlation between disease activity and damage scores and consolidated the concept of damage as an independent domain in the assessment of SLE [12–14].

With consideration of sensitivity to change, members of the SLICC followed damage scores for patients in their centres for up to 10 years, demonstrating SDI scores' ability to increase over time, with higher scores in patients who passed away [15].

## Predicative Ability

The risks of mortality and damage accrual are significantly higher in individuals with higher damage scores at baseline and over time, supported by several prospective and retrospective studies. In a cohort of 263 patients followed at the Toronto Lupus Clinic, 25% of patients who exhibited damage on first assessment died within

10 years compared to a 7.3% 10-year mortality in those who had no early damage. Patients who died within 10 years were more likely to have renal damage and a trend towards cardiovascular disease [16]. These results corroborated other studies, including a prospective study that showed SDI scores were predictive of hospitalization and death, and a separate study that noted more rapid damage accrual in deceased patients as compared to survivors over a 3-year span [17, 18].

Another 10-year retrospective study of 80 SLE patients supported these findings, revealing renal damage at 1 year is predictive of ESRD and that pulmonary damage at 1 year is predictive of death at year 10 of follow-up [19].

Additionally, glucocorticoid treatment has been shown to predict damage. A study of patients with childhood-onset SLE suggested that high-dose glucocorticoids, though highly effective for controlling disease features, can be an important cause of damage. In this study, it was further suggested that immunosuppressive agents may have a protective effect against disease damage [20].

## Critical Appraisal and Overall Value of SDI

Several key factors are important to consider when choosing a specific metric beside its psychometric properties on reliability and validity—ease of use, associated administrative burden and cost, score calculation, and interpretability. The SDI confers several advantages, including ease of administration and scoring and accessibility within the clinical setting. The index takes a maximum of 15 minutes to complete and is scored on the basis of clinical judgement and easily accessible tests such as urinalysis or chest radiography. Furthermore, the index has garnered widespread acceptance in the research community given it can reflect change over time, proving useful when comparing accumulated damage in different arms of randomized trials.

With consideration of pediatric populations, the current index may not reflect developmental damage such as pubertal delay and growth abnormalities. The applicability of the index in pediatric populations has been further called into question given the majority of items are specific to adult populations (lack of face validity in pediatric populations), including myocardial infarction, malignancies, cataracts, and claudication—sequelae of damage rarely seen in children. Additionally, the irreversibility of damage in children has been challenged for several items, as avascular necrosis may have potential for regeneration in pediatric populations. Given these challenges, a pediatric version of the SDI (Ped-SDI) has been developed. This modified index includes items specific to pubertal delay and reduced final height and delineates new height- and weight-based proteinuria cutoffs for younger children. However, it should be noted that regular use of the Ped-SDI may jeopardize the translation and applicability of long-term pediatric to adult studies [21].

With regard to the descriptors associated with the SDI, one area of potential improvement may lie in the definition of damage proposed. The current index specifies that items may only score after the diagnosis of SLE is made—however, this definition may exclude damage attributable to disease that occurred prior to official diagnosis. As such, the index may not accurately reflect damage early in disease course. Venous thrombosis may be an example of early damage occurring prior to the diagnosis, with the first event not prompting a full autoimmune workup and the diagnosis made some time after this inciting event. As a result, the SDI final score may not accurately reflect accrued damage from SLE. The SLICC Frailty Index (FI), a novel measure in SLE, may address these concerns by incorporating damage incurred prior to diagnosis, serving as a useful prognosticator early in disease. The index is comprised of 48 items relating to damage, disease activity, comorbidities, and functional status. Preliminary studies demonstrate internal validity and suggest the tool may be used to predict future mortality risk [22].

Individual items in the SDI may benefit from further standardization to reflect current clinical guidelines and evidence-based medicine. For example, the psychiatric and cognitive impairment descriptors may benefit from inclusion of neurocognitive batteries recommended by the European League Against Rheumatism (EULAR) and the ACR. Additionally, the pulmonary component of the index, which is presently scored on the basis of a loud P2 or right ventricular prominence, may benefit from standardization by inclusion of echocardiogram results which are used to establish the diagnosis in practice. Similarly, the pulmonary section of the SDI may be expanded to include computed tomography (CT) results, as this readily available imaging modality is superior to chest radiography in detecting pulmonary fibrosis. With regard to the cardiovascular component, one potential area for improvement may be the definition of myocardial infarction (content validity), which requires corroboration by EKG and cardiac enzymes—this definition may benefit from further clarification regarding scoring of acute coronary syndrome and whether NSTEMI qualifies for scoring as myocardial infarction. Additionally, the peripheral vascular section may benefit from inclusion of the ankle-brachial index (ABI) to further corroborate claudication, which the descriptor currently scores solely on the basis of clinical history. With consideration of the musculoskeletal section descriptor, the osteomyelitis descriptor in particular may benefit from removal of culture results, as the diagnosis is often made on the basis of clinical judgement and imaging modalities, particularly magnetic resonance imaging (MRI). Finally, the endocrinology section may benefit from a definition of diabetes on the basis of HbA1c and blood glucose cutoffs, commonly accessible tests used to confirm diagnosis and initiate treatment and the addition of thyroid disease.

Returning to the definition of damage as irreversible organ dysfunction, the 6-month cutoff to score items may require further examination. For example, in the current index, renal damage is scored by presence of proteinuria for at least 6 months. Current literature reveals proteinuria recovery can be slow and not necessarily irreversible, with a study from Touma et al. revealing recovery can take up to 2 years with approximately additional 20% of patients recovering by year 5. As such, the persistence of proteinuria for 6 months may not be necessarily representative of irreversible damage as currently documented in the SDI [23]. Of note, proteinuria associated with membranous nephropathy may take even longer to recover than proliferative subtypes with a more unfavourable prognosis, calling into question the face validity of this renal item [24]. In a larger sense, several SDI descriptors, such as nephrotic range of proteinuria, may lack sufficient face validity and require further studies to confirm validity of psychometric properties.

One of the fundamental aims of the SDI is to differentiate between active SLE disease and damage. While this is straightforward and clearly elucidated with the majority of its items, the definition of chronic peritonitis may require further examination. This item is defined on the basis of persistent abdominal pain and irritation on examination, which can also be related to lupus serositis (active disease). Within this particular descriptor, it would be important to clarify that peritonitis should be scored under damage only if the pain and irritation are not attributable to SLE disease activity. Similarly, another item that may benefit from further examination is renal damage as defined by a GFR < 50%. While it is not very common to have a GFR < 50% for 6 months followed by normalisation of kidney function or improvement in GFR above this cutoff, it is crucial to clarify the content and face validity of this item. This item may benefit from parameters specifying that this item should not be scored in the context of active lupus nephritis during induction and maintenance therapy, whereby patients may experience improvement with time. As the SDI is a weighted index, one potential solution may lie in designating lower scores to items that can improve over time, such as GFR. Pulmonary hypertension is another example of this, as it is often responsive to glucocorticoids and immunosuppressants in SLE patients when related to vasculitis as opposed to pulmonary embolism. It is critical to clarify if transient pulmonary hypertension lasting 6–12 months or longer is associated with permanent damage.

Finally, the index may benefit from inclusion of additional items that reflect damage associated with SLE. The cardiovascular section can be expanded to include arrhythmogenic sequelae associated with pericarditis and myopericarditis, particularly if such events necessitate the use of anti-arrhythmic medications which may confer organ damage (such as in the case of amiodarone). With further consideration of medication-related damage, glucocorticoid damage is indirectly captured by items such as cataracts, osteoporotic fractures, avascular necrosis, and diabetes mellitus. The SDI may be expanded to capture damage as it relates to other antimalarial and immunosuppressants/biologic agents. As an example, hydroxychloroquine administration can be associated with ophthalmologic (retinopathy, corneal changes), otic (hearing impairment, tinnitus), cardiomyopathy, neuromuscular, and dermatologic toxicity that can be captured in the index as additional items. Similarly, mycophenolate mofetil therapy has been associated with herpes zoster involvement—this can result in persistent and painful postherpetic neuralgia that can be captured in a revised version of the damage index.

## Next Steps

Despite areas for further improvement, the SDI is the most widespread tool used to assess damage in SLE given the number of studies confirming several of its psychometric properties. Future studies should focus on updating the SDI with the following amendments in mind: (1) identification of novel descriptors that can be added to SDI—descriptors that can be identified through systematic reviews of the literature, surveys of experts in the field, etc.; (2) assessment of the face validity and content validity of SDI descriptors and their association with damage (e.g. nephrotic proteinuria, chronic peritonitis, and transient pulmonary hypertension); (3) revisiting the weighted scoring approach of SDI particularly for items where improvement over time is possible (e.g. GFR < 50%); and (4) as several items are significantly related to the use of glucocorticoids, it would be important to derive a system that would allow raters to attribute damage to either SLE activity, glucocorticoids use, both, or miscellaneous. This would provide meaningful information within both a clinical and research setting and further our understanding of damage in SLE.

## References


1. Gladman DD, Urowitz MB. Morbidity in systemic lupus erythematosus. J Rheumatol Suppl. 1987;14(Suppl 13):s223–6.
2. Urowitz MB, et al. Biomodal mortality pattern of SLE. Am J Med. 1976;60:221–5.
3. Touma Z, Gladman DD, Urowitz MB. Clinical measures, metrics, and indices. In: Wallace DJ, Hahn BH, editors. Dubois' lupus erythematosus. 8th ed. Saunders: Lippincott Williams & Wilkins; 2012.
4. Bombardier C, et al. Derivation of the SLEDAI. A disease activity index for lupus patients. The Committee on Prognosis Studies in SLE. Arthritis Rheum. 1992;35:630–40.
5. Gladman DD, Ginzler E, Goldsmith C, et al. Workshop report: systemic lupus international collaborative clinics (SLICC): development of a damage index in SLE. J Rheumatol. 1992;19:1820–1.
6. Gladman DD, Ginzler E, Goldsmith C, et al. Developemental and validation SLICC/ACR for SLE. Arthritis Rheum. 1996;39:363–9.
7. Kuriya B, et al. Quality of life over time in patients with systemic lupus erythematosus. Arthritis Rheum. 2008;59:181–5.
8. Petri M, Purvey S, Fang H, Magder LS. Predictors of organ damage in systemic lupus erythematosus: the Hopkins' Lupus Cohort. Arthritis Rheum. 2012;64:4021–8.
9. Costenbader KH, Khamashta M, Ruiz-Garcia S, et al. Development and initial validation of the self-assessed lupus damage index questionnaire (LDIQ). Arthritis Care Res (Hoboken). 2010;62:559–68.
10. Stoll T, Stucki G, Malik J, Pyke S, Isenberg DA. Association of the Systemic Lupus International Collaborating Clinics/American College of Rheumatology Damage Index with measures of disease activity and health status in patients with systemic lupus erythematosus. J Rheumatol. 1997;24:309–13.
11. Gladman DD, Urowitz MB, Goldsmith CH, et al. The reliability of the Systemic Lupus International Collaborating Clinics/American College of Rheumatology Damage Index in patients with systemic lupus erythematosus. Arthritis Rheum. 1997;40:809–13.
12. Gorgos L, Goldman D, Petri M. The ACR=SLICC damage index in systemic lupus erythematosus (SLE). Arthritis Rheum. 1993;36(Suppl 9):S68. (abstract).
13. Fortin PR, Fraenkel L, Danoff D, Abrahamowicz M. Clinical predictors of function in systemic lupus erythematosus. Arthritis Rheum. 1994;37(Suppl 9):S326. (abstract).
14. Gladman D, Urowitz M, Ong A, et al. Lack of correlation among 3 outcome measures in SLE: disease activity, damage and quality of life. Clin Exp Rheumatol. 1996;14:305–8.

15. Gladman DD, Goldsmith CH, Urowitz MB, et al. The Systemic Lupus International Collaborating Clinics/American College of Rheumatology (SLICC/ACR) Damage Index for Systemic Lupus Erythematosus International Comparison. J Rheumatol. 2000;27:373–6.
16. Rahman P, Gladman DD, Urowitz MB, Hallett D, Tam LS. Early damage as measured by the SLICC=ACR damage index is a predictor of mortality in systemic lupus erythematosus. Lupus. 2001;10:93–6.
17. Fortin PR, Feland D, Clarke AE, et al. Activity and damage predict later flares in lupus. Arthritis Rheum. 1997;40(Suppl 9):S207.
18. Bastian HM, Mickail I, Straatpm KV, et al. Factors associated with early death in African-American and Hispanic patients with SLE. Arthritis Rheum. 1997;40(Suppl 9):S160.
19. Stoll T, Seifert B, Isenberg DA. SLICC=ACR Damage Index is valid, and renal and pulmonary organ scores are predictors of severe outcome in patients with systemic lupus erythematosus. Br J Rheumatol. 1996;35:248–54.
20. Brunner HI, Silverman ED, To T, Bombardier C, Feldman BM. Risk factors for damage in childhood-onset systemic lupus erythematosus: cumulative disease activity and medication use predict disease damage. Arthritis Rheum. 2002;46:436–44.
21. Lattenzi B, et al. Measures of disease activity and damage in pediatric systemic lupus erythematosus: British Isles Lupus Assessment Group (BILAG), European Consensus Lupus Activity Measurement (ECLAM), Systemic Lupus Activity Measure (SLAM), Systemic Lupus Erythematosus Disease Activity Index (SLEDAI), Physician's Global Assessment of Disease Activity (MD Global), and Systemic Lupus International Collaborating Clinics/American College of Rheumatology Damage Index (SLICC/ACR DI; SDI). Arthritis Care Res (Hoboken). 2011;63(Suppl 11):S112–7.
22. Legge A, et al. Evaluating the properties of a frailty index and its association with mortality risk among patients with systemic lupus erythematosus. Arthritis Rheumatol. 2019;71:1297–307.
23. Touma Z, Urowitz MB, Ibañez D, Gladman DD. Time to recovery from proteinuria in patients with lupus nephritis receiving standard treatment. J Rheumatol. 2014;41:688–97. https://doi.org/10.3899/jrheum.130005.
24. Schieppati A, Mosconi L, Perna A, Mecca G, Bertani T, Garattini S, Remuzzi G. Prognosis of untreated patients with idiopathic membranous nephropathy. N Engl J Med. 1993;329(2):85–9.

# Chapter 8
# Metrics and Outcome Measures of Disease Activity and Damage in Childhood-Onset Systemic Lupus Erythematosus

**Pinar Ozge Avar-Aydin, Katherine Schultz, and Hermine I. Brunner**

## Abbreviations

| | |
|---|---|
| ACR | American College of Rheumatology |
| BILAG | British Isles Lupus Assessment Group |
| CHILI | Childhood Lupus Improvement Index |
| CHQ | Child Health Questionnaire |
| CHQ-P50 | 50-item parent-proxy report of CHQ |
| CLASI | Cutaneous Lupus Erythematosus Disease Area and Severity Index |
| CRI | Clinically relevant improvement |
| cSLE | Childhood-onset systemic lupus erythematosus |
| ECLAM | European Consensus Lupus Activity Measurement |
| FDI | Functional Disability Inventory |
| GFR | Glomerular filtration rate |
| HRQoL | Health-related quality of life |
| LN | Lupus nephritis |
| PedANAM | Pediatric Automated Neuropsychological Assessment Metrics |
| PedsQL | Pediatric Quality of Life Inventory |
| PedsQL-MFS | Pediatric Quality of Life Multidimensional Fatigue Scale |
| PedsQL-GC | Pediatric Quality of Life 4.0 Generic Core Scale |
| PedsQL-RM | Pediatric Quality of Life 3.0 Rheumatology Module |
| PGA | Physician global assessment |

P. O. Avar-Aydin
Department of Pediatric Rheumatology, Ankara University School of Medicine, Ankara, Turkey
e-mail: pinar.ozge.avar.aydin@ankara.edu.tr

K. Schultz · H. I. Brunner (✉)
Department of Rheumatology, Cincinnati Children's Hospital Medical Center, Cincinnati, OH, USA
e-mail: katherine.schultz@cchmc.org; hermine.brunner@cchmc.org



Z. Touma (ed.), *Outcome Measures and Metrics in Systemic Lupus Erythematosus*, https://doi.org/10.1007/978-3-030-73303-2_8

| | |
|---|---|
| PhS | Physical summary score |
| PRINTO | Pediatric Rheumatology International Trials Organization |
| PRO | Patient-reported outcome |
| PROMIS | Patient-Reported Outcomes Measurement Information System |
| pSkindex-27 | Pediatric Skindex-27 |
| PsS | Psychosocial summary score |
| QoL | Quality of life |
| RAIL | Renal Activity Index for Lupus Nephritis |
| SDI | Systemic Lupus International Collaborating Clinics/American College of Rheumatology Damage Index |
| SELENA | Safety of Estrogens in Lupus National Assessment |
| SLAM | Systemic Lupus Activity Measure |
| SLAQ | Systemic Lupus Activity Questionnaire |
| SLE | Systemic lupus erythematosus |
| SLEDAI | Systemic Lupus Erythematosus Disease Activity Index |
| SMILEY | Simple Measure of Impact of Lupus Erythematosus in Youngsters |
| SRI | Systemic Lupus Erythematosus Responder Index |

## Introduction

Childhood-onset systemic lupus erythematosus (cSLE) is a complex, chronic autoimmune disease with relapsing and remitting episodes of inflammation. The disease continues to pose diagnostic and therapeutic challenges, especially during episodes of uncontrolled disease activity. A multidisciplinary approach to develop individualized treatment strategies is essential to successfully manage cSLE, prevent damage, and, by extension, improve patient outcomes. To characterize the disease status and the course of cSLE and its impact on patients' daily lives, global and organ-specific indices or scales have been developed. Patient-reported outcome (PRO) measures are used to capture the effects of cSLE on patient health-related quality of life (HRQoL), i.e., everyday functioning and physical, emotional, and social well-being. This chapter discusses global and organ-specific disease activity and damage measures, measures of change in disease activity and response to therapy, pediatric-specific measures of clinically relevant change, and HRQoL measures that have been validated for use in cSLE.

## Disease Measures of Global Disease Activity

Given the absence of a laboratory test or clinical features to measure the degree of inflammation from systemic lupus erythematosus (SLE), a series of disease activity measures have been developed for adults with SLE and subsequently validated for use in children (Table 8.1).

**Table 8.1** Measures of global disease activity validated for use in cSLE

| | Time frame | Number of items | Summary score | Strengths | Cautions | Key reference for use in cSLE |
|---|---|---|---|---|---|---|
| SLEDAI/ SLEDAI-2000 (or 2K) | 10 days/30 days | 24 | 0–105 | Ease of use<br>SLEDAI-2K score ≤4 is often considered as controlled cSLE<br>Can identify flare in cSLE<br>Renal domain score can be used to assess LN disease activity clinically | No important cautions | [7, 12, 20] |
| SLAM | 4 weeks | 23 | 0–81 | Ease of use<br>Able to capture degree of disease activity per organ system | Relies on subjective patient reporting of symptoms<br>Has more items to measure than other tools | [12] |
| pBILAG-2004 | 3 months | 8 | A, B, C, D, E | Provides detailed information on specific organ involvement<br>Commonly used in clinical trials of cSLE | Complex and requires significant time to score<br>BILAG flare tool validated in cSLE but not recommended for routine use | [12, 18] |
| ECLAM | 4 weeks | 15 | 0–10 | No important advantages over other disease activity tools | Some items lack strict definitions | [19, 20] |

*SLEDAI/SLEDAI-2K* Systemic Lupus Erythematosus Disease Activity Index, *SLAM* Systemic Lupus Activity Measure, *pBILAG-2004* pediatric British Isles Assessment Group, *ECLAM* European Consensus Lupus Activity Measurement, *cSLE* childhood-onset systemic lupus erythematosus

## *Systemic Lupus Erythematosus Disease Activity Index*

One of the most recognized and utilized disease activity measure is the Systemic Lupus Erythematosus Disease Activity Index (SLEDAI), developed in 1985 and revised in 2002 [1–3]. As a measure of global disease activity, the 24 items are all objectively measurable clinical and laboratory features of a patient during the 10 days preceding the scoring of the SLEDAI [2, 4]. The SLEDAI items can be categorized into nine organ domains; they are rated as present or absent based on the provided item definitions, without further grading by severity [5]. Item scores of 8 points are given for central nervous system and vascular, 4 points for renal and musculoskeletal, 2 for serosal/dermatologic/immunologic, and 1 point for constitutional and hematologic items, respectively [3]. The SLEDAI summary score ranges from 0 to 105, though in practice few cSLE patients reach scores over 20–45 [3–5]. In terms of clinical parameters, the initial SLEDAI only counted proteinuria, rash, alopecia, and mucous membrane lesions at their first occurrence or upon recurrence; this was done to separate out acute from chronic lesions, with the thought that chronic lesions may represent damage from the disease rather than the disease itself [2]. In 2002, the SLEDAI was modified to allow for these features to be counted more than once. Known as the SLEDAI-2000 (or SLEDAI-2K, referred to as SLEDAI from here on), persistent active alopecia, inflammatory mucous membrane lesions, inflammatory rash, and proteinuria >0.5 g/24 hour are all scored [6]. Laboratory measures in the SLEDAI include autoantibodies, complement, and renal and hematologic parameters. Based on the SLEDAI summary score, SLE may be defined as inactive (SLEDAI = 0), mildly active (SLEDAI = 1–5), moderately active (SLEDAI = 6–10), highly active (SLEDAI = 11–19), and of very high activity (SLEDAI = ≥20) [5]. SLEDAI scores of ≤4 in cSLE are considered to reflect controlled disease. The SLEDAI is responsive to worsening and improvement of cSLE disease activity, and recent literature demonstrates that it can help to identify flare in cSLE. The SLEDAI is easy to complete and simple to score, making it ideal for use in both clinical and research purposes [7].

## *Safety of Estrogens in Lupus National Assessment-Systemic Lupus Erythematosus Disease Activity Index and Flare Tool*

Adapted from the SLEDAI, the Safety of Estrogens in Lupus National Assessment-Systemic Lupus Erythematosus Disease Activity Index (SELENA-SLEDAI) was created for evaluation in the Safety of Estrogens in Lupus National Assessment study [8]. This global disease index was intended to account for persistently active disease and therefore modified the SLEDAI to include rash, alopecia, and mucocutaneous lesions if they were ongoing [8]. It also specified that hematuria that could be attributed to menstrual bleeding did not count in the scoring system [8]. The measurement properties of the SELENA-SLEDAI are comparable to those of the

SLEDAI when used in cSLE [9]. While the SELENA-SLEDAI was initially thought to be advantageous as it could define flares, studies in cSLE did not demonstrate the efficacy of the tool; in fact, its efficacy was found to be <50% [10]. Therefore, this tool and its subsequent SELENA flare index are not recommended in cSLE.

## *Systemic Lupus Activity Measure*

The Systemic Lupus Activity Measure (SLAM) is a global disease measurement tool that scores disease activity over a 4-week period, originally created in 1988 and revised in 1991 [4, 8]. The SLAM also considers subjective features of cSLE, such as fatigue, arthralgias, and myalgias. The SLAM considers 23 clinical manifestations grouped in 9 different organ systems and 7 laboratory features. SLAM summary scores range from 0 to 81 and reflect the sum of the SLAM item scores which range from 0 to 3, depending on whether there are new manifestations or if the severity within the last month increased [8]. A change of SLAM summary score exceeding 7 is considered clinically relevant in cSLE [11, 12]. When compared to the SLEDAI and the British Isles Lupus Assessment Group (BILAG; see below) in a pediatric population, the SLAM possessed similarly strong psychometric properties [12, 13].

The strength of the SLAM is that the degree of disease activity per organ system can be captured [8]. A shortcoming might be that there is a reliance on subjective patient reporting of symptoms and the measure has more items than the SLEDAI [8, 13]. Despite this, the SLAM is user-friendly and may have more granularity when monitoring cSLE in clinical settings [13].

## *Systemic Lupus Activity Questionnaire*

The Systemic Lupus Activity Questionnaire (SLAQ) is a measure of disease activity based on patient self-report, requiring about 10 minutes for completion [14]. It serves as an initial screening method to identify patients with increased disease activity who may need clinical evaluation. The 29 SLAQ items were adapted from those used in the SLAM. Items are grouped in nine organ systems where symptoms of disease activity are scored on a 4-point Likert scale (no problem, mild, moderate, and severe) and item weighting is aligned with those used in the SLAM. There is also a single numerical rating scale (range 0–10) of patient self-reported disease activity in the preceding 3 months. The SLAQ summary score ranges from 0 to 44. It correlates well with the physician-completed SLAM. The SLAQ has excellent reliability and construct validity in population studies, which found that SLAQ scores are significantly higher during an SLE flare and correlate strongly with general measures of health status [15]. A SLAQ score of 9 or higher has 83% sensitivity and 70% specificity for capturing clinically relevant disease activity in adults with

SLE [14, 16]. However, the responsiveness to change of the SLAQ seems lower than that of other disease activity tools in SLE [14, 15].

Although the SLAQ has not been compared head-to-head to other disease activity measures in cSLE, the SLAQ summary score is moderately to strongly correlated with Child Health Questionnaire (CHQ) health concept scores when used in cSLE [17]. Taken together, the SLAQ may be useful for home monitoring of cSLE activity by the parents and older patients with cSLE to alert physicians for further assessments when SLAQ summary scores are worsening.

## British Isles Lupus Assessment Group Index

The BILAG Index is the most comprehensive lupus assessment measurement [13]. The BILAG was initially developed with the idea of incorporating the physician's intention to treat principle. Items are scored as on a 4-point Likert scale (new, same, worse, or improving) [13]. The BILAG was updated in 2004 and subsequently modified for use in cSLE (pBILAG); an assessment time frame of 3 months was also used. The pBILAG-2004 consists of alphabetical scores (A–E) assigned to eight organ domains, where A = severe disease requiring change in corticosteroids or disease-modifying immunosuppression; B = moderate disease activity; C = stable disease activity not requiring treatment alterations; D = inactive disease but with history of organ involvement; and E = no history of organ involvement [18]. Alphabetical scores were further categorized into numerical values, where A = 9, B = 3, C = 1, and D/E = 0 [18]. The BILAG has been validated for use in cSLE [10, 12]. The pBILAG-2004 is advantageous as it provides quite detailed information on specific organ involvement when compared against the SLEDAI [18]. Nonetheless, the BILAG and pBILAG are rarely used in clinical settings due to the time needed for scoring. However, the BILAG is commonly used in clinical trials of SLE and cSLE and is a component of response measures used in clinical trials.

## European Consensus Lupus Activity Measurement

The European Consensus Lupus Activity Measurement (ECLAM) is a global disease measurement examining 15 clinical and serological items, each scoring 0–10, over the preceding month [4]. It has been shown to have strong validity in predicting disease damage, the need for steroids, and disease improvement [13]. The ECLAM seems comparable to the SLEDAI for predicting disease damage and response to therapy in a 6-month period and actually may be more responsive to clinically relevant change in cSLE activity than the SLEDAI [13, 19]. Further evidence supports the use of ECLAM in cSLE, with a strong correlation of it to the modified SLEDAI-2K [20].

Arguably, the ECLAM is preferable to the SLEDAI and SLAM due to its superior psychometric properties, but critics point out that vague definitions of some of the ECLAM items by far outweigh any such advantage [13]. Examples of vague item definitions include a lack of a clearly defined time frame during which symptom changes must occur or "evolve" and what counts as a "significant" drop in complement levels [13].

## Disease Measure of Global Damage in cSLE

With the introduction of immunosuppression, patients with SLE are living longer and facing increasing morbidity due to disease activity. Damage in SLE can be from current clinical inflammation or medication side effects or accumulated after long-standing inflammation [21, 22]. There have been numerous risk factors for damage found in adults with SLE, including age and disease activity at diagnosis, duration of SLE, ethnicity (African, Caribbean, or Asian), and steroid use [23]. In children, the presence of antiphospholipid antibodies or thrombocytopenia and therapy with corticosteroids have been found to be risk factors for increased predisposal to damage [22]. There is only one measure of disease damage for use in adults, the Systemic Lupus International Collaborating Clinics/American College of Rheumatology Damage Index (SDI). For cSLE, a pediatric adaptation has been suggested (Ped-SDI) [24]. This means there are strictly spoken two damage indices that may be used to capture irreversible organ and tissue scarring for use in children with cSLE.

### *Systemic Lupus International Collaborating Clinics/American College of Rheumatology Damage Index*

As a means of capturing the damage wrought by SLE, the SDI was created in 1991 by a group of rheumatologists [21]. It consists of 12 different organ systems and 41 items, with each system scoring up to 6 points [25]. The SDI includes damage that has been developed over time or from medicines [21]. It was initially validated in adults in 1991 [21], and further evaluation has demonstrated that the SDI is sensitive at detecting differences among patients with good agreement between observers [21, 26].

The SDI has also been evaluated as an index for cSLE with concern that the items need to be weighted and defined differently, especially important as children have been found to accumulate disease damage more rapidly than adults [22, 27]. A modified SDI, the Ped-SDI, was proposed in 2006 by Ravelli et al. which consisted of the original items in the SDI plus the addition of growth failure and delayed puberty [24]. The authors further clarified that proteinuria should be adjusted for height and weight. Thus, the Ped-SDI consists of 43 items divided into 14 organ systems or domains for a maximum score of 49 [24].

## Measures of Flare and Response to Therapy for Use in cSLE

An international consensus approached a definition of global disease flare in cSLE as follows: "A flare of disease is a measurable worsening of SLE disease activity in at least one organ system, involving new or worse signs of disease that may be accompanied by new or worse SLE symptoms; depending on the severity of the flare, more intensive therapy may be required." [28]. After more intensive drug therapy, a disease remission can be observed. Clinically relevant improvement was defined with a reduction in disease signs without any increased lupus activity in major organ systems. Symptoms should be stable or decreased [29].

### *BILAG Flare Tool*

Based on the BILAG, the BILAG flare tool has been developed and validated in cSLE [7]. Nonetheless, it is not recommended for use in cSLE, as international consensus among pediatric rheumatologists states that the scores of a disease activity measure alone are not sufficient enough to measure cSLE flares [28].

### *Systemic Lupus Erythematosus Responder Index*

The Systemic Lupus Erythematosus Responder Index (SRI) was created to assess therapeutic efficacy in clinical trials and validated with high specificity but modest sensitivity for cSLE in 2014 [4, 9]. It is composed of the SELENA-SLEDAI (to monitor global disease improvement or worsening), the BILAG (to monitor organ-specific disease improvement or worsening), and physician global assessment (PGA; to serve as validity) [9]. Participants are considered responders if they fulfill all of the following: (1) SELENA-SLEDAI score reduction by ≥4; (2) no new BILAG A and no more than one new BILAG B domain score; and (3) no worsening of PGA by ≥0.3 points [4]. The SRI is a highly specific tool, but because it was found to be only modestly sensitive for capturing clinical improvement, it is considered a conservative estimate of the clinical efficacy of therapeutic agents in cSLE [9]. A post hoc analysis of data from the Phase III belimumab trials in SLE demonstrated that SRI response was associated with meaningful improvements in the clinical, laboratory, and patient-reported outcomes [30]. With the Phase II belimumab trial in cSLE, it was revised and is now known as the SRI4 [31, 32]. Newer data also suggests that the SRI response is associated with a global benefit [32]. Despite this, the SRI is challenging to use in the individual patient in daily clinical practice [4].

## Pediatric-Specific Measures of Clinically Relevant Change in SLE Course

Clinically relevant improvement (CRI) of cSLE is defined as (1) no change or improvement in MD global or disease activity index score and (2) no new organ involvement in neuropsychiatric, hematologic, gastrointestinal, renal, ophthalmologic, or cardiopulmonary systems [29]. This was decided to be the measure against which the Pediatric Rheumatology International Trials Organization provisional criteria (PRINTO/ACR) and the Childhood Lupus Improvement Index (CHILI) were compared (see below).

### *Pediatric Rheumatology International Trials Organization Provisional Criteria of Response to Therapy*

The PRINTO/ACR provisional criteria of response to therapy was developed by experts in pediatric rheumatology using consensus methodology and created to evaluate clinical response to therapy specifically in cSLE [33]. It is composed of an algorithm that evaluates five core set parameters and the percentage change in those parameters [33]. The parameters include the scores of global disease activity, physician assessment of overall disease activity, parent assessment of overall well-being, proteinuria, and the patient HRQoL measure [33]. The definition of improvement includes a score improvement of at least 50% or more from baseline in two core measures, and no more than one of the remaining worsening by more than 30% [34].

The PRINTO/ACR provisional criteria of response to therapy have been found to have high levels of specificity but varying levels of sensitivity [33]. When evaluated for CRI, the PRINTO/ACR provisional criteria were found to have fair accuracy for capturing CRI [29]. The PRINTO/ACR provisional criteria were found to be superior in determining improvement in cSLE when compared to the SRI [29].

### *Childhood Lupus Improvement Index*

A shortcoming of the PRINTO/ACR criteria may be that it is not well suited to capture mild or moderate improvement in cSLE. The CHILI scores range from 0 to 100, with a minimum score of 54 showing 89.5% sensitivity and 92.6% specificity for capturing CRI status correctly. The CHILI also has high accuracy for capturing mild, moderate, and major improvement of cSLE. An advantage of the CHILI compared to the PRINTO/ACR provisional criteria is that it better captures patient perspectives [29].

## Organ-Specific Measures

### *Lupus Nephritis,Response to Therapy and Lupus Nephritis Flare*

A renal biopsy remains the gold standard method for the diagnosis of lupus nephritis (LN) in children, and a lack of clinical improvement or even worsening of LN may prompt a repeat kidney biopsy [35–37]. Despite the advances in procedures, cSLE is still considered a risk factor for complications after kidney biopsy [38]. Kidney involvement in children is more common than among adults and constitutes a potentially fatal complication of cSLE, creating a pressing need for alternative noninvasive methods [39]. Proteinuria, creatinine clearance, and urine sediment have been identified as core renal parameters to define renal response and renal flare during the development of consensus treatment plans for induction therapy of proliferative LN in cSLE [40]. However, the urine sediment is not often used in practice given that urine casts are highly unstable and necessitate urine analysis to be read within 15 minutes. Thus, it is likely that in pediatric LN trials, as already done in adult LN trials, hematuria alone will be used as a reflection of active urine sediment.

Urine proteomic profiling provides a promising noninvasive approach for disease activity, damage, and response to therapy in LN [41]. In addition, urine biomarkers correlate well with the renal composite scores, discriminate proliferative and membranous histologic classes and active LN from inactive LN, and predict LN flares [42–46].

### *Renal Activity Index for Lupus Nephritis*

To improve the accuracy to quantify LN activity without a kidney biopsy, the Renal Activity Index for Lupus Nephritis (RAIL) was developed. The RAIL is a composite measure calculated from the log-transformed and creatinine-standardized urine concentrations of the six urine biomarkers (neutrophil gelatinase-associated lipocalin, ceruloplasmin, monocyte chemoattractant protein-1, adiponectin, hemopexin, and kidney injury molecule-1). The RAIL measures LN activity with high sensitivity and accuracy irrespective of coexisting LN chronicity or medication use. Besides differentiating LN activity as seen histologically in kidney biopsies, the RAIL has an excellent ability to anticipate response to LN therapy [47, 48].

Although repeat kidney biopsies are still required to evaluate the histologic classification, LN activity, and the degree of renal structural destruction in LN, the RAIL seems promising to identify patients at risk and to monitor early renal changes and provides a personalized approach in improving long-term outcome in LN.

## *Cutaneous Lupus Erythematosus Disease Area and Severity Index*

Mucocutaneous involvement is common with cSLE [49, 50]. The Cutaneous Lupus Erythematosus Disease Area and Severity Index (CLASI) was developed to quantitatively measure activity and damage of cutaneous lupus-associated lesions in adults with SLE or cutaneous lupus [51]. It has been recently validated in cSLE and in pediatric cutaneous lupus erythematosus (CLE) and demonstrated excellent inter- and intra-rater reliability and superior measurement properties [52, 53].

The CLASI scores both activity and damage of lupus-related mucocutaneous lesions. There are two separate summary scores: a CLASI activity summary score and a CLASI damage summary score. The activity score includes the assessment of erythema and scale/hypertrophy on 13 different body parts (scalp, ears, nose including malar area, rest of the face, (frontal) V-area neck, posterior neck and shoulders, chest, abdomen, back and buttocks, arms, hands, legs, and feet), mucous membrane lesions, and non-scarring alopecia; it is calculated by simple addition of all scores on each section. The damage score is measured by dyspigmentation and scarring/atrophy/panniculitis on the same anatomical locations as in the activity score and scarring alopecia. The item score for dyspigmentation is doubled if present for >12 months [51, 54]. Total activity scores are used to categorize disease severity and responsiveness to therapy [52, 55].

The CLASI provides an objective comprehensive evaluation of both active and chronic mucocutaneous lesions in cSLE. It is a valid, reliable, and accurate outcome measure that is sensitive to change. Moreover, about 5 minutes is needed to score the CLASI supporting its feasibility and ease of use.

## *Pediatric Automated Neuropsychological Assessment Metrics*

Neuropsychiatric involvement is common among children and adolescents with cSLE and it is associated with poor outcomes [56]. In children, neuropsychiatric symptoms mostly arise within the first year after diagnosis, and neurocognitive dysfunction is seen frequently [57]. As cognitive ability is considered a measure of overall brain health, recording the cognitive ability of a child with cSLE seems essential to monitor cSLE-associated brain disease. Formal neurocognitive testing is the gold standard method to assess neurocognitive impairment [58].

The Pediatric Automated Neuropsychological Assessment Metrics (PedANAM) is a computerized library of tests that have been designed to assess neurocognitive function in children and adolescents in an age-appropriate way. The PedANAM can be completed by children as young as 9 years of age without an upper age limit, meaning it can also be used to measure cognitive ability in adults. Although it was originally developed in English, it has been translated into several different languages.

The PedANAM is a generic tool that has been validated for use in cSLE [59–61]. The test is administered on a computer without any special training or equipment that takes 20–30 minutes to complete. In contrast to the formal neurocognitive testing, it can be repeated within short time intervals without any apparent practice effects. The battery includes measures of simple reaction time, procedural reaction time, code substitution learning and memory, logical reasoning, spatial processing, continuous performance (sustained attention), mathematical processing, matching grids, matching to sample, and (Sternberg) memory search. Each subtest produces three age-corrected standardized scores: percent correct, mean response time for correct responses, and throughput (correct responses/minute) [60].

Vega-Fernandez et al. developed Cognitive Performance Scores as a summary measure of the overall cognitive ability considering all of the subtests of the PedANAM performance. The PedANAM Cognitive Performance Scores are 97% sensitive to identify neurocognitive dysfunction in cSLE [62].

## Health-Related Quality of Life and Other Patient-Reported Outcomes

According to the Public Health Agency of Canada, health is "a positive concept that emphasizes social and personal resources, as well as physical capacities" [63]. There are both generic and disease-specific measures of HRQoL that have been validated for use in cSLE (Table 8.2).

### *Child Health Questionnaire*

The Child Health Questionnaire (CHQ) is a generic patient-reported outcome measure that assesses overall HRQoL in physical, emotional, and social aspects for children and adolescents between 5 and 17 years of age [64]. Although both parent-completed forms (CHQ-PF) for children over 5 years of age and child self-reports (CHQ-CF) over 10 years of age of varying lengths have been developed [65], only the 50-item parent-proxy report of CHQ (CHQ-P50) has been cross-culturally validated for use in cSLE [66]. The CHQ-P50 includes 15 subscales and 2 summary scores, the physical summary score (CHQ-PhS) and the psychosocial summary score (CHQ-PsS). Each item is scored on a Likert scale and higher scores indicate better HRQoL. The CHQ-P50 takes about 15 minutes to complete, but scoring cannot be easily done by hand. Rather a computer program is needed. Both CHQ-PhS and CHQ-PsS correlate well with disease activity, but only the CHQ-PhS correlates with disease damage [67]. The CHQ-PhS has been used in a core set to define improvement after a cSLE flare. Mean changes of CHQ-PhS were found significantly decreased among patients with flare, and they were included in the flare

**Table 8.2** Measures of health-related quality of life for use in cSLE

| | Purpose | Score interpretation | Strengths | Cautions | Key reference for use in cSLE |
|---|---|---|---|---|---|
| CHQ | Generic pediatric HRQoL measure | Higher scores indicate better HRQoL on a Likert scale | Ease of use<br>A comprehensive evaluation of HRQoL<br>PhS is responsive to change in disease status | PsS is unable to capture changes in disease status<br>The minimal clinically important difference in cSLE not defined | [28, 33, 66, 67] |
| SMILEY | Disease-specific HRQoL measure in cSLE | Higher total scores indicate better HRQoL on a 1–100 scale | Only disease-specific HRQoL measure in cSLE<br>Ease of use | Not adequate to detect change | [71, 72] |
| PedsQL-GC | Generic pediatric HRQoL measure | Higher scores indicate better HRQoL on a Likert scale | Minimal clinically important difference defined in the pediatric population<br>Ease of use | Limited responsiveness to change | [76–78, 80] |
| PedsQL-RM | Pediatric rheumatology-specific HRQoL measure | Higher scores indicate better HRQoL on a Likert scale | Able to detect change<br>Ease of use | Normative values for cSLE not defined | [76–78, 80] |
| FDI | Generic pediatric measure for functional disability | Higher scores indicate higher levels of functional disability | Categorized levels of disability according to its severity available<br>A reliable outcome measure of functional limitations for patients with cSLE<br>Good psychometric properties when used in cSLE | Additional studies in cSLE needed | [76, 80] |

(continued)

**Table 8.2** (continued)

| | Purpose | Score interpretation | Strengths | Cautions | Key reference for use in cSLE |
|---|---|---|---|---|---|
| pSkindex-27 | Skin-specific HRQoL measure | Higher scores indicate the more negative impact of skin disease on HRQoL on a Likert scale | Responsive to change in mucocutaneous activity and damage in cSLE<br>Excellent agreement between child self-reports and parent-proxy reports<br>Ease of use | Additional validation studies in cSLE needed | [52, 83, 85] |
| Pediatric PROMIS-SFs | Generic pediatric HRQoL measure | Item-level calibrations preferred for scoring; higher scores equal more of concept being measured | Strong correlation with other HRQoL tools when used in cSLE | Not responsive to change in cSLE<br>Weak correlation with disease activity and damage indices in cSLE | [87] |

*CHQ* Child Health Questionnaire, *cSLE* childhood-onset systemic lupus erythematosus, *FDI* Functional Disability Inventory, *HRQoL* health-related quality of life, *PedsQL-GC* Pediatric Quality of Life 4.0 Generic Core Scale, *PedsQL-RM* Pediatric Quality of Life 3.0 Rheumatology Module, *PhS* physical summary score, *PROMIS-SFs* Patient-Reported Outcomes Measurement Information System Short Forms, *pSkindex-27* pediatric Skindex-27, *PsS* psychosocial summary score, *SMILEY* Simple Measure of Impact of Lupus Erythematosus in Youngsters

algorithm [28]. However, in a single study, CHQ-PhS was not found responsive to change of disease activity in cSLE [33]. The CHQ-PhS seems more profoundly correlated with the level of disease activity in cSLE. This may be expected as cSLE flares often involve worsening of arthritis, with an expected decrease in physical function which is captured by the CHQ-PhS.

## *Simple Measure of Impact of Lupus Erythematosus in Youngsters*

The Simple Measure of Impact of Lupus Erythematosus in Youngsters (SMILEY) is the only cSLE-specific HRQoL assessment tool. It uses a visual 5-point Likert scale with different facial expressions for responses. It has a total number of 26 items in 4 domains: effect of self, limitations, social, and burden of SLE. All items and domains are included in parent-proxy reports and child self-reports that are in parallel. Around 10 minutes is needed to complete with around the same time needed for manual scoring. The first two items questioning current SLE status and HRQoL status are not included in the SMILEY domain or overall summary score, ranging from 0 to 100 (best possible score) [68]. The SMILEY was translated into multiple languages and cross-culturally validated [69, 70]. SMILEY scores, especially the limitation and the burden of SLE domains, reversely correlate with disease activity and damage scores. The SMILEY scores and changes in cSLE disease activity over time are only weakly correlated [71, 72].

## *Pediatric Quality of Life Inventory*

The Pediatric Quality of Life Inventory (PedsQL) measures a generic HRQoL that uses an age-appropriate way available in a wide age range for children and includes a parallel child self-report for ages 5–18 years and a proxy report for ages 2–18 years [73]. In contrast to the PedsQL 4.0 Generic Core Scale (PedsQL-GC), the PedsQL 3.0 Rheumatology Module (PedsQL-RM) is a pediatric rheumatology-specific measure of HRQoL, and it is generally used in combination with the PedsQL-GC. Both measures are relatively brief and easily administered. The PedsQL-GC is composed of 23 items in 4 domains, physical, emotional, social, and school functioning, whereas the PedsQL-RM assesses HRQoL with 22 items in 5 domains: pain and hurt, daily activities, treatment, worry, and communication, respectively. Items are scored on a 5-point Likert scale from 0 (never) to 4 (almost always) and reversely transformed to a 0–100 scale. Physical and psychosocial health summary scores can be calculated for the PedsQL-GC with higher scores indicating better HRQoL [74, 75]. A 4.4 change in the PedsQL-GC total score for child self-reports and a 4.5 change for parent-proxy reports are considered minimal clinically meaningful in diverse pediatric populations [75].

Patients with cSLE have lower scores on the PedsQL-GC than healthy children [76, 77]. Higher levels of disease activity, increase in disease activity, and the presence of disease damage in cSLE are all risk factors for poor HRQoL measured by the PedsQL-GC and PedsQL-RM [77]. Compared to the PedsQL-RM, the PedsQL-GC has limited ability to capture changes in HRQoL with changing disease activity over time [77, 78].

The PedsQL Multidimensional Fatigue Scale (PedsQL-MFS) designed to measure fatigue in pediatric patients includes 18 items in 3 domains: general fatigue, sleep/rest fatigue, and cognitive fatigue [79]. Significantly lower PedsQL-MFS scores than healthy pediatric populations have been observed among patients with cSLE that show significant correlations with the PedsQL-GC and PedsQL-RM scores [76]. Because increased fatigue is associated with lower HRQoL in cSLE, routine use of the PedsQL-MFS may assist with identifying at-risk patients with persistently poor HRQoL in cSLE [80].

## *Functional Disability Inventory*

The Functional Disability Inventory (FDI) is a generic measure of physical and psychological functional difficulty and perceived limitation in activity. The FDI serves as a reliable outcome measure of functional limitations for patients with cSLE with its good psychometric properties. The FDI can be used in children as young as 8 years of age and consists of 15 items, each rated on a 5-point Likert scale. The total FDI score reflects the sum of all item scores [81]. An FDI score of 0–12 defines no or minimal, 13–20 mild, 21–29 moderate, and ≥30 severe levels of disability, respectively [82]. In a previous study in adolescents with mostly well-controlled cSLE, many reported no more than minimal functional disability; moderate to high functional disability was reported in a subset of cSLE patients with high levels of anxiety and pain [76, 80].

## *Pediatric Skindex-27*

The Skindex-29 captures skin-related HRQoL, which has been shown to be reliable, to have construct validity and responsiveness to change in cutaneous lupus erythematosus and SLE [52, 83, 84]. It includes 30 items where 29 items are scored. The item about side effects of treatment is not included in scoring for it is different from HRQoL effects of the skin diseases. Similar to the Skindex-29, the items of the pSkindex-27 are rated on a 5-point Likert-type scale probing in three health domains: emotions, symptoms, and functioning. The adaptation of the Skindex-29 for use in children (pSkindex-27) omitted 2 items questioning sex life and affection difficulty in functioning domain [52]. Item responses are transformed into a range of scores from 0 (never) to 100 (effect experienced all the time). A domain score is the unweighted average of responses to the items in the particular domain, and a summary score can be calculated from the unweighted average of the three domain scores. A higher score reflects a higher impact of skin disease on HRQoL [85]. Patient self-reports and parent-proxy reports showed an excellent agreement [52]. The Skindex-27 is an easy tool to use by children and their caregivers which takes 5 minutes to complete.

## *Patient-Reported Outcomes Measurement Information System*

The Patient-Reported Outcomes Measurement Information System (PROMIS) is a generic PRO measure developed to assess multiple HRQoL domains. The PROMIS development has been supported by the National Institutes of Health to help to standardize and improve PRO measurement for use in a variety of diseases [86]. PROMIS measures can be applied through static forms, short forms (PROMIS-SFs), and computer-adaptive testing in pediatric populations. A total of 64 items in 8 domains (anger, anxiety, depression, fatigue, peer relationships, physical function-mobility, physical function-upper extremity, and pain interference) provided by the PROMIS-SFs were studied in cSLE. Patients respond to each item on a 5-point Likert scale considering the preceding 7 days. The questionnaire takes about 5 minutes and less than 1 minute is needed for each domain. The pediatric PROMIS-SFs showed outstanding feasibility, construct validity, high internal consistency, and moderate to high correlation with other validated HRQoL instruments when used in cSLE; however, the PROMIS-SFs responses demonstrated no more than weak correlation with cSLE disease activity and damage [87]. Potentially, this is due to the fact that cSLE affects many organ systems with diverse impacts on HRQoL while the PROMIS-SF strictly measures a single HRQoL concept.

## Summary

Measures to capture the degree of disease activity and damage as well as the course of cSLE over time have been developed and/or validated for use in cSLE. Furthermore, a toolbox of measure to capture PRO with cSLE has become available. Together, these measures can be used to capture the impact and changes of cSLE in pediatric populations with lupus, both in the setting of clinical trial and treat to target strategies as part of clinical care.

## References

1. Uribe AG, Vilá LM, McGwin G, Sanchez ML, Reveille JD, Alarcón GS. The systemic lupus activity measure-revised, the Mexican Systemic Lupus Erythematosus Disease Activity Index (SLEDAI), and a modified SLEDAI-2K are adequate instruments to measure disease activity in systemic lupus erythematosus. J Rheumatol. 2004;31:1934–40.
2. Gladman DD, Ibañez D, Urowitz MB. Systemic lupus erythematosus disease activity index 2000. J Rheumatol. 2002;29:288–91.
3. Bombardier C, Gladman DD, Urowitz MB, et al. Derivation of the SLEDAI. A disease activity index for lupus patients. The Committee on Prognosis Studies in SLE. Arthritis Rheum. 1992;35:630–40.
4. Luijten KMAC, Tekstra J, Bijlsma JWJ, Bijl M. The Systemic Lupus Erythematosus Responder Index (SRI); a new SLE disease activity assessment. Autoimmun Rev. 2012;11:326–9.
5. Mosca M, Merrill JT, Bombardieri S. Chapter 2 – assessment of disease activity in systemic lupus erythematosus. In: Syst. Lupus Erythematosus: Mosby; 2007. p. 19–23.
6. Isenberg DA. BILAG, SLEDAI, SIS, ECLAM, WAM, SLAM .... thank you MAM. Lupus. 2007;16:849–51.
7. Brunner HI, Holland M, Beresford MW, et al. American College of Rheumatology provisional criteria for global flares in childhood-onset systemic lupus erythematosus. Arthritis Care Res (Hoboken). 2018;70:813–22.
8. Mikdashi J, Nived O. Measuring disease activity in adults with systemic lupus erythematosus: the challenges of administrative burden and responsiveness to patient concerns in clinical research. Arthritis Res Ther. 2015;17:183.

9. Mina R, Klein-Gitelman MS, Nelson S, et al. Validation of the systemic lupus erythematosus responder index for use in juvenile-onset systemic lupus erythematosus. Ann Rheum Dis. 2014;73:401–6.
10. Brunner HI, Mina R, Pilkington C, et al. Preliminary criteria for global flares in childhood-onset systemic lupus erythematosus. Arthritis Care Res. 2011;63:1213–23.
11. Brunner HI, Higgins GC, Klein-Gitelman MS, Lapidus SK, Olson JC, Onel K, Punaro M, Ying J, Giannini EH. Minimal clinically important differences of disease activity indices in childhood-onset systemic lupus erythematosus. Arthritis Care Res (Hoboken). 2010;62:950–9.
12. Brunner HI, Feldman BM, Bombardier C, Silverman ED. Sensitivity of the Systemic Lupus Erythematosus Disease Activity Index, British Isles Lupus Assessment Group Index, and Systemic Lupus Activity Measure in the evaluation of clinical change in childhood-onset systemic lupus erythematosus. Arthritis Rheum. 1999;42:1354–60.
13. Lattanzi B, Consolaro A, Solari N, Ruperto N, Martini A, Ravelli A. Measures of disease activity and damage in pediatric systemic lupus erythematosus: British Isles Lupus Assessment Group (BILAG), European Consensus Lupus Activity Measurement (ECLAM), Systemic Lupus Activity Measure (SLAM), Systemic Lupus Erythematosus Disease Activity Index (SLEDAI), Physician's Global Assessment of Disease Activity (MD Global), and Systemic Lupus International Collaborating Clinics/American College of Rheumatology Damage Index (SLICC/ACR DI; SDI). Arthritis Care Res (Hoboken). 2011;63(Suppl 11):S112–7.
14. Karlson EW, Daltroy LH, Rivest C, Ramsey-Goldman R, Wright EA, Partridge AJ, Liang MH, Fortin PR. Validation of a systemic lupus activity questionnaire (SLAQ) for population studies. Lupus. 2003;12:280–86.
15. Yazdany J, Yelin EH, Panopalis P, Trupin L, Julian L, Katz PP. Validation of the systemic lupus erythematosus activity questionnaire in a large observational cohort. Arthritis Rheum. 2008;59:136–43.
16. Abrahamowicz M, Fortin PR, Du Berger R, Nayak V, Neville C, Liang MH. The relationship between disease activity and expert physician's decision to start major treatment in active systemic lupus erythematosus: a decision aid for development of entry criteria for clinical trials. J Rheumatol. 1998;25(2):277–84.
17. Levy DM, Peschken CA, Tucker LB, et al. Association of health-related quality of life in childhood-onset systemic lupus erythematosus with ethnicity: results from a multiethnic multicenter Canadian cohort. Arthritis Care Res. 2014;66:1767–74.
18. Watson L, Leone V, Pilkington C, et al. Disease activity, severity, and damage in the UK juvenile-onset systemic lupus erythematosus cohort. Arthritis Rheum. 2012;64:2356–65.
19. Brunner HI, Silverman ED, Bombardier C, Feldman BM. European Consensus Lupus Activity Measurement is sensitive to change in disease activity in childhood-onset systemic lupus erythematosus. Arthritis Rheum. 2003;49:335–41.
20. Sato JO, Corrente JE, Saad-Magalhães C. Correlation between the Modified Systemic Lupus Erythematosus Disease Activity Index 2000 and the European Consensus Lupus Activity Measurement in juvenile systemic lupus erythematosus. Lupus. 2016;25:1479–84.
21. Gladman D, Ginzler E, Goldsmith C, et al. The development and initial validation of the Systemic Lupus International Collaborating Clinics/American College of Rheumatology damage index for systemic lupus erythematosus. Arthritis Rheum. 1996;39:363–69.
22. Brunner HI, Silverman ED, To T, Bombardier C, Feldman BM. Risk factors for damage in childhood-onset systemic lupus erythematosus: cumulative disease activity and medication use predict disease damage. Arthritis Rheum. 2002;46:436–44.
23. Ravelli A, Duarte-Salazar C, Buratti S, et al. Assessment of damage in juvenile-onset systemic lupus erythematosus: a multicenter cohort study. Arthritis Rheum. 2003;49:501–7.
24. Gutiérrez-Suárez R, Ruperto N, Gastaldi R, Pistorio A, Felici E, Burgos-Vargas R, Martini A, Ravelli A. A proposal for a pediatric version of the systemic lupus international collaborating clinics/American College of Rheumatology Damage Index based on the analysis of 1,015 patients with juvenile-onset systemic lupus erythematosus. Arthritis Rheum. 2006;54:2989–96.
25. Romero-Diaz J, Isenberg D, Ramsey-Goldman R. Measures of adult systemic lupus erythematosus: updated version of British Isles Lupus Assessment Group (BILAG 2004), European

Consensus Lupus Activity Measurements (ECLAM), Systemic Lupus Activity Measure, Revised (SLAM-R), Systemic Lupus Activity Questionnaire for Population Studies (SLAQ), Systemic Lupus Erythematosus Disease Activity Index 2000 (SLEDAI-2K), and Systemic Lupus International Collaborating Clinics/American College of Rheumatology Damage Index (SDI). Arthritis Care Res (Hoboken). 2011;63 Suppl 11:S37–46.
26. Gladman DD, Urowitz MB, Goldsmith CH, et al. The reliability of the Systemic Lupus International Collaborating Clinics/American College of Rheumatology Damage Index in patients with systemic lupus erythematosus. Arthritis Rheum. 1997;40:809–13.
27. Holland MJ, Beresford MW, Feldman BM, et al. Measuring disease damage and its severity in childhood-onset systemic lupus erythematosus. Arthritis Care Res (Hoboken). 2018;70:1621–9.
28. Brunner HI, Klein-Gitelman MS, Higgins GC, et al. Toward the development of criteria for global flares in juvenile systemic lupus erythematosus. Arthritis Care Res. 2010;62:811–20.
29. Brunner HI, Holland MJ, Beresford MW, et al. American College of Rheumatology Provisional Criteria for clinically relevant improvement in children and adolescents with childhood-onset systemic lupus erythematosus. Arthritis Care Res (Hoboken). 2019;71:579–90.
30. Furie R, Petri MA, Strand V, Gladman DD, Zhong ZJ, Freimuth WW, BLISS-52 and BLISS-76 Study Groups. Clinical, laboratory and health-related quality of life correlates of Systemic Lupus Erythematosus Responder Index response: a post hoc analysis of the phase 3 belimumab trials. Lupus Sci Med. 2014;1:e000031.
31. Furie R, Wang L, Illei G, Drappa J. Systemic Lupus Erythematosus (SLE) Responder Index response is associated with global benefit for patients with SLE. Lupus. 2018;27:955–62.
32. Brunner HI, Abud-Mendoza C, Viola DO, et al. Safety and efficacy of intravenous belimumab in children with systemic lupus erythematosus: results from a randomised, placebo-controlled trial. Ann Rheum Dis. 2020;79:1340-48.
33. Brunner HI, Higgins GC, Wiers K, Lapidus SK, Olson JC, Onel K, Punaro M, Ying J, Klein-gitelman MS, Giannini EH. Prospective validation of the provisional criteria for the evaluation of response to therapy in childhood-onset systemic lupus erythematosus. Arthritis Care Res (Hoboken). 2010;62:335–44.
34. Ruperto N, Ravelli A, Oliveira S, et al. The Pediatric Rheumatology International Trials Organization/American College of Rheumatology provisional criteria for the evaluation of response to therapy in juvenile systemic lupus erythematosus: prospective validation of the definition of improvement. Arthritis Rheum. 2006;55:355–63.
35. Silva CA, Avcin T, Brunner HI. Taxonomy for systemic lupus erythematosus with onset before adulthood. Arthritis Care Res. 2012;64:1787–93.
36. Hahn BH, McMahon MA, Wilkinson A, et al. American College of Rheumatology guidelines for screening, treatment, and management of lupus nephritis. Arthritis Care Res (Hoboken). 2012;64:797–808.
37. Bertsias GK, Tektonidou M, Amoura Z, et al. Joint European League Against Rheumatism and European Renal Association-European Dialysis and Transplant Association (EULAR/ERA-EDTA) recommendations for the management of adult and paediatric lupus nephritis. Ann Rheum Dis. 2012;71:1771-82.
38. Wenderfer SE, Lane JC, Shatat IF, Von Scheven E, Ruth NM. Practice patterns and approach to kidney biopsy in lupus: a collaboration of the Midwest Pediatric Nephrology Consortium and the Childhood Arthritis and Rheumatology Research Alliance. Pediatr Rheumatol Online J. 2015;13:26.
39. Ardoin SP, Daly RP, Merzoug L, et al. Research priorities in childhood-onset lupus: results of a multidisciplinary prioritization exercise. Pediatr Rheumatol Online J. 2019;17:32.
40. Mina R, von Scheven E, Ardoin SP, et al. Consensus treatment plans for induction therapy of newly diagnosed proliferative lupus nephritis in juvenile systemic lupus erythematosus. Arthritis Care Res (Hoboken). 2012;64:375–83.
41. Aljaberi N, Bennett M, Brunner HI, Devarajan P. Proteomic profiling of urine: implications for lupus nephritis. Expert Rev Proteomics. 2019;16:303–13.

42. Brunner HI, Mueller M, Rutherford C, Passo MH, Witte D, Grom A, Mishra J, Devarajan P. Urinary neutrophil gelatinase-associated lipocalin as a biomarker of nephritis in childhood-onset systemic lupus erythematosus. Arthritis Rheum. 2006;54:2577-84.
43. Hinze CH, Suzuki M, Klein-Gitelman M, et al. Neutrophil gelatinase-associated lipocalin is a predictor of the course of global and renal childhood-onset systemic lupus erythematosus disease activity. Arthritis Rheum. 2009;60:2772-81.
44. Singh RG, Usha, Rathore SS, Behura SK, Singh NK. Urinary MCP-1 as diagnostic and prognostic marker in patients with lupus nephritis flare. Lupus. 2012;21:1214-18.
45. Abd-Elkareem MI, Al Tamimy HM, Khamis OA, Abdellatif SS, Hussein MRA. Increased urinary levels of the leukocyte adhesion molecules ICAM-1 and VCAM-1 in human lupus nephritis with advanced renal histological changes: preliminary findings. Clin Exp Nephrol. 2010;14:548-57.
46. Brunner HI, Bennett MR, Mina R, et al. Association of noninvasively measured renal protein biomarkers with histologic features of lupus nephritis. Arthritis Rheum. 2012;64:2687-97.
47. Brunner HI, Bennett MR, Abulaban K, et al. Development of a novel renal activity index of lupus nephritis in children and young adults. Arthritis Care Res (Hoboken). 2016;68:1003-11.
48. Brunner HI, Bennett MR, Gulati G, et al. Urine biomarkers to predict response to lupus nephritis therapy in children and young adults. J Rheumatol. 2017;44:1239-48.
49. Santiago-Casas Y, Vilá LM, McGwin G, Cantor RS, Petri M, Ramsey-Goldman R, Reveille JD, Kimberly RP, Alarcón GS, Brown EE. Association of discoid lupus erythematosus with clinical manifestations and damage accrual in a multiethnic lupus cohort. Arthritis Care Res (Hoboken). 2012;64:704–12.
50. Chiewchengchol D, Murphy R, Morgan T, et al. Mucocutaneous manifestations in a UK national cohort of juvenile-onset systemic lupus erythematosus patients. Rheumatol (United Kingdom). 2014;53:1504–12.
51. Albrecht J, Taylor L, Berlin JA, et al. The CLASI (cutaneous lupus erythematosus disease area and severity index): an outcome instrument for cutaneous lupus erythematosus. J Invest Dermatol. 2005;125:889–94.
52. Ale'Ed A, Aydin POA, Al Mutairi N, Alsaleem A, Sonmez HE, Henrickson M, Huggins JL, Ozen S, Al-Mayouf SM, Brunner HI. Validation of the cutaneous lupus erythematosus disease area and severity index and pSkindex27 for use in childhood-onset systemic lupus erythematosus. Lupus Sci Med. 2018;5:e000275.
53. Kushner CJ, Tarazi M, Gaffney RG, et al. Evaluation of the reliability and validity of the cutaneous lupus erythematosus disease area and severity index (CLASI) in paediatric cutaneous lupus among paediatric dermatologists and rheumatologists. Br J Dermatol. 2019;180:165–71.
54. Albrecht J, Werth VP. Development of the CLASI as an outcome instrument for cutaneous lupus erythematosus. Dermatol Ther. 2007;20:93–101.
55. Klein R, Moghadam-Kia S, LoMonico J, Okawa J, Coley C, Taylor L, Troxel AB, Werth VP. Development of the CLASI as a tool to measure disease severity and responsiveness to therapy in cutaneous lupus erythematosus. Arch Dermatol. 2011;147:203-8.
56. Muscal E, Brey RL. Neurologic manifestations of systemic lupus erythematosus in children and adults. Neurol Clin. 2010;28:61-73.
57. Benseler SM, Silverman ED. Neuropsychiatric involvement in pediatric systemic lupus erythematosus. Lupus. 2007;16:564–71.
58. AlE'ed A, Vega-Fernandez P, Muscal E, et al. Challenges of diagnosing cognitive dysfunction with neuropsychiatric systemic lupus erythematosus in childhood. Arthritis Care Res. 2017;69:1449–59.
59. Christopher Daniel J, Olesniewicz MH, Reeves DL, Tam D, Bleiberg J, Thatcher R, Salazar A. Repeated measures of cognitive processing efficiency in adolescent athletes: implications for monitoring recovery from concussion. Neuropsychiatry Neuropsychol Behav Neurol. 1999;12(3):167–9.
60. Brunner HI, Ruth NM, German A, Nelson S, Passo MH, Roebuck-Spencer T, Ying J, Ris D. Initial validation of the Pediatric Automated Neuropsychological Assessment Metrics for childhood-onset systemic lupus erythematosus. Arthritis Rheum. 2007;57:1174–82.

61. Brunner HI, Klein-Gitelman MS, Zelko F, et al. Validation of the Pediatric Automated Neuropsychological Assessment Metrics in childhood-onset systemic lupus erythematosus. Arthritis Care Res (Hoboken). 2013;65:372-81.
62. Vega-Fernandez P, Vanderburgh White S, Zelko F, et al. Cognitive Performance Scores for the Pediatric Automated Neuropsychological Assessment Metrics in childhood-onset systemic lupus erythematosus. Arthritis Care Res (Hoboken). 2015;67:1119-27.
63. Public Health Agency of Canada (2017) What is health?
64. Landgraf JM, Maunsell E, Speechley KN, Bullinger M, Campbell S, Abetz L, Ware JE. Canadian-French, German and UK versions of the Child Health Questionnaire: methodology and preliminary item scaling results. Qual Life Res. 1998;7:433-45.
65. Landgraf JM, van Grieken A, Raat H. Giving voice to the child perspective: psychometrics and relative precision findings for the Child Health Questionnaire self-report short form (CHQ-CF45). Qual Life Res. 2018;27:2165–76.
66. Ruperto N, Ravelli A, Pistorio A, Malattia C, Cavuto S, Gado-West L, Tortorelli A, Landgraf JM, Singh G, Martini A. Cross-cultural adaptation and psychometric evaluation of the Childhood Health Assessment Questionnaire (CHAQ) and the Child Health Questionnaire (CHQ) in 32 countries. Review of the general methodology. Clin Exp Rheumatol. 2001;19(4 Suppl 23):S1–9.
67. Ruperto N, Buratti S, Duarte-Salazar C, et al. Health-related quality of life in juvenile-onset systemic lupus erythematosus and its relationship to disease activity and damage. Arthritis Rheum. 2004;51:458–64.
68. Moorthy LN, Peterson MGE, Baratelli M, Harrison MJ, Onel KB, Chalom EC, Haines K, Hashkes PJ, Lehman TJA. Multicenter validation of a new quality of life measure in pediatric lupus. Arthritis Rheum. 2007;57:1165-73.
69. Moorthy LN, Weiss E, Peterson MGE, et al. An update on cross-cultural adaptation of US English SMILEY. Lupus. 2012;21:1450-54.
70. Moorthy NN, Roy E, Kurra V, et al. Health related quality of life measure in systemic pediatric rheumatic diseases and its translation to different languages: an international collaboration. Pediatr Rheumatol Online J. 2014;12:49.
71. Moorthy LN, Peterson MGE, Hassett AL, Baratelli M, Chalom EC, Hashkes PJ, Hong S, Reiff A, Lehman TJA. Relationship between health-related quality of life and SLE activity and damage in children over time. Lupus. 2009;18:622–9.
72. Moorthy LN, Baldino ME, Kurra V, Puwar D, Llanos A, Peterson MGE, Hassett AL, Lehman TJA. Relationship between health-related quality of life, disease activity and disease damage in a prospective international multicenter cohort of childhood onset systemic lupus erythematosus patients. Lupus. 2017;26:255–65.
73. Varni JW, Seid M, Kurtin PS. PedsQL 4.0: reliability and validity of the Pediatric Quality of Life Inventory version 4.0 generic core scales in healthy and patient populations. Med Care. 2001;39:800-12.
74. Varni JW, Seid M, Rode CA. The PedsQL: measurement model for the pediatric quality of life inventory. Med Care. 1999;37:126-39.
75. Varni JW, Burwinkle TM, Seid M, Skarr D. The PedsQL 4.0 as a pediatric population health measure: feasibility, reliability, and validity. Ambul Pediatr. 2003;3:329–41.
76. Jones JT, Cunningham N, Kashikar-Zuck S, Brunner HI. Pain, fatigue, and psychological impact on health-related quality of life in childhood-onset lupus. Arthritis Care Res. 2016;68:73–80.
77. Brunner HI, Higgins GC, Wiers K, Lapidus SK, Olson JC, Onel K, Punaro M, Ying J, Klein-Gitelman MS, Seid M. Health-related quality of life and its relationship to patient disease course in childhood-onset systemic lupus erythematosus. J Rheumatol. 2009;36:1536–45.
78. Moorthy LN, Harrison MJ, Peterson M, Onel KB, Lehman TJA. Relationship of quality of life and physical function measures with disease activity in children with systemic lupus erythematosus. Lupus. 2005;14:280–7.
79. Varni JW, Burwinkle TM, Szer IS. The PedsQL Multidimensional Fatigue Scale in pediatric rheumatology: reliability and validity. J Rheumatol. 2004;31:2494–500.

80. Donnelly C, Cunningham N, Jones JT, Ji L, Brunner HI, Kashikar-Zuck S. Fatigue and depression predict reduced health-related quality of life in childhood-onset lupus. Lupus. 2018;27:124–33.
81. Walker LS, Greene JW. The functional disability inventory: measuring a neglected dimension of child health status. J Pediatr Psychol. 1991;16:39–58.
82. Kashikar-Zuck S, Flowers SR, Claar RL, Guite JW, Logan DE, Lynch-Jordan AM, Palermo TM, Wilson AC. Clinical utility and validity of the functional disability inventory among a multicenter sample of youth with chronic pain. Pain. 2011;152:1600–7.
83. Chren MM, Lasek RJ, Quinn LM, Mostow EN, Zyzanski SJ. Skindex, a quality-of-life measure for patients with skin disease: reliability, validity, and responsiveness. J Invest Dermatol. 1996;107:707–13.
84. Klein R, Moghadam-Kia S, Taylor L, Coley C, Okawa J, Lomonico J, Chren MM, Werth VP. Quality of life in cutaneous lupus erythematosus. J Am Acad Dermatol. 2011;64:849–58.
85. Chren MM, Lasek RJ, Flocke SA, Zyzanski SJ. Improved discriminative and evaluative capability of a refined version of Skindex, a quality-of-life instrument for patients with skin diseases. Arch Dermatol. 1997;133:1433–40.
86. Cella D, Yount S, Rothrock N, Gershon R, Cook K, Reeve B, Ader D, Fries JF, Bruce B, Rose M. The Patient-Reported Outcomes Measurement Information System (PROMIS): progress of an NIH Roadmap cooperative group during its first two years. Med Care. 2007;45(5 Suppl 1):S3–S11.
87. Jones JT, Carle AC, Wootton J, Liberio B, Lee J, Schanberg LE, Ying J, Morgan DeWitt E, Brunner HI. Validation of patient-reported outcomes measurement information system short forms for use in childhood-onset systemic lupus erythematosus. Arthritis Care Res. 2017;69:133–42.

# Chapter 9
# Pregnancies in Lupus: Monitoring and Metrics

**Evelyne Vinet and Stephanie Ensworth**

## Pregnancy Outcomes in SLE

SLE predominantly affects women during their reproductive years, occurring in about 1/1000 women aged between 15 and 45 years [1]. SLE is associated with substantial maternal and fetal morbidity during pregnancy. Compared with the non-SLE population, SLE has been shown to be associated with an increased risk of preterm birth, cesarean delivery, preeclampsia, low birth weight, intrauterine growth restriction (IUGR), congenital heart block (CHB), and intrauterine and neonatal death [2–5]. Preterm birth is the most common adverse pregnancy outcome in women with SLE, with incidence ranging from 15% to 50% (as opposed to 10% in unaffected women), with increased risk in women with lupus nephritis, lupus anticoagulant, or high disease activity. In the general population, preterm birth is the leading cause of neonatal death and the second most common cause of death (after pneumonia) in children younger than 5 years [6].

SLE has a waxing and waning course. It has been shown that if women conceive during a period of disease quiescence, this will minimize the risk of flare in pregnancy, but will not eliminate it, with rates of flare still ranging between 20% and 40% of pregnancies that are conceived during remission [7–10]. In addition to a greater frequency of pregnancy complications, the SLE disease course itself can be negatively affected by pregnancy, with a greater number of women developing an SLE flare in the peripartum period [11–13].

E. Vinet (✉)
Divisions of Rheumatology & Clinical Epidemiology, McGill University Health Centre, Montreal, QC, Canada
e-mail: evelyne.vinet@mcgill.ca

S. Ensworth
Division of Rheumatology, Department of Medicine, Faculty of Medicine, University of British Columbia, Vancouver, BC, Canada



Z. Touma (ed.), *Outcome Measures and Metrics in Systemic Lupus Erythematosus*, https://doi.org/10.1007/978-3-030-73303-2_9

To date, research has mainly focused on assessing the risk of immediate complications during SLE pregnancies, such as preterm births and small for gestational age (SGA) infants. However, until recently, little was known regarding the long-term health of children born to affected women. SLE offspring are potentially exposed in utero to maternal autoantibodies, cytokines, and drugs, as well as obstetrical complications. This might result in developmental anomalies, congenital defects, and/or increased autoimmune disease susceptibility. In the past few years, observational studies have suggested an increased risk of adverse health outcomes, including neurodevelopmental disorders, congenital heart defects (CHDs), and autoimmune diseases in offspring born to mothers with SLE [14–16].

Because SLE pregnancies are associated with higher maternal and fetal morbidity and mortality, they are considered "high-risk." Although the majority of SLE pregnancies end with live births, active disease and major organ involvement can mandate close maternal follow-up during pregnancy as well as in the postpartum period. In addition, major fetal issues such as IUGR and neonatal SLE syndromes make monitoring imperative in SLE pregnancies [17]. Finally, some symptoms of SLE can be silent, such as renal flare or thrombocytopenia, emphasizing the need for closer monitoring in pregnancy; these silent flares can still increase the chance of adverse pregnancy outcomes [18].

## Monitoring

Quality indicators pertaining to reproductive health in SLE have been developed but are limited only to the recommendation that anti-SSA/anti-SSB and antiphospholipid (aPL) antibodies be documented in the chart, prior to conception [19]. Optimal quality indicators remain undefined, and topics to be addressed include not only laboratory monitoring but also newer imaging modalities for monitoring high-risk pregnancies, such as umbilical and uterine artery Doppler studies. These are believed to be useful in monitoring pregnancies at high risk of placental insufficiency, which include SLE pregnancies [20]. Because the issue of how best to follow disease activity, and how often to monitor for disease flares, has not been systematically addressed in the literature, current practice is heterogeneous and not necessarily evidence-based [21].

A 2018 systematic review of the literature revealed there is no evidence to guide the frequency of routine monitoring of complete blood count, chemistry profile including liver enzymes, and urinalysis (routine or microscopy) or urine protein to creatinine levels, during pregnancy with SLE [22]. There is some evidence for a role for measuring anti-Ro (SSA) and anti-La (SSB) antibodies prior to conception or early in SLE-related pregnancy to risk-stratify pregnancies regarding the development of complete CHB. Similarly, the presence of aPL is predictive of poor outcomes, particularly preeclampsia and fetal loss, and so may be reasonable to measure prior to conception or early in pregnancy. Monitoring SLE disease activity should be done, potentially with a validated scoring system such as the SLEDAI because it relies on assessment of different clinical aspects of the disease (i.e., clinical manifestations and specific blood tests). Of note, disease activity scoring systems modified to account for the physiologic changes of pregnancy, such as the SLE in Pregnancy Disease Activity Index [23] and the Lupus Activity Index in Pregnancy [24], have never been formally validated. If a flare is suspected, measuring anti-dsDNA antibodies and complement levels may be helpful. One expanding area of monitoring in SLE pregnancies relates to the role of uterine and umbilical artery Doppler studies. Absent end-diastolic velocities in the umbilical artery predict early pregnancy-induced hypertension/preeclampsia and fetal or neonatal death in non-SLE pregnancies [25, 26]. Abnormalities demonstrating increased resistive indices, notching of the arteries, or, in very severe cases, reversal of end-diastolic flow are highly predictive of poor fetal outcomes in SLE pregnancies [27, 28]. Women with SLE should be considered for referral to an expert in maternal-fetal medicine for fetal monitoring with umbilical artery Doppler studies, given that Doppler abnormalities are predictive of adverse outcomes; among pregnant populations without SLE, this monitoring modality has improved fetal outcomes.

## Metrics in Observational Studies of SLE Pregnancies

Because of the relative infrequency of pregnancies in SLE women, collecting datasets of sufficient size with reliable data can be challenging. Administrative databases, registers, and multicenter prospective cohort studies can be interesting data sources to address important research questions on reproduction in women with SLE. There are many different types of observational datasets worldwide, and it is important to understand the type of data present and those which are unavailable in each dataset, validity and potential misclassification of variables, and the ability to perform mother-child linkage.

### *Administrative Databases*

Administrative databases used in epidemiological research are large datasets collected as part of the billing and administrative components of clinical care that can be used to study healthcare delivery and outcomes. The collection of these data is not primarily for research purposes. However, the increased availability of such data has fuelled research by allowing for more rapid collection of data on subjects with rare diseases in sufficiently large numbers. Some administrative data sources (such as population-based registers) are representative of a large population of individuals, unlike subjects who may voluntarily participate in a clinical cohort or subjects who are seen exclusively at tertiary care medical centers and must often provide informed consent to be included. Similarly, large numbers of control subjects can be identified within the dataset who may represent non-diseased individuals as comparators whose data are collected in the same fashion as cases of interest. Additionally, as the data are generated at the time of the encounter, it is systematic and prospectively collected without the inherent biases of recall of past exposures, or self-selection by volunteer status. Of course, differences in healthcare utilization may affect the appropriate selection of control populations. Similarly, confounding by indication may influence the extent of resources used based on the individual's underlying disease status. For example, a SLE patient may be more likely to be hospitalized than a similarly aged healthy individual for a given set of symptoms.

## Claim-Based Databases

Because the United States does not have a nationwide health system or systematic capture of medical data, the ability to collect comprehensive medical data on a truly population-based cohort is necessarily limited. However, several datasets are available that may be relevant to research into pregnancy outcomes in SLE populations. Perhaps the most commonly used are administrative data based on medical claims, either by publicly funded insurers (e.g., Medicaid) or private insurers (e.g., MarketScan commercial databases). These data are quite valuable in that they often contain inpatient and outpatient visits listing diagnoses and procedures and prescription drug data linked to individuals. Unfortunately, because of the fragmentation of health care in the United States, individuals may not retain extended enrolment with any specific insurer, making long-term evaluation across multiple pregnancies more difficult. Numerous algorithms are currently used to maximize sensitivity and specificity of diagnoses made on claims data [29, 30]. Additionally, important variables may not be captured in claims data, including lifestyle variables (e.g., smoking, alcohol, exercise), reproductive history, results of laboratory studies, and variables on disease activity or severity.

More detailed individual-level data may be obtained by using electronic medical record (EMR) data which can complement administrative datasets with laboratory and imaging data. Access to EMR for research purposes can vary considerably across institutions. Additionally, data fields and key word searches may include information regarding vital signs, body mass index, lifestyle variables, reproductive history, and even data regarding gestational age and other antepartum pregnancy variables. In general, patient-reported outcomes and standardized assessments of disease activity and severity remain unavailable. Using such datasets is complex and requires sophisticated analyses and cautious interpretation, thus increasing the cost, time, and required expertise of performing such studies.

## Population-Based Registers

Population-based registers are a type of administrative database that offer a systematic data collection on specific outcomes, usually based on mandatory reporting within a country or region. These may contain data on all outpatient visits, hospitalizations, deaths, and filled drug prescriptions for a given population over some period of time. Such registers may also be supplemented with self-reported information, which may capture important potential confounders, exposures of interest, and comorbidities. Regions with such registers also often collect data on vital statistics, census, employment, immigration, and emigration.

One example of population-based surveillance registers is the Nordic Birth Registers, which cover Denmark, Finland, Iceland, Norway, and Sweden, encompassing approximately 25 million births [31, 32]. Each of the Nordic countries has kept medical birth registers for decades, all with compulsory notification with identifiers for mother and neonate and, in some cases, for fathers. Linkage to other registers and national healthcare databases is possible, often using a personal identification number, such as outpatient, hospitalization, and prescription databases. Collectively, this means that researchers can potentially identify some exposures of interest and outcomes from women with SLE and a representative comparator sample of births.

The Canadian administrative healthcare databases can also be considered a population-based surveillance register, with each Canadian province having its own register. For example, Quebec's administrative databases cover all residents in the province (>8 million) and collect information on all hospitalizations, physician visits, and procedures. In addition, they include data on drug prescriptions filled for residents on the public drug plan which covers recipients of social assistance and workers and their families without access to a private drug plan, representing about a third of the population. Quebec's Institute of Statistics monitors important vital statistics, including live birth and stillbirth rates, with a mandatory reporting of gestational age at birth (based on date of last menstrual period) and cause of stillbirth. All these databases can be linked to provide a rich source of information to assemble a population-based cohort of pregnancies or deliveries, with available mother and child linkage, creating a cohort of offspring with prenatal exposure of interest. One such cohort, the Offspring of Systemic Lupus Erythematosus (SLE) Mother Registry (OSLER), has been assembled to assess the risk of long-term health outcomes and stillbirths in children born to women with SLE [14, 15].

## Advantages of Administrative Databases for Reproductive Studies in SLE

Administrative databases offer several advantages for the study of reproductive issues in women with SLE. The large sample size makes it possible to study outcomes associated with rare exposures, such as SLE, which only affects 0.1% of women of childbearing age [33, 34]. This is particularly true for the assessment of rare outcomes (such as neurodevelopment disorders in SLE offspring), which is not easily feasible in prospective cohort studies. Such data have been collected in a systematic manner, facilitating the conduct of observational studies rapidly and at relatively low cost. Population-based register data cover the entire population of a geographic region, thereby improving the generalizability of findings. Because informed consent is generally not required for selection of subjects in a study, study designs using these data sources are less prone to selection bias from nonresponse. Moreover, the use of administrative databases also eases the selection of a control group from the same source population. In the case of population-based registers, data are available to estimate the baseline risks of the outcomes of interest to estimate and understand the true general population risks.

## Prospective Pregnancy Cohorts

Prospective pregnancy cohorts, which can be assembled during routine clinical care, can provide a wealth of information beyond what can be collected from administrative databases. Single-site lupus cohorts, such as the Hopkins Lupus Cohort and the Toronto Lupus Cohort, provided the first data suggesting SLE women could have safe pregnancies. In 1980, the Toronto Lupus Cohort published data from 24 pregnancies in SLE women, showing that disease is quiescent during pregnancy if the disease is inactive at conception [35], whereas in 1991, findings from the first 40 pregnancies from the Hopkins Lupus Cohort were published, showing an increased risk of flare in pregnancy [36]. Single-site pregnancy cohorts are limited by the rate of enrolment, limiting their power to answer study questions assessing infrequent outcomes. In addition, they often lack a healthy control comparison group, as nonaffected subjects are not usually followed by the research team. Additionally, these cohorts are limited to the subset of patients who have access to specialty clinics (often tertiary centers), and findings may not be generalizable to the general SLE population.

Multicenter prospective cohorts may be able to overcome some of these limitations. By having pregnancies collected at multiple sites, pregnancy accrual is usually easier and faster, and outcomes may be somewhat more generalizable, though they will still be managed, most likely, at specialized centers. The Predictors of Pregnancy Outcome: Biomarkers in Antiphospholipid Antibody Syndrome and Systemic Lupus Erythematosus (PROMISSE) study is an excellent example of a multicenter prospective cohort of SLE pregnancies with subjects enrolled from nine sites across North America [2]. Despite its multi-site design, accrual was relatively slow, taking a decade to enrol almost 350 pregnancies, and was perhaps hampered by the strict inclusion criteria that limited enrolment to the first trimester and a protocol that required frequent follow-ups and blood samples. However, PROMISSE succeeded in assembling very rich data from a specific and relatively uniform SLE patient population, as well as an extensive biorepository to fuel many translational research efforts.

## Limitations in Observational Studies of Reproductive Outcomes in SLE: Differences Between Pregnancy and Birth

Several published studies examining pregnancy complications and outcomes in women with SLE use data from birth registers and birth certificates, as well as labor and delivery admissions. These data sources require that a birth be registered, therefore missing information on first and second trimester pregnancy losses. In some instances, losses after 20 gestational weeks are registered as stillbirths and therefore can be found, but this is not always the case. When reviewing the literature or conducting a study, it is thus important to determine how the data were identified. For instance, were only pregnancies that lasted at least 20 weeks included in the analysis, or were pregnancies early in the first trimester identified?

Most administrative databases have access to delivery admissions and birth characteristics. However, some initiatives, such as the Swedish Pregnancy Register, are collecting data from the first trimester visit to capture clinically recognized pregnancies [37]. Using EMR, it may also be possible to search clinic notes, human chorionic gonadotropin testing, genetic testing, ultrasound records, and other clinical interactions which might identify a pregnancy in its early stages.

The distinction is crucial because if a study investigates adverse pregnancy outcomes and only includes births, certain adverse pregnancy outcomes (i.e., early fetal loss) might be excluded, underestimating the true prevalence of the outcome. This could lead to an invalid conclusion that no fetal loss was associated with the exposure of interest when in fact the investigators selected a study population (i.e., births) that did not have losses. Interpretation of these data and the underlying selection of patients must be carefully considered.

## Early Pregnancy Complications and Loss

Just as pregnancy onset is challenging to define precisely using administrative data, complications of early pregnancy can be difficult to ascertain. Approximately 99% of fetal deaths occurring at greater than 20 weeks' gestational age identified in administrative databases using International Classification of Diseases, Ninth Revision (ICD-9) codes were confirmed by medical record review; however, it is unknown how many cases were not ascertained within the datasets [38]. Furthermore, pregnancy losses that occur before 12 weeks are likely not captured in administrative datasets, as many of these losses do not require hospitalization, surgical intervention, or even medical attention if uncomplicated and early in gestation. Indeed, some early pregnancy losses may not even be clinically recognized, particularly in women who are not actively attempting to conceive. To date, there are no validation studies to understand the degree of incomplete ascertainment of early pregnancy losses in SLE.

## Timing of Pregnancy

Understanding the timing of gestation using administrative data presents its own set of challenges, particularly as it relates to the onset of pregnancy (i.e., conception) and exposures related to specific gestational ages. This can be critical when considering issues of potential teratogenicity, in which there is often a specific time window during organogenesis when embryos are most vulnerable in early pregnancy. Given that SLE women often need medications to control disease activity, some of which are teratogenic (e.g., mycophenolate mofetil), accurately identifying the timing of pregnancy can be extremely important to ascertain certain outcomes.

To estimate onset of pregnancy, several algorithms have been developed to maximize accuracy, and the algorithm is selected based on the availability of variables within the dataset [39]. The simplest algorithm assigns a uniform length based on the date of delivery – 270 days for full-term delivery and 245 days for a preterm delivery. Onset of pregnancy is dated by subtracting the appropriate number of days from the delivery date. This method is convenient due to its simplicity but subject to misclassification of extremely premature or post-term pregnancies. More complicated algorithms might include all available data from EMR, for instance, assigning first trimester of pregnancy to the first prenatal visit, using birth weight from birth certificates to assign gestational age based on race and sex-specific standards, using standardized prenatal testing (e.g., α-fetoprotein screening usually done at 11–14 weeks), and dating by ultrasound during pregnancy.

## Parity and Repeated Events

Because pregnancy outcomes, as well as the decision to proceed with additional pregnancies, depend on the outcome of previous pregnancies, appropriately classifying parity to each birth (e.g., first birth versus subsequent births) is critical [3, 40]. Pregnancy outcome studies have very different results when the analysis is restricted to first births only compared with analyses including subsequent births, even in cases in which only one birth per woman is included. Some administrative databases do not include information about parity, and it cannot be assumed (in most circumstances) that the first pregnancy during the study period is necessarily the first pregnancy for a given woman as enrolment periods in health insurance might not cover the entire reproductive history. In these cases, stratifying data on first versus subsequent births may lead to misclassification.

Additional complications in analysis and interpretation arise when multiple births per woman are included in the dataset, as each birth is not independent of the others. The generalized estimating equation approach can be used to account for this lack of independence as long as the pregnancies can be appropriately clustered according to mother [41]. If correlation in the data is not appropriately accounted for, effect estimate will appear more precise than they actually are (e.g., narrower confidence intervals).

## Measuring Drug Exposures

Most administrative databases capture drug exposure based on a filled prescription. As with all pharmacoepidemiologic studies, filling a prescription does not guarantee compliance as the patient might not actually take the drug, leading to some drug exposure misclassifications. However, as patients often need to pay a minimal portion of their medications in most public drug plans, it is likely that patients who fill their prescriptions intend to take at least some of the prescribed drug. Unfortunately, data are rarely collected on over-the-counter medications. This is a particular concern for the study of vitamins (such as folic acid), aspirin, and/or nonsteroidal anti-inflammatory drugs (NSAIDs) in pregnancy, as these are frequently obtained without a prescription. Furthermore, most administrative databases include data only on outpatient-prescribed drugs and do not provide information on drugs dispensed during hospitalizations or administered as infusions. Thus, if pregnant women are hospitalized during pregnancy (and most are at least for delivery), drug exposures during the hospitalization cannot be measured, producing what is called an immeasurable period of exposure [42]. This can lead to differential misclassification of exposure in mothers with SLE as opposed to unaffected mothers, as women with SLE are more likely to be hospitalized during pregnancy and have longer hospitalization stays for delivery. As an example, the mean length of stay for delivery within the OSLER cohort was 5.4 ± 6.7 days for SLE mothers as opposed to 3.3 ± 2.6 days for mothers from the general population [14, 15]. Studies of pregnancy outcomes in the United States similarly find more frequent prenatal hospitalizations and increased length of stay for delivery hospitalizations for mothers with SLE [43]. Statistical methods have been described by Suissa [42], which use a time-varying exposable period to circumvent this potential limitation.

## Ascertaining Congenital Malformations

With increasing use of polypharmacy (inadvertently or intentionally to treat maternal illness) during the periconceptional period and into pregnancy comes increasing concerns for identifying any associations with congenital malformations and medication exposure. The large numbers of subjects available through administrative datasets can be ideal for studying rare outcomes of uncommon prenatal exposures. However, several issues regarding the use of administrative datasets for teratogenicity studies must be addressed. The first issue is the ability to link each mother's records to those of her infant. In the United States, state birth certificate data are often the only infant data available to determine infant outcomes, and the ability and ease of linking these data to maternal data depend on the specific datasets and user access to such data [44]. Neonatal outcomes are limited to those that could be diagnosed at birth. In other cases, infant medical records can be linked to maternal records. Comprehensive medical records for infants will contain more detailed data on neonatal outcomes and complications identified beyond the delivery period than will data obtained solely from birth certificates. As described above, there are inherent difficulties in accurately determining the onset of pregnancy to a precision of days to weeks, which makes a precise determination of when early prenatal exposure to medications occurred with respect to conception.

Once maternal medical records are linked to infant data, the diagnostic accuracy and completeness of ascertainment of congenital anomalies from these records is critical. A major concern of using administrative databases is related to the validity of the diagnostic information because diseases are primarily coded for billing and not for research purposes. One can try to use previously validated case definitions. However, they are not always available, and, when available, none are 100% sensitive and specific. One recent study comparing birth certificate data with administrative health plan data found a high positive predictive value (PPV) for demographic and some pregnancy outcome data on birth certificates, including gestational age, birth weight, race/ethnicity, and prior maternal obstetric history [45]. Unfortunately, PPVs for selected congenital anomalies were much lower for both birth certificate data and administrative claims data. For example, using medical record review as the gold standard, the PPV for cardiac defects in the Tennessee Medicaid population was only 35.7% for birth certificate data, increasing to 74.5% for claims data [46]. Arguably, this is unacceptably low to make meaningful interpretations regarding teratogenicity.

To address the issue of imperfect case ascertainment, one can use Bayesian latent class models, which use various case definitions with each contributing some information about the latent case status of each individual instead of trying to identify a disease case (or outcome) with certainty [47]. Subjects are thus assigned a probability of being a disease case. This method can be used to correct for all sources of uncertainty related to case ascertainment.

## Unmeasured Confounders

As with all observational research, unmeasured confounders may be present. For instance, administrative databases may not record information on smoking, alcohol use, and obesity, which all have been associated with adverse reproductive outcomes. To account for this, one can use sensitivity analyses of unmeasured confounders using previously developed formulas [48].

As an example, if we wanted to study the effect of maternal SLE on the risk of birth defects in the offspring, maternal alcohol intake could be an important unmeasured confounder. Using previously described formulas, one can determine how large the maternal SLE-alcohol association in the cohort would have to be so that adjusting for the presence of the maternal confounder (i.e., alcohol intake) during pregnancy would remove an apparent maternal SLE-birth defect association [48].

## Immortal Time Bias

Observational studies using administrative databases might also be plagued by immortal time bias. Immortal time refers to a period over cohort follow-up, during which, by design, subjects could not have died (or have the outcome/event). As an example, Daniel and colleagues [49] described the potential for immortal time bias in assessing the effect of maternal NSAID exposure in pregnancy on fetal death before 20 weeks of gestation. If NSAID exposure is based on at least one prescription filled before 20 weeks of gestation, exposed fetuses are necessarily immortal during the time span between conception and exposure. By contrast, fetuses in the unexposed group have no such advantage because they could have had the outcome of fetal death at any time during follow-up [49]. To avoid introducing immortal time in our analysis, the solution is simply to categorize follow-up time for each subject according to exposure category.

## Timing of SLE Diagnosis in Relation to Pregnancy

The timing of SLE onset (or diagnosis) with respect to pregnancy is another important issue to consider when conducting some types of studies of SLE in pregnancy. If the onset of disease falls between pregnancies, then one or more of a woman's pregnancies will have occurred prior to SLE, and subsequent pregnancies will have occurred in the presence of the disease. The date of onset of SLE symptoms or date of diagnosis of SLE may not be available in some datasets; in fact, it may not even be recorded in some EMR. This could result in inaccurate data with pregnancies that occurred in women prior to SLE disease onset being included with their other pregnancies that occurred after the onset or diagnosis of SLE. If studying the influence of SLE disease activity on pregnancy outcome, each SLE woman's pregnancies would have to be categorized as prior to onset of SLE symptoms/diagnosis or after, whereas if performing an heritability study, the timing of the maternal SLE onset or diagnosis would not be as relevant. In addition, when SLE presents for the first time during a pregnancy, identifying the precise time of onset of SLE may be difficult as the initial symptoms of SLE may be difficult to distinguish from symptoms or complications of pregnancy unassociated with SLE (e.g., proteinuria and hypertension may be initially diagnosed as preeclampsia rather than lupus nephritis). Further, in such a situation as this, it has not been established when fetal exposure to SLE begins (i.e., throughout the entire pregnancy or only following the diagnosis of SLE).

## Conclusion

SLE is associated with adverse outcomes in pregnancy both for the mother and the fetus with the most common adverse outcome being preterm birth. Preterm birth can have significant impact on the health and survival of the neonate. Women with SLE who conceive during times of disease quiescence have better pregnancy outcomes compared to those pregnancies conceived when the disease is active. Thus, it is very important that women with SLE have low disease activity or remission on medications and dosages that are compatible with pregnancy well prior to conception. Even when these guidelines are followed, there is still a risk for adverse pregnancy outcomes and SLE disease flare during pregnancy. Therefore, SLE pregnancies need careful and close monitoring by the rheumatologist beginning well prior to pregnancy and continuing throughout the pregnancy and postpartum period and by a maternal-fetal medicine specialist throughout pregnancy in order to optimize pregnancy outcome while preventing harm to the mother. There are some clinical guidelines as to what should be assessed and measured prior to conception or early in pregnancy and what should be followed throughout pregnancy, but more research is needed in order to provide more precise recommendations. Multiple data sources are available to study reproductive outcomes in women with SLE. However, they all present some potential methodological considerations that need to be carefully addressed in order to obtain valid findings.

## References

1. Fessel WJ. Epidemiology of systemic lupus erythematosus. Rheum Dis Clin N Am. 1988;14(1):15–23. PMID: 3041487
2. Buyon JP, Kim MY, Guerra MM, Laskin CA, Petri M, Lockshin MD, Sammaritano L, Branch DW, Porter TF, Sawitzke A, Merrill JT, Stephenson MD, Cohn E, Garabet L, Salmon JE. Predictors of pregnancy outcomes in patients with lupus: a cohort study. Ann Intern Med. 2015;163(3):153–63. https://doi.org/10.7326/M14-2235. PMID: 26098843
3. Wallenius M, Salvesen KÅ, Daltveit AK, Skomsvoll JF. Systemic lupus erythematosus and outcomes in first and subsequent births based on data from a national birth registry. Arthritis Care Res (Hoboken). 2014;66(11):1718–24. https://doi.org/10.1002/acr.22373. PMID: 24839126
4. Clowse ME, Jamison M, Myers E, James AH. A national study of the complications of lupus in pregnancy. Am J Obstet Gynecol. 2008;199(2):127.e1–6. https://doi.org/10.1016/j.ajog.2008.03.012. Epub 2008 May 5. PMID: 18456233
5. Lockshin MD, Sammaritano LR. Lupus pregnancy. Autoimmunity. 2003;36(1):33–40. https://doi.org/10.1080/0891693031000067313. PMID: 12765469
6. World Health Organization. Preterm birth. [Internet. Accessed July 21, 2020]. Available from: https://www.who.int/en/news-room/fact-sheets/detail/preterm-birth.
7. Zhang W, Chen SL. An overview on systemic lupus erythematosus pregnancy. Mod Rheumatol. 2003;13(4):293–300. https://doi.org/10.3109/s10165-003-0254-5. PMID: 24387249
8. Koh JH, Ko HS, Kwok SK, Ju JH, Park SH. Hydroxychloroquine and pregnancy on lupus flares in Korean patients with systemic lupus erythematosus. Lupus. 2015;24(2):210–7. https://doi.org/10.1177/0961203314555352. Epub 2014 Oct 10. PMID: 25305214

9. Clowse ME, Wallace DJ, Weisman M, James A, Criscione-Schreiber LG, Pisetsky DS. Predictors of preterm birth in patients with mild systemic lupus erythematosus. Ann Rheum Dis. 2013;72(9):1536–9. https://doi.org/10.1136/annrheumdis-2012-202449. Epub 2013 Jan 29. PMID: 23361085
10. Ko HS, Ahn HY, Jang DG, Choi SK, Park YG, Park IY, Lee G, Park SH, Shin JC. Pregnancy outcomes and appropriate timing of pregnancy in 183 pregnancies in Korean patients with SLE. Int J Med Sci. 2011;8(7):577–83. https://doi.org/10.7150/ijms.8.577. Epub 2011 Oct 1. PMID: 22022210
11. Singh AG, Chowdhary VR. Pregnancy-related issues in women with systemic lupus erythematosus. Int J Rheum Dis. 2015;18(2):172–81. https://doi.org/10.1111/1756-185X.12524. Epub 2014 Dec 25. PMID: 25545844
12. Yasmeen S, Wilkins EE, Field NT, Sheikh RA, Gilbert WM. Pregnancy outcomes in women with systemic lupus erythematosus. J Matern Fetal Med. 2001;10(2):91–6. https://doi.org/10.1080/714904302. PMID: 11392599
13. Molad Y, Borkowski T, Monselise A, Ben-Haroush A, Sulkes J, Hod M, Feldberg D, Bar J. Maternal and fetal outcome of lupus pregnancy: a prospective study of 29 pregnancies. Lupus. 2005;14(2):145–51. https://doi.org/10.1191/0961203305lu2072oa. PMID: 15751819
14. Vinet É, Pineau CA, Scott S, Clarke AE, Platt RW, Bernatsky S. Increased congenital heart defects in children born to women with systemic lupus erythematosus: results from the offspring of Systemic Lupus Erythematosus Mothers Registry Study. Circulation. 2015;131(2):149–56. https://doi.org/10.1161/CIRCULATIONAHA.114.010027. Epub 2014 Oct 29. PMID: 25355915
15. Vinet É, Pineau CA, Clarke AE, Scott S, Fombonne É, Joseph L, Platt RW, Bernatsky S. Increased risk of autism spectrum disorders in children born to women with systemic lupus erythematosus: results from a large population-based cohort. Arthritis Rheumatol. 2015;67(12):3201–8. https://doi.org/10.1002/art.39320. PMID: 26315754
16. Couture J, Bernatsky S, Scott S, Pineau CA, Vinet E. Brief Report: Risk of Childhood Rheumatic and Nonrheumatic Autoimmune Diseases in Children Born to Women With Systemic Lupus Erythematosus. Arthritis Rheumatol. 2018;70(11):1796–1800.
17. Lateef A, Petri M. Managing lupus patients during pregnancy. Best Pract Res Clin Rheumatol. 2013;27(3):435–47. https://doi.org/10.1016/j.berh.2013.07.005. PMID: 24238698; PMCID: PMC3834352
18. Liu J, Zhao Y, Song Y, Zhang W, Bian X, Yang J, Liu D, Zeng X, Zhang F. Pregnancy in women with systemic lupus erythematosus: a retrospective study of 111 pregnancies in Chinese women. J Matern Fetal Neonatal Med. 2012;25(3):261–6. https://doi.org/10.3109/14767058.2011.572310. Epub 2011 Apr 19. PMID: 21504337
19. Gillis JZ, Panopalis P, Schmajuk G, Ramsey-Goldman R, Yazdany J. Systematic review of the literature informing the systemic lupus erythematosus indicators project: reproductive health care quality indicators. Arthritis Care Res (Hoboken). 2011;63(1):17–30. https://doi.org/10.1002/acr.20327. PMID: 20734353
20. Campbell S, Diaz-Recasens J, Griffin DR, Cohen-Overbeek TE, Pearce JM, Willson K, Teague MJ. New Doppler technique for assessing uteroplacental blood flow. Lancet. 1983;1(8326 Pt 1):675–7. https://doi.org/10.1016/s0140-6736(83)91970-0. PMID: 6132039
21. Demas KL, Costenbader KH. Disparities in lupus care and outcomes. Curr Opin Rheumatol. 2009;21(2):102–9. https://doi.org/10.1097/BOR.0b013e328323daad. PMID: 19339919
22. McDonald EG, Bissonette L, Ensworth S, Dayan N, Clarke AE, Keeling S, Bernatsky S, Vinet E. Monitoring of systemic lupus erythematosus pregnancies: a systematic literature review. J Rheumatol. 2018;45(10):1477–90. https://doi.org/10.3899/jrheum.171023. Epub 2018 Jul 15. PMID: 30008450
23. Ruiz-Irastorza G, Khamashta MA. Evaluation of systemic lupus erythematosus activity during pregnancy. Lupus. 2004;13(9):679–82. https://doi.org/10.1191/0961203304lu1099oa. PMID: 15485102
24. Ruiz-Irastorza G, Khamashta MA, Gordon C, Lockshin MD, Johns KR, Sammaritano L, Hughes GR. Measuring systemic lupus erythematosus activity during pregnancy: validation

of the lupus activity index in pregnancy scale. Arthritis Rheum. 2004;51(1):78–82. https://doi.org/10.1002/art.20081. PMID: 14872459
25. Alfirevic Z, Neilson JP. Doppler ultrasonography in high-risk pregnancies: systematic review with meta-analysis. Am J Obstet Gynecol. 1995;172(5):1379–87. https://doi.org/10.1016/0002-9378(95)90466-2. PMID: 7755042
26. Chavez M, Guzman ER, Benito C, Yeo L, Vintzileos A. The clinical significance of absence of end-diastolic velocities of the umbilical artery detected in the severely preterm fetus. Obstet Gynecol. 2001;97:S45.
27. Farine D, Granovsky-Grisaru S, Ryan G, Seaward PG, Teoh TG, Laskin C, Ritchie JW. Umbilical artery blood flow velocity in pregnancies complicated by systemic lupus erythematosus. J Clin Ultrasound. 1998;26(8):379–82. https://doi.org/10.1002/(sici)1097-0096(199810)26:8<379::aid-jcu1>3.0.co;2-f. PMID: 9783243
28. Le Thi Huong D, Wechsler B, Vauthier-Brouzes D, Duhaut P, Costedoat N, Andreu MR, Lefebvre G, Piette JC. The second trimester Doppler ultrasound examination is the best predictor of late pregnancy outcome in systemic lupus erythematosus and/or the antiphospholipid syndrome. Rheumatology (Oxford). 2006;45(3):332–8. https://doi.org/10.1093/rheumatology/kei159. Epub 2005 Oct 25. PMID: 16249242
29. Moores KG, Sathe NA. A systematic review of validated methods for identifying systemic lupus erythematosus (SLE) using administrative or claims data. Vaccine. 2013;31(Suppl 10):K62–73. https://doi.org/10.1016/j.vaccine.2013.06.104. PMID: 24331075
30. Hanly JG, Thompson K, Skedgel C. Identification of patients with systemic lupus erythematosus in administrative healthcare databases. Lupus. 2014;23(13):1377–82. https://doi.org/10.1177/0961203314543917. Epub 2014 Jul 23. PMID: 25057038
31. Langhoff-Roos J, Krebs L, Klungsøyr K, Bjarnadottir RI, Källén K, Tapper AM, Jakobsson M, Børdahl PE, Lindqvist PG, Gottvall K, Colmorn LB, Gissler M. The Nordic medical birth registers--a potential goldmine for clinical research. Acta Obstet Gynecol Scand. 2014;93(2):132–7. https://doi.org/10.1111/aogs.12302. PMID: 24237585
32. Furu K, Wettermark B, Andersen M, Martikainen JE, Almarsdottir AB, Sørensen HT. The Nordic countries as a cohort for pharmacoepidemiological research. Basic Clin Pharmacol Toxicol. 2010;106(2):86–94. https://doi.org/10.1111/j.1742-7843.2009.00494.x. Epub 2009 Dec 4. PMID: 19961477
33. Dall'Era M, Cisternas MG, Snipes K, Herrinton LJ, Gordon C, Helmick CG. The incidence and prevalence of systemic lupus erythematosus in San Francisco County, California: the California Lupus Surveillance Project. Arthritis Rheumatol. 2017;69(10):1996–2005. https://doi.org/10.1002/art.40191. Epub 2017 Sep 10. PMID: 28891237
34. Izmirly PM, Wan I, Sahl S, Buyon JP, Belmont HM, Salmon JE, Askanase A, Bathon JM, Geraldino-Pardilla L, Ali Y, Ginzler EM, Putterman C, Gordon C, Helmick CG, Parton H. The incidence and prevalence of systemic lupus erythematosus in New York County (Manhattan), New York: the Manhattan lupus surveillance program. Arthritis Rheumatol. 2017;69(10):2006–17. https://doi.org/10.1002/art.40192. Epub 2017 Sep 10. PMID: 28891252
35. Tozman EC, Urowitz MB, Gladman DD. Systemic lupus erythematosus and pregnancy. J Rheumatol. 1980;7(5):624–32. PMID: 7441654
36. Petri M, Howard D, Repke J. Frequency of lupus flare in pregnancy. The Hopkins Lupus Pregnancy Center experience. Arthritis Rheum. 1991;34(12):1538–45. https://doi.org/10.1002/art.1780341210. PMID: 1670196
37. Palmsten K, Simard JF, Chambers CD, Arkema EV. Medication use among pregnant women with systemic lupus erythematosus and general population comparators. Rheumatology (Oxford). 2017;56(4):561–9. https://doi.org/10.1093/rheumatology/kew448. PMID: 28013193; PMCID: PMC5850850
38. Likis FE, Sathe NA, Carnahan R, McPheeters ML. A systematic review of validated methods to capture stillbirth and spontaneous abortion using administrative or claims data. Vaccine. 2013;31(Suppl 10):K74–82. https://doi.org/10.1016/j.vaccine.2013.03.076. PMID: 24331077

39. Margulis AV, Palmsten K, Andrade SE, Charlton RA, Hardy JR, Cooper WO, Hernández-Díaz S. Beginning and duration of pregnancy in automated health care databases: review of estimation methods and validation results. Pharmacoepidemiol Drug Saf. 2015;24(4):335–42. https://doi.org/10.1002/pds.3743. Epub 2015 Jan 28. PMID: 25627986
40. Hernández-Díaz S, Toh S, Cnattingius S. Risk of pre-eclampsia in first and subsequent pregnancies: prospective cohort study. Version 2. BMJ. 2009;338:b2255. https://doi.org/10.1136/bmj.b2255. PMID: 19541696
41. Ziegler A, Vens M. Generalized estimating equations. Notes on the choice of the working correlation matrix. Methods Inf Med. 2010;49(5):421–5. https://doi.org/10.3414/ME10-01-0026. discussion 426–32. Epub 2010 Sep 22. PMID: 20871939
42. Suissa S. Immeasurable time bias in observational studies of drug effects on mortality. Am J Epidemiol. 2008;168(3):329–35. https://doi.org/10.1093/aje/kwn135. Epub 2008 May 30. PMID: 18515793
43. Chakravarty EF, Nelson L, Krishnan E. Obstetric hospitalizations in the United States for women with systemic lupus erythematosus and rheumatoid arthritis. Arthritis Rheum. 2006;54(3):899–907. https://doi.org/10.1002/art.21663. PMID: 16508972
44. Johnson KE, Beaton SJ, Andrade SE, Cheetham TC, Scott PE, Hammad TA, Dashevsky I, Cooper WO, Davis RL, Pawloski PA, Raebel MA, Smith DH, Toh S, Li DK, Haffenreffer K, Dublin S. Methods of linking mothers and infants using health plan data for studies of pregnancy outcomes. Pharmacoepidemiol Drug Saf. 2013;22(7):776–82. https://doi.org/10.1002/pds.3443. Epub 2013 Apr 18. PMID: 23596095
45. Andrade SE, Scott PE, Davis RL, Li DK, Getahun D, Cheetham TC, Raebel MA, Toh S, Dublin S, Pawloski PA, Hammad TA, Beaton SJ, Smith DH, Dashevsky I, Haffenreffer K, Cooper WO. Validity of health plan and birth certificate data for pregnancy research. Pharmacoepidemiol Drug Saf. 2013;22(1):7–15. https://doi.org/10.1002/pds.3319. Epub 2012 Jul 3. PMID: 22753079
46. Cooper WO, Hernandez-Diaz S, Gideon P, Dyer SM, Hall K, Dudley J, Cevasco M, Thompson AB, Ray WA. Positive predictive value of computerized records for major congenital malformations. Pharmacoepidemiol Drug Saf. 2008;17(5):455–60. https://doi.org/10.1002/pds.1534. PMID: 18081215
47. Joseph L, Gyorkos TW, Coupal L. Bayesian estimation of disease prevalence and the parameters of diagnostic tests in the absence of a gold standard. Am J Epidemiol. 1995;141(3):263–72. https://doi.org/10.1093/oxfordjournals.aje.a117428. PMID: 7840100
48. Greenland S. Basic methods for sensitivity analysis of biases. Int J Epidemiol. 1996;25(6):1107–16. PMID: 9027513
49. Daniel S, Koren G, Lunenfeld E, Levy A. Immortal time bias in drug safety cohort studies: spontaneous abortion following nonsteroidal antiinflammatory drug exposure. Am J Obstet Gynecol. 2015;212(3):307.e1–6. https://doi.org/10.1016/j.ajog.2014.09.028. Epub 2014 Oct 12. PMID: 25265406

# Chapter 10
# Digital Data in Lupus: Metrics and Future Directions

**Julia F. Simard, Yashaar Chaichian, and Titilola Falasinnu**

## Introduction

The forms of digital data are growing, and computer science and other technology will continue building more tools to leverage and learn from these data. The ultimate hope is that these data can be opportunistically used to answer questions around the causes and consequences of SLE. We first describe some major categories of digital data to understand how these data are generated and what they represent. We then highlight the promising potential and important caveats of digital data.

J. F. Simard (✉)
Department of Epidemiology & Population Health, and Division of Immunology & Rheumatology, Department of Medicine, Stanford University School of Medicine, Stanford, CA, USA
e-mail: jsimard@stanford.edu

Y. Chaichian
Division of Immunology & Rheumatology, Department of Medicine, Stanford University School of Medicine, Stanford, CA, USA
e-mail: Ychaich@stanford.edu

T. Falasinnu
Department of Epidemiology & Population Health, and Department of Anesthesiology, Perioperative and Pain Medicine, Stanford University School of Medicine, Stanford, CA, USA
e-mail: lola.falasinnu@stanford.edu

 
Z. Touma (ed.), *Outcome Measures and Metrics in Systemic Lupus Erythematosus*, https://doi.org/10.1007/978-3-030-73303-2_10

## Section I: Major Types of Digital Data

### *Electronic Health Records*

Electronic health records (EHR), which serve as the digital warehouse of a patient's medical history, have transformed how medical information is recorded and shared for clinical decision-making. EHR have supplanted paper records in the vast majority of clinic and office-based practices [1]. Since the adoption of the Health Information Technology for Economic and Clinical Health Act of 2009, EHR use has climbed fivefold, being employed by 90% of office-based and 100% of hospital-based physicians in the USA [2]. The increased digitization of health information requires novel techniques for extracting and standardizing data from EHR systems [3]. Beyond its clinical applications, EHR data mining has played an essential role in advancing research starting with the critical step of reliably identifying patients with SLE. Case definitions, and phenotypes, may be constructed from combinations of diagnostic and procedure codes, text words, medications, and laboratory results.

Using clinical notes or free text in the EHR is gradually becoming widespread with the adoption of natural language processing (NLP) and often useful for obtaining supplementary information. For example, notes may be the only way to identify specific lupus phenotypes such as classes of lupus nephritis. Jorge et al. constructed a novel machine learning coded algorithm using both coded and NLP-derived data, which outperformed existing rule-based algorithms [4]. Murray et al. used a new technique involving "noisy labeling" which has previously been applied to type 2 diabetes and myocardial infarction and found that constructing a final model that incorporated both structured data and text processing of clinical notes improved the ability to identify SLE cases compared to all prior algorithms [5]. The improvement in yield in combination with structured data is unknown and is a ripe area for future research.

Benefits of EHR as a research data source include the degree of detail available within clinical notes. This can provide access to valuable clinical information that may be unavailable using other data sources. However, there are also several limitations related to the use of EHR data for clinical research. It is important to remember that EHR data is not designed to facilitate research. As discussed in more detail later, there are concerns over the issues of incompleteness and missingness. The data presented are only as thorough as the provider inputting the data. Records from outside hospitals and/or clinics may not be available, or, if present, may not be as detailed as those derived from the home institution. The more fragmented a patient's care, the less likely the data represented in the EHR will represent the entire clinical picture. Selection bias is another concern. For example, despite increasing recognition regarding the importance of patient-reported outcomes, these may not be recorded within the EHR, or, if they are, may not be formally codified making retrieval more challenging [6]. Lastly, medication data may be less valid when obtained from EHR records limited to pharmacy prescription data rather than dispensation data [7].

## Administrative Data

Administrative data has also been used in SLE research. Perhaps the most commonly used form of administrative data is health insurance claims data, which involves data coded during billing of healthcare services to insurers. This type of data includes, but is not limited to, diagnosis codes, procedure codes, and dispensed prescriptions.

Data from Medicaid, the largest public health insurance program in the USA, has been well-studied in SLE. Medicaid, which covers health costs for individuals with low income, is comprised of a high proportion of racial and ethnic minorities contributing a significant burden of chronic disease compared to the general population (The Henry J. Kaiser Foundation. State Health Facts 2011. URL: www.statehealthfacts.org/index.jsp). Nationwide Medicaid claims data have been used to study sociodemographic differences in the incidence and prevalence of SLE and lupus nephritis among US adults, as well as serious infections in both adults and children with SLE [8–10]. Data from Medicare, the public insurance program for individuals aged 65 years and older, as well as young people with disability status, have also been used to characterize the prevalence and burden of SLE [11].

There are various strengths associated with health insurance claims data. First, these data may provide population-level information. Second, medication data obtained from claims data captures filled prescriptions, rather than only written prescriptions. Third, all data elements are recorded as structured fields, facilitating retrieval for research with less difficulty. However, limitations include the inability to contact patients for additional clinical information due to the anonymized nature of the data, as well as limited lifestyle factors data such as cigarette smoking, which may increase the risk of bias due to confounding [7].

Vital statistics data such as birth and death certificates are another form of administrative data largely disconnected from specific billing procedures. Depending on the source, birth data may include or exclude stillbirths and is most likely de-identified. Data may include maternal and paternal race/ethnicity, marital status, and education, as well as maternal health and medical information, features of labor and delivery, and limited data on the newborn. Similarly, death certificate data provides background about the decedent and reported causes of death. Reliability of defining SLE on the basis of documentation in these vital statistics data is variable [12, 13] (Table 10.1).

## Registries

Due to disease heterogeneity, complexity, and the relatively rare nature of SLE, adequately powering studies is a challenge. In addition to administrative data, using large national registries to create patient cohorts can enhance study power in SLE. Population-based registries, such as those in Scandinavian countries and

**Table 10.1** Systemic lupus erythematosus case definition elements and performance

| First author | Database | ICD code visits | Medication | Specialist diagnosed | Problems list | Lab results | Free text | Classification criteria | SN | SP | PPV | NPV |
|---|---|---|---|---|---|---|---|---|---|---|---|---|
| Katz 1997 [39] | Rheumatology practices[A,B] | X | | | | | | | 85% | NA | 90% | NA |
| Costenbader 2002 [40] | Brigham and Women's Hospital patients[A] | | | | | X | | X | 88–93% | 65–69% | 83–84% | 74–85% |
| Sanchez 2003 [41] | Rheumatology Outpatient Clinic in Alabama[A] | X | | | | | | X | 87–90% | 60–72% | 71–77% | NA |
| Arbuckle 2003 [42] | US military database[A] | X | | | | | | X | NA | NA | NA | NA |
| Naleway 2005 [43] | Marshfield clinic in Wisconsin[A] | X | | | | | | | NA | NA | NA | NA |
| Bernatsky 2007 [44] | Quebec physicians claims and hospital data[B] | X | | | | | | | 42–68% | 100% | NA | NA |
| Klein 2010 [45] | Kaiser Permanente Northern California[A] | X | | X | | | X | | NA | NA | NA | NA |
| Chibnik 2010 [46] | Medicaid and Brigham and Women's Hospital patients[A] | X | | | | | | | NA | NA | 89–92% | NA |

| First author | Database | ICD code visits | Medication | Specialist diagnosed | Problems list | Lab results | Free text | Classification criteria | SN | SP | PPV | NPV |
|---|---|---|---|---|---|---|---|---|---|---|---|---|
| Bernastsky 2011 [32] | Nova Scotia health claims and billing databases[B] | X | | X | | | | | 98% | 73% | 58% | NA |
| Broder 2011 [47] | Montefiore Medical Center[A,B] | X | | X | | | | X | NA | NA | 43% | NA |
| Arkema 2016 [14] | Swedish Lupus Linkage cohort[C] | X | X | X | | | | | 97–99% | 99–100% | 97–98% | 100% |
| Barnado 2016 [35] | Vanderbilt's Synthetic Derivative[A] | X | X | | X | X | | | 86% | NA | 89–94% | NA |
| Rees 2016 [24] | Clinical Practice Research Datalink in UK[A] | X | X | | | X | | | NA | NA | NA | NA |
| Jorge 2019 [4] | Partners HealthCare in Massachusetts[A] | X | X | | | X | X | | 64% | 97% | 90% | NA |
| Murray 2019 [5] | UCSF health system[A] | X | | | | X | X | | 83–97% | 91–93% | 85–98% | NA |

*A* Electronic health records, *B* administrative data, *C* registry-based data

Canada, can be linked internally to study an individual's movement through health-care systems including hospitalizations, medication dispensations, births, deaths, sick leave, and disability pensions. One such well-characterized registry linkage is in Sweden, which has been a rich source of epidemiologic data in SLE. Outlining the methodology behind their case definitions using this registry, the investigators considered a range of definitions for SLE in register data and used supervised machine learning methods to identify a case definition with minimal misclassification [14–16].The Danish National Patient Registry is another prominent nationwide registry to facilitate identification of SLE cases, including studies of the incidence of SLE and lupus nephritis, hospitalization rates among SLE patients, and concordance of SLE incidence among twins [17, 18]. Similar types of register linkages have been conducted in Canadian provinces including British Columbia [19, 20] and Quebec [21]. In addition to large study populations facilitated by linkage of population registers, some registries have been developed through international and multi-site collaborations leading to efforts such as the SLICC Cohort and the RELESSER Registry in Spain [22].

Strengths of registry data include the detailed and highly standardized nature of the data collection and the ability to incorporate patient-reported outcomes when incorporating clinical sites or specialized data such as through linkage to EHR or other data sources. Challenges in interpreting data from registries, similar to other datasets, include variability in case definitions of SLE as some registries use ICD coding to define SLE while others include only well-characterized clinical populations with abstracted data on classification criteria. There is great variability in the types of data that are included in registries, and investigators should consider how the data are generated and how the underlying healthcare system informs these efforts. These may not represent routine care experiences as well as EHR or claims data, and variables collected are often fixed and cannot be modified [7]. Perhaps the main limitation of registry data is the intensive burden in terms of time and resources to establish and maintain such a comprehensive data source.

## *Biobank Data with Linkage*

Biobanks are repositories of biological samples which may be complemented with some clinical metadata. Linkage of biobank data with other sources of data, such as registers or characterized clinical populations, may allow researchers to identify SLE and facilitate studies of biomarkers relevant to disease etiology or outcomes. This type of data, for example, may link to various health records to provide a multifaceted portfolio of medical data.

The Clinical Practice Research Datalink (CPRD), established in 1987 in the UK, is an open-access population-based database of ~660 general practices across all 4 countries in the UK [23]. In addition to descriptive epidemiology studies of SLE [24], linkage to UK biobank data was the first to characterize the evolution of symptoms from onset to SLE diagnosis in a prospective manner using primary care data [25]. With biobanking efforts growing internationally, linkage of preexisting clinical or registry data to biobanks will likely be instrumental to future research efforts for a rare disease like SLE.

## *Social Media*

Social media has become a central means of communication and information sharing worldwide. Over 1.5 billion individuals use Facebook, and of the 2.5 million monthly posts related to skin disease, approximately 20% are related to lupus [26]. Patients increasingly use social media to obtain and disseminate medical information in online communities like patient support groups [27]. It is incumbent to recognize how this is transforming the way patients interface with their health and use this to facilitate improved outcomes. Clinical care and research can be both informed and facilitated by social media through qualitative analysis of online discussions, recruitment and survey dissemination, or even as part of an intervention. A recent pilot study investigated the impact of a social media component on medication adherence among adolescents and young adults with SLE using Web-based education [28]. Those who additionally received the social media intervention in combination with Web-based education had significantly improved adherence to hydroxychloroquine, as well as increased self-efficacy, sense of agency, sense of community, and empowerment compared to subjects who received only the Web-based education.

There is growing interest within the medical research community, including among lupus researchers, to harness the power of social media to gain insight into the patient perspective. One recent study globally marketed an online pilot survey using social media platforms to patients with SLE seeking to ascertain triggers for disease flares [26]. Another study used social media and a lupus charity website to advertise an online survey assessing the ease of creating patient opinion data for specific scientific research projects, along with identifying the topics most relevant to patients with SLE and/or antiphospholipid antibody syndrome [29]. Research topics ranked highest among respondents were related to treatment, genetics, triggers, diagnosis, and mechanistic research.

The primary advantage of using social media for SLE research is that it has the potential to reach patients that may not be as apt to engage in traditional forms of media but who are active members of the online community. This may be particularly true for younger patients. Working online also allows patients to connect remotely, decreasing barriers around transportation, and can facilitate global recruitment. At the same time, the use of social media for research is not without limitations. This type of research inherently self-selects for patients who have regular internet access. Those without such access, whether due to socioeconomic barriers or other reasons, are less likely to be recruited in studies or have their experiences represented in the online narrative. Further, even among regular users, there is variability of frequency of social media use. Therefore, research should consider platform or instrument specific user characteristics to evaluate the generalizability or potential selection bias – for example, who are the most active consumers of social media? Lastly, as with some other types of data, patients are often identified via self-diagnosis, which can contribute to potential misclassification that needs to be taken into account when interpreting results. Nevertheless, with the increasing ubiquity of the internet in everyday life, research incorporating social media seems not only savvy but also practical.

## *Wearables*

Wearables are externally applied mobile health devices that can capture health data remotely and continuously. These devices, such as watches with pedometers, GPS tracking, and heart rate monitors, collect copious real-time data that may provide important insights into energy, cardiovascular health, and lifestyle. Policy changes in healthcare highlighting the importance of the patient perspective in disease, along with advances in medical technology, have driven the rise in wearables as a clinical research tool [30]. The Institute for Healthcare Improvement (IHI) has endorsed the "Triple Aim framework" to enhance system-level performance [31]. Beyond the aims of improving population health and reducing the cost per capita of healthcare, the IHI has advocated for improving the patient-reported experience. Wearables are a means to help achieve this goal.

Studies using wearable technology are only just emerging in SLE. A recently completed multicenter randomized clinical trial (results not yet published), RAYOS, incorporated electronic patient-reported outcome measures (ePROM) data to determine whether delayed-release prednisone (RAYOS) improves fatigue and morning stiffness compared to immediate-release prednisone in the treatment of SLE (ClinicalTrials.gov identifier NCT03098823). Self-reported outcome measures were measured throughout the duration of the study, using a smartphone and smartwatch with ePRO tools.

There is increasing interest in the use of ePROM – including those obtained through wearables – and determining their validity in SLE. If shown to be reliable, this will enhance the value and range of SLE patient data that can be collected, as it will no longer need to occur solely at the clinic visit. Indeed, wearables allow patients to document self-reported outcome measures on a smartwatch, smartphone, or other electronic device at any time as well as collect relevant data passively. Integration of ePROM data with that contained within the EHR is an integral step to maximizing its clinical and research applications in SLE. However, at present, there is minimal integration of this data with the EHR.

## Section II: Caveats

### *Defining SLE*

Of fundamental importance when labeling patients as having SLE is ensuring that they indeed carry that diagnosis. Identification of SLE cases using solely diagnosis codes has limitations, with a positive predictive value of only 50–60% for one or two SLE ICD-9 codes [32, 33]. There is often no way to check who has SLE in administrative data unless there is a sample that is captured in an EHR system to conduct the validation. Ideally, gold standard validation should be performed in a blinded manner and in a random sample of the patient charts. The algorithm should also be validated in separate EHR systems (not involved in the development) to test for generalizability. The range of the performance metrics varied: sensitivity (42–100%), specificity (60–100%), PPV (43–100%), and NPV (74–100%). Arkema et al. was the only study that reported on all four performance metrics because of their sampling strategy and found high levels of performance metrics (~97–100%) using the following definition: ≥1 hospitalization or outpatient visit with diagnosis codes for SLE [14]. Another high-yield algorithm the authors found was ≥1 visit in a specialist clinic, hospitalization or outpatient visit [14]. Validation of these algorithms in additional settings needs to be conducted to ensure generalizability.

Further, many studies used the international classification of disease codes (ICD-9 or ICD-10) as discharge, diagnostic, or billing codes. The ICD-9 code for SLE was 710.0 with no way to identify the SLE subtype and no way to exclude drug-induced lupus. Figure 10.1 compares the anatomy of ICD-9 and ICD-10 codes for SLE. The expansion of characters in ICD-10 compared with ICD-9 allows for increased character length and allows for laterality, severity, and complexity of

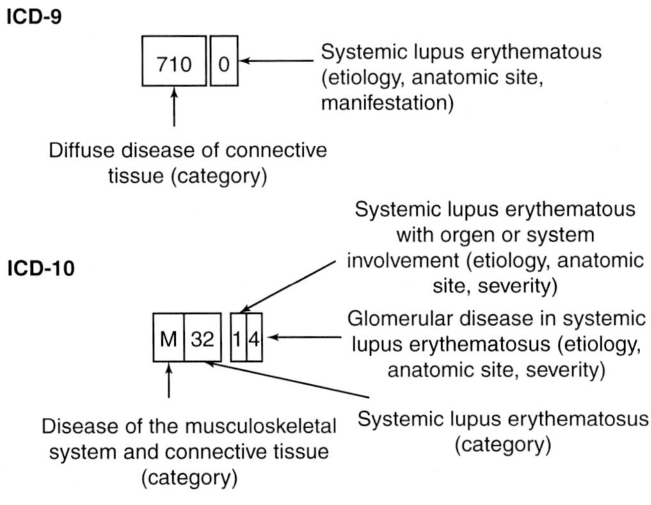


**Fig. 10.1** Comparison of the anatomy of International Classification of Diseases (ICD) codes for systemic lupus erythematosus. (*Note that the expansion of characters in ICD-10 compared with ICD-9 allows for increased character length and allows for laterality, severity, and complexity of disease conditions, which will enable more precise identification and tracking of specific conditions. **Adapted from Pendergrass and Crawford (2018))

disease conditions, which enables more precise identification and tracking of specific conditions [34]. Specifically, ICD-10 now includes SLE with the different subtypes of kidney and cardiovascular manifestations, as well as one expansion for lung involvement. However, neuropsychiatric lupus is absent from ICD-10. The combination of ICD codes for SLE and neuropsychiatric ICD codes could be used to identify these patients in the EHR. There are no studies examining whether clinicians and other providers regularly enter these ICD-10 subtypes into the EHR, and it is unknown whether these subtypes are used in clinical research. The extraction of diagnoses from the problem list may provide some yield, and in situations where the incidence of SLE is under study, it may be helpful for excluding patients with longstanding disease if these patients are new to the EHR system but were diagnosed at another institution.

Given the complexity of SLE as a diagnosis, accuracy can be improved using rule-based algorithms that utilize pre-specified combinations of ICD-9 codes, medications, and laboratory tests [35], but may not always be easily applied between institutions. Requiring specialist care may inadvertently restrict the study population to a subset of SLE phenotypes, limiting generalizability and potentially introducing selection bias (see below). Care should be taken when including medications in algorithms to avoid similarly restricting on disease severity or certain subtypes of SLE. In addition, many medications used in the management of SLE are also used widely in other rheumatic diseases. Some algorithms require that the diagnosis codes be given by specific subspecialists including rheumatologists, dermatologists, nephrologists, and internists. More recent studies included clinical laboratory data in their algorithms, specifically antinuclear antibody (ANA). Positive ANA tests are notoriously nonspecific, but a few studies used more restrictive titer levels (e.g., >1:160) to get around this problem [35].

## *Incomplete Information*

Missingness is a challenge in all aspects of research, but this issue is especially salient in EHR where missing values may often be more frequent than observed or recorded values and what elements may be missing is often unknown [36]. Accuracy of data in the EHR relies on correct and careful documentation of patient care by clinicians, but this is not always top priority due to the busy nature of clinical practices and the complexity of care in SLE. EHR are designed primarily for improving care and billing; thus the secondary use for research can be challenging. A distinction should be made between closed and open systems in EHR. For example, in a referral or tertiary care center, there may be missingness in all clinic visits unrelated to rheumatology, including primary and acute care visits. In outpatient health systems, missingness of acute care visits and hospitalizations also presents challenges, and although some of this may be captured in clinical notes, it may not be recoverable for research purposes. There may also be records from outside hospitals and/or clinics that may not be available, or, if present, not to the same degree as those of the home institution. Thus, the more fragmented a patient's care, the less likely the data represented in the EHR will represent the entire clinical picture.

EHR do not always tell a complete patient story depending on the clinical setting. Missingness often spans inaccurate or incorrect data. However, lack of documentation does not always denote the absence of an event that warranted documentation and often depends on the clinical context and culture. For example, if a medication is prescribed for an acute condition such as pain, diarrhea, or rash, there may be various scenarios that reflect the eventual outcome of this situation (Fig. 10.2). Knowledge of how these four scenarios unfold in the EHR, as detailed in the figure, may be helpful in determining whether missingness is random or systematic, or, for example, whether the patient is recorded as lost to follow-up. In addition, there is often no way to determine whether data elements are self-reported by the patient or whether they are assumed. For example, race/ethnicity is sometimes assumed by medical assistants and may not reflect the self-identity of the patient or capture mixed race individuals.

Routine data quality checks on EHR data may address data quality issues. Error checks can include assessing whether certain related data elements agree. Data entry logs should also be reviewed to examine whether practices varied by time or individuals. The distribution of summary characteristics related to the clinical management of SLE could be compared to the expected distribution. For example, the prevalence and incidence ratio of females to males with SLE is often cited to be 9–13:1, and this ratio could be evaluated in the EHR of interest as a quality check. Finally, researchers may compare the distribution of certain elements to published population-based studies in SLE.

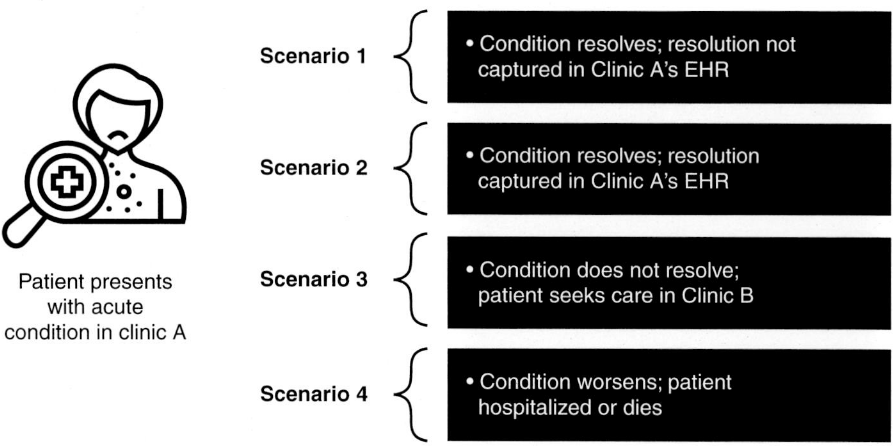


**Fig. 10.2** Hypothetical scenarios depicting the possible outcomes of an acute condition in electronic health records (EHR)

## *Misclassification and Measurement Error*

As described above, leveraging digital data such as EHR and administrative claims requires defining what constitutes SLE and making assumptions about the underlying world from which these data are derived. In addition to robust and valid case definitions, reliable data on comorbid conditions, outcomes, medications, and the timing of all of the above is critical to the estimation of risks and rates. In countries such as Sweden and Canada with national registers and universal access to healthcare, an individual's observable trajectory through the healthcare system facilitates constructing a timeline of their disease, even if only crudely. In other systems without such data, it is often the first visit in a specific clinic or first time with a specific diagnosis in a specific clinic that is used as a proxy for diagnosis. This can overestimate (artificially delay) the true timing for patients with complex conditions like SLE who transfer care, seek second opinions, or have changes in insurance access. The degree to which this may be misclassified depends on the structural and social constructs of the world from which these data originate.

The same challenges exist for pharmacoepidemiologic studies in these types of data. From a timing perspective, do the available data accurately reflect if and when a medication is started? If relying only on clinical documentation or pharmacy orders to define exposure, then researchers are likely to overestimate the number of users. In contrast, when data are available on the dispensing of medication, only those who fill prescriptions are assumed to be exposed. Nevertheless, although dispensing of a medication may represent a patient's intention to take a medication, both actual adherence and duration of use are often unknown. Further when defining medication exposure solely on the basis of whether a medication is dispensed from the pharmacy, we may inadvertently struggle with bias. This can be due to confounding by (1) indication – those who are prescribed a medication have a different risk profile than those who are not prescribed that medication – and (2) adherence, because those who do not fill a prescription are both individuals who were never prescribed the medication *and* individuals who were prescribed the medication but chose not to fill it.

Generally, misclassification and measurement error are classified as either differential or non-differential, sometimes referred to as systematic or random, respectively. This type of bias can impact any variable of interest, and is not remedied by simply increasing the sample size, and the degree and direction of bias may be unpredictable [37]. In the context of digital data, understanding the origins of the data is therefore critical.

## *Selection Bias*

There are "natural" selection forces around us, such as survival, and secondary selection processes that influence how data are obtained or populations are defined. Selection bias is an underappreciated threat to the validity of a study and has been discussed in more detail elsewhere [38]. Survivor bias, a form of selection bias, arises when those who survive and are eligible to be included in a study are systematically different from the full population at risk. When using a prevalent SLE population, this is an important consideration because prevalence is determined by two things: incidence (the occurrence of SLE) and disease duration (surviving with the diagnosis). Some questions are well-suited for prevalent populations, while others, such as estimating the 5-year survival after diagnosis, are not. Identifying prevalent cases in many sources of digital data may be easier than incident cases because one is looking for related healthcare utilization, but the type of data matter here. Are we operating in a system such as the Danish registers where individuals can be identified from birth and one can follow their interactions with the healthcare system? Or are we using tertiary care center clinical data from one specialty that coincides with when individuals were eligible to enroll because of their employment and insurance status?

Selection bias can also be artificially introduced by making unnecessary constraints when putting together a study population. Conditioning on, or requiring, specific events to occur for an SLE case to be defined can inadvertently contribute to selection bias. Numerous validation studies among SLE decedents have found that a considerable proportion of individuals with SLE who die do not have this diagnosis listed as a main or contributory cause of death [12, 13]. At the other end of the spectrum, using birth certificate data for research on pregnancy outcomes implicitly conditions on a birth, which excludes pregnancy losses before 20 weeks of gestation.

As described earlier, some case definitions require patients to be seen by specialists, which may translate to restricting on severity and access to certain healthcare and may result in an overrepresentation of certain phenotypes such as kidney involvement. The potential generalizability may also be influenced by the underlying healthcare system and whether universal healthcare is available. In some situations, SLE may be managed in primary care, especially if the presentation is mild, and in some settings (e.g., rural communities) where access to rheumatologists is limited. Therefore, the completeness of the available data may be related to geography, finances, and myriad socioeconomic factors. Any or all of these factors can be related to exposures of interest, access to treatment, and risk of numerous outcomes.

## Future Directions

Some of the data sources discussed in part one of this chapter describe past research in growing digital data sources. Online data via social media forums such as Reddit, Quora, Facebook, and Twitter provide access to publicly available commentary while also serving as a potential source population for research studies and a medium for innovative interventions. Patients, caregivers, and other stakeholders self-identify, may take on pseudonyms to maintain anonymity, and engage in online discussion about their experiences with SLE. Wearables and other devices may provide real-time data on biometrics, location, and activity. As technology continues to advance the capabilities of these devices, this will continue to add to the richness of data that can inform research and clinical care. Natural language processing (NLP) and the growing world of artificial intelligence/machine learning continues to advance how we can use unstructured data. As these tools advance, what can be learned from different forms of data and how they can be used to inform research will only grow. We have highlighted some biases and how they may manifest in different forms of digital data, and this list is by no means exhaustive.

When thinking about using EHR and other clinically derived data for research, it is important to keep in mind that every healthcare institution, department, and provider has habits and cultures that dictate how things are recorded that may not be easily extractable or knowable. The clinical encounter is about care, first and foremost, and leveraging it for the purposes of research has a number of important considerations around its origins and interpretation. The same is true for many other data sources discussed in this chapter – reconciling the original purpose from the research use of these data requires thoughtful consideration and attention to the caveats and data quality issues identified.

**Disclosures** YC is a sub-investigator on ClinicalTrials.gov identifier NCT03098823.

## References


1. Rasmussen LV. The electronic health record for translational research. J Cardiovasc Transl Res. 2014; https://doi.org/10.1007/s12265-014-9579-z.
2. Henry J., Pylypchuk Y. ST& P V. Adoption of Electronic Health Record Systems among U.S. Non-Federal Acute Care Hospitals: 2008–2015. ONC Data Brief, no. 35. 2016.
3. Manion FJ, Harris MR, Buyuktur AG, Clark PM, An LC, Hanauer DA. Leveraging EHR data for outcomes and comparative effectiveness research in oncology. Curr Oncol Rep. 2012; https://doi.org/10.1007/s11912-012-0272-6.
4. Jorge A, Castro VM, Barnado A, et al. Identifying lupus patients in electronic health records: development and validation of machine learning algorithms and application of rule-based algorithms. Semin Arthritis Rheum. 2019; https://doi.org/10.1016/j.semarthrit.2019.01.002.
5. Murray SG, Avati A, Schmajuk G, Yazdany J. Automated and flexible identification of complex disease: building a model for systemic lupus erythematosus using noisy labeling. J Am Med Informatics Assoc. 2019; https://doi.org/10.1093/jamia/ocy154.
6. Raman SR, Curtis LH, Temple R, et al. Leveraging electronic health records for clinical research. Am Heart J. 2018;202:13–9. https://doi.org/10.1016/j.ahj.2018.04.015.
7. Desai RJ, Solomon DH. Use of large healthcare databases for rheumatology clinical research. Curr Opin Rheumatol. 2017;29(2):138–43. https://doi.org/10.1097/BOR.0000000000000363.
8. Feldman CH, Hiraki LT, Liu J, et al. Epidemiology and sociodemographics of systemic lupus erythematosus and lupus nephritis among US adults with Medicaid coverage, 2000-2004. Arthritis Rheum. 2013; https://doi.org/10.1002/art.37795.
9. Hiraki LT, Feldman CH, Marty FM, Winkelmayer WC, Guan H, Costenbader KH. Serious infection rates among children with systemic lupus erythematosus enrolled in Medicaid. Arthritis Care Res. 2017; https://doi.org/10.1002/acr.23219.
10. Feldman CH, Hiraki LT, Winkelmayer WC, et al. Serious infections among adult Medicaid beneficiaries with systemic lupus erythematosus and lupus nephritis. Arthritis Rheumatol. 2015; https://doi.org/10.1002/art.39070.

11. Garris C, Shah M, Farrelly E. The prevalence and burden of systemic lupus erythematosus in a Medicare population: retrospective analysis of Medicare claims. Cost Eff Resour Alloc. 2015; https://doi.org/10.1186/s12962-015-0034-z.
12. Calvo-Alén J, Alarcón GS, Campbell R, Fernández M, Reveille JD, Cooper GS. Lack of recording of systemic lupus erythematosus in the death certificates of lupus patients. Rheumatology (Oxford). 2005;44(9):1186–9. https://doi.org/10.1093/rheumatology/keh717.
13. Falasinnu T, Rossides M, Chaichian Y, Simard JF. Do death certificates underestimate the burden of rare diseases? The example of systemic lupus erythematosus mortality, Sweden, 2001-2013. Public Health Rep. 2018; https://doi.org/10.1177/0033354918777253.
14. Arkema EV, Jönsen A, Rönnblom L, Svenungsson E, Sjöwall C, Simard JF. Case definitions in Swedish register data to identify systemic lupus erythematosus. BMJ Open. 2016;6(1) https://doi.org/10.1136/bmjopen-2015-007769.
15. Arkema EV, Simard JF. Cohort profile: systemic lupus erythematosus in Sweden: the Swedish lupus linkage (SLINK) cohort. BMJ Open. 2015; https://doi.org/10.1136/bmjopen-2015-008259.
16. Simard JF, Sjöwall C, Rönnblom L, Jönsen A, Svenungsson E. Systemic Lupus Erythematosus Prevalence in Sweden in 2010: what do National Registers say? Arthritis Care Res. 2014;66(11) https://doi.org/10.1002/acr.22355.
17. Hermansen MLF, Lindhardsen J, Torp-Pedersen C, Faurschou M, Jacobsen S. Incidence of systemic lupus erythematosus and lupus nephritis in Denmark: a nationwide cohort study. J Rheumatol. 2016; https://doi.org/10.3899/jrheum.151221.
18. Busch RW, Kay SD, Voss A. Hospitalizations among Danish SLE patients: a prospective study on incidence, causes of admission and risk factors in a population-based cohort. Lupus. 2018; https://doi.org/10.1177/0961203317734919.
19. Li L, Xie H, Lu N, Esdaile JM, Aviña-Zubieta JA. The impact of systemic lupus erythematosus on the risk of newly diagnosed hip fracture. a general population-based study. Arthritis Care Res (Hoboken). 2019:acr.24112. https://doi.org/10.1002/acr.24112.
20. Aviña-Zubieta JA, Vostretsova K, De Vera MA, Sayre EC, Choi HK. The risk of pulmonary embolism and deep venous thrombosis in systemic lupus erythematosus: a general population-based study. Semin Arthritis Rheum. 2015;45(2):195–201. https://doi.org/10.1016/j.semarthrit.2015.05.008.
21. Ng R, Bernatsky S, Rahme E. Disease characterization of systemic lupus erythematosus (SLE) patients in Quebec. Lupus. 2017;26(9):1005–11. https://doi.org/10.1177/0961203317692435.
22. Riveros Frutos A, Casas I, Rúa-Figueroa I, et al. Systemic lupus erythematosus in Spanish males: a study of the Spanish rheumatology society lupus registry (RELESSER) cohort. Lupus. 2017; https://doi.org/10.1177/0961203316673728.
23. Walley T, Mantgani A. The UK general practice research database. Lancet. 1997;350(9084):1097–9. https://doi.org/10.1016/S0140-6736(97)04248-7.
24. Rees F, Doherty M, Grainge M, Davenport G, Lanyon P, Zhang W. The incidence and prevalence of systemic lupus erythematosus in the UK, 1999-2012. Ann Rheum Dis. 2016; https://doi.org/10.1136/annrheumdis-2014-206334.
25. Nightingale AL, Davidson JE, Molta CT, Kan HJ, McHugh NJ. Presentation of SLE in UK primary care using the clinical practice research datalink. Lupus Sci Med. 2017; https://doi.org/10.1136/lupus-2016-000172.
26. Updyke KM, Urso B, Beg S, Solomon J. Developing a continuous quality improvement assessment using a patient-centered approach in optimizing systemic lupus erythematosus disease control. Cureus. 2017; https://doi.org/10.7759/cureus.1762.
27. Smailhodzic E, Hooijsma W, Boonstra A, Langley DJ. Social media use in healthcare: a systematic review of effects on patients and on their relationship with healthcare professionals. BMC Health Serv Res. 2016; https://doi.org/10.1186/s12913-016-1691-0.
28. Scalzi LV, Hollenbeak CS, Mascuilli E, Olsen N. Improvement of medication adherence in adolescents and young adults with SLE using web-based education with and without a

social media intervention, a pilot study. Pediatr Rheumatol. 2018; https://doi.org/10.1186/s12969-018-0232-2.
29. McDonnell TCR, Wincup C, Rahman A, Giles I. Going viral in rheumatology: using social media to show that mechanistic research is relevant to patients with lupus and antiphospholipid syndrome. Rheumatol Adv Pract. 2018; https://doi.org/10.1093/rap/rky003.
30. DeVore AD, Wosik J, Hernandez AF. The future of wearables in heart failure patients. JACC Hear Fail. 2019; https://doi.org/10.1016/j.jchf.2019.08.008.
31. Stiefel M, Nolan K. A guide to measuring the triple aim: population health, experience of care, and per capita costs. IHI Innov Ser white Pap. 2012;
32. Bernatsky S, Linehan T, Hanly JG. The accuracy of administrative data diagnoses of systemic autoimmune rheumatic diseases. J Rheumatol. 2011; https://doi.org/10.3899/jrheum.101149.
33. Moores KG, Sathe NA. A systematic review of validated methods for identifying systemic lupus erythematosus (SLE) using administrative or claims data. Vaccine. 2013; https://doi.org/10.1016/j.vaccine.2013.06.104.
34. Pendergrass SA, Crawford DC. Using electronic health records to generate phenotypes for research. Curr Protoc Hum Genet. 2018:e80. https://doi.org/10.1002/cphg.80.
35. Barnado A, Casey C, Carroll RJ, Wheless L, Denny JC, Crofford LJ. Developing electronic health record algorithms that accurately identify patients with systemic lupus erythematosus. Arthritis Care Res. 2017; https://doi.org/10.1002/acr.22989.
36. Beaulieu-Jones BK, Lavage DR, Snyder JW, Moore JH, Pendergrass SA, Bauer CR. Characterizing and managing missing structured data in electronic health records: data analysis. JMIR Med Inform. 2018; https://doi.org/10.2196/medinform.8960.
37. van Smeden M, Lash TL, Groenwold RHH. Reflection on modern methods: five myths about measurement error in epidemiological research. Int J Epidemiol. 2020;49(1):338–47. https://doi.org/10.1093/ije/dyz251.
38. Choi HK, Nguyen US, Niu J, Danaei G, Zhang Y. Selection bias in rheumatic disease research. Nat Rev Rheumatol. 2014; https://doi.org/10.1038/nrrheum.2014.36.
39. Katz JN, Barrett J, Liang MH, et al. Sensitivity and positive predictive value of Medicare part B physician claims for rheumatologic diagnoses and procedures. Arthritis Rheum. 1997; https://doi.org/10.1002/art.1780400908.
40. Costenbader KH, Karlson EW, Liang MH, Mandl LA. Defining lupus cases for clinical studies: the Boston weighted criteria for the classification of systemic lupus erythematosus. J Rheumatol. 2002;29:12.
41. Sanchez ML, Alarcón GS, McGwin G, Fessler BJ, Kimberly RP. Can the weighted criteria improve our ability to capture a larger number of lupus patients into observational and interventional studies? A comparison with the American College of Rheumatology Criteria. Lupus. 2003; https://doi.org/10.1191/0961203303lu369oa.
42. Arbuckle MR, James JA, Dennis GJ, et al. Rapid clinical progression to diagnosis among African-American men with systemic lupus erythematosus. Lupus. 2003; https://doi.org/10.1191/0961203303lu334oa.
43. Naleway A, Davis ME, Greenlee RT, Wilson DA, McCarty DJ. Epidemiology of systemic lupus erythematosus in rural Wisconsin. Lupus. 2005; https://doi.org/10.1191/0961203305lu2182xx.
44. Bernatsky S, Joseph L, Pineau CA, Tamblyn R, Feldman DE, Clarke AE. A population-based assessment of systemic lupus erythematosus incidence and prevalence - results and implications of using administrative data for epidemiological studies. Rheumatology. 2007; https://doi.org/10.1093/rheumatology/kem233.
45. Klein NP, Ray P, Carpenter D, et al. Rates of autoimmune diseases in Kaiser Permanente for use in vaccine adverse event safety studies. Vaccine. 2010; https://doi.org/10.1016/j.vaccine.2009.10.115.
46. Chibnik LB, Massarotti EM, Costenbader KH. Identification and validation of lupus nephritis cases using administrative data. Lupus. 2010; https://doi.org/10.1177/0961203309356289.
47. Broder A, Khattri S, Patel R, Putterman C. Undertreatment of disease activity in systemic lupus erythematosus patients with endstage renal failure is associated with increased all-cause mortality. J Rheumatol. 2011; https://doi.org/10.3899/jrheum.110571.

# Chapter 11
# Patient-Reported Outcomes in SLE

**Lily McMorrow, Jerik Leung, Vibeke Strand, and Alfred H. J. Kim**

Patient-reported outcome (PRO) measures are a means to quantitatively gauge patients' perceptions of their overall health. Health-related quality of life (HRQoL) is increasingly recognized as an important metric to measure in randomized controlled trials (RCTs) and longitudinal observational studies (LOS) as well as practice, particularly in rheumatologic diseases such as SLE. Quantitatively gauging HRQoL through PROs enriches the clinical assessment of health status and engages patients as stakeholders in their health. This evaluation includes perceived burdens of disease, such as fatigue, pain, and physical function, as well as factors affecting HRQoL, including anxiety and depression [1]. Typically, these factors characterize three facets of health: physical, mental, and social.

Both generic and disease-specific questionnaires have been used to assess HRQoL in SLE populations in RCTs, LOS, and clinical practice [2]. These PROs have distinct advantages and disadvantages. Generic PROs have been validated across a wide range of diseases and have demonstrated responsiveness to changes in patient-reported physical, social, and mental aspects of health [3]. Utilization of generic instruments allows comparisons of the impact of disease between SLE patients and normative as well as different disease populations, including assessment of health status in the context of comorbid conditions. Yet, the wide range of

L. McMorrow · A. H. J. Kim (✉)
Division of Rheumatology, Department of Medicine, Washington University School of Medicine, St. Louis, MO, USA
e-mail: lmcmorrow@wustl.edu; akim@wustl.edu

J. Leung
Department of Behavioral Science and Health Education, College for Public Health and Social Justice, Saint Louis University, St. Louis, MO, USA
e-mail: jerik.leung@slu.edu

V. Strand
Division of Immunology & Rheumatology, Department of Medicine, Stanford University School of Medicine, Palo Alto, CA, USA



Z. Touma (ed.), *Outcome Measures and Metrics in Systemic Lupus Erythematosus*, https://doi.org/10.1007/978-3-030-73303-2_11

SLE-specific impacts on patients limits the ability of generic PROs to reflect burden of disease, thus the development of disease-specific PROs [4]. Inclusion of unique factors, such as body image and burden to others, creates a more relevant and sensitive measure of HRQoL in SLE. Patient input is essential in the development process; patient involvement ensures selection of pertinent items and focuses on the feasibility of PRO utilization. What follows is a review of some of the most widely used generic and disease-specific PROs in SLE, including descriptions of performance characteristics, indications for use, content coverage, and interpretation guidelines (Table 11.1).

**Table 11.1** Key features of commonly used PROs in SLE

| Questionnaire | Generic or disease-specific | Patient involvement | Key characteristics |
|---|---|---|---|
| SF-36 | Generic | Patient input during development | Legacy PRO, well-validated in SLE populations |
| FACIT-F | Generic (fatigue specific) | Patient and expert input during development | Specific measure of fatigue, legacy PRO |
| PROMIS | Generic | No patient input | Aimed at comparison of HRQoL between disease populations, CAT formatting |
| LupusQoL | Disease-specific | Developed from patient interviews | Legacy PRO, paired with SF-36 |
| LupusPRO | Disease-specific | Patient input during development and evaluation | Includes health-related and non-health-related items |
| LIT | Disease-specific | Patient input during development and evaluation | Designed for real-world clinic use |
| SLEQOL | Disease-specific | Patient input included in development and evaluation | Significant patient input, real-world use in Singapore |
| L-QoL | Disease-specific | Patient input during evaluation | Based on needs-based ideological model |
| **Cost-utility analysis questionnaire** | **Generic or disease-specific** | **Patient involvement** | **Key characteristics** |
| EQ-5D | Generic | Patient input during validation | Required by NICE for RCTs |
| SF-6D | Generic | Derived from SF-36 which included patient input | Contains relevant questions to rheumatologic populations, linked to SF-36 |

## Overview of Current PRO Measures

### *Generic Patient-Reported Outcomes*

#### Medical Outcomes Survey Short Form 36 (SF-36)

The SF-36 is a well-validated, generic measure of HRQoL that is sensitive to the effects of disease activity across a broad spectrum of health conditions [5]. In SLE RCTs, this questionnaire has been most frequently used because of its demonstrated sensitivity to changes in physical and emotional health across a variety of rheumatic diseases [6]. This is, in part, due to the broad content coverage, including measures of physical, social, and mental health, with individual items addressing fatigue and depression. Because of the prevalence of such symptoms in SLE and its demonstrated efficacy in terms of discrimination and sensitivity to change, the SF-36 was one of three instruments recently recommended for use as supportive measures in RCTs and LOS by the international consensus group, Outcome Measures in Rheumatology (OMERACT) [1, 7]. This reflects strong discrimination and demonstrated sensitivity to change in HRQoL in SLE patients. Despite its widespread use and validation, SF-36 has limitations because of its generic nature. Aspects of HRQoL specific to SLE, such as intimate relationships and body image, are omitted in SF-36, and thus it is recommended for use in conjunction with SLE-specific measures of HRQoL, such as the LupusQoL, which is discussed further in this review.

SF-36 has demonstrated validity in SLE populations, and its credibility is enhanced because of substantial patient input during initial development [3, 8]. Extensive use of this questionnaire in RCTs has resulted in the establishment of minimum clinically important differences (MCIDs) for patient-reported improvements and/or deterioration. Useful at a group level, extrapolation of MCIDs to patients' individual reported scores in a real-world setting may be an overvaluation, as discussed further in this review. Scoring is facilitated by collection of data on personal electronic devices (such as a tablet or phone), which can then readily generate a score or spydergram, illustrating changes in SF-36 domain scores. The ability of these visuals to illustrate changes has been an important aid to interpretation of SF-36 results in a variety of clinical settings and has been adapted for use in a real-world clinic.

#### The Functional Assessment of Chronic Illness Therapy-Fatigue (FACIT-F) Scale

FACIT-F is a generic PRO questionnaire specifically developed, with a combination of expert and patient input, to assess fatigue as a component of HRQoL. Originally developed to evaluate fatigue in cancer patients, it has been used in a variety of rheumatic diseases [9–11]. Because an estimated 90% of SLE patients experience fatigue, this questionnaire is well-validated and has found great traction in evaluation of this population [12]. Due to the high prevalence of fatigue and its negative impact on HRQoL, OMERACT SLE Working Group recommended its utilization in lupus RCTs [1, 13]. This measure has already been employed in several SLE RCTs, including combined analysis of BLISS-52 and BLISS-76, where it discriminated between HRQoL of medication responders and nonresponder with statistically significant differences and has closely correlated with the vitality domain of SF-36 [13–17].

#### National Institute of Health Initiative Patient-Reported Outcome Measurement Information System (PROMIS) Global Health

This comprehensive PRO was developed in 2004 as a generic measure of health status by compiling items from a variety of existing instruments. An emphasis is placed on the ability of this questionnaire to compare HRQoL profiles across disease populations [18]. To enable this, standardized scoring of this questionnaire is centered around the US general population, and disease scores can be transformed for easy comparison to specific disease populations [19].

Compared to existing generic PROs, PROMIS intends to reduce burden on the patient through flexible administration and survey brevity, in addition to increasing precision [19]. In an effort to facilitate this, computer-adaptive testing (CAT) guides patients through a unique survey path, altering questions posed according to previous responses [19]. Although this measure has demonstrated adequate ability among different disease populations in early evaluation, PROMIS is only beginning to be employed in SLE studies [18, 20–22]. Most recently, responsiveness of the PROMIS Global Short Form was examined in SLE LOS [23].

Early evaluation has highlighted multiple challenges to the use of PROMIS and demonstrates a need to further examine its use in SLE LOS, RCTs, and clinical management. Currently, there is no clear definition of clinically meaningful changes in scores, limiting the ability to interpret results in RCTs and ultimately its functionality. Additionally, the integration of CAT poses challenges to the standardization of this questionnaire, which is especially important when envisioning application in RCTs, as the FDA does not currently accept CAT. Most significantly, this PRO lacks foundational patient input, which may pose limitations to future applicability.

### *Disease-Specific PROs*

#### LupusQoL

The LupusQoL survey was designed in the United Kingdom as an SLE-specific measure of HRQoL to be used in parallel with the SF-36 [24]. Items in this questionnaire were elucidated by thematic analysis of patient interviews, anchoring this measure in the patient experience [24]. The foundational role of patient input also enhanced its specificity to SLE because of the inclusion of distinctive factors of

HRQoL, such as body pain and burden to others, alongside traditional domains of health [24]. Thus, this questionnaire may be more reflective of fluctuations in disease activity in SLE patients [1, 24, 25]. The LupusQoL has demonstrated validity, responsiveness, and close correlation with SF-36 in longitudinal studies and RCTs, with increased sensitivity at intervals of 1 month [2, 24, 26].

The demonstrated reliability, short length, and SLE specificity have resulted in its recent use in SLE trials [1, 4]. In addition, this questionnaire has clearly established MCID values and has become a recommended PRO in SLE RCTs alongside SF-36 [24].

### LupusPRO

LupusPRO is a disease-specific PRO, notable for the inclusion of QoL factors that are both health-related (i.e., pain and sleep) and non-health-related (i.e., coping and goals/desires) [27]. The intentional patient involvement in the evolution of this PRO is understood to have influenced the inclusion of non-HRQoL items in an effort to better represent the patient experience. However, non-HRQoL items have complicated the reliability and consistency of this questionnaire, limiting its applicability in SLE studies. Although this questionnaire was designed to be administered in clinic every 3 months, to put this measure into practice, clinicians must be attentive to the various understandings of the complex non-HRQoL concepts. Further, utilization of this measure in RCTs becomes especially challenging without clearly established MCID values [18].

### Lupus Impact Tracker (LIT)

The LIT was developed from the LupusPRO for use as a routine clinical questionnaire, aimed at evaluating HRQoL in SLE on a regular basis [28]. Because this survey is intended for use in clinical practice, consideration of the patient was central in the design, with patient input included at multiple steps in the development and approval [28]. Despite this, there are still potential drawbacks to this questionnaire. The short form, although more practical for clinical use, reduces content coverage by excluding items addressing SLE symptoms [28]. Thus, depending on a patient's primary symptoms, a more comprehensive questionnaire may be more appropriate given the poorer correlation of LIT with effects of disease activity compared to the SF-36 [29]. As a result, this questionnaire may be most valuable in fostering conversations regarding HRQoL between patients and physicians [28].

### Additional PROs

There are additional SLE-specific measures that have not been as thoroughly evaluated as the previously mentioned PROs and thus have been used sparingly in RCTs. As a result, these measures would not translate well to clinical practice in the United States without further, intentional analysis. Nevertheless, these questionnaires hold a few distinguishing characteristics. The SLE-Specific Quality of Life (SLEQOL) was developed in Singapore and is notable for the patient role during development and evaluation of the survey [30]. This is consistent with increasing emphasis on patient inclusion in the PRO development process. Although this PRO is routinely used in clinics in Singapore, further evaluation of its efficacy in other SLE populations is necessary.

Following this trend of patient involvement, the SLE Quality of Life (L-QoL) also incorporated patient input during the evaluation of the questionnaire [31]. In addition to patient evaluation of validity, L-QoL bases the questionnaire in a needs-based ideological model, focusing on patient capacity and ability to satisfy needs [31]. Although these measures have not had significant traction in SLE studies, they nonetheless illustrate important, patient-centered trends in PRO development.

## *Use as Cost-Utility Measures*

### SF-6D

The SF-6D utilizes items from the eight domains of the SF-36 to formulate an equation of cost-utility. The condensed domains included in the SF-6D include physical functioning, role limitations, social functioning, pain, mental health, and vitality with evaluation from 0 (death) to 1.0 (excellent health) [32, 33]. Thus, this measure retains the robust characterization of HRQoL of the SF-36 and incorporates the measure of quality-adjusted life years (QALYs) in terms of cost-utility analyses [34]. This quantification of health status is an important part of the evaluation of new therapies and is of particular interest to policy makers [35]. The SF-6D has demonstrated validity in SLE populations, and its credibility is enhanced because it is derived from the SF-36, which had significant patient contribution during development and includes questions that are very relevant to rheumatologic populations [36].

### Euro-QoL 5D

The EQ-5D is a generic health questionnaire initially developed in the United Kingdom, and it has been subsequently employed in RCTs in various disease populations, including SLE [37]. Much like the SF-6D, this questionnaire is commonly used because it generates a health-utility measure which allows quantification of QALYs [35].

In considering the applicability of this preference-based measure of health, there are a few factors to highlight. The EQ-5D is broadly used in RCTs, as the National Institute for Health and Care Excellence (NICE) in the United Kingdom requires this evaluation in order for new therapies to be considered for approval. However, it is often used in conjunction with the SF-36 or a disease-specific PRO in order to create a more complete representation of patient HRQoL. It is important to highlight that, although patient input was included during validation, the content of this instrument is derived from professional input [37, 38].

## Application of PROs

As the use of PROs in clinical settings expands, there are opportunities to leverage the administration of surveys in novel ways. The potential for longitudinal use and integration into EMRs, as well as the shift in clinical appreciation of patient perspective, intimates an unrealized capacity in clinical use. This is, however, contingent upon mitigation of logistical and cultural barriers among healthcare providers and clinics. The ability to overcome the current obstacles facing PRO usage is dependent upon increasing utilization in a broad range of clinics; to develop experientially based solutions and identify unforeseen challenges, PROs must be presently implemented in clinical practice.

### *Logistical Considerations for Implementation*

Perhaps the most immediate barriers to PRO integration are operational concerns, as implementation can be disruptive to clinical flow. Indeed, traditional use of these questionnaires requires time for patients to fill out surveys and for scores to be processed, increasing the time each patient spends in the clinic. However, by leveraging electronic administration of PROs, much of the logistical burden can be easily mitigated.

Integration of PROs into clinic flow also has the potential to increase the efficiency of appointments and health evaluation while giving patients more authority in their health care. In-office administration of PROs can be facilitated using tablets or other electronic devices, enabling rapid scoring and connection to EMRs. Initiating out-of-office administration of PROs, such as through a patient portal accessed using a smartphone or other personal electronic device, will reduce the in-office time burden and allow the provider to review the data prior to the office visit. This will also enable patients to identify their main questions and concerns, streamlining clinical conversations by bringing patients' points of interest to the table early in the appointment. Depositing this data into EMRs and giving patients access to their own PRO data will enable clinicians and patients to monitor changes in scores over time and identify patterns and fluctuations in HRQoL. Moreover, this will allow patients to return to the data and reabsorb information that may not have been clearly conveyed during the appointment, fostering a deeper understanding of health and making it easier to participate in treatment decisions and care plans. This is especially important for patients with SLE, as "brain fog" or other cognitive disturbances are commonly experienced and can impact the information processed during an appointment [39].

### *Interpretation of PROs*

The ability of PRO results to determine action is another issue that may limit use in the clinic. This issue is twofold, pertaining to (1) the ability of clinicians to properly interpret scores and (2) the availability of sufficient resources for an effective intervention.

Regarding the interpretation of PROs, defining the point at which changes in PRO scores become actionable can be challenging on an individual basis. MCIDs have been defined for several PROs for use in RCTs as an interpretation guide, but their functionality as a point of score comparison in a clinic setting is limited [39]. MCIDs represent the smallest change in score that corresponds to a perceptible change in health status to a patient, but the extrapolation of these values to the real-world setting oversimplifies the interpretation of PROs [40, 41]. Each patient's health status must be measured against the patient's normative health state, tolerance of symptoms, disease activity, and goals for therapy, all of which constitute status of well-being [41]. These components are best reflected as changes relative to baseline or even normative scores, which are more applicable on an individual basis. Thus, although they may be useful touchstones, this consideration prevents MCIDs from being effective general interpretation guidelines. Alternative ways of interpreting scores in order to better suit clinical use, such as the spydergrams described in the following section, are gaining traction, providing an easily comprehensible platform for comparing scores over time, and increasing accessibility for patients. This further contextualizes findings and aids interpretation on an individual scale, which can then inform action.

Moreover, the known discordance between physician- and patient-reported outcomes in SLE can be emphasized by PRO utilization [42–45]. The disease activity indices were not designed to reflect HRQoL, and may not always correspond well with the intensity of symptoms experienced by patients. Symptoms of SLE have recently been characterized as type I and type II symptoms depending upon their relation to disease activity [46]. Type I refers to symptoms that may reflect SLE disease activity, such as joint pain, rash, and chest pain [46]. In comparison, type II refers to symptoms such as fatigue, widespread pain from fibromyalgia, cognitive function, and sleep disturbance [46]. The effects of type II symptoms are not completely captured by SLE disease activity indices, and, thus, do not correlate as closely to measured disease activity as type I symptoms. As a result, providers may underestimate the severity and impact of type II symptoms in SLE. This discordance is important to measure in order to work toward a common understanding of the disease impact.

In SLE, this is particularly relevant to adverse effects of therapy: although disease activity may decrease upon switching to a new treatment option, side effects may prevent HRQoL from improving to the same degree. This discord may contribute to medication nonadherence among patients with SLE, demonstrating the necessity of decreasing this discord [47, 48]. PROs can be instrumental in the effort to decrease discord by increasing recognition of factors that contribute to type II SLE symptoms, thus acknowledging them as a distinct and important aspect of SLE symptomatology. By reducing this discord, symptoms that broadly impact HRQoL will be more readily identified, encouraging interdisciplinary treatment that extends past care from a physician, such as improving self-management skills and setting treatment goals whenever treatment is adjusted.

## *Illustration of Potential Clinical Use: Spydergrams*

The adoption of spydergrams as a means to visually portray SF-36 scores facilitates interpretation in RCTs, LOS, and real-world practice [15]. Spydergrams display SF-36 domains across eight different axes, which are linked to form octagonal polygons [42] (Figs. 11.1 and 11.2). Thus, the change in shape corresponds to changes in score values. The order in which domain scores are represented around the ring remains constant, enabling rapid assessment of changes in domain scores [42]. This visual is paired with a summary metric as a reflection of overall health status [42].

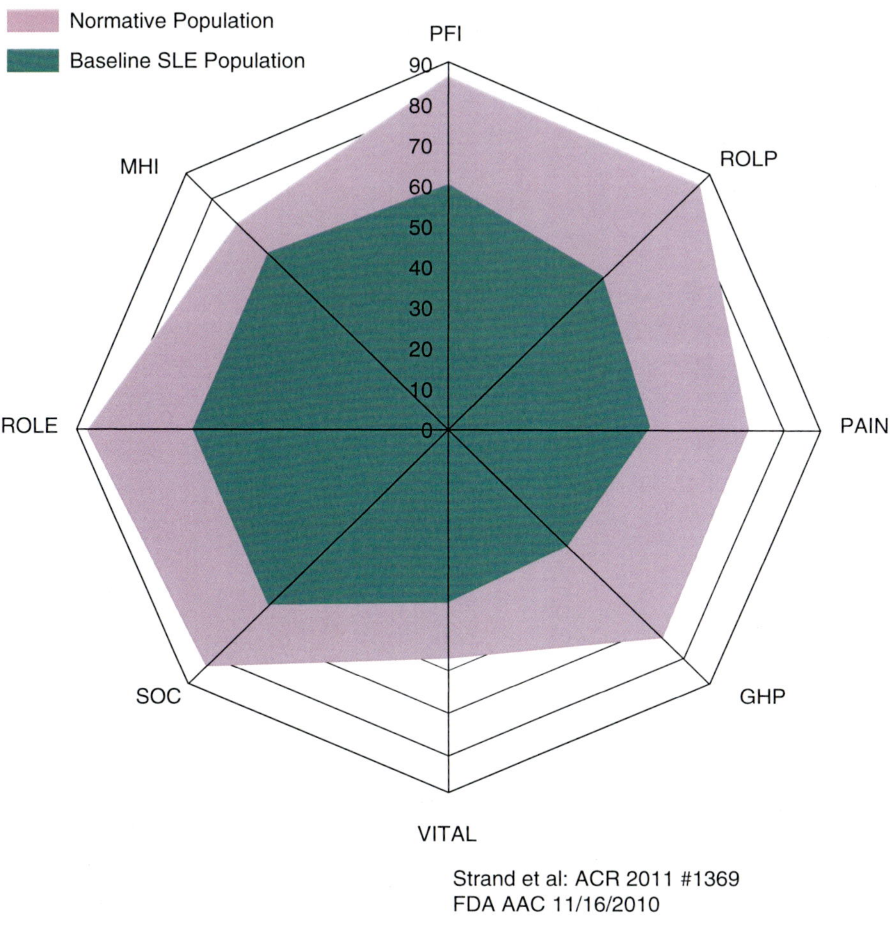


**Fig. 11.1** Visualization of the layering of normative, baseline, and treatment populations in SLE BLISS trials, demonstrating differences in SF-36 scores [data set: 15, 16]. As HRQoL improves, SF-36 scores improve and the area of the shape increases. Normative populations have greater SF-36 scores overall, but statistically significant improvements in scores were seen in medication responders versus the baseline SLE population

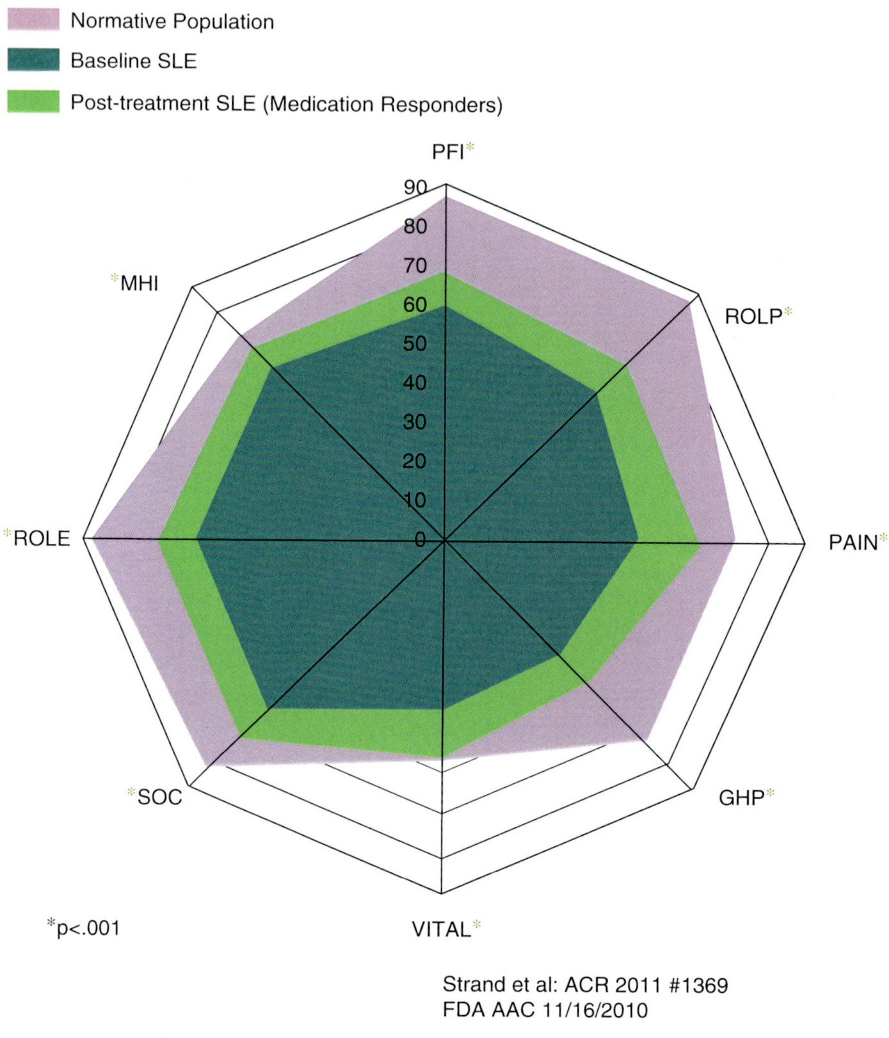


**Fig. 11.1** (continued)

Because these spydergrams reflect SF-36 domain scores, the SF-6D can be utilized to quantify the changes across all domains and present a single score to facilitate comparison between baseline and subsequent visits while offering cost-utility analyses [42].

As opposed to traditional bar charts or tabular data, this geometric representation has the benefit of providing a more intuitive display of HRQoL by leveraging visual cues. Spydergrams spanning multiple visits can be layered to provide a visual comparison of baseline scores and changes across domains over time, revealing patterns of progression or deterioration in HRQoL [42] (Fig. 11.1). In addition, scores from a normative population can also be compared, providing a useful contrast in

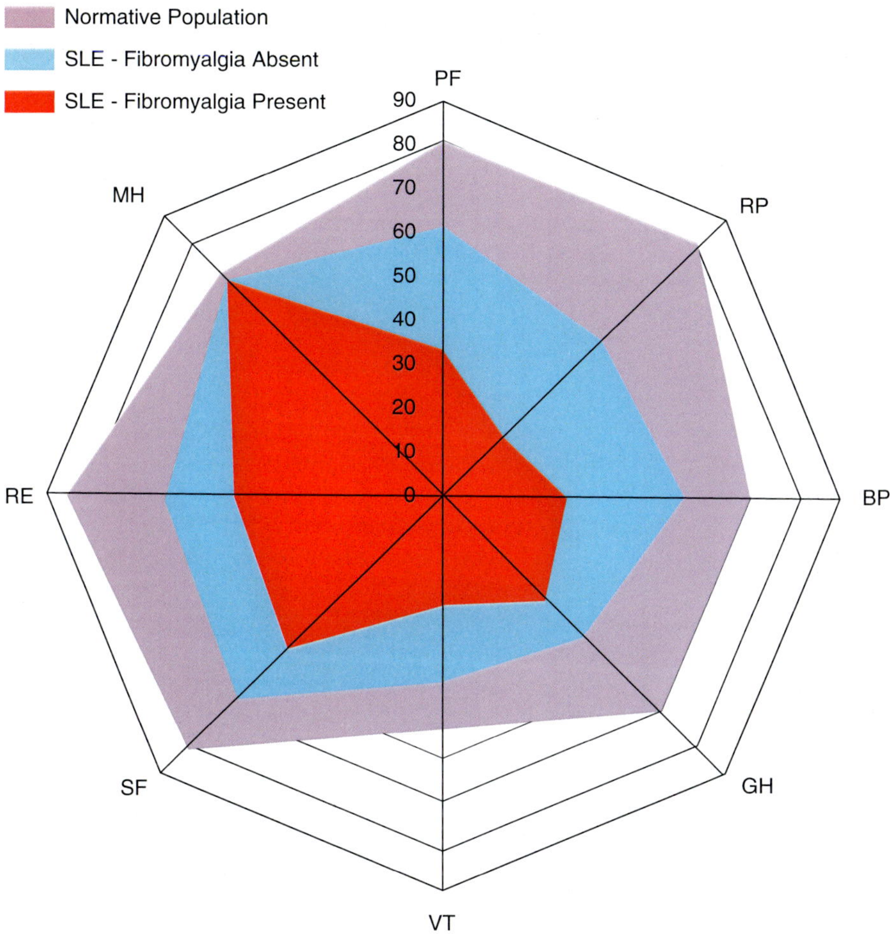


**Fig. 11.2** Spydergrams aid discernment between SLE patients with and without fibromyalgia, with lower overall SF-36 scores and a particular deficit in vitality scores for patients with fibromyalgia. Vitality, encompassing symptoms such as fatigue, is not well-represented by disease activity indices; thus, fibromyalgia may be readily identifiable by PROs. This PRO data presents clinicians and patients with an effective opportunity to distinguish type I (responsive to immunosuppression, such as pleurisy) versus type II SLE (not responsive to immunosuppression, such as fatigue) symptoms [46, 49] [data set: 53]

evaluating scores [42]. Due to the unique way the data are presented, initial training will be required to facilitate patient and provider familiarity with the graphic, but the intuitive nature makes it easy for patients and healthcare providers to rapidly assess stabilization and/or improvements. Spydergrams can then become a dynamic clinical tool that can track changes in HRQoL over long periods of time. In this sense, spydergrams facilitate the use of PROs by enhancing interpretation. This fosters communication by giving patients the language and tools to express any concern and ask questions about treatment and the effect on HRQoL. Thus, the use of spydergrams, as an avenue through which PROs are communicated in clinic, can bridge the gap between patient and provider understanding of health status by reflecting the effects of disease activity. This can be particularly effective in distinguishing SLE signs and symptoms responsive to immunosuppression (type I SLE symptoms) from those nonresponsive to immunosuppression (type II SLE symptoms) [46, 49] (Fig. 11.2).

## *Increasing Actionability*

Deciding the best way to address unmet needs identified using PROs is highly dependent on both provider and clinic capacities, as HRQoL is frequently impacted by factors that cannot be addressed by medical treatment. For example, patients with SLE frequently experience insufficient social support [50, 51]. While PROs can assist in assessing the severity and impact of eroded support in these patients, most providers are not trained to offer effective solutions.

An effective response to low PRO scores requires leveraging interdisciplinary health resources. In addition to the availability of specialists for various organs (i.e., nephrology), liaisons to physical therapy, psychiatric and psychotherapy services, dieticians, and occupational therapy should be used in response to improve HRQoL. Additionally, patient support groups and the provision of education and guidance through social services could improve HRQoL in ways medical treatment may not. Increasing availability and accessibility of these resources to be used in response to PRO scores will be key in maximizing the impact of PROs [52].

Despite the variance in clinic and provider capacities, implementation of PROs can be beneficial in any clinic setting, simply because it may catalyze conversations about HRQoL between physicians and patients and work toward building a path for shared decision-making and understanding of disease burden. This strengthened communication and mutual understanding is conducive to productive conversations about potential therapies, health perception, and resource usage. PROs change the delivery and perspective of healthcare evaluation for the better. The provision of a continuous measure of HRQoL, as opposed to discrete assessments, creates an unprecedented opportunity to identify patterns in health fluctuations and engage patients in their care. Patient feedback will be valuable in improving PRO usage and innovation, and this requires present implementation. Because the goal of PRO use in practice is different from that of RCTs, there remains significant flexibility when deciding how PROs should contribute to clinical conversations, and this can be influenced by patient input. PROs may be beneficial as part of a formalized process that facilitates patient selection of resources that suit changes in health status. In this way, PROs are used to enable patients as stakeholders in their own health while recognizing the multifactorial nature of HRQoL and potential improvements. This reflects an increased awareness of the past marginalization of patients' voices in evaluation of their health, especially within the context of SLE, seen in the absence of patient perspectives during the creation of health outcome measures. As PROs seek to re-center evaluation of health around the patient, using measures that have been authenticated by patient populations will be paramount.

## References


1. Strand V, Simon L, Meara A, Touma Z. Measurement properties of selected patient-reported outcome measures for use in randomised controlled trials in patients with systemic lupus erythematosus: a systematic review. Lupus Sci Med. 2020;7(1):e000373.
2. Smolen JS, Strand V, Cardiel M, Edworthy S, Furst D, Gladman D, et al. Randomized clinical trials and longitudinal observational studies in systemic lupus erythematosus: consensus on a preliminary core set of outcome domains. J Rheumatol. 1999;26(2):504–7.
3. Strand V, Aranow C, Cardiel M, Alarcon-Segovia D, Furie R, Sherrer Y, et al. Improvement in health-related quality of life in systemic lupus erythematosus patients enrolled in a randomized clinical trial comparing LJP 394 treatment with placebo. Lupus. 2003;12(9):677–86.
4. Touma Z, Gladman DD, Ibañez D, Urowitz MB. Is there an advantage over SF-36 with a quality of life measure that is specific to systemic lupus erythematosus. J Rheumatol. 2011;38(9):1898–905.
5. Ware JE, Sherbourne CD. The MOS 36-item short-form health survey (SF-36). I. Conceptual framework and item selection. Med Care. 1992;30(6):473–83.
6. Jolly M. How does quality of life of patients with systemic lupus erythematosus compare with that of other common chronic illnesses. J Rheumatol. 2005;32(9):1706–8.
7. Strand V, Gladman D, Isenberg D, Petri M, Smolen J, Tugwell P. Endpoints: consensus recommendations from OMERACT IV. Outcome measures in rheumatology. Lupus. 2000;9(5):322–7.
8. Hays R, Sherbourne C, Mazel R. The rand 36-item health survey 1.0. Health Econ. 1993;2(3):217–27.
9. Yellen S, Cella D, Webster K, Blendowski C, Kaplan E. Measuring fatigue and other anemia-related symptoms with the Functional Assessment of Cancer Therapy (FACT) measurement system. J Pain Symptom Manag. 1997;13(2):63–74.
10. Cella D, Yount S, Sorensen M, Chartash E, Sengupta N, Grober J. Validation of the functional assessment of chronic illness therapy fatigue scale relative to other instrumentation in patients with rheumatoid arthritis. J Rheumatol. 2005;32(5):811–9.
11. Chandran V, Bhella S, Schentag C, Gladman D. Functional assessment of chronic illness therapy-fatigue scale is valid in patients with psoriatic arthritis. Ann Rheum Dis. 2007;66(7):936–9.
12. Cleanthous S, Tyagi M, Isenberg DA, Newman SP. What do we know about self-reported fatigue in systemic lupus erythematosus. Lupus. 2012;21(5):465–76.
13. Kwan A, Strand V, Touma Z. The role of patient-reported outcomes in systemic lupus erythematosus. Curr Treat Option Rheumatol. 2017;3(4):308–21.
14. Furie R, Petri M, Strand V, Gladman D, Zhong Z, Freimuth W. Clinical, laboratory and health-related quality of life correlates of systemic lupus erythematosus responder index response: a post hoc analysis of the phase 3 belimumab trials. Lupus Sci Med. 2014;1(1):e000031.
15. Strand V, Levy R, Cervera R, Petri M, Birch H, Freimuth W, et al. Improvements in health-related quality of life with belimumab, a B-lymphocyte stimulator-specific inhibitor, in patients with autoantibody-positive systemic lupus erythematosus from the randomised controlled BLISS trials. Ann Rheum Dis. 2013;73(5):838–44.
16. Strand V, Berry P, Lin X, Asukai Y, Punwaney R, Ramachandran S. Long-term impact of Belimumab on health-related quality of life and fatigue in patients with systemic lupus erythematosus: six years of treatment. Arthritis Care Res. 2019;71(6):829–38.

17. Strand V, Chu A. Measuring outcomes in systemic lupus erythematosus clinical trials. Expert Rev Pharmacoecon Outcomes Res. 2011;11(4):455–68.
18. Mahieu M, Yount S, Ramsey-Goldman R. Patient-reported outcomes in systemic lupus erythematosus. Rheum Dis Clin N Am. 2016;42(2):253–63.
19. Cella D, Riley W, Stone A, Rothrock N, Reeve B, Yount S, et al. The Patient-Reported Outcomes Measurement Information System (PROMIS) developed and tested its first wave of adult self-reported health outcome item banks: 2005–2008. J Clin Epidemiol. 2010;63(11):1179–94.
20. Ow YL, Thumboo J, Cella D, Cheung YB, Yong Fong K, Wee HL. Domains of health-related quality of life important and relevant to multiethnic English-speaking Asian systemic lupus erythematosus patients: a focus group study. Arthritis Care Res (Hoboken). 2011;63(6):899–908.
21. Oude Voshaar MA, ten Klooster PM, Glas CA, Vonkeman HE, Taal E, Krishnan E, et al. Calibration of the PROMIS physical function item bank in Dutch patients with rheumatoid arthritis. PLoS One. 2014;9(3):e92367.
22. Fries JF, Cella D, Rose M, Krishnan E, Bruce B. Progress in assessing physical function in arthritis: PROMIS short forms and computerized adaptive testing. J Rheumatol. 2009;36(9):2061–6.
23. Kasturi S, Szymonifka J, Berman J, Kirou K, Levine A, Sammaritano L, et al. Responsiveness of the patient-reported outcomes measurement information system Global Health short form in outpatients with systemic lupus erythematosus. Arthritis Care Res. 2020;72(9):1282–8.
24. McElhone K, Abbott J, Shelmerdine J, Bruce I, Ahmad Y, Gordon C, et al. Development and validation of a disease-specific health-related quality of life measure, the LupusQol, for adults with systemic lupus erythematosus. Arthritis Rheum. 2007;57(6):972–9.
25. McElhone K, Burnell J, Sutton C, Abbott J, Lanyon P, Rahman A, et al. Is the disease-specific Lupusqol sensitive to changes of disease activity in systemic lupus erythematosus patients after treatment of a flare? Value Health. 2014;17(7):A538.
26. González-Rodríguez V, Peralta-Ramírez MI, Navarrete-Navarrete N, Callejas-Rubio JL, Santos Ruiz AM, Khamashta M. Adaptation and validation of the Spanish version of a disease-specific quality of life measure in patients with systemic lupus erythematosus: the Lupus quality of life. Med Clin (Barc). 2010;134(1):13–6.
27. Azizoddin DR, Weinberg S, Gandhi N, Arora S, Block JA, Sequeira W, et al. Validation of the LupusPRO version 1.8: an update to a disease-specific patient-reported outcome tool for systemic lupus erythematosus. Lupus. 2018;27(5):728–37.
28. Jolly M, Garris CP, Mikolaitis RA, Jhingran PM, Dennis G, Wallace DJ, et al. Development and validation of the lupus impact tracker: a patient-completed tool for clinical practice to assess and monitor the impact of systemic lupus erythematosus. Arthritis Care Res (Hoboken). 2014;66(10):1542–50.
29. Jolly M, Kosinski M, Garris CP, Oglesby AK. Prospective validation of the lupus impact tracker: a patient-completed tool for clinical practice to evaluate the impact of systemic lupus erythematosus. Arthritis Rheumatol. 2016;68(6):1422–31.
30. Leong K, Kong K, Thong B, Koh E, Lian T, Teh C, et al. Development and preliminary validation of a systemic lupus erythematosus-specific quality-of-life instrument (SLEQOL). Rheumatology. 2005;44(10):1267–76.
31. Doward LC, McKenna SP, Whalley D, Tennant A, Griffiths B, Emery P, et al. The development of the L-QoL: a quality-of-life instrument specific to systemic lupus erythematosus. Ann Rheum Dis. 2009;68(2):196–200.
32. Ara R, Brazier J. Populating an economic model with health state utility values: moving toward better practice. Value Health. 2010;13(5):509–18.
33. Ara R, Brazier J. Using health state utility values from the general population to approximate baselines in decision analytic models when condition-specific data are not available. Value Health. 2011;14(4):539–45.
34. Brazier J, Roberts J, Deverill M. The estimation of a preference-based measure of health from the SF-36. J Health Econ. 2002;21(2):271–92.
35. Wang S, Wu B, Zhu L, Leng L, Bucala R, Lu L. Construct and criterion validity of the euro Qol-5D in patients with systemic lupus erythematosus. PLoS One. 2014;9(6):e98883.

36. Harrison M, Ahmad Y, Haque S, Dale N, Teh L, SNOWDEN N, et al. Construct and criterion validity of the short form-6D utility measure in patients with systemic lupus erythematosus. J Rheumatol. 2012;39(4):735–42.
37. Wolfe F, Michaud K, Li T, Katz R. EQ-5D and SF-36 quality of life measures in systemic lupus erythematosus: comparisons with rheumatoid arthritis, noninflammatory rheumatic disorders, and fibromyalgia. J Rheumatol. 2009;37(2):296–304.
38. EuroQol – a new facility for the measurement of health-related quality of life. Health Policy. 1990;16(3):199–208.
39. Mackay M. Lupus brain fog: a biologic perspective on cognitive impairment, depression, and fatigue in systemic lupus erythematosus. Immunol Res. 2015;63(1–3):26–37.
40. Nantes S, Strand V, Su J, Touma Z. Comparison of the sensitivity to change of the 36-item short form health survey and the lupus quality of life measure using various definitions of minimum clinically important differences in patients with active systemic lupus erythematosus. Arthritis Care Res. 2017;70(1):125–33.
41. Strand V, Boers M, Idzedza L, Kirwan J, Kvien T, Tugwell P, et al. It's good to feel better but It's better to feel good and even better to feel good as soon as possible for as long as possible. Response criteria and the importance of change at OMERACT 10: figure 1. J Rheumatol. 2011;38(8):1720–7.
42. Strand V, Crawford B, Singh J, Choy E, Smolen J, Khanna D. Use of "spydergrams" to present and interpret SF-36 health-related quality of life data across rheumatic diseases. Ann Rheum Dis. 2009;68(12):1800–4.
43. Yen JC, Abrahamowicz M, Dobkin PL, Clarke AE, Battista RN, Fortin PR. Determinants of discordance between patients and physicians in their assessment of lupus disease activity. J Rheumatol. 2003;30(9):1967–76.
44. Golder V, Ooi JJY, Antony AS, Ko T, Morton S, Kandane-Rathnayake R, et al. Discordance of patient and physician health status concerns in systemic lupus erythematosus. Lupus. 2018;27(3):501–6.
45. Aranow C, Askanase A, Oon S, Huq M, Calderone A, Morand E et al. Laboratory investigation results influence Physician's Global Assessment (PGA) of disease activity in SLE. Ann Rheumat Dis. 2020;:annrheumdis-2019-216753.
46. Pisetsky D, Clowse M, Criscione-Schreiber L, Rogers J. A novel system to categorize the symptoms of systemic lupus erythematosus. Arthritis Care Res. 2019;71(6):735–41.
47. Mosley-Williams A, Lumley M, Gillis M, Leisen J, Guice D. Barriers to treatment adherence among African American and white women with systemic lupus erythematosus. Arthritis Rheum. 2002;47(6):630–8.
48. Leung J, Baker EA, Kim AHJ. Exploring intentional medication non-adherence in patients with systemic lupus erythematosus: the role of physician–patient interactions. Rheumatology Advances in Practice [Internet]. 2021;5(1).
49. Rogers J, Eudy A, Pisetsky D, Criscione-Schreiber L, Sun K, Doss J, et al. Using clinical characteristics and patient-reported outcome measures to categorize lupus subtypes. Arth Care Res. 2020;73(3):386–93.
50. Leung J, Ra J, Baker E, Kim A. "…Not having the real support that we need": patients' experiences with ambiguity of systemic lupus erythematosus and Erosion of social support. ACR Open Rheumatol. 2019;1(3):135–44.
51. Mazzoni D, Cicognani E. Social support and health in patients with systemic lupus erythematosus: a literature review. Lupus. 2011;20(11):1117–25.
52. Hale ED, Treharne GJ, Lyons AC, Norton Y, Mole S, Mitton DL, et al. "Joining the dots" for patients with systemic lupus erythematosus: personal perspectives of health care from a qualitative study. Ann Rheum Dis. 2006;65(5):585–9.
53. Kiani AN, Strand V, Fang H, Jaranilla J, Petri M. Predictors of self-reported health-related quality of life in systemic lupus erythematosus. Rheumatology (Oxford). 2013;52(9):1651–7.

# Chapter 12
# Assessment of Health-Related Quality of Life in Systemic Lupus Erythematosus

**Lee-Suan Teh, Madhura Castelino, Kathleen McElhone, and Janice Abbott**

## Abbreviations

| | |
|---|---|
| ACR | American College of Rheumatology |
| AIMS | Arthritis Impact Measurement Scale |
| BILAG | British Isles Lupus Assessment Group |
| EuroQoL | European Quality of Life |
| FDA | Food and Drug Administration |
| HRQoL | Health-related quality of life |
| LFA | Lupus Foundation of America |
| LIT | Lupus Impact Tracker |
| L-QoL | Systemic Lupus Erythematosus Quality of Life |
| LupusPRO | Lupus Patient-Reported Outcome |
| LupusQoL | Lupus Quality of Life |
| PGA | Physician Global Assessment |
| QoL | Quality of life |

L.-S. Teh (✉)
Department of Rheumatology, Royal Blackburn Teaching Hospital, Blackburn, UK

Faculty of Clinical and Biomedical Sciences, University of Central Lancashire (UCLan), Preston, UK

M. Castelino
Department of Rheumatology, University College London Hospital NHS Foundation Trust, London, UK

Centre for Musculoskeletal Research, University of Manchester, Manchester, UK

K. McElhone
Division of Musculoskeletal and Dermatological Sciences, University of Manchester, Manchester, UK

J. Abbott
School of Psychology, University of Central Lancashire, Preston, UK


Z. Touma (ed.), *Outcome Measures and Metrics in Systemic Lupus Erythematosus*, https://doi.org/10.1007/978-3-030-73303-2_12

| | |
|---|---|
| QOL-S | Quality of Life Scale |
| SF-20 | Short Form-20 |
| SF-36 | Short Form-36 |
| SIP | Sickness Impact Profile |
| SLE | Systemic lupus erythematosus |
| SLEDAI | Systemic Lupus Erythematosus Disease Activity Index |
| SLEQOL | Systemic Lupus Erythematosus Quality of Life |
| SLICC/ACR DI | Systemic Lupus International Collaborating Clinics/American College of Rheumatology Damage Index |
| SSC | SLE Symptom Checklist |
| VAS | Visual Analogue Scale |
| WHOQOL-BREF | World Health Organisation Quality of Life – Abbreviated version |

## Introduction

Systemic lupus erythematosus (SLE) is a chronic autoimmune multisystem disorder which varies in severity and clinical features depending on the spectrum of which organs/systems are involved and the differing antibody profiles. For example, renal and central nervous system involvement can be potentially life-threatening, whereas skin or joint involvement may lead to disfigurement or deforming arthritis. In addition, non-specific clinical features such as fevers, fatigue, weight loss and lymphadenopathy can also be debilitating [5] (Table 12.1). Clinically, the disease course can be unpredictable with remissions and relapses. The disease may be mild and patients can lead a fairly normal life; some patients experience infrequent flares, and other patients can have frequent flares which are life-threatening requiring hospitalisation and sometimes prolonged critical care. It can also be an evolving disease with patients developing new organ/system manifestations over time.

Diagnosis of SLE is based on a combination of clinical and laboratory features [3, 29, 54, 59]. However, a non-specific symptom or single organ involvement at initial presentation can result in a delay in the diagnosis. Management of SLE includes treating the affected organ systems, prevention and reduction of flares, early detection of relapses and prevention of disease-related damage (e.g. osteoporosis, cardiovascular disease). Medications used to treat SLE are of two main types: symptomatic drugs (e.g. topical steroids, non-steroidal anti-inflammatories, antidepressants, anti-epileptics) and immunosuppressive drugs (e.g. antimalarials, steroids, cytotoxics, biologics). All these medications, although essential in disease control, can have undesirable and potentially toxic side effects.

**Table 12.1** Prevalence of non-specific clinical manifestations in SLE [5]

| Non-specific clinical features | Overall prevalence in % |
|---|---|
| Fatigue | 74–100 |
| Fever | 40–80 |
| Weight loss | 44–60 |
| Lymphadenopathy | 21–50 |

The severity of SLE is assessed by measuring three components: the disease activity, damage as a result of the disease or treatment and the impact of the disease and/or treatment on the patient's quality of life. Disease activity and damage are assessed by the clinician, whereas the quality of life is self-reported by the patient. Disease activity and damage have been assessed using standardised and validated SLE-specific measures for decades; however, use of SLE-specific quality of life measures is relatively new. It is important to capture all three components as (a) disease activity measures help to identify reversible organ involvement that should be targeted by treatment; (b) damage indices are prognostic indicators and inversely related to survival; and (c) quality of life measures provide the patient's perspective of the effect of the disease/treatment on their life. As the survival of patients with SLE has significantly improved [62], quality of life as an outcome measure has increased in importance.

## *How Can Systemic Lupus Erythematosus Affect the Patient's Quality of Life?*

SLE and its treatment can have a significant impact on the patients' lives [45]. Diagnostic delay due to the lack of awareness of SLE by some health professionals or single organ/system presentation to different specialties could lead to the patient losing confidence in their healthcare team and lead to feelings of isolation. Beyond an initial relief experienced on receiving the diagnosis of SLE that would validate the symptoms they suffer, for some, the knowledge of the chronicity of the disease could result in feelings of anger, frustration, despair and fear [47]. The paucity of information around the pathogenesis of the disease, the lack of clarity on the role of hormones in disease activity and the unpredictability of the course of SLE can have a significant impact on the patient's life.

Patients with SLE are often young women in the prime of their lives who by their own expectations should be leading productive lives at work, at home and socially. Pregnancy has to be carefully planned after the control of active disease because active disease can be detrimental. In addition, the presence or absence of certain autoantibodies (lupus anticoagulant or anti-phospholipid antibodies) may adversely affect the survival of the foetus, and other autoantibodies (anti-Ro/SSA, anti-La/SSB) may be associated with foetal and neonatal abnormalities, some of which can be permanent (heart block). The lack of autonomy in personal decisions may result in the loss of self-confidence and a feeling of lack of control over their bodily functions and helplessness at a loss of choice over the timing and their ability to fall pregnant [24, 47].

The multi-organ involvement in SLE can not only affect the physical, mental and social health of an individual [50] but can also impact on the patient's ability to function as a mother, wife, friend or co-worker. This may have financial implications as well as lead to marital or relationship problems. Emotional health and their perception of body image and sexuality may be affected by reproductive complications and musculoskeletal and skin involvement. Uncertainty of the course of disease and the possibility of its progression in severity may take its toll on their emotional health. Anxiety about whether their children will be affected by SLE may be tinged with fear and guilt. Non-specific clinical features such as fatigue are prevalent in SLE patients and can be so disabling that day-to-day activities and social commitments may not be fulfilled (summarised by [45]). This may then have a domino effect on the patient's social circle such as spouses, partners, children, the wider family, friends, classmates, co-workers and acquaintances.

## *Why Is It Important to Measure Health-Related Quality of Life in Systemic Lupus Erythematosus?*

There is general consensus that HRQoL is a multidimensional concept and related to the impact of the disease and its treatment 'on an individual's ability to function and his or her perceived well-being in physical, mental and social domains of life' [20]. The collection of HRQoL data alongside clinical measures of disease activity and damage will give a more comprehensive and holistic picture of the patient and their disease. This is especially important in chronic diseases such as SLE where there is no cure and management is based on a balance between controlling the signs and symptoms of the disease and reducing the side effects of the medications. Even if disease activity is suppressed, the side effects of some treatment may potentially cause deterioration in the patient's perceived health. Therefore, measuring HRQoL together with assessing disease activity and damage may prove to be better indicator of treatment outcomes than assessing only the latter two [58]. In addition, HRQoL data may help inform the health professionals caring for the patients by providing a platform to facilitate discussions around issues that are important to the patient and provide them with an opportunity to participate more fully in their own management and planning of their future care. This improved communication between patients and health professionals [19], in turn, may result in better patient concordance with management strategies and thus may have a positive influence on the outcome of the disease. From the health service perspective, assessing HRQoL may be useful for the evaluation of the relative efficacy of interventions including new therapies. The Food and Drug Administration (FDA) agency has advocated that HRQoL should be an essential outcome measure for the assessment of all new treatments [1].

The main aim of measuring HRQoL is to appreciate the patient's perspective. If a particular HRQoL domain is impacted, deficiencies in the health service provision would be highlighted, and contingency plans or services could be put in place to try and address this and thus improve the HRQoL. This may, however, not be easy to implement due to time and manpower constraints in the clinical setting for HRQoL data collection and/or financial limitations for change in health service delivery [16]. Nevertheless, it is something that we should strive to achieve. To facilitate and enable the use of HRQoL measures in routine clinical care, instruments that are valid, reliable, responsive and easy to use/interpret for the clinician and those acceptable (in terms of number and nature of questions) and least burdensome to patients would be better choices.

## Measures Used for Assessing Health-Related Quality of Life in Systemic Lupus Erythematosus and Comparisons Between These Measures

It is generally agreed that HRQoL is a multidimensional concept, and thus unidimensional measures assessing only one aspect of health such as the Stanford Health Assessment Questionnaire (HAQ) which assesses only physical health or the Hospital Anxiety and Depression Scale (HADS) which assesses only mental health are not truly HRQoL measures. Although these measures have been used in SLE patients, they will not be discussed further.

HRQoL questionnaires are designed to be completed unaided by the patient (self-administered), but some can be administered by interview provided the method of asking the questions is standardised to avoid bias. The measure should also be acceptable to the patients in terms of the *number* and *nature* of the items and time to completion as it may affect the willingness of patients to complete it. In addition, questionnaires assessing HRQoL should fulfil three main psychometric properties: validity, reliability and responsiveness.

The validity of the questionnaire includes evaluation of content, construct (convergent/divergent), discriminant (known groups) and criterion validity. Content validity ensures that the measure is sensible and relevant and comprehensively covers all aspects of the condition assessed. The involvement of experts (doctors, nurses and social scientists) as well as patients at the stage of questionnaire development is advocated. Construct validity evaluates the robustness of the scale structure and determines the subscales of the questionnaire. Convergent validity was judged to be adequately demonstrated if there were high positive correlations between scales and divergent validity, if correlations were low or if they were negative. Known groups validity involves hypothesis testing to predict the expected differences between groups (e.g. higher HRQoL scores in less severe patient groups). Assessment of the instrument against the true value or against a gold standard is termed concurrent (criterion) validity.

Internal reliability measures the extent to which items within a subscale are conceptually related and the acceptable statistical value is Cronbach's a $\geq 0.7$ [61]. Test-retest reliability measures the stability of a questionnaire and is gauged by the intraclass correlation coefficient (ICC). An ICC $> 0.7$ is considered adequate [61]. Responsiveness is the ability of the scale to detect changes within the same patient in longitudinal studies. An instrument is considered to have floor or ceiling effects if >15% of respondents scored at the extreme ends of the scale.

## Generic and Condition-Specific Measures Used in Adults with SLE

It is generally accepted that there are three main types of HRQoL measures: generic, condition-specific and disease-specific. Generic measures are applicable to those with any conditions or disease and even where there is absence of disease, condition-specific measures address a disease group (e.g. arthritis, cancer, skin conditions), and disease-specific measures relate to just one disease (e.g. ankylosing spondylitis, rheumatoid arthritis or psoriasis).

Generic measures can be used to compare HRQoL between patients and normal controls or between patients with different diseases allowing for population surveys which are not possible by using either condition- or disease-specific scales.

Generic and condition-specific measures (e.g. the Arthritis Impact Measurement Scale) have been used to assess HRQoL in SLE patients (summarised in [45, 60]). The Medical Outcome Survey Short Form-36 (MOS SF-36) is the most commonly used generic measure in SLE. Table 12.2 provides the number of items, factor structure (domains measured), mode of administration, average completion time, internal reliability and test-retest reliability of these measures. Table 12.3 summarises the concepts assessed.

## SLE-Specific Health-Related Quality of Life Measures for Use in Adults

Generic measures lack specificity and thus may not identify issues important to patients with a particular disease. Therefore, using disease-specific measures may give a more appropriate, comprehensive and unique picture of the disease allowing for important and meaningful data to be collected [40]. Thus, these measures may be more sensitive to subtle changes in HRQoL [12] compared to generic measures.

Body image impairment has been reported to be a major concern for patients with SLE [28] but is missing from the major generic measures used in SLE [57]. In addition, SLE patients have a higher rate of sexual dysfunction compared to controls [11], and sleep disturbances are also common which may impact on fatigue [13] which in turn can affect HRQoL. Neither of these important concepts of sleep and sexual functioning is captured by generic measures [63]. This deficiency in generic measures has led to the development of the following disease-specific questionnaires for patients with SLE. Table 12.4 summarises the number of items, factor structure (domains assessed), administration mode, time to completion, internal reliability and test-retest reliability and Table 12.5 the concepts assessed in the different disease-specific measures.

**Table 12.2** Adult generic and condition-specific measures of HRQoL used in SLE

| Measure | Number of items | Domains assessed (number of domains) | *Administration* Time to completion | Internal reliability mean (range) | Test-retest reliability |
|---|---|---|---|---|---|
| MOS SF-36 | 36 | Physical functioning, role limitations due to physical problems, bodily pain, general health, social functioning, mental health, role limitations due to emotional problems, vitality (8) | *Self- or interview-administered* <10 minutes | 0.85 (0.71–0.95) $n = 150$ | Not assessed |
| MOS SF-20 | 20 | Physical functioning, role functioning, social functioning, mental health, health perception, pain [SF-20+ has a question on fatigue] (6) | *Self- or interview-administered* 5 minutes | Not assessed in SLE | Not assessed in SLE |
| EuroQoL | 5 and one VAS scale | Mobility, self-care, usual activity, pain/discomfort, anxiety/depression VAS for overall general health (5) | *Self-administered* 2–5 minutes | Not assessed in SLE | Not assessed in SLE |
| WHOQoL-BREF | 26 | Physical health, psychological, social relationships, environmental, overall quality of life and general health (6) | *Self-administered* 10 minutes | Not assessed in SLE | Not assessed in SLE |
| SIP | 136 | Sleep and rest; eating; work; home management; recreation and pastimes; ambulation; mobility; body care and movement; social interaction; alertness behaviour; emotional behaviour; communication (12) | *Self- or interview-administered* 20–30 minutes | Not assessed in SLE | Not assessed in SLE |
| QOL-S (QoL rather than HRQoL measure) | 16 | Material goods, health, interpersonal relationships, self, recreational activities and independence (6) | *Self-administered* 2–3 minutes | Time 1: 0.85 Time 1: 0.91 | 0.86 $n$ = not specified $t$ = 4 weeks |
| AIMS | 78 | Mobility, physical activity, dexterity, household activity, social activities, activities of daily living, pain, depression and anxiety, arm function, social support, work (11) | *Self-administered* 20–30 minutes | Not assessed in SLE | Not assessed in SLE |

*AIMS* Arthritis Impact Measurement Scale, *EuroQoL* European Quality of Life, *HRQoL* health-related quality of life, *MOS* SF-36 Medical Outcome Survey Short Form-36, *MOS SF-20* Medical Outcome Survey Short Form-20, *n* number of patients, *QoL* quality of life, *QOL-S* Quality of Life Scale, *SIP* Sickness Impact Profile, *t* time interval between test and retesting, *VAS* Visual Analogue Scale, *WHOQoL-BREF* World Health Organisation Quality of life – Abbreviated version

**Table 12.3** Concepts assessed by adult generic and condition-specific measures of HRQoL used in SLE

| Concepts assessed | SF-36 (36 items) | SF-20 (20 items) | EuroQoL (5 items) | WHOQOL-BREF (26 items) | SIP (136 items) | QOL-S (16 items) | AIMS (78 items) |
|---|---|---|---|---|---|---|---|
| Disease-related symptoms | | | | | | | ✓ |
| Treatment-related symptoms | | | | | | | |
| Burden to patient/ self-care | ✓ | | ✓ | | ✓ | | ✓ |
| Physical functioning/ activities/health/ vitality | ✓ | ✓ | ✓ | ✓ | ✓ | ✓ | ✓ |
| Emotional health/ functioning | ✓ | ✓ | ✓ | ✓ | ✓ | | |
| Self-esteem/body image | | | | ✓ | | | ✓ |
| Pain | ✓ | ✓ | ✓ | ✓ | | | ✓ |
| Planning | | | | | | | |
| Social functioning | ✓ | ✓ | ✓ | ✓ | ✓ | ✓ | ✓ |
| Occupational activities/desires/ goals | | | ✓ | | ✓ | ✓ | ✓ |
| Intimate relationship/ relationship | | | | ✓ | | ✓ | |
| Burden to others/ support from others | | | | | | | ✓ |
| Fatigue/sleep | ✓ | | | ✓ | ✓ | | |
| Cognition | | | | ✓ | ✓ | ✓ | |
| Procreation | | | | | | ✓ | |
| General health | ✓ | ✓ | ✓ | | | ✓ | ✓ |

**Table 12.4** Adult SLE-specific health-related quality of life measures

| Measure | Number of items | Domains assessed (number of domains) | *Administration* Time to completion | Internal consistency Cronbach's α mean (range) | Test-retest reliability ICC (unless stated) mean (range) |
|---|---|---|---|---|---|
| L-QoL | 25 | Unidimensional measure (1) | *Self-administered* (Duration not mentioned) | Time 1: 0.91 ($n = 93$) Time 2: 0.92 ($n = 76$) | 0.95 ($n = 76$) ($t = 2$ weeks) |
| SSC | 38 | List of disease- and treatment-related symptoms and their burden on the patient (1) | *Self-administered* <10 minutes | SSC: 0.89 TDL: 0.89 | Pearson's correlation coefficient ($n = 28$) ($t = 1$ month) SSC, 0.78; TDL, 0.87 |

**Table 12.4** (continued)

| Measure | Number of items | Domains assessed (number of domains) | *Administration* Time to completion | Internal consistency Cronbach's α mean (range) | Test-retest reliability ICC (unless stated) mean (range) |
|---|---|---|---|---|---|
| SLEQOL | 40 | Physical functioning, activities, symptoms, treatment, mood, self-image (6) | *Self-administered* Duration not mentioned | Overall 0.95 ($n = 275$) For subsections, 0.87 (0.76–0.93) | ($n = 51$) ($t = 2$ weeks) Summary score: 0.83 For subsections: 0.63 (0.57–0.80) |
| LupusQoL | 34 | Physical health, pain, planning, intimate relationships, burden to others, body image, emotional health, fatigue (8) | *Self-administered* <10 minutes | 0.93 (0.88–0.96) ($n = 160$) | 0.83 (0.72–0.93) ($n = 83$) ($t = 4$ weeks) |
| LupusPRO *Version 1.6* | 44 | HRQoL (9) – lupus symptoms, lupus medications, physical health, pain-vitality, emotional health, body image, cognition, procreation, general health NHRQoL (4) – relationship/social support, coping, desires-goals, satisfaction with medical care | *Self-administered* <10 minutes | NA (0.68–0.92) ($n = 323$) | ($n = 67$) ($t = 12$ weeks) [NA (0.55–0.92)] |
| *Version 1.7* | 43 | HRQoL as *Version 1.6* with General health removed (8) NHRQoL (4) – as *Version 1.6* | *Self-administered* <10 minutes | NA | NA |
| *Version 1.8* | 49 | HRQoL as *Version 1.6* with Sleep, Pain, vitality separate domains (10) NHRQoL (4) as *Version 1.6* | *Self-administered* <10 minutes | HRQoL 0.96 (0.68–0.97) NHRQoL 0.81(0.69–0.97) | ($n = 16$) ($t = 2$ weeks) Score equivalence of the two time points – data NA |
| LIT | 10 | HRQoL (6) – cognition, lupus medications, physical health, pain/fatigue impact, emotional health, body image NHRQoL (1) – planning/desires/goals | *Self-administered* *<5 minutes* | Time 1: 0.91 Time 2: 0.92 | 0.86 ($n = 300$) ($t = 7$–14 days) 0.88 ($n = 195$; stable sample) ($t = 7$ days) |

*HRQoL* Health-related quality of life, *ICC* intraclass correlation coefficient, *LIT* Lupus Impact Tracker, *LupusPRO* Lupus Patient-Reported Outcome, *LupusQoL* Lupus Quality of Life, *L-QoL* Lupus Quality of Life, *n* number of patients involved, *NA* not available, *NHRQoL* non-health-related quality of life, *SLEQOL* Systemic Lupus Erythematosus Quality of Life, *SSC* SLE Symptom Checklist, *t* time interval between test and retesting, *TDL* total distress level

**Table 12.5** Concepts assessed by adult SLE-specific health-related quality of life measures

| Concepts assessed | L-QoL (25 items) | SSC (38 items) | SLEQOL (40 items) | LupusQoL (34 items) | LupusPRO (43 items) | LIT (10 items) |
|---|---|---|---|---|---|---|
| Disease-related symptoms | | ✓ | ✓ | | ✓ | |
| Treatment-related symptoms | | ✓ | ✓ | | ✓ | ✓ |
| Burden to patient/ self-care | ✓ | ✓ | | | ✓ | |
| Physical functioning/ activities/health/ vitality | ✓ | | ✓ | ✓ | ✓ | ✓ |
| Emotional health/ functioning | ✓ | | ✓ | ✓ | ✓ | ✓ |
| Self-esteem/body image | ✓ | | ✓ | ✓ | ✓ | ✓ |
| Pain | | | ✓ | ✓ | ✓ | ✓ |
| Planning | | | | ✓ | ✓ | ✓ |
| Social functioning | | | ✓ | | | |
| Occupational activities/desires/ goals | | | ✓ | | ✓ | |
| Intimate relationship/ relationship | | | ✓ | ✓ | | |
| Burden to others/ support from others | ✓ | | | ✓ | ✓ | |
| Fatigue/sleep | ✓ | | ✓ | ✓ | ✓ | ✓ |
| Cognition | | | ✓ | | ✓ | ✓ |
| Procreation | | | | | ✓ | |
| General health | | | | | ✓ | |

## Systemic Lupus Erythematosus Quality of Life (L-QoL)

The L-QoL is a unidimensional measure and the content was derived from in-depth qualitative interviews with 50 SLE patients [17]. Face and content validity were confirmed by semi-structured cognitive debriefing interviews. The first version was evaluated by a postal survey of 95 patients (76% response) and the items reduced and retested by 93 patients (63% response), again by postal survey. Rasch analysis was used for item reduction and to confirm the unidimensionality of the measure. There is good test-retest reliability. The L-QoL is able to distinguish between groups according to self-perceived severity of disease, current flare of symptoms and general health. It corresponds moderately to the Nottingham Health Profile. There is no sensitivity to change data for the original L-QoL. The Turkish L-QoL-TR has been demonstrated to be valid and reliable [18], and the website (www.galen-research.

com) [21] states that there are also Estonian, Hungarian and Russian versions of the L-QoL but no mention of the validity of these versions.

## Systemic Lupus Erythematosus Symptom Checklist (SSC)

The SSC [26] is a list of disease- and treatment-related symptoms and their burden. The items were derived from the literature and interviews with physicians and patients. It is a unidimensional measure and was tested in 157 outpatients demonstrating good internal reliability, good test-retest reliability, moderate concurrent validity with the SF-36, as expected poor correlation to the disease activity measure, SLEDAI and the physician's assessment of the disease activity by VAS. There was also good responsiveness in patients treated with pulse cyclophosphamide for lupus nephritis when comparing the SSC at the start of treatment and after 1 year, but this was based on a small sample size [27]. The most frequently scored symptoms were fatigue, musculoskeletal complaints and mental symptoms with fatigue being the most debilitating. Strictly speaking, the SSC is not a true HRQoL measure as it only consists of a list of symptoms. It is validated for Dutch speakers in the Netherlands and cross-culturally adapted to and valid in Brazilian Portuguese [22].

## Systemic Lupus Erythematosus Quality of Life (SLEQOL)

In 2005, the SLEQOL [44] was developed in Singapore. The items were derived from interviews of 16 physicians and specialist nurses. These items were confirmed by the 12 'concepts of relevance' to SLE patients derived from the qualitative work conducted in the USA with 20 female SLE patients [65]. One hundred SLE patients also reviewed these items. Rasch and factor analyses were employed to reduce the number of items, and the items covered six subsections (physical functioning, activities, symptoms, treatment, mood and self-image). It was then tested in 275 outpatients and demonstrated good internal reliability, moderate to good test-retest reliability and poor concurrent validity with the SF-36. As expected, the SLEQOL was also poorly correlated to disease activity measured by the Systemic Lupus Erythematosus Disease Activity Index (SLEDAI), the Systemic Lupus Activity Measure (SLAM) and the damage index, the Systemic Lupus International Collaborating Clinics/American College of Rheumatology Damage Index (SLICC/ACR DI). The authors stated that the SLEQOL was more sensitive but less specific to change in HRQoL than the SF-36 and had significant floor effects while the SF-36 had ceiling effects. Thus, the authors suggested that the SLEQOL should be used alongside the SF-36 when assessing HRQoL in SLE patients which would also allow for comparisons with other diseases. The SLEQOL has been cross-culturally adapted for use in Chinese-speaking SLE patients in Singapore, and this version, the SLEQOL-C, has been evaluated for content validity and has semantic, idiomatic and conceptual equivalence to the SLEQOL [43] and is reliable for use in SLE patients in mainland China [34]. The SLEQOL has also been translated, cross-culturally adapted and validated in Brazilian Portuguese [23] and Thai [41].

## LupusQoL

The LupusQoL is a SLE-specific HRQoL measure developed in the UK [46]. The items were derived from semi-structured interviews with 30 patients with SLE. The interviews were informed by the literature and from interviews with ten clinicians who specialised in looking after patients with SLE. Cognitive debriefing with a further 20 patients with SLE was conducted before the first version of the LupusQoL was devised. It was evaluated in over 600 outpatients with the 3 versions of the questionnaire which were either handed out in clinic or posted to the patients. Factor analysis was utilised to examine the construct validity of the three versions of the questionnaire and the third and final version of the LupusQoL. The LupusQoL was found to have good internal reliability, good test-retest reliability and good concurrent validity with the comparable domains of the SF-36, and good discriminant validity was demonstrated for different levels of disease activity, measured by the British Isles Lupus Assessment Group (BILAG) index and damage (SLICC/ACR DI) but not for all domains. The fatigue domain changed little regardless of the levels of disease activity and damage. It has acceptable ceiling effects and minimal floor effects. Some of its limitations include the lack of men in its initial development phase. However, in the subsequent phases, approximately 6% of all the patients recruited were men, and this is representative of the SLE population in the UK. Furthermore, there is a section at the end of the LupusQoL to allow patients to provide comments. At all development stages, these comments were carefully studied and suggestions incorporated into the next stage of development. Thus, those men who took part had the opportunity to suggest additional areas of importance to them. The LupusQoL is sensitive to change and there is data on the minimal important difference [48]. In 2015, Meacock and colleagues developed a mapping algorithm to provide a practical solution for researchers seeking to use existing data sets where the LupusQoL but no preference-based utility measure is collected for economic evaluation [49].

The LupusQoL has been cross-culturally adapted and evaluated for use in the United States (US) [35] in a cohort of 161 patients with SLE. The results show that the LupusQoL-US has good internal reliability. Principal component analysis revealed five factors, and although the factor structure was different from the UK version, the US version supported the eight domains of the original UK version. There was moderate to good concurrent validity to relevant domains of the SF-36. Only four domains demonstrated good discriminant validity to different degrees of disease activity (SLEDAI) and six domains to different degrees of damage (SLICC/ACR DI). Again, the fatigue domain showed little change to different degrees of disease activity and damage. The differences between the UK and US LupusQoL and could be due to ethnic, disease severity and medical care variations between the patients. The LupusQoL has been translated into and linguistically validated in over

50 languages (www.lupusqol.com), and many of these are available in electronic (ePRO) and/or paper versions. In addition to US English, the LupusQoL has also been validated in a number of other languages, traditional Chinese [64], Iranian [31], Turkish [53], Italian [10] and French [14].

## Lupus Patient-Reported Outcome (LupusPRO)

The LupusPRO was developed and evaluated in the USA [36]. The item pool was derived from semi-structured interviews with 18 outpatients (16 females, 2 males) inquiring their perceptions on how SLE and/or its treatment affected their health and quality of life. Additionally, focus group feedback informed the measure. Several iterations of the measure have been noted making the development of the instrument and evaluations of psychometric properties difficult to follow. The first version (1.6) was administered to 323 SLE patients in multiple centres with a recall period of 4 weeks. Internal consistency was moderate to good. However, this estimate is based on the use of the Cronbach's α statistic inappropriately in domains comprising of two items, so it may be inaccurate. Test-retest reliability ranged from poor to very good, but the 12-week test-retest interval used is potentially influenced by recall bias. Correlations between corresponding domains of the LupusPRO and SF-36 ranged from moderate to strong. Weak negative correlations between LupusPRO domains and disease activity and damage were observed. There were significant floor effects for some domains but acceptable ceiling effects.

Minor changes were made (general health removed) to produce version 1.7. The recall period for non-HRQOL domains was extended to 3 months, and although the authors argue that this was based on patient and expert feedback, it is unlikely that recall is accurate after 3 months and also does not concur with the FDA (Food and Drug Administration) agency patient-reported recommendations for PROs. This version of the LupusPRO (1.7) has been evaluated in several different languages/countries: Tagalog (Philippines), English (Canada), Spanish (Spain), Turkish (Turkey), French (Canada and France), Chinese (Hong Kong), Hindi (India), Japanese (Japan) [6, 7, 15, 32, 38, 42, 51, 52, 55] and Arabic (Egypt) [personal communication]. However, consistent psychometric issues emerged across the evaluations in different cultures. Several countries reported poor internal reliability for the lupus symptoms domain (e.g. Tagalog, Turkish, Canadian French and English) indicating that further developmental work would be useful. Where ceiling/floor effects were reported, some countries demonstrated massive effects for some domains (e.g. between 50% and 70% of the sample). Careful interpretations of data are required when comparing data from different countries, and including different cultural versions of the instrument in the same sample should be avoided.

In 2018, the tool underwent another revision (version 1.8), where the HRQoL domain of pain-vitality was separated into three distinct domains (sleep, pain, vitality). This was done to facilitate longitudinal tracking of these concepts individually. Six items were added to this version without information on derivation. The psychometric properties of this version were tested in 131 consecutive SLE outpatients at two centres [4]. The factor analysis was underpowered, but seven HRQoL factors were derived, with sleep, fatigue and pain loading as a single factor. However, these concepts are strongly associated with one another, and this needs to be considered in longitudinal tracking. Generally, the internal reliability of the instrument appears acceptable, but Cronbach's α coefficients are not an appropriate statistic where there are only two items in the domain. Test-retest reliability was established by examining 'score equivalence' (≤2 weeks between visits) and was undertaken with only 16 patients. Acceptable correlations (indicating convergent validity) were observed between LupusPRO domains and appropriate corresponding domains of the SF-36, FACIT-Fatigue scale, Patient Health Questionnaire-9 (depression) and the Insomnia Severity Index. Discriminant validity measured using the self-reported first item of the SF-36 was good (people were asked to rate their health as either excellent/very good, good or poor). However, known groups validity was not established with clinical 'objective' measures.

Throughout the various versions of the LupusPRO, non-HRQoL items and domains have been presented. It is assumed that aspects such as ways of coping, social support issues and satisfaction with care spontaneously emerged in the patient interviews. However, these are complex concepts, and the coping domain comprises two items both of which consist of optimistic coping strategies which can only provide a biased perception of the ways in which people with SLE cope with their disease.

## Lupus Impact Tracker (LIT)

Jolly et al. [37, 38] developed the Lupus Impact Tracker (LIT) as a unidimensional measure identifying ten items from LupusPRO version 1.6. The LIT is a short patient-report measure to monitor the impact of SLE in routine clinical practice. The selection of items was based on 3 distinct methods: factor analysis and regression analyses (data from previous studies) indicated the 15 most 'significant' items. Most importantly, patient focus groups were asked to rate the most important 15 items from the LupusPRO. Twenty-six patients contributed to this task although there are no demographic or clinical data reported for this sample. Agreement across the three methods was found for only seven items, of which four were retained in the LIT. The authors selected the remaining six items. Of the ten selected items, patients had rated only six of them as 'most important'. The psychometric properties were evaluated from retrospective data, from two previous studies where the LupusPRO was administered. Internal reliability was acceptable, and although test-retest reliability appears acceptable, it was derived from a study with a 3-month time interval. There were moderate associations between the domains of the SF-36 and LIT and weak correlations with the disease activity measures (SELENA-SLEDAI total score and PGA). Known groups validity was demonstrated according to flare severity (Lupus Foundation of America [LFA] physician-rated flare) and SELENA-SLEDAI total scores indicating that those with greater disease severity scored higher on the LIT than those with low disease activity. The authors report 'responsiveness' of the measure using changes in patient-reported health ratings.

Subsequently, the LIT underwent prospective multicentre evaluation among 325 SLE patients [39]. It appears there was no further patient involvement or feedback concerning the items. However, the measure was accepted by both patients and physicians. Nearly 80% of patients and nearly 70% of physicians reported that the LIT helped them discuss the impact of SLE on the patient's life. Similarly, nearly 75% of patients and 50% of physicians reported that the LIT improved communication between them. Confirmatory factor analysis confirmed the unidimensional nature of the scale. Internal reliability and test-retest reliability (1–2 weeks apart) were good. Convergent validity against the SF-36 and LupusQoL was strong apart from with LupusQoL intimate relationship. Discriminant and known groups validity against self-reported health status and disease activity (PGA, SELENA flare index) were observed. Many of the patients had mild disease, but subsequent evaluation of an African American population with more severe disease demonstrated an association with disease activity and organ damage [8]. There is a suggested minimal important difference for the LIT of 2–4 points (from a 100-point scale) [25] although this needs confirmation from robust methodological work as it is likely that a change of 2 points in a 100-point scale is within the region of error. A well-designed evaluation of the LIT across five European countries (France, Germany, Italy, Spain and Sweden) demonstrated similar psychometric results as in the USA [56], and similar evaluation data have been observed in a multi-ethnic Australian cohort [2]. Evaluations of the uptake of the LIT in clinical practice and the value of its use are awaited.

## *Comparison of Psychometric Properties of Adult Health-Related Quality of Life Measures in Systemic Lupus Erythematosus*

In order to assess health-related quality of life accurately, questionnaires used to measure HRQoL, whether generic or disease-specific, should be valid, reliable and responsive to change. These have been reviewed previously [9, 30, 33].

Table 12.6 summarises the degree of evidence for the various psychometric properties for the different HRQoL measures used for adults with systemic lupus erythematosus which has been described in the previous sections.

**Table 12.6** Schematic representation of the level of evidence for psychometric properties of HRQoL measures validated for use in adults with SLE

| Instrument | Content validity | Construct validity | Known groups validity | Internal consistency | Test-retest reliability | Responsiveness | Absence of floor/ceiling effect |
|---|---|---|---|---|---|---|---|
| SF-36 (UK) | NA | + | ++ | +++ | NA | NA | NA |
| QOLS-S | ++ | + | + | ++ | ? | NA | NA |
| SF-6D | NA | + | + | NA | NA | + | ++ |
| EQ-5D | NA | ++ | ++ | NA | NA | + | ++ |
| SSC | ++ | ++ | + | ++ | + | 0 | NA |
| SLEQOL | +++ | ++ | ++ | +++ | ++ | + | +++ |
| LupusQoL [UK] | +++ | ++ | ++ | +++ | ++ | +++ | +++ |
| L-QoL | +++ | ++ | + | +++ | +++ | NA | ? |
| LupusPRO 1.6 | +++ | ++ | 0 | ++ | + | NA | + |
| LupusPRO 1.7 | +++ | ? | 0 | 0 | 0 | NA | + |
| LupusPRO 1.8 | ++ | ++ | + | ++ | ? | NA | NA |
| LIT | ++ | ++ | ++ | +++ | ++ | ? | NA |

+++ signifies strong evidence for measurement property [consistent findings in multiple studies of good methodological quality *or* in one study of excellent methodological quality]; ++ shows moderate evidence for measurement property [consistent findings in multiple studies of fair methodological quality *or* in one study of good methodological quality]; + shows limited evidence for measurement property [one study of fair methodological quality]; ? reports that interpretation is difficult [only studies of poor methodological quality]; 0 indicates no evidence for measurement property; and NA indicates the psychometric property is not assessed (or reported)

## Conclusion

SLE is a multisystem disease that has a significant negative impact on the patients' quality of life. Although, health-related quality of life is a difficult concept to define and measure, major strides have been undertaken in assessing it in many diseases including SLE in the last 20 years. Some manuscripts are unclear regarding scale development and aspects of psychometric evaluation. Yet researchers and clinicians have to be able to independently understand what is being measured and how to interpret the results. Hence, our interpretation may differ from what authors have intended.

The SF-36 is the most commonly employed generic HRQoL measure in SLE studies. It has some disadvantages, common to all generic measures, in that domains specific and important to patients with SLE may not be addressed. This has to some extent been overcome by the newly developed and validated SLE-specific HRQoL questionnaires. However, there remains the question of the choice of questionnaire to use in a study, whether it should be generic or disease-specific scales or both types together and which particular generic or disease-specific scale. Given the various pros and cons of the different scales of the robustness of the validity, reliability and responsiveness, the questionnaire to be chosen should also depend on the research question to be answered and on the population in which it is studied. If HRQoL comparisons are to be made between different diseases or with normal controls, then a generic scale should be used, and the SF-36 would be the best one. If, however, SLE-specific issues are being examined in SLE patients in Singapore, then the SLEQOL may be the optimal choice, whereas the LupusQoL-UK or LupusQoL-US may be preferable in multicentre international studies, and if non-HRQoL issues are being studied, then the LupusPRO or LIT would be more favoured.

The increasing importance of measuring HRQoL in SLE patients has culminated in the development of validated SLE-specific HRQoL measures over the last 15 years. However, there is still some way to go to integrate HRQoL measurement into routine clinical care and to set in place interventions which may positively improve HRQoL. Nevertheless, these important strides have paved the way for improving the care of patients with SLE in the future.

## References

1. US Department of Health and Human Services, Food and Drug Administration, Center for Drug Evaluation and Research, Center for Biologics Evaluation and Research, Center for Devices and Radiological Health. Guidance for industry patient-reported outcome measures: use in medical product development to support labeling claims. Health Qual Life Outcomes. 2006;4:79. http://www.fda.gov/cder/guidance/5460dft.htm.
2. Antony A, Kandane-Rathnayake RK, Ko T, Boulos D, Hoi AY, Jolly M, Morand EF. Validation of the lupus impact tracker in an Australian patient cohort. Lupus. 2017;26:98–105.
3. Aringer M, Costenbader K, Daikh D, Brinks R, Mosca M, Ramsey-Goldman R, Smolen JS, Wofsy D, Boumpas DT, Kamen DL, Jayne D, Cervera R, Costedoat-Chalumeau N, Diamond B, Gladman DD, Hahn B, Hiepe F, Jacobsen S, Khanna D, Lerstrøm K, Massarotti E, McCune J, Ruiz-Irastorza G, Sanchez-Guerrero J, Schneider M, Urowitz M, Bertsias G, Hoyer BF, Leuchten N, Tani C, Tedeschi SK, Touma Z, Schmajuk G, Anic B, Assan F, Chan TM, Clarke AE, Crow MK, Czirják L, Doria A, Graninger W, Halda-Kiss B, Hasni A, Izmirly PM, Jung M, Kumánovics G, Mariette X, Padjen I, Pego-Reigosa JM, Romero-Diaz J, Rúa-Figueroa Fernández I, Seror R, Stummvoll GH, Tanaka Y, Tektonidou MG, Vasconcelos C, Vital EM, Wallace DJ, Yavuz S, Meroni PL, Fritzler MJ, Naden R, Dörner T, Johnson SR. 2019 European league against rheumatism/American College of Rheumatology classification criteria for systemic lupus erythematosus. Arthritis Rheumatol. 2019;71:1400–12.
4. Azizoddin DR, Weinberg S, Gandhi N, Arora S, Block JA, Sequeira W, Jolly M. Validation of the LupusPRO version 1.8: an update to a disease-specific patient-reported outcome tool for systemic lupus erythematosus. Lupus. 2018;27:728–37.
5. Bickerstaff MCM, Isenberg DA. Systemic lupus erythematosus. CPD Rheumatol. 1999;1:3–12.
6. Bourré-Tessier J, Clarke AE, Mikolaitis-Preuss RA, Kosinski M, Bernatsky S, Block JA, Jolly M. Cross-cultural validation of a disease-specific patient-reported outcome measure for systemic lupus erythematosus in Canada. J Rheumatol. 2013;40:1327–33.

7. Bourré-Tessier J, Clarke AE, Kosinski M, Mikolaitis-Preuss RA, Bernatsky S, Block JA, Jolly M. The French-Canadian validation of a disease-specific, patient-reported outcome measure for lupus. Lupus. 2014;23:1452–9.
8. Brandt JE, Drenkard C, Kan H, Bao G, Dunlop-Thomas C, Pobiner B, Chang DJ, Jolly M, Lim SS. External validation of the lupus impact tracker in a Southeastern US longitudinal cohort with systemic lupus erythematosus. Arthritis Care Res. 2017;69:842–8.
9. Castelino M, Abbott J, McElhone K, Teh LS. Comparison of the psychometric properties of health-related quality of life measures used in adults with systemic lupus erythematosus: a review of the literature. Rheumatology. 2013;52:684–96.
10. Conti F, Perricone C, Reboldi G, Gawlicki M, Bartosiewicz I, Pacucci VA, Massaro L, Miranda F, Truglia S, Alessandri C, Spinelli FR, Teh LS, Ceccarelli F, Valesini G. Validation of a disease-specific health-related quality of life measure in adult Italian patients with systemic lupus erythematosus: LupusQoL-IT. Lupus. 2014;23:743–51.
11. Curry SL, Levine SB, Corty E, Jones PK, Kurit DM. The impact of systemic lupus erythematosus on women's sexual functioning. J Rheumatol. 1994;21:2254–60.
12. Curtis TL, Deyo RA, Hudson LD. Pulmonary rehabilitation in chronic respiratory insufficiency. 7. Health-related quality of life among patients with chronic obstructive pulmonary disease. Thorax. 1994;49:162–70.
13. DaCosta D, Bernatsky S, Dritxa M, Clarke AE, Dasgupta K, Keshani A, Pineau C. Determinants of sleep quality in women with systemic lupus erythematosus. Arthritis Care Res. 2005;53:272–8.
14. Devilliers H, Amoura Z, Besancenot JF, Bonnotte B, Pasquali JL, Wahl D, Maurier F, Kaminsky P, Pennaforte JL, Magy-Bertrand N, Arnaud L, Binquet C, Guillemin F. LupusQoL-FR is valid to assess quality of life in patients with systemic lupus erythematosus. Rheumatology. 2012;51:1906–15.
15. Devilliers H, Jolly M, Samson M, et al. Validation of the French version of Lupus Patient Reported Outcome (LupusPRO), a disease-specific patient reported outcome for lupus patients. ACR/ARHP annual meeting; A1419; 2016.
16. Donaldson MS. Applying the Institute of medicine's report, Crossing the Quality Chasm, to QOL assessment in clinical practice. Clin Ther. 2003;25(Suppl D):49–50, (short communication).
17. Doward LC, McKenna SP, Whalley D, Tennant A, Griffiths B, Emery P, Veale DJ. The development of the L-QoL: a quality-of-life instrument specific to systemic lupus erythematosus. Ann Rheum Dis. 2009;68:196–200.
18. Duruöz MT, Unal C, Toprak CS, Sezer I, Yilmaz F, Ulutatar F, Atagündüz P, Baklacioglu HS. The validity and reliability of systemic lupus erythematosus quality of life questionnaire (L-QoL) in a Turkish population. Lupus. 2017;26:1528–33.
19. Fayers PM, Machin D. In: Fayers PM, Machin D, editors. Quality of life assessment, analysis and interpretation. Chichester, New York, Weinheim, Brisbane, Singapore, Toronto: Wiley; 2000. p. 3–27.
20. Ferrans CE. In: Lipscomb J, Gotay CC, Snyder C, editors. Outcome assessment in cancer. Measures, methods, and applications. Cambridge, New York, Melbourne, Madrid, Cape Town: Cambridge University Press; 2005. p. 14–30.
21. http://www.galen-research.com/measures-database/.
22. Freire EA, Guimarães E, Maia I, Ciconelli RM. Systemic lupus erythematosus symptom checklist cross-cultural adaptation to Brazilian Portuguese language and reliability evaluation. Acta Reumatol Port. 2007;32:341–4.
23. Freire EAM, Bruscato A, Leite DRC, Sousa TTS, Ciconelli RM. Translation into Brazilian Portuguese, cultural adaptation and validation of the systemic lupus erythematosus quality of life questionnaire (SLEQOL). Acta Reumatol Port. 2010;35:334–9.
24. Gallop K, Nixon A, Swinburn P, Sterling KL, Naegeli AN, Silk MET. Development of a conceptual model of health-related quality of life for systemic lupus erythematosus from the patient's perspective. Lupus. 2012;21:934–43.

25. Giangreco D, Devilliers H, Annapureddy N, Block JA, Jolly M. Lupus impact tracker is responsive to physician and patient assessed changes in systemic lupus erythematosus. Lupus. 2015;24:1486–91.
26. Grootscholten C, Ligtenberg G, Derksen RHWM, Schreurs KMG, de Glas-Vos JW, Hagen EC, van den Wall Bake AW, Huizinga TW, van den Hoogen FH, Bijl M, van Houwelingen JC, Snoek FJ, Berden JH. Health-related quality of life in patients with systemic lupus erythematosus: development and validation of a lupus specific symptom checklist. Qual Life Res. 2003;12:635–44.
27. Grootscholten C, Snoek FJ, Bijl M, van Houwelingen JC, Derksen RHWM, Berden JHM. Health-related quality of life and treatment burden in patients with proliferative lupus nephritis treated with cyclophosphamide or azathioprine/methylprednisolone in a randomized controlled trial. J Rheumatol. 2007;34:1699–707.
28. Hale ED, Treharne GJ, Norton Y, Lyons AC, Douglas KMJ, Erb N, Kitas GD. 'Concealing the evidence': the importance of appearance concerns for patients with systemic lupus erythematosus. Lupus. 2006;15:532–40.
29. Hochberg MC. Updating the American College of Rheumatology revised criteria for the classification of systemic lupus erythematosus. Arthritis Rheum. 1997;40:1725.
30. Holloway L, Humphrey L, Heron L, Pilling C, Kitchen H, Højbjerre L, Strandberg-Larsen M, Hansen BB. Patient-reported outcome measures for systemic lupus erythematosus clinical trials: a review of content validity, face validity and psychometric performance. Health Qual Life Outcomes. 2014;12:116.
31. Hosseini N, Bonakdar ZS, Gholamrezaei A, Mirbagher L. Linguistic validation of the LupusQoL for the assessment of quality of life in Iranian patients with systemic lupus erythematosus. Int J Rheumatol. 2014;2014:151530.
32. Inoue M, Shiozawa K, Yoshihara R, Yamane T, Shima Y, Hirano T, Jolly M, Makimoto K. The Japanese LupusPRO: a cross-cultural validation of an outcome measure for lupus. Lupus. 2017;26:849–56.
33. Izadi Z, Gandrup J, Katz PP, Yazdany J. Patient-reported outcome measures for use in clinical trials of SLE: a review. Lupus Sci Med. 2018;5:e000279.
34. Jiang H-Z, Lin Z-G, Li H-J, Du Q, Tian W, Wang S-Y, Guan S-Q, Mei Y-F. The Chinese version of the SLEQOL is a reliable assessment of health-related quality of life in Han Chinese patients with systemic lupus erythematosus. Clin Rheumatol. 2018;37:151–60.
35. Jolly M, Pickard AS, Wilke C, Mikolaitis RA, Teh LS, McElhone K, Fogg L, Block J. Lupus-specific health outcome measure for US patients: the LupusQoL-US version. Ann Rheum Dis. 2010;69:29–33.
36. Jolly M, Pickard AS, Block JA, Kumar RB, Mikolaitis RA, Wilke CT, Rodby RA, Fogg L, Sequeira W, Utset TO, Cash TF, Moldovan I, Katsaros E, Nicassio P, Ishimori ML, Kosinsky M, Merrill JT, Weisman MH, Wallace DJ. Disease-specific patient reported outcome tools for systemic lupus erythematosus. Semin Arthritis Rheum. 2012;42:56–65.
37. Jolly M, Garris CP, Mikolaitis RA, Jhingran PM, Dennis G, Wallace DJ, Clarke A, Dooley MA, Parke A, Strand V, Alárcon GS, Kosinski M. Development and validation of the Lupus Impact Tracker: a patient-completed tool for clinical practice to assess and monitor the impact of systemic lupus erythematosus. Arthritis Care Res (Hoboken). 2014;66(10):1542–50. https://doi.org/10.1002/acr.22349.
38. Jolly M, Toloza S, Block J, Mikolaitis R, Kosinski M, Wallace D, Durran-Barragan S, Bertoli A, Blazevic I, Vilá L, Cooray D, Moldovan I, Katsaros E, Weisman M, Torralba KM, Alarcón G. Spanish LupusPRO: cross-cultural validation study for lupus. Lupus. 2013;22:431–6.
39. Jolly M, Kosinski M, Garris CP, Oglesby AK. Prospective validation of the lupus impact tracker: a patient-completed tool for clinical practice to evaluate the impact of systemic lupus erythematosus. Arthritis Rheumatol. 2016;68:1422–31.
40. Jones PW. Quality of life measurement: the value of standardisation. Eur Respir Rev. 1997;7:46–9.
41. Kasitanon N, Wangkaew S, Puntana S, Sukitawut W, Leong KP, Tan Tock Seng Hospital Lupus Study Group, Louthrenoo W. The reliability, validity and responsiveness of the Thai

version of Systemic Lupus Erythematosus Quality of Life (SLEQOL-TH) instrument. Lupus. 2013;22:289–96.
42. Kaya A, Goker B, Cura ES, Tezcan ME, Tufan A, Mercan R, Bitik B, Haznedaroglu S, Ozturk MA, Mikolaitis-Preuss RA, Block JA, Jolly M. Turkish LupusPRO: Crosscultural validation study for lupus. Clin Rheumatol. 2014;33:1079–84.
43. Kong KO, Ho HJ, Howe HS, Thong BY, Lian TY, Chng HH, Leong KP, Tan Tock Seng Hospital Systemic Lupus Erythematosus Study Group. Cross-cultural adaptation of the Systemic Lupus Erythematosus Quality of Life Questionnaire into Chinese. Arthritis Rheum. 2007;57:980–5.
44. Leong KP, Kong KO, Thong BYH, Koh ET, Lian TY, Teh CL, Cheng YK, Chng HH, Badsha H, Law WG, Lau TC, Chew LC, Ho HJ, Pong LY, Hoi LS, Sangeetha N, Chan SP, Howe HS. Development and preliminary validation of a systemic lupus erythematosus-specific quality-of-life instrument (SLEQOL). Rheumatology. 2005;44:1267–76.
45. McElhone K, Abbott J, Teh L-S. A review of health related quality of life in systemic lupus erythematosus. Lupus. 2006;15:633–43.
46. McElhone K, Abbott J, Shelmerdine J, Ahmad Y, Bruce IN, Gordon C, Peers K, Isenberg DA, Ferenkeh-Koroma A, Griffiths B, Akil M, Maddison P, Teh L-S. Development and validation of a disease-specific health-related quality of life measure, the LupusQoL for adults with systemic lupus erythematosus. Arthritis Care Res. 2007;57:972–9.
47. McElhone K, Abbott J, Gray J, Williams A, Teh LS. Patient perspective of systemic lupus erythematosus in relation to health-related quality of life concepts: a qualitative study. Lupus. 2010;19:1640–7.
48. McElhone K, Abbott J, Sutton C, Mullen M, Lanyon P, Rahman A, Yee C-S, Akil M, Bruce IN, Ahmad Y, Gordon C, Teh LS. Sensitivity to change and minimal important differences of the LupusQoL in patients with systemic lupus erythematosus. Arthritis Care Res. 2016;68:1505–13.
49. Meacock R, Harrison M, McElhone K, Abbott J, Haque S, Bruce I, Teh LS. Mapping the disease-specific LupusQoL to the SF-6D. Qual Life Res. 2015;24:1749–58.
50. Maeshima E, Maeshima S, Mizobata R, Goda M, Sakagashira M, Otani H, Mune M. Life-style activities in systemic lupus erythematosus. Clin Exp Rheumatol. 2007;25:189–94.
51. Mok CC, Kosinski M, Ho LY, Chan KL, Jolly M. Validation of the LupusPRO in Chinese patients from Hong Kong with systemic lupus erythematosus. Arthritis Care Res. 2015;67:297–304.
52. Navarra SV, Tanangunan RM, Mikolaitis-Preuss RA, Kosinkski M, Block JA, Jolly M. Cross-cultural validation of a disease specific patient-reported outcome measure for lupus in Philippines. Lupus. 2013;22:262–7.
53. Pamuk ON, Onat AM, Donmez S, Mengüs C, Kisacik B. Validity and reliability of the lupus QoL index in Turkish systemic lupus erythematosus patients. Lupus. 2015;24:816–21.
54. Petri M, Orbai A-M, Alarcón GS, Gordon C, Merrill JT, Fortin PR, Bruce IN, Isenberg D, Wallace DJ, Nived O, Sturfelt G, Ramsey-Goldman R, Bae SC, Hanly JG, Sánchez-Guerrero J, Clarke A, Aranow C, Manzi S, Urowitz M, Gladman D, Kalunian K, Costner M, Werth VP, Zoma A, Bernatsky S, Ruiz-Irastorza G, Khamashta MA, Jacobsen S, Buyon JP, Maddison P, Dooley MA, van Vollenhoven RF, Ginzler E, Stoll T, Peschken C, Jorizzo JL, Callen JP, Lim SS, Fessler BJ, Inanc M, Kamen DL, Rahman A, Steinsson K, Franks AG Jr, Sigler L, Hameed S, Fang H, Pham N, Brey R, Weisman MH, McGwin G Jr, Magder LS. Derivation and validation of the systemic lupus international collaborating clinics classification criteria for systemic lupus erythematosus. Arthritis Rheum. 2012;64:2677–86.
55. Pinto B, Jolly M, Dhooria A, Grover S, Raj JM, Devilliers H, Sharma A. Hindi LupusPRO: cross cultural validation of disease specific patient reported outcome measure of lupus. Lupus. 2019;28(13):1534–40.
56. Schneider M, Mosca M, Pego-Reigosa JM, Gunnarsson I, Maurel F, Garofano A, Perna A, Porcasi R, Devilliers H. Cross-cultural validation of lupus impact tracker in five European clinical practice settings. Rheumatology. 2017;56:818–28.
57. Stamm TA, Bauernfeind B, Coenen M, Feierl E, Mathis M, Stucki G, Smolen JS, Machold KP, Aringer M. Concepts important to persons with systemic lupus erythematosus and

their coverage by standard measures of disease activity and health status. Arthritis Rheum. 2007;57:1287–95.
58. Strand V, Aranow C, Cardiel M, Alarcón-Segovia D, Furie R, Sherrer Y, Tumlin J, Wallace DJ, Crawford B, LJP 394 Investigator Consortium. Improvement in health-related quality of life in systemic lupus erythematosus patients enrolled in a randomized clinical trial comparing LJP 394 treatment with placebo. Lupus. 2003;12:677–86.
59. Tan EM, Cohen AS, Fries JF, Masi AT, McShane DJ, Rothfield NF, Schaller JG, Talal N, Winchester RJ. The 1982 revised criteria for the classification of systemic lupus erythematosus. Arthritis Rheum. 1982;25:1271–7.
60. Teh L-S, McElhone K, Abbott J. Chapter on "Health-related quality of life in adults with systemic lupus erythematosus". In: Preedy VR, Watson RR, editors. Handbook of disease burdens and quality of life measures. New York: Springer-Verlag; 2010., Part 3, 3.7. p. 3261–79.
61. Terwee CB, Bot SD, de Boer MR, van der Windt DA, Knol DL, Dekker J, Bouter LM, de Vet HC. Quality criteria were proposed for measurement properties of health status questionnaires. J Clin Epidemiol. 2007;60:34–42.
62. Urowitz MB, Gladman DD, Tom BDM, Ibañez D, Farewell VT. Changing patterns in mortality and disease outcomes for patients with systemic lupus erythematosus. J Rheumatol. 2008;35:2152–8.
63. Wang C, Mayo NE, Fortin PR. The relationship between health related quality of life and disease activity and damage in systemic lupus erythematosus. J Rheumatol. 2001;28:525–32.
64. Wang SL, Wu B, Leng L, Bucala R, Lu LJ. Validity of LupusQoL-China for the assessment of health related quality of life in Chinese patients with systemic lupus erythematosus. PLoS One. 2013;8:e63795.
65. Wiginton KL. Illness representations: mapping the experience of lupus. Health Educ Behav. 1999;26:443–53.

# Chapter 13
# Assessment of Cognitive Function in Systemic Lupus Erythematosus

**Kimberley Yuen, Mahta Kakvan, Oshrat E. Tayer-Shifman, Nathalie Rozenbojm, Kathleen Bingham, and Zahi Touma**

## Overview of Cognition in Patients with SLE

Systemic lupus erythematosus (SLE) is a systemic autoimmune disease that can affect multiple organ systems, including the brain. As a result, cognition in patients with SLE may be affected and can lead to cognitive impairment (CI). Cognitive impairment-related symptoms are commonly experienced by patients with SLE, which can include but are not limited to difficulty with thinking clearly, reasoning, and remembering things such as facts, events, and memories. The American College of Rheumatology (ACR) defined cognitive dysfunction (synonymously used in this

K. Yuen
Queen's University School of Medicine, Kingston, ON, Canada
e-mail: kyuen@qmed.ca

M. Kakvan · N. Rozenbojm · Z. Touma (✉)
University of Toronto Lupus Clinic, Centre for Prognosis Studies in Rheumatic Diseases, Toronto Western Hospital, Toronto, ON, Canada
e-mail: mahta.kakvan@uhnresearch.ca; Nathalie.Rozenbojm1@uhn.ca; Zahi.Touma@uhn.ca

O. E. Tayer-Shifman
Department of Internal Medicine and Rheumatology Service, Meir Medical Center, Kfar Saba, Israel
e-mail: oshrat.shifman@clalit.org.il

K. Bingham
Centre for Mental Health, University Health Network, Department of Psychiatry, University of Toronto, Toronto, ON, Canada
e-mail: kathleen.bingham@uhn.ca



Z. Touma (ed.), *Outcome Measures and Metrics in Systemic Lupus Erythematosus*, https://doi.org/10.1007/978-3-030-73303-2_13

chapter as cognitive impairment), as 1 of the 19 different neurological and neuropsychiatric syndromes (NPSLE) of SLE. It is defined as "significant deficits in any or all of the following main cognitive functions: memory (learning and recall), simple attention, complex attention, executive skills (planning, organizing, and sequencing), visual-spatial processing, language (e.g. verbal, fluency), reasoning/problem solving and psychomotor speed" [1]. To measure deficits in the cognitive functions described, a neuropsychological battery (NB) (a collection of tests assessing different cognitive domains), is often used as the gold standard. The ACR developed a NB consisting of ten tests measuring cognitive domains such as manual motor speed, attention, processing speed, language processing, learning and memory (visuospatial and verbal), and executive functioning [1]. The ACR also provided a definition of CI along with their battery, which was ≥2 standard deviations (SD) below the estimated population mean in domains of attention, memory, and psychomotor speed [2]. Furthermore, they coined the term "focal" to refer to the condition where ≥1 test within an individual domain was impacted and "multifocal" if ≥2 domains were affected [3].

The overall assessment of cognitive function in patients with SLE is complex and multifactorial. This chapter covers several topics that contribute to the assessment of cognitive functioning in patients with SLE, including the definition and prevalence of CI, instruments for measuring cognitive function, the existing heterogeneity of CI definitions and cognitive assessment, changes in cognition overtime, comorbidities such as depression and anxiety, cognition and patient health-related quality of life, and the role of cytokines and antibodies in relation to cognition (Fig. 13.1).

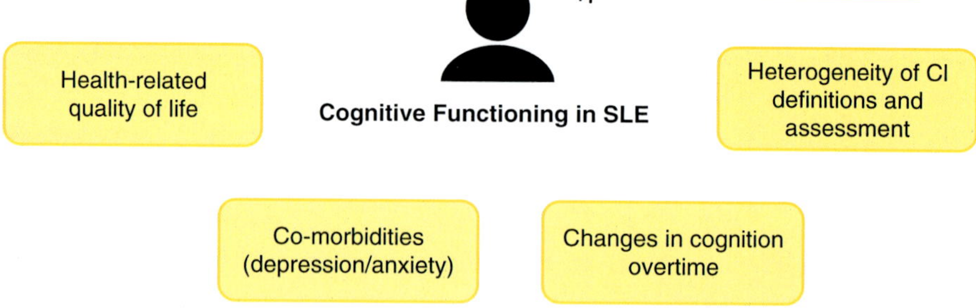


**Fig. 13.1** Various topics related to cognitive function in patients with SLE covered in this chapter

### *The Prevalence of Patients with SLE Presenting with Cognitive Impairment*

Cognitive impairment is a common manifestation in patients with SLE. A recent systematic review assessing the prevalence of CI in SLE reported a range of 3–81% from studies that described the use of a CI measurement tool [3] and a pooled prevalence of 38% (95% confidence interval: 33–43%) from 35 studies and 2419 patients with SLE that used a comprehensive NB [3]. In patients with NPSLE, the prevalence of CI was similarly widespread, ranging from 4% to 83% with a pooled prevalence of 39% (95% confidence interval: 24–55%) from 12 studies of 647 patients with NPSLE [3]. In 10 case-control studies with 483 patients with SLE and 266 healthy controls, CI was identified in 37.7% of patients with SLE and 15.4% in healthy controls [3]. Patients with SLE were at a higher risk for developing CI compared to the healthy controls with a risk ratio (RR) of 2.80 (95% confidence interval: 2.06–3.81) [3]. Patients with SLE were also found to be at higher risk for developing CI compared to patients with rheumatoid arthritis, with a RR of 1.80 (95% confidence interval: 1.30–2.49) [3].

The wide-ranging prevalence of CI in patients with SLE and NPSLE could be due in part because SLE is a complex autoimmune disease that is often associated with many factors that can influence cognitive function. Patient's demographics, neuropsychiatric conditions, and medication use are just some factors that can influence cognitive function [3]. As a result, patients with NPSLE are often found to be associated with increased prevalence of CI, especially in those with depression, anxiety, mood disorders, and stroke [3]. Another explanation for the variability in CI prevalence could be due to the heterogeneity in CI assessment in SLE which will be discussed later in this chapter.

Currently, there is no specific CI phenotype for domains impaired in patients with SLE, but some studies have shown verbal and nonverbal learning and working memory to be the most affected domains, followed by deficits in simple attention and psychomotor speed [3]. Executive functions such as planning and higher-level organization are also commonly affected in patients with SLE [3]. Studies have found both direct effects (e.g., ischemic and inflammatory phenotypes) and indirect effects such as demographic data or the presence of psychiatric conditions to be relevant for CI in SLE, which will be discussed later in this chapter. However, the causal mechanism behind the development of CI in patients with SLE is unclear. Thus, CI in patients with SLE is common, but the development of CI in SLE is complex and difficult to define due to the complicated nature of both CI and SLE.

## Measurement Instruments for Assessing Cognitive Function in Patients with SLE

Measurement instruments that evaluate cognitive function and detect CI in patients with SLE can be categorized into two main categories: *patient-reported and objective* (Fig. 13.2).

## *Patient-Reported Tests*

*Patient-reported tests* are measurement tools that are completed by the patient and collect subjective information. For example, self-report cognition questionnaires are commonly employed in cognitive assessment and are based on the patient's own perception of their cognitive function. Along with cognition, other self-reported questionnaires are often administered to assess a variety of dimensions (constructs) such as depression, anxiety, personality disorders, and fatigue, which can interfere with a patient's reported perspective on cognitive tasks or overall cognition [4]. Therefore, it is very important when assessing cognitive function to also gather information on all these dimensions (depression, anxiety, pain, fatigue, sleep, etc.) to understand the patient's perspective and the factors potentially influencing their cognition. An example of patient-reported tests to assess different constructs is presented in Table 13.1. This list is not exhaustive and is presented solely as an example of different patient-reported tests.

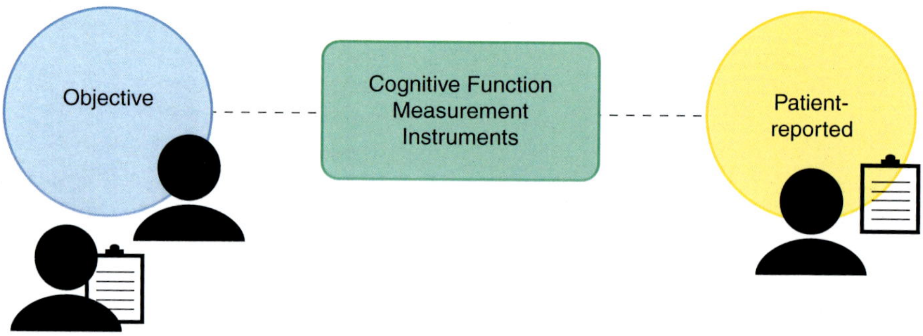


**Fig. 13.2** Two categories of cognitive function measurement instruments: patient-reported and objective tests

**Table 13.1** An example of some patient-reported tests

| Patient-reported tests | Constructs measured |
|---|---|
| Beck Anxiety Inventory (BAI) [5] | Anxiety |
| Beck Depression Inventory (BDI) [6] | Depression |
| Fatigue Severity Scale (FSS) or Functional Assessment of Chronic Illness Therapy-Fatigue (FACIT-F) [7] | Fatigue |
| Lupus Quality of Life (QoL) Questionnaire [8] | Affecting factors related by lupus |
| Medical Outcomes Study Short Form (SF-36) Health Survey [9, 10] | Patient's view about their health |
| Perceived Deficits Questionnaire (PDQ) [11] | Patient's view about their cognitive function |
| Work Productivity and Activity Impairment Questionnaire-Specific Health Problem v2.0 (WPAI:SHP) [12] | Factors affecting patients' work performance and regular activity |
| Minnesota Multiphasic Personality Inventory (MMPI-2) Restructured Form [13] or Personality Assessment Inventory (PAI) [14] | Personality and psychopathology |

## Self-Report Cognition Questionnaires

Self-report cognition questionnaires are a type of patient-reported tests that collect subjective CI information. The subjective CI tools reported in the literature in SLE include the Cognitive Failures Questionnaire (CFQ), Cognitive Symptom Inventory (CSI), Multiple Assessment Questionnaire (MAQ), Perceived Deficits Questionnaire (PDQ) and its short form (PDQ-SF) [3], and others. Most of these tools measure CI based on a Likert scale with values representing a range from never (0) to very often (4) and a series of questions capturing everyday cognitive aspects. The **CSI** consists of 21 questions screening for the patient's ability to perform cognitive tasks during daily activities, based on the domains of memory, attention, and executive function [2, 15, 16]. The maximum score on the CSI is 84 points with each question scored on a scale of 0–4; a higher score indicates more severe CI [17]. To define CI with the CSI, 6 out of 21 questions indicating a cognitive difficulty that is present most or all the time are required. The Ad Hoc Committee on Lupus Response Criteria: Cognition Sub-committee recommended the CSI as a screening test for CI in SLE, in both clinical and research contexts [2].

The **Perceived Deficits Questionnaire** (PDQ) 5-item (PDQ-5) or 20-item (PDQ-20) was developed to assess the patient's perceived CI [11, 18] in multiple sclerosis (MS). Few studies have evaluated its performance in patients with SLE. To complete the PDQ, patients rank their cognitive performance on a 4-point Likert scale (ranging from 0 (never) to 4 (almost always)), for each of the four main subscales: attention and concentration, retrospective memory, prospective memory, and planning/organization [11].

The rationale for collecting this subjective data is to evaluate the patient's self-report of their cognitive function and to investigate any probable discrepancies compared to the objective cognitive assessment. It has been shown that perceived cognitive deficits reported by patients are often incongruent with the cognitive deficits detected with objective testing [19], however, it is critical to explore cognitive deficits perceived by patients, as these perceptions can adversely impact their cognitive performance [19]. Therefore, the administration of subjective CI measurement tools is highly recommended to supplement objective cognitive assessment.

## Psychological Measurement

Psychological measurement involves standardized psychological tests, such as personality tests, that have been designed to capture patient behavior in order to detect psychopathological syndromes or behavioral manifestations. Collecting information on personality disorders is important as behavioral abnormalities may influence cognitive function [20]. To detect psychopathological syndromes and the possible influence of behavioral abnormalities on CI, patients often complete a personality questionnaire prior to cognitive assessment. Among the personality assessment instruments, the **Minnesota Multiphasic Personality Inventory** (MMPI-2) Restructured Form [13] has been used to assess personality in patients with SLE

[20–22]. The MMPI-2 consists of 567 items and takes approximately 60–90 minutes to complete. Items on the MMPI-2 yield several evaluations of personality and psychopathology. The scoring process is based on six of the MMPI-2 scales including depression, psychopathic deviate, paranoia, psychasthenia, schizophrenia, and hypomania [23]. Results of studies using the MMPI-2 for evaluating mood disorders and their influence on CI in SLE are mixed. One study reported that the MMPI-2 is not an optimal battery for assessing mood disorders; however the depression scale of the MMPI-2 confirmed the presence of depression in the same patients that were previously clinically diagnosed [20]. Another study investigating MMPI-2 profiles in patients with rheumatoid arthritis (RA) and SLE found that higher scores on the neurotic triad scales may reflect comorbid psychiatric disorders, although MMPI-2 characteristics appeared to be a consequence of the disease [21]. Another study found that patients with SLE, with and without behavioral abnormalities based on the MMPI-2, did not differ in global cognitive dysfunction scores [22].

Another widely employed and validated personality assessment used in studying cognitive function is the **Personality Assessment Inventory** (PAI), although literature on its use in SLE is lacking [14]. The PAI includes 344 items comprising 22 individual and nonoverlapping scales that cover a broad range of mental disorders such as anxiety, major depression, obsessive-compulsive disorder, and phobia. Normalized adult data is available for the PAI in a variety of clinical and community settings, which allows PAI patient reports to be compared with both normal and clinical populations.

## *Objective Tests*

*Objective* tests are based on standardized assessment procedures which include brief cognitive screening tests and different neuropsychological batteries (NBs) which are comprised of neuropsychological tests [3]. Objective tests are often completed by pencil and paper and administered by a trained health-care personnel; however computerized tests are also available. These assessments are administered by trained personnel such as psychologists or trained psychometrists.

### Neuropsychological Batteries

A comprehensive NB is conventionally used to investigate cognitive function. However, a long NB imposed limitations on its applicability by consuming immense amounts of time for completion and requiring a high financial budget to administer the tests. Consequently, a multidisciplinary committee, formed by the ACR Research Committee in, proposed a brief standard 1–2-hour NB for the assessment of cognitive function in patients with SLE in 1999 [1]. In addition, the ACR committee developed standard nomenclature for NPSLE, such as cognitive dysfunction, that provided recommendations for diagnostic examination in neuropsychology. The definitions for 19 neuropsychiatric syndromes were generated followed by experiential evaluation of diagnostic agreement [1].

In a study validating the American College of Rheumatology Neuropsychological Battery (ACR-NB) compared to a longer, comprehensive NB, the comprehensive NB used as the reference standard consisted of a set of neuropsychological tests examining eight cognitive domains including intelligence, attention, reasoning, learning, recall, fluency, language, and psychomotor and required 2–4 hours to administer and interpret results [24] (Fig. 13.3).

The cognitive tests selected for the ACR-NB demonstrated validity evidence against the traditional NB as findings from Kozora et al.'s 2004 study revealed 90% agreement between the two [24]. The ACR-NB consists of the Wechsler Adult Intelligence Scale-Revised (WAIS-R) Digit Symbol Substitution Test (Digit Symbol) [26] which measures psychomotor speed and concentration; the WAIS (Third Edition) Letter-Number Sequencing [27] which examines auditory working memory; the Trail Making Test (Parts A and B) [28] which examines psychomotor speed, attention, and cognitive sequencing; the Stroop Color and Word Test [29] which assesses complex and switching attention by naming color print for words written in different colors; the Controlled Oral Word Association Test (COWAT) and Animal Naming Test [30] which measure phonemic and semantic verbal fluency, respectively, by asking participants to produce as many words as possible beginning with a specific stated letter (e.g., F, A, S) or naming as many animals as possible within 60 seconds; the Finger Tapping Test [28] which measures motor speed bilaterally (dominant and nondominant hands); the Rey-Osterrieth Complex

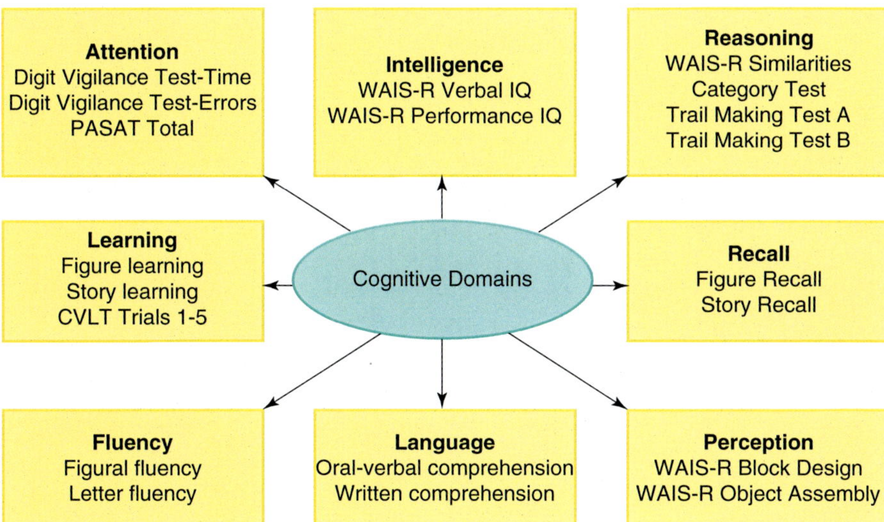


**Fig. 13.3** Cognitive domains examined by the comprehensive NB from Kozora et al. 2004 validation study of the ACR-NB [24, 25]. Abbreviations: WAIS-R Wechsler Adult Intelligence Scale-Revised, PASAT Paced Auditory Serial Addition Test, CVLT California Verbal Learning Test, IQ intelligence quotient, ACR-NB American College of Rheumatology Neuropsychological Battery

Figure Test (RCFT) [31] which assesses immediate and 30-minute delayed recall and recognition of visual learning and memory; and the California Verbal Learning Test (CVLT) [32] which measures verbal learning and memory and consists of five trials followed by immediate or short delayed recall and 20-minute delayed recall and recognition of verbal memory.

Although the ACR-NB has been conventionally used to assess CI in patients with SLE and is widely regarded as the gold standard, many studies have substituted certain neuropsychological tests, creating variability among utilized batteries [24]. Some recent studies from the Toronto Lupus Clinic [33, 34] have proposed a slightly different NB with an attempt to improve the efficiency of the ACR-NB. The CVLT was substituted with a shorter version – the Hopkins Verbal Learning Test-Revised (HVLT-R) – while maintaining the validity of the test [34]. The HVLT-R is a brief word-learning and memory test consisting of a list of 12 nouns with 4 words belonging to each of 3 specific semantic categories [35]. Like the CVLT, the HVLT-R measures verbal learning efficiency, recall, and recognition. The validity of HVLT-R has been examined against ACR-NB by phone interview [36] and has demonstrated 100% sensitivity and 89% specificity in screening for CI in patients with SLE [37]. Table 13.2 demonstrates the NB domains and tests used from the Toronto Lupus Clinic, adapted from the ACR-NB.

## Brief Cognitive Screening Tests

Some studies rely on brief screening tools rather than NBs to detect CI in SLE. One of these short cognitive screening tests is the **Mini Mental State Examination** (MMSE) [38]. The MMSE was originally designed to examine CI in those with dementia or delirium and evaluates cognitive domains such as orientation, learning-evocation, attention, language, and visuospatial construction. The results of the MMSE indicate no deterioration in cognitive functions if scores fall within the range of 26–30 points, possible deterioration with 25 points, mild to moderate dementia between 10 and 24 points, moderate to severe dementia between 6 and 9, and severe dementia for <6 points [17]. In a recent systematic review, the MMSE was used in 11 studies and 821 patients with SLE with a pooled prevalence of CI of 23%, although the heterogeneity among those studies was high ($I^2$ of 89% (95% confidence interval: 82.3–93.2%)). In a comparison of screening tests for CI in 98 patients with SLE using the HVLT-R as the reference test, the MMSE had a lower sensitivity (27%) and higher specificity (90%) than the Montreal Cognitive Assessment (MoCA) which had a sensitivity of 73% and specificity of 63% [37]. Generally, the utility and support for the MMSE as a screening tool for CI in SLE has not been well established; however it does have its advantages; it is brief, requires no trained personnel for administration, and is easy to use [2, 39]. Its largest pitfall is the lack of sensitivity for detecting mild CI [3].

Similarly, the **Montreal Cognitive Assessment** (MoCA) [40] was developed as a brief screening test to detect mild CI. The MoCA measures several cognitive domains including attention, concentration, executive functions, memory, language,

**Table 13.2** Cognitive domains and tests in the NB used at the Toronto Lupus Clinic

| NB domains | NB tests |
|---|---|
| 1. Manual motor speed and dexterity | Finger Tapping Test: dominant hand and nondominant hand |
| 2. Simple attention and processing speed | Trail A, Stroop color naming, Stroop word reading |
| 3. Visuospatial construction | RCFT copy |
| 4. Verbal fluency | COWAT and ANIMALS |
| 5. Learning and memory | |
| Visuospatial | RCFT delay recall and RCFT delay recognition |
| Verbal | HVLT-R learning, HVLT-R delayed recall, HVLT-R recognition, HVLT-R total recall |
| 6. Executive functioning | |
| Untimed | Stroop (interference score), WAIS Letter-Number, consonant trigrams (used lower value from 18 seconds or 36 seconds) |
| Executive timed | WAIS-III Digit Symbol, Trail B |

Abbreviations: *COWAT* Controlled Oral Word Association Test, *HVLT-R* Hopkins Verbal Learning Test-Revised, *RCFT* Rey Complex Figure Test, *WAIS-III* Wechsler Adult Intelligence Scale, Third Edition

visuospatial skills, abstraction, calculation, and orientation. The MoCA is a paper-and-pencil test and requires approximately 10 minutes to administer. The total score is 30 points, and the conventional cutoff for CI is ≤26, although in some studies the score ≤25 is considered to be positive for CI. The MoCA has been recognized as a valid tool for detecting mild CI in patients with Alzheimer's disease and other diseases who scored within the normal range on the MMSE [41]. The MoCA's ability to detect CI in Parkinson's disease, Huntington's disease, and SLE has been empirically well documented [41]. A recent systematic review reported two studies that used the MoCA in patients with SLE with a different CI prevalence (61% in 54 patients with SLE [42], 29.5% in 44 patients with SLE [39]). In the study with 44 patients with SLE, the MoCA demonstrated a sensitivity and specificity of 83% and 73%, respectively, compared against the Automated Neuropsychological Assessment Metrics (ANAM) as the reference test [39]. Findings from a study exploring and comparing the efficacy of the MMSE, MoCA, and CSI against a NB found the MoCA to have the greatest efficacy and to be the most efficient screening tool among the three tests [17]. The MoCA showed the highest correspondence with the NB (area under the curve (AUC) of 99.4%, 84% sensitivity, 100% specificity) followed by the MMSE (AUC of 92.6%, 55% sensitivity, 100% specificity) and the CSI (AUC of 31%, 55% sensitivity, 31% specificity) [17]. As previously mentioned, Nantes et al. found the MoCA to have a higher sensitivity but a lower specificity than the MMSE when compared to HVLT-R as the reference test for CI. Results from their study also suggest that level of education should be considered when interpreting the results of the MoCA, as education was a contributing factor to patients' performance on MoCA, and those with higher years of education were less likely to have CI [37]. However, another study from the same center comparing the MoCA to NB found that CI was not accurately predicted by the MoCA (AUC of

65%, sensitivity of 50%, specificity of 70%) and thus could not recommend the MoCA as a screening tool for CI in SLE [43]. Thus, results surrounding the utility of the MoCA as a screening tool for CI in patients with SLE are mixed; however the MoCA has been found to yield better results than the MMSE as a brief CI screening tool.

Standalone neuropsychological tests such as the **Hopkins Verbal Learning Test-Revised** (HVLT-R) [44] and the **Controlled Oral Word Association Test** (COWAT) [45] have also been used as screening tools to assess cognition [36, 37, 46, 47]. The HVLT-R is similar to the CVLT, as they both assess verbal learning and memory, but is a briefer test available for repeated testing and more feasible to use when comprehensive testing is not possible [35]. The HVLT-R consists of three learning trials and a fourth delayed recall trial. It takes approximately 5 minutes to complete but can take up to 35 minutes if the delayed recall trial is administered. A total recall score, learning measure, retention score, and recognition of true and false positives are recorded. Raw scores are converted to t- or z-scores and compared to normative data. The HVLT-R was found to have a sensitivity and specificity of 95% and 83%, respectively, when using a cutoff of 1 SD in patients with dementia and 67% sensitivity and 98% specificity when the cutoff was 2 SD [35]. Julian et al. showed a sensitivity of 74% and specificity of 68% in the learning trial using a cutoff of ≤26 and a sensitivity of 47% and specificity of 85% in the delayed recall trial when using a cutoff of ≤9 [36] in patients with SLE [36].

The COWAT is another popular neuropsychological test used for screening CI in SLE and evaluates phonemic and semantic verbal fluency [36, 47]. Patients are asked to list as many words as possible beginning with one of the letters F, A, S or C, F, L for a total of three trials. For semantic fluency, patients are asked to name as many items as possible from a specific category, typically animals. The COWAT has been shown to have a sensitivity of 79% (95% confidence interval: 0.62–0.91) and specificity of 67% (95% confidence interval: 0.56–0.76) for detecting CI in SLE patients when compared to a NB [36]. The HVLT-R and COWAT are both widely used in clinical environments as a brief cognitive assessment tool and are feasible to use due to its low administrative and patient burden. Both the HVLT-R and COWAT have been studied in patients with SLE with promising psychometric evidence [48]. However, both tools assess limited cognitive domains, and other tests should be used to provide a comprehensive cognitive evaluation.

## Automated Tests

The time-consuming NB and costs associated with administering assessments are viewed as limitations of objective tests. These limitations have motivated researchers to consider other options, such as automated tests for CI assessment in patients with SLE. *Automated* tests are electronic-based cognitive assessments and often require patients to use a mouse and press the space bar or touchscreen to respond to stimuli on the screen. These tests, as the name implies, do not require an administrator.

One of the most popular automated tests is the **Automated Neuropsychological Assessment Metrics** (ANAM), which has validity evidence for CI screening compared to a NB [34]. The ANAM was originally designed as a self-administered, computer-based program consisting of automated tasks that assess variety aspect of cognitive functions. The longest battery of the ANAM (v4) General Neuropsychological Screening (GNS) (ANAM (v4) GNS) consists of 15 subtests, with each test representing an individual domain of the total 7 cognitive domains of attention and concentration, working memory, mental flexibility, spatial processing, cognitive processing efficiency, memory recall, mood, fatigue level, and psychomotor performance [49]. The ANAM takes approximately 30–40 minutes to complete and includes the following subtests: *tapping right hand, tapping left hand, running memory, procedural reaction time, two-choice reaction time, simple reaction time, simple reaction time repeated, spatial processing, logical relations, code substitution learning, code substitution delayed, match to sample, math processing, go/no go, and tower puzzle*. The ANAM also includes a demographics/history module, mood scale, post-traumatic stress assessment, sleep scale, and symptoms scale. All of the tests within the ANAM produce a consistent set of scores, including percentage of correct responses, mean response time for all responses, mean response time for correct responses, standard deviation of the mean response time for all responses, standard deviation of the mean response time for correct responses, median response time for all responses, median response time for correct responses, throughput (the calculated number of correct responses per minute), response omissions, and premature responses (responses <130 ms) [49]. Not all scores are reported for each test, as some tests have their own specific scores. The ANAM Performance Report (APR) reports the tests results and compares previous results along with normative data [50].

Prior to each actual test in any domain, instructions on how to complete a specific test followed by a trial practice appears on the screen. This allows participants to understand and practice each test before proceeding to the actual test. After completion of all tasks, the program generates scores for interpretation. The ANAM has been applied to screen cognitive performance in various clinical populations including SLE [49, 51].

The main advantage of ANAM in comparison to the NB is its short duration, as the entire GNS battery can be completed within 30–40 minutes depending on the patient's performance speed [52]. Another advantage of ANAM is its ability to generate enormous amounts of data. The ANAM produces scores automatically with no requirement for manual data entry while applying a complex directory for data reduction and simplification [34].

Findings from several studies on the efficiency of ANAM in screening patients with SLE are promising [53], and the ANAM has been shown to be a valid screening tool for detecting CI in SLE [34]. The ANAM was compared against a battery similar to the ACR-NB in 211 patients with SLE and was found to be able to accurately detect CI [34]. The study created six models based on different combinations of ANAM scores, and the most discriminatory ANAM subtests for detecting CI were selected [34]. The best models included different score types (percentage of correct responses, mean reaction time scores, coefficient of variation of reaction time scores, throughput) and reported AUCs of 81% and 84% [34]. Furthermore, composite indices with cutoff scores were derived to improve the interpretation of ANAM scores in clinical settings and demonstrated a sensitivity of 78–80% and specificity of 70% [34].

Some limitations of ANAM can be prominent under circumstances that patients require assistance on some of the tests. For instance, to properly perform the Finger Tapping Test of the ANAM (a dexterity task), patients are required to hold their hands and finger in a specific position. While there is a brief description and demonstration of hand position during this task, patients often report the instructions to be vague. Another limitation is its task response dependency on the mouse. This can be extremely challenging for patients with arthritis, pain in the joints, limitation in the range of motion, or deformities of joints. Consequently, patients may be unable to perform optimally on such tasks. This becomes problematic when interpreting results, as the results are based on accuracy and speed. Thus, decreased speed in response to stimuli, due to physical disability or weakness of fingers, can be misinterpreted as CI rather than physical impairment. Therefore, the ANAM may be unable to accurately reflect the cognitive functioning of these patients with SLE, and results should be interpreted with caution or controlled for. See Table 13.3.

Another automated test is the **Cambridge Neuropsychological Test Automated Battery** (CANTAB), which was originally developed at the University of Cambridge in the 1980s. The CANTAB measures general memory and learning, working memory, executive function, visual memory, attention and reaction time (RT), semantic and verbal memory, decision-making, and response control. These domains are examined by the following tasks: motor screening (MOT), big/little circle (BLC), paired associates learning (PAL), stockings of Cambridge (SOC), and graded naming tests (GNT) [54].

The CANTAB tests are scored based on expressed difficulty. MOT results are expressed as standard score of mean latency and mean error, BLC is expressed as a standard score of percentage of correct actions, PAL is expressed as the standard score of total errors, SOC is expressed as a standard score of mean initial and subsequent thinking time and problems solved in minimum moves, and GNT is expressed as the standard score of percentage of correct answers [54]. The CANTAB provides a database of normative data from healthy individuals from ages 4 to 90 across four different estimated IQ bands. Results from the CANTAB tests are thus automatically referred to the age- and gender-matched norms and standard scores, where CI is defined by results <0.5 of the standard score [54]. Findings from recent studies show a moderate correlation between the results of CANTAB subtests and those of conventional subtests from neuropsychological batteries [55]. Overall, the efficacy of CANTAB in assessing cognitive functions and detecting CI in patients with SLE has not been empirically well documented.

The advantage of both the ANAM and CANTAB is that both are culture and language independent, as they utilize nonverbal stimuli and require nonverbal responses. This is of a significant relevance for patients with SLE who suffer from language impairment or have limited English proficiency.

**Table 13.3** Cognitive domains and tests in ANAM [34]

| Cognitive domains | ANAM tests |
|---|---|
| 1. Fine motor processing | 1. Tapping right hand<br>2. Tapping left hand |
| 2. Attention and processing speed | 3. Running memory<br>4. Procedural reaction time<br>5. Two-choice reaction time<br>6. Simple reaction time<br>7. Simple reaction time repeated |
| 3. Visuospatial perception | 8. Spatial processing |
| 4. Abstract language function | 9. Logical relations |
| 5. Learning | 10. Code substitution learning |
| 6. Memory | 11. Code substitution delayed<br>12. Match to sample |
| 7. Executive functioning | 13. Math processing<br>14. Go-no-go hits<br>15. Tower test |

The **NIH Toolbox Cognition Battery** (developed by the National Institutes of Health (NIH)) is a free, automated battery of tests measuring different cognitive constructs including attention, executive functioning, episodic memory, working memory, language, and processing speed [56, 57]. Although it is an automated battery, an examiner is required to present instructions to the patient and to ensure valid results [56]. The NIH Toolbox Cognition Battery consists of seven tests: Flanker Inhibitory Control and Attention Test, Picture Sequence Memory Test, List Sorting Working Memory Test, Picture Vocabulary Test, Oral Reading Recognition Test, Dimensional Change Card Sort Test, and Pattern Comparison Processing Speed Test, and takes approximately 30 minutes to complete [56, 57]. There are also two supplemental measures to the battery: the Rey Auditory Verbal Learning Test for immediate recall and Oral Symbol Digit Test which assess processing speed and require 6 minutes to complete. All the tests in the battery provide individual and summary scores. The NIH Toolbox Cognition Battery has been validated as a research tool in cognitively normal adults and against "gold standard" neuropsychological tests [56]; however it has not been routinely used for assessing CI in SLE and requires further research for use in patients with SLE.

## Heterogeneity of CI Definitions and Assessment in SLE

The topic of cognition in SLE has grown in popularity over the years, as reflected by the growing number of studies and CI measurement tools. However, a lack of consistency in defining and measuring CI in patients with SLE among studies remains [37]. Similarly, while the ACR-NB remains to be the gold standard for assessing CI in patients with SLE, discrepancies continue to exist among the use of CI measurement tools. Due to the wide range of tools available for CI assessment including subjective questionnaires, brief screening tools, NB, and automated methods, the use of different tools across studies increases the variability of CI prevalence in SLE.

## *Heterogeneity of CI Definitions in SLE*

Cognitive impairment identification is conventionally based on the performance on a comprehensive NB, and the interpretation of test results is based on existing normative data for sex, age, education, and ethnicity. Studies often compare patient results against normative data for each test to decide whether the patient's performance falls within the impaired range, while other studies compare the patient to a control group. Thus, the definition of CI is difficult to pinpoint and has been shown to vary between studies. The definition of CI typically consists of three components: the score (raw score, z-score, or t-score), the standard deviation, and the number of domains involved. As previously mentioned, the definition of CI according to the ACR is ≥2 SD below the estimated population mean in domains of attention, memory, and psychomotor speed based on their 1-hour battery [1, 2]. A review of the literature showed that studies that used a comprehensive NB and reported a CI definition had definitions that varied between the use of raw scores, t-scores, or z-scores. Cutoffs for CI ranged from 1 SD to 3 SD, below the mean compared to age-matched normative data or control group in one or more cognitive domains or tests [58–76]. Many studies reported different definitions of CI including different standard deviation cutoffs, differing impairment levels (e.g., mild, moderate, severe), and varying numbers of cognitive domains impairment. For example, Tayer-Shifman et al. classified patients into three groups: non-CI, indeterminate, and CI. Classification is based on the following criteria: (a) non-CI, z-scores in all domains greater than $-1.5$; (b) indeterminate, a z-score of $\leq -1.5$ in only one domain; and (c) CI, a z-score of $\leq -1.5$ in two or more domains [34]. Studies conducted by Kozora and colleagues used a CI definition based on their own CI index which was calculated using 12 of the selected tests scores from the ACR-NB. Each score was then converted to t-scores using demographically corrected normative data. Impairment was considered for t-scores <40 [24]; and the CI index had a range of 0–12 with higher numbers representing greater CI [24, 25, 77–82]. Appenzeller et al. also included a classification system: deficits in <3 dimensions constituted mild CI, 3–4 dimensions moderate, and ≥5 dimensions severe [66–68, 70]. Brey and Holliday provided a 4-point clinical impairment rating scale ranging from 0 (no impairment) to 4 (severe impairment) for specific domains such as attention/concentration, visuomotor, executive function and memory, as well as global impairment as reviewed by a board-certified clinical neuropsychologist [51, 83]. Tomietto et al. derived raw scores which were converted into z-scores and percentiles, where the z-scores were grouped in 15 different summary scores, each representing a different cognitive process due to tests assessing more than 1 domain [84]. The 15 scores were then grouped into the 8 domains defined by the ACR committee, to which they also followed an impairment rating scale: normal, mildly impaired (<3 functions impaired in ≤2 domains), and moderately/severely impaired (≥3 impaired functions in ≥2 domains) [84]. It is clear that different definitions of CI are being used and there is a lack of consistency among studies.

## *Heterogeneity of CI Assessment in SLE*

As covered earlier in the section "Measurement Instruments for Assessing Cognitive Function in Patients with SLE", it is evident that the metrics used to investigate CI in SLE can vary widely. The CI assessment tools highlighted in a recent systematic review examining the prevalence of CI in SLE included the NB, ANAM, MMSE, MoCA, HVLT-R, COWAT, CSI, and PDQ, demonstrating a mix of objective and subjective instruments [3].

As previously mentioned, the ACR-NB was first proposed in 1999 to be used as a standard assessment battery for CI in patients with SLE. It was validated in 2004 and has since been widely regarded as the "gold standard" battery for assessing CI in SLE. However, it has been over a decade since its inception and inconsistencies persist regarding the use of the ACR-NB whereby studies have been shown to acknowledge the ACR-NB but opt to use other tests or make substitutions [24, 51, 58, 62, 65, 77–82, 85–90]. The literature has shown that cognition studies in SLE that state the use of the ACR-NB frequently substitute neuropsychological tests or use batteries similar to the recommendations of the ACR committee [24, 51, 58, 62, 65, 77–82, 85–90]. For example, following the validation of the ACR-NB in Kozora's 2004 study, they modified the ACR-NB in their studies by adding four tests that showed sensitivity in patients with SLE: The Paced Auditory Serial Addition Test (PASAT), Digit Vigilance Test, WAIS Block Design, and Category Test [4, 77–79, 81, 82]. Another example, as previously mentioned, includes the substitution of the CVLT for the HVLT-R [33, 34].

However, deviations from the ACR-NB could be due to accessibility, in terms of similar tests that measure the same cognitive domains such as the CVLT and HVLT-R. It may also be difficult to follow guidelines for the ACR-NB due to limited funding, or the lack of trained personnel to administer the tests that have this requirement. Furthermore, the ACR-NB requires approximately 1–2 hours to administer, which may not be feasible in some research or clinical settings. This could explain the increasing use of computerized batteries such as the ANAM, or the use of screening tools such as the MoCA or MMSE. In summary, it is evident that the batteries used to measure CI as well as the definition of CI in SLE vary between studies, and the need for a new consensus is warranted to standardize CI assessment within SLE.

## Changes in Cognition Over Time in SLE

Several longitudinal studies have addressed the course of CI in patients with SLE [20, 48, 58, 73, 91–99]. Seven of these studies assessed intraindividual CI course over time showing persistence of CI in some patients and fluctuation of CI (including resolution or evolution) in others (Table 13.4). In these studies 34 to 755 patients were reassessed after 1–10 years. CI persisted in 4–29% of all patients with SLE examined and fluctuated in 10–41% of patients. In the majority of patients, CI was stable and did not progress over time [73, 92–95] with worsening in only 10% of subjects over a 10-year period [20].

The association of CI with NPSLE is controversial. Hanly et al. suggested that in some patients, previous neuropsychiatric events were associated with a small but significant deterioration in selected aspects of cognitive function after 5 years of follow-up [92]. Similarily, Gao et al. found that NPSLE patients had significantly worse and persistently impaired memory and learning deficits compared to non-NPSLE patients over a 12-month period [58]. Denburg et al. showed that endorsement of minor neuropsychiatric symptoms by patients with SLE related significantly to objectively assessed cognitive function over time. However, other studies failed to show any association between CI persistence and NPSLE [93, 98].

The association between CI and psychiatric status has been described, and an improvement in cognitive function in patients whose psychiatric disorder had

**Table 13.4** Studies of interindividual course of CI in SLE

| Study | Cognitive assessment tool | Reassessment period | No. of patients | Persistence of CI of follow-up | Fluctuation of CI of follow-up |
|---|---|---|---|---|---|
| Hanly et al. [91] | WAIS-R, WMS-R, CVLT, NART-R | 12 months | 59 | 5% | 39% |
| Carlomagno et al. [93] | Battery of tests | 12 months | 51 | 27% | 10% |
| Tayer-Shifman et al. [97] | ACR-NB | 6 and 12 months | 111 | 14% | 41% |
| Hay et al. [73] | WAIS, VFT, BVRT, WMS | 2 years | 38 | 29% | 39% |
| Hanly et al. [92] | WAIS-R, WMS-R, CVLT, NART-R | 1 and 5 years | 53 | 4% | 32% |
| Ceccarelli et al. [20] | Battery of 18 tests | 10 years | 34 | 9% | 14% |
| Touma et al. [48] | HVLT-R | Yearly up to 7 years | 755 | 28% | Not reported |

Abbreviations: *WAIS-R* Wechsler Adult Intelligence Scale-Revised, *WMS-R* Wechsler Memory Scale-Revised, *CVLT* California Verbal Learning Test, *NART-R* National Adult Reading Test-Revised, *ACR-NB* American College of Rheumatology Neuropsychological Battery, *WAIS* Wechsler Adult Intelligence Scale shortened version, *VFT* Verbal Fluency Test, *BVRT* the Benton Visual Retention Test A, *WMS* the Wechsler Memory Scale, *HVLT-R* Hopkins Verbal Learning Test-Revised resolved was suggested by Hay et al. [73]. Tayer-Shifman et al. identified higher level of fatigue, pain, and anxiety among patients with persistent CI, and Gao et al. showed an association of the mental component measures of the SF-36 with CI in patients with NPSLE. However, other studies could not show a clear association between CI and psychiatric disorders [20, 58, 91, 93, 94].

Antiphospholipid syndrome (APLS) and antiphospholipid (aPL) antibodies are associated in a couple of studies with CI persistence. Patients with SLE with persistently elevated IgG anticardiolipin (aCL) values over a 2–3-year period, as opposed to patients with negative or inconsistently raised titers, were found to have significantly poorer performance on cognitive tasks. Persistently increased aCL levels were associated with problems of word fluency, concentration, attention, and reaction time [99]. A significant correlation between SLE anticoagulant positivity and worsening in visuospatial functions was identified in the Ceccarelli cohort as well [20]. This association was not found in other cohorts [73, 94, 98].

Other factors that were shown anecdotally to be associated with CI persistence included SLE activity, cumulative damage, and dyslipidemia [20], as well as Black ethnicity and male sex [98]. The Ceccarelli cohort followed patients with SLE for 10 years and described the association of dyslipidemia with CI in all the domains, except for attention, and significantly correlated with worsening of visuospatial functions. Association with disease activity and chronic damage was also suggested by this cohort. Specifically, occurrence of flares was significantly associated with a worsening in the memory domain, implying that prevention of disease relapse could attenuate cognitive function deterioration [20]. The discrepancy between these findings and other studies who failed to show an association between disease activity and CI persistence or progression could be explained by the different follow-up lengths or factors related to study design such as patient's characteristics and heterogeneity of CI metrics and definitions [58, 73, 95, 98, 99].

Although some studies have approached the topic of CI persistence over time and its associations with different factors such as patients' demographics, SLE disease manifestations, other comorbidities (e.g., fibromyalgia), medication use (corticosteroid, immunosuppression, hydroxychloroquine, antiplatelets, and anticoagulation), and immunological profile, future research will help to better understand these complex relationships [20, 91–94, 98].

Several studies investigated the change in the affected cognitive domains over time. In a study of 111 patients with SLE followed over 1 year using the ACR-NB, the most affected domain over time in patients with persistent CI was *learning and memory* followed by *visuospatial construction* and *simple attention and processing* with no marked change over time in the domains involved. The same domains were affected in patients with fluctuating CI; however, fluctuating patients displayed less severe CI, as determined by average z-scores of the domains, with more variation in the affected domains over time [97]. Similarly, the changes of different neuropsychological tests after 5 years of follow-up in a cohort of 28 patients identified a stable pattern in 8 of 11 tests but improvement in 3 tests measuring *attention* and *psychomotor speed* domains [94]. In another study of 43 patients assessing cognitive function by a battery of tests over a 10-year period, all the domains showed an improvement over time, yet the pattern of domains involved was similar, with the exception of the *executive function* domain which showed significant improvement [20]. Similarly, in a study investigating 51 patients with SLE over 1 year, performance was consistent across subtests of the cognitive battery, with the most sensitive and reliable tests being those measuring *visuospatial reasoning* and *visuoconstructive function* [93]. In a study comparing 13 patients with NPSLE and 13 patients with non-NPSLE over a period of 12 months, using a battery of cognitive tests, patients with NPSLE were stable in all cognitive tests, while patients with non-NPSLE showed improvement in some tests measuring *abstract reasoning* and *visuospatial processing* [58].

The impact of persistent CI over time on employment and disability was studied in 167 patients with SLE. The likelihood of being unemployed or temporarily/permanently disabled after 3 years of follow-up correlated with the presence of impairment in *attention*, *memory*, and *executive functions* when compared with patients with other cognitive domains impairment [96].

## How Is Cognition Associated with Other Comorbidities (Depression/Anxiety)?

Like CI, mood and anxiety symptoms are common in SLE [100, 101]. Although estimates vary depending on the study population and measurement used, the prevalence of depression in SLE is about 35%, and the prevalence of anxiety is about 26% [101]. There is a clear and consistent relationship between CI and depression in SLE [101, 102], and together these conditions represent among the most common and disabling neuropsychiatric symptoms associated with SLE [103].

In a study examining a number of sociodemographic and clinical predictors of CI in SLE (age, education, neuropsychiatric involvement, disease duration, disease activity, current corticosteroid use, depression and anxiety), Monastero et al. found that depression was the only clinical variable associated with CI in a multiple regression model [104]. Aside from the study by Monastero et al., which did not find a relationship between anxiety and CI, there are no data regarding the relationship between anxiety and CI in SLE [104]. However, this study had a relatively small sample size ($n = 75$), and participants generally had low levels of anxiety. Given that anxiety and depression are typically highly comorbid [105], it would be surprising if such a relationship did not exist.

Less is known about the relationship between depression and specific cognitive domains in SLE, though two cross-sectional studies have investigated this question. Higher levels of depression and anxiety have been found to be associated with lower scores on the cognitive domains of attention, processing speed, visuospatial abilities, reaction time, and memory [102, 106]. Although studies are limited, evidence suggests that change in depression and anxiety is associated with change in cognitive scores. A 2-year prospective study comparing change in a depressive or anxiety disorder with change in cognitive scores at two time points identified that resolution of psychiatric disorder was associated with improvement in memory and verbal fluency [73]. Another prospective study indicated that, in patients with SLE followed for at least 3 years, higher depressive symptom score was associated with decline in overall cognitive score [107]. Although these observational studies suggest depression treatment as a target for improving cognition, randomized controlled trials are required to determine whether treating depression improves cognitive function in SLE and, if so, whether all cognitive domains improve equally.

The relationship between depression and CI in SLE is likely multifactorial, with biological and psychosocial influences. Depression itself is associated with CI, independent of additional comorbidities [108], and impaired concentration is part of the *Diagnostic and Statistical Manual of Mental Disorders, 5th Edition* (DSM-5) diagnostic criteria for depression [109].

Both depression and CI are associated with inflammation. Specifically, patients with major depression have been shown to have increased levels of inflammatory markers TNF-alpha, C-reactive protein (CRP), interleukin (IL)-1, and IL-6 [110, 111]. There is a well-established relationship between systemic inflammation and aging-related cognitive decline, with IL-6, TNF-alpha, and CRP levels found to be associated with overall cognitive decline [112]. In SLE specifically, IL-6 and IL-10 have been found to be associated with depression scores [113], and IL-6 has been shown to be related to learning and attention [114], suggesting a potential common role for IL-6 in both CI and depression in SLE.

Neuroanatomical changes may also contribute to both CI and depression in SLE. Certainly, major pathology such as stroke (for which patients with SLE are at increased risk) can contribute to both depression and CI [47, 115]. However, more subtle microstructural abnormalities in the brain's white matter (bundles of neuron fibers connecting different brain regions) have been observed in SLE, including decreased white matter volume and disruption in white matter microstructure within several white matter tracts [116, 117]. White matter abnormalities can contribute to neuropsychiatric symptoms such as CI and depression via a number of mechanisms, such as reduced connectivity and communication among pertinent brain cells and regions and reduced neuroplasticity [118]. White matter microstructural abnormalities have been demonstrated in major depression [119], and white matter microstructure is associated with cognitive performance in healthy adults [120]. In SLE specifically, both CI and mood disorder have been found to be related to white matter microstructural abnormalities [121]. Note that white matter abnormalities may be related to structural damage from inflammation, meaning that white matter dysfunction may partially mediate the relationship between inflammation and neuropsychiatric symptoms in SLE [122].

Medication side effects may also contribute to both CI and depression in patients with SLE. Corticosteroids in particular are well-known cause of a variety of neuropsychiatric symptoms, including depression and CI [123]. Other immunosuppressant medications have also been associated with neuropsychiatric symptoms [124]. From a clinical perspective, fatigue is commonly seen in patients with SLE in conjunction with depression and CI and is also thought to be immune-mediated [125].

Fatigue may contribute to frequent complaint of "brain fog" in patients with SLE and is also a core symptom of depression [109]. Thus, while a separate construct, fatigue may explain some of the overlap observed when measuring symptoms of CI and depression in patients with SLE.

In summary, CI and psychiatric symptoms, particularly depression, are commonly comorbid in SLE, likely due to a shared underlying mechanism such as inflammation and its effect on pertinent brain structures. Further research investigating this shared relationship will illuminate pathways for interventions targeting both of these disabling conditions.

## The Effects on Health-Related Quality of Life (HRQoL) in Patients with SLE with Cognitive Impairment

Health-related quality of life (HRQoL) is the physical, mental, and social aspect of health that is influenced by an individual's life experiences and expectations [126] (Fig. 13.4). Physical health includes but is not limited to fatigue, pain, sleep, and energy. Mental health encompasses the individual's emotions, including self-esteem, anxiety, depression, cognition, perception, and more. Social health involves interpersonal relationships, social support, and their social role.

Currently, there are few studies exploring the relationship between HRQoL and CI in patients with SLE. Overall, in SLE, studies have found lower HRQoL in patients with SLE than in patients with other common chronic conditions such as hypertension, depression, diabetes mellitus, rheumatoid arthritis, and more [127, 128]. A recent study by Dobrowolski et al. in 171 patients with SLE showed that CI is associated with significantly lower HRQoL scores [129]. Results from the Medical Outcomes Study Short Form 36 (SF-36) showed a decrease in mental health, social functioning, and planning domains, as well as a decrease in the physical component summary (PCS) score and lower scores in planning from the Lupus Quality of Life (LupusQoL).

Of the many different factors affecting HRQoL, CI has been often reported by patients with SLE to impact their HRQoL [127, 130–132]. Four studies explored the relationship between cognition and HRQoL and found a negative relationship between CI and HRQoL, although the strength of the relationship varied from small to large among the studies [16, 128, 133–135]. Moreover, social role participation has been found to be a fundamental aspect of HRQoL affected by CI [3, 136, 137]. Social role participation can be defined as experiences in human life that include being involved in close relationships, interacting with one's social network and community, being a member of professional groups, and/or pursuing leisure activities [138]. In other words, social role participation can encompass activities that are related to a life situation or life role, for example, employment or academic activities [132, 139–144]. In adults with SLE, employment has been a primary area of study with a recent review estimating employment rates to be 26–54% which are well below employment rates of adults without a chronic health condition [132]. Additionally, academics including school attendance and performance have been

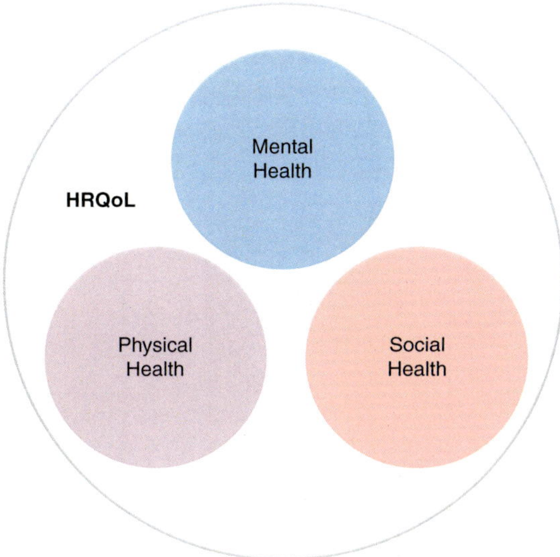


**Fig. 13.4** Components of HRQoL influenced by a patient's life experiences and expectations

found to be influenced by SLE – especially in the pediatric cohort of patients with SLE [142, 143, 145]. Activities of daily living (ADLs) are another aspect of social role participation impacted by CI. For example, it was determined that a patient's HRQoL decreased when they were unable to complete basic chores such as grooming or household activities [3].

In summary, the existing small body of literature suggests there is a negative relationship between CI and HRQoL in patients with SLE, where social role participation has been found to be greatly affected by CI. However more research is needed to provide a comprehensive understanding of this relationship.

## Pathogenesis of Cognitive Impairment in SLE: Antibodies and Cytokines

The pathogenesis of CI in SLE is poorly understood. A variety of mechanisms have been proposed as potential mediators of CI in SLE including antibodies and cytokines.

### *Antibodies*

Autoantibodies formation is one of the hallmarks of SLE. Several autoantibodies are linked to NPSLE manifestations and are believed to contribute to the pathogenesis of CI in particular. Of these, antiphospholipid (aPL) antibodies are thought to be directly related to focal NPSLE via autoantibody-mediated thrombosis; others, such as anti-NMDAR and anti-ribosomal P protein antibodies, are considered to target specific brain parenchymal structures and might explain diffuse NPSLE presentations.

## Antiphospholipid (aPL) Antibodies

Antiphospholipid syndrome (APLS) is characterized by arterial, venous, or small vessel thromboembolic events and/or pregnancy morbidity in the presence of persistently elevated titers of one or more aPL antibodies including lupus anticoagulant, anticardiolipin antibodies, and anti-β2-glycoprotein I antibodies [146]. The exact role of aPL antibodies in thrombus formation is still not fully identified, although they are known to activate endothelial cells, platelets, and monocytes, which are then thought to shed prothrombic microparticles [147]. APLS accompanies approximately 30% of patients with SLE, and the combination of these two conditions can amplify the risk of aPL-mediated cerebrovascular disease (CVD) [148]. aPL antibody-positive patients with SLE are about twice as likely as aPL antibody-negative patients to develop NPSLE [149]. The increased risk for cerebrovascular ischemia seen in aPL antibody-positive patients is caused by the susceptibility of the CNS to thrombus formation in addition to accelerated atherosclerosis, an independent risk factor for CVD [147]. Local scarring or damage from a thrombotic event can be associated with CI; however, apparently, these autoantibodies have a pathogenic role beyond their prothrombotic effects [147, 150]. In vitro, aPL antibodies bind to neurons and other CNS cells, and intrathecal transfer of immunoglobulins from aPL antibody-positive patients induces cognitive deficits in recipient mice, thereby supporting a direct effect of these antibodies on the brain [147, 151]. Clinically, the presence of aPL antibodies in patients with SLE has also been linked to NPSLE manifestations other than cerebrovascular ischemia, including CI [22, 47, 84, 107, 152–154]. A meta-analysis from 2016 by Ho et al. [149] showed that positivity of serum aPL antibodies had a pooled odds ratio of 2.01 ($p < 0.001$) for CI. Nevertheless, other studies have failed to confirm this association [155–157]. Cognitive domains which were described as impaired in aPL-positive patients include executive functioning, simple attention and memory, learning and memory (visual and verbal), verbal fluency, and visuospatial construction [81, 158, 159].

## Anti-N-methyl-d-aspartate Receptor (NMDAR) Antibodies

The NMDARs are glutamate receptor subtypes and ligand-gated ion channels that mediate a $Ca^{2+}$-permeable component of excitatory neurotransmission in the CNS. They are expressed throughout the CNS and play key physiological roles in synaptic function, such as synaptic plasticity, learning, and memory [160]. Anti-NMDAR antibodies are subsets of anti-dsDNA antibodies which cross-reacts with the NR2A and NR2B subunits of NMDARs [147]. Animal models exhibited induction of NPSLE including CI in healthy mice after passive transfer of sera containing anti-NMDAR antibodies from patients with SLE following disruption of the blood-brain barrier (BBB). Once the antibody penetrates the brain parenchyma, it binds the NMDAR leading to neuronal death, primarily via increased neuronal calcium influx [161, 162]. Beyond direct neuronal excitotoxic effects, a second phase of pathology is characterized by microglial activation and dendritic pruning of the surviving neurons which induced deficiencies in spatial recognition. This effect is dependent on locally activated microglia and the presence of complement component C1q [163, 164]. These cross-reactive anti-NMDAR antibodies are frequently associated with NPSLE in general and CI in particular, with reported deficits in attention, spatial cognition, learning, and memory [165–167]. Although serum levels of anti-NMDAR antibodies are not consistently correlated with CI [62, 168–171], CSF titers of these antibodies are higher in patients with diffuse NPSLE, and patients with CI, in particular, comparing to patients with focal NPSLE or noninflammatory CNS disease CI [172–175].

## *Anti-ribosomal P Protein Antibodies*

Anti-ribosomal P protein antibodies are highly specific for SLE and 80% specific for NPSLE [176, 177]. These antibodies recognize three specific ribosomal P proteins, P0, P1, and P2, located in the large ribosome's subunit [178]. They cross-react with a P epitope found exclusively on neuronal surface P antigen (NSPA), which regulates the function of NMDAR at the synaptic region. NSPA is also involved in synaptic transmission and plasticity related to memory in the hippocampus and mediates the deleterious effects of anti-ribosomal P protein antibodies on these processes [147]. In vitro, anti-ribosomal P proteins react with activated human peripheral blood monocytes and induce Th1 responses causing production of tumor necrosis factor-α and interleukin-6 [179]. The release of TNF could promote local CNS inflammation and result in BBB impairment, which enables infiltration of the antibodies into the CNS where they cause direct neuronal damage [147]. Anti-ribosomal P protein antibodies from patients with SLE injected to mice impaired hippocampal-dependent memory when the blood-brain barrier was disrupted [180]. These antibodies have been found in one study to be associated with CI with deficits in spatial recognition and attention [166]; however another study failed to show that these antibodies were associated with neither neuropsychiatric syndromes nor with CI [181].

## *Cytokines*

Cytokines function as inflammation mediators as well as neuromodulators [182]. Serum and CSF cytokine environments have been studied and have been linked to NPSLE manifestations and CI specifically, including interferon alpha (IFNα) and interleukin-6 (IL-6). Other candidate cytokines, such as IL-8, IL-10, TNF-like weak inducer of apoptosis (TWEAK), and IFNγ, might also play a role [183].

## IFNα

IFNα has been implicated as a leading effector of SLE as well as NPSLE pathogenesis. Increased CSF levels of IFNα were found in patients with NPSLE, as well as evidence of IFNα production within the CNS [147]. Patients receiving therapeutic IFNα frequently exhibit a number of neuropsychiatric side effects including CI with confusion, psychomotor slowing, impaired memory, and executive function [184, 185]. Neuropsychiatric changes have also been observed in healthy volunteers and SLE-prone mice peripherally administered IFNα [185, 186] However, anti-IFN-receptor antibody treatment did not reverse neuropsychiatric disease in lupus model mice [187], and studies examining clinical associations between IFNα expression and NPSLE manifestations have reported mainly negative results [157, 188, 189].

## IL-6

Increase of IL-6 in the older population is independently associated with an increased rate of cognitive decline in both executive function and memory [190]. Elevated intrathecal levels of IL-6 and intrathecal production of IL-6 have been demonstrated in patients with NPSLE as compared with non-NPSLE and non-autoimmune diseases control patients [147, 183, 191–193]. One study identified a relationship between serum IL-6 production and learning deficits in patients with SLE [114], and another showed that cognitive function was independently associated with higher levels of IL-6 [194]. Yet, other studies could not show an association between serum or CSF IL-6 levels and CI [157, 195].

## Others

Various other cytokines have also been linked to the development of NPSLE, including IL-8, IFNγ, IL-10, and TWEAK [147, 183]. IL-8 and IL-10 were found to be elevated in CSF of patients with NPSLE compared to patients with non-NPSLE [147, 192, 193]. Additionally, TWEAK has shown promise in mouse models of NPSLE, and intracerebroventricular administration of TWEAK induced depression-like behavior and cognitive dysfunction in non-autoimmune mice [147, 196, 197]. There are no studies linking these cytokines with CI specifically.

## Conclusion

This chapter addressed the many different components that contribute to cognition in SLE. Cognitive impairment has been found to be quite common in patients with SLE although its prevalence is wide ranging. Patient-reported measurement tools provide subjective CI information and are important to collect alongside objective CI information. Objective tools encompass the NB, standalone neuropsychological tests, and automated batteries such as the ANAM and CANTAB. Within the assessment of CI, studies of CI in SLE have shown ongoing heterogeneity with respect to CI definitions and assessment methods, warranting a new consensus to harmonize the field and provide updated standardized criteria. Overtime, cognition in patients with SLE have predominantly remained stable, and CI did not progress overtime; however some studies have shown a CI persistence up to 29% with fluctuations up to 41%. Cognitive impairment in patients with SLE has also been found to be associated with comorbidities such as anxiety and depression, patient health-related quality of life, and cytokines and antibodies. It is evident that cognition is influenced by a myriad of factors, making it a fascinating but complex construct to define and assess in patients with SLE.

## References

1. The American College of Rheumatology nomenclature and case definitions for neuropsychiatric lupus syndromes. Arthritis Rheum. 1999;42(4):599–608.
2. Mikdashi JA. Proposed response criteria for neurocognitive impairment in systemic lupus erythematosus clinical trials. Lupus. 2007;16(6):418–25.
3. Rayes HA, Tani C, Kwan A, Marzouk S, Colosimo K, Medina-Rosas J, et al. What is the prevalence of cognitive impairment in lupus and which instruments are used to measure it? A systematic review and meta-analysis. Semin Arthritis Rheum. 2018;48(2):240–55.
4. Kozora E, Ellison MC, West S. Depression, fatigue, and pain in systemic lupus erythematosus (SLE): relationship to the American College of Rheumatology SLE neuropsychological battery. Arthritis Care Res. 2006;55(4):628–35.
5. Beck AT, Epstein N, Brown G, Steer RA. An inventory for measuring clinical anxiety: Psychometric properties. J Consult Clin Psychol. 1988;56:893–7.
6. Beck AT, Ward CH, Mendelson M, Mock J, Erbaugh J. An inventory for measuring depression. Arch Gen Psychiatry. 1961;4:561–71.
7. Krupp L, LaRocca N, Muir-Nash J, Steinberg A. The Fatigue Severity Scale. Application to patients with multiple sclerosis and systemic lupus erythematosus. Arch Neurol. 1989;46(10):1121–3.
8. Yazdany J, Yelin E. Health-related quality of life and employment among persons with systemic lupus erythematosus. Rheum Dis Clin N Am. 2010;36(1):15–32.
9. Tarlov AR, Ware JE Jr, Greenfield S, Nelson EC, Perrin E, Zubkoff M. The Medical Outcomes Study. An application of methods for monitoring the results of medical care. JAMA. 1989;262(7):925–30.
10. Ware JJ, Sherbourne C. The MOS 36-Item Short-Form Health Survey (SF-36). I. Conceptual framework and item selection. Med Care. 1992;30(6):473–83.

11. Sullivan M, Edgley K, DeHousx E. A survey of multiple sclerosis, part 1: perceived cognitive problems and compensatory strategy use. Can J Rehabil. 1990;4:7.
12. Reilly MC, Zbrozek AS, Dukes EM. The validity and reproducibility of a work productivity and activity impairment instrument. PharmacoEconomics. 1993;4(5):353–65.
13. Ben-Porath YS, Tellegen A. MMPI-2-RF user's guide for reports. Minneapolis: University of Minnesota Press; 2008.
14. Morey LC. The personality assessment inventory professional manual. Psychological Assessment Resources: Odessa; 1991.
15. Hanly JG, Fisk JD, McCurdy G, Fougere L, Douglas JA. Neuropsychiatric syndromes in patients with systemic lupus erythematosus and rheumatoid arthritis. J Rheumatol. 2005;32(8):1459–6.
16. Alarcón GS, Cianfrini L, Bradley LA, Sanchez ML, Brooks K, Friedman AW, et al. Systemic lupus erythematosus in three ethnic groups. X. Measuring cognitive impairment with the cognitive symptoms inventory. Arthritis Care Res. 2002;47(3):310–9.
17. Paez-Venegas N, Jordan-Estrada B, Chavarria-Avila E, Perez-Vazquez F, Gómez-Bañuelos E, Medina-Dávalos R, et al. The Montreal Cognitive Assessment test: a useful tool in screening of cognitive impairment in patients with systemic lupus erythematosus. J Clin Rheumatol. 2019;25(8):325–8.
18. Vogel A, Bhattacharya S, Larsen JL, Jacobsen S. Do subjective cognitive complaints correlate with cognitive impairment in systemic lupus erythematosus? A Danish outpatient study. Lupus. 2011;20(1):35–43.
19. Engel L, Su J, Nalder E, Goverover Y, Gignac M, Tartaglia MC, et al. Patient-reported cognitive screen does not identify cognitive sub-domains: exploration of the subscale structure of the perceived deficits questionnaire in a systemic lupus erythematosus cohort [abstract]. In: 2018 ACR/ARHP annual meeting. Chicago, IL: Arthritis Rheumatology. p. 2018.
20. Ceccarelli F, Perricone C, Pirone C, Massaro L, Alessandri C, Mina C, et al. Cognitive dysfunction improves in systemic lupus erythematosus: results of a 10 years prospective study. PLoS One. 2018;13(5):e0196103.
21. Csókási K, Hargitai R, Járai R, Nagy L, Czirják L, Kiss EC. MMPI-2 profiles in groups of systemic autoimmune disease – rheumatoid arthritis and systemic lupus erythematosus – patients. Psychiatr Hung. 2015;30(4):409–17.
22. Conti F, Alessandri C, Perricone C, Scrivo R, Rezai S, Ceccarelli F, et al. Neurocognitive dysfunction in systemic lupus erythematosus: association with antiphospholipid antibodies, disease activity and chronic damage. PloS One. 2012;7(3):e33824.
23. Crighton AH, Tarescavage AM, Gervais RO, Ben-Porath YS. The generalizability of over-reporting across self-report measures: an investigation with the Minnesota multiphasic personality inventory-2-restructured form and the personality assessment inventory in a civil disability sample. Assessment. 2017;24(5):555–74.
24. Kozora E, Ellison MC, West S. Reliability and validity of the proposed American College of Rheumatology neuropsychological battery for systemic lupus erythematosus. Arthritis Rheum. 2004;51(5):810–8.
25. Kozora E, Thompson LL, West SG, Kotzin BL. Analysis of cognitive and psychological deficits in systemic lupus erythematosus patients without overt central nervous system disease. Arthritis Rheum. 1996;39(12):2035–45.
26. Weschler D. Wechsler adult intelligence scale—revised manual. San Antonio: The Psychological Corporation; 1981.
27. Wechsler D. Wechsler adult intelligence scale, third addition. San Antonio: The Psychological Corporation; 1997.
28. Reitan RM, Wolfson D. The Halstead-Reitan neuropsychological test battery: theory and clinical interpretation: Reitan neuropsychology. Tucson: Neuropsychology Press; 1985.
29. Golden CJ, Freshwater SM. Stroop color and word test. Chicago; 1978.
30. Borkowski JG, Benton AL, Spreen O. Word fluency and brain damage. Neuropsychologia. 1967;5(2):135–40.

31. Corwin J, Bylsma FW. Psychological examination of traumatic encephalopathy. Clin Neuropsychol. 1993;7(1):3–21.
32. Delis DC, Kramer JH, Kaplan E, Ober BA. CVLT, California verbal learning test: adult version: manual. San Antonio: Psychological Corporation; 1987.
33. Touma Z, Green R, Tartaglia MC, Ruttan L, Lombardi S, Anderson N, et al. Does cognitive function change over-time in systemic lupus erythematosus? [abstract]. In: 2018 ACR/ARHP annual meeting. Chicago, IL: Arthritis Rheumatology. p. 2018.
34. Tayer-Shifman EO, Green R, Beaton D, Ruttan L, Wither JE, Tartaglia MC, et al. Validity evidence supports the use of automated neuropsychological assessment metrics (ANAM) as a screening tool for cognitive impairment in patients with systemic lupus erythematosus. Arthritis Care Res (Hoboken). 2020;72:1809–19.
35. Shapiro AM, Benedict RH, Schretlen D, Brandt J. Construct and concurrent validity of the Hopkins verbal learning test–revised. Clin Neuropsychol. 1999;13(3):348–58.
36. Julian LJ, Yazdany J, Trupin L, Criswell LA, Yelin E, Katz PP. Validity of brief screening tools for cognitive impairment in rheumatoid arthritis and systemic lupus erythematosus. Arthritis Care Res. 2012;64(3):448–54.
37. Nantes SG, Su J, Dhaliwal A, Colosimo K, Touma Z. Performance of screening tests for cognitive impairment in systemic lupus erythematosus. J Rheumatol. 2017;44(11):1583.
38. Folstein MF, Folstein SE, McHugh PR. "Mini-mental state". A practical method for grading the cognitive state of patients for the clinician. J Psychiatr Res. 1975;12(3):189–98.
39. Adhikari T, Piatti A, Luggen M. Cognitive dysfunction in SLE: development of a screening tool. Lupus. 2011;20(11):1142–6.
40. Nasreddine ZS, Phillips NA, Bédirian V, Charbonneau S, Whitehead V, Collin I, et al. The Montreal Cognitive Assessment, MoCA: A brief screening tool for mild cognitive impairment. J Am Geriatr Soc. 2005;53(4):695–9.
41. Julayanont P, Phillips N, Chertkow H, Nasreddine ZS. Montreal Cognitive Assessment (MoCA): concept and clinical review. Cognitive screening instruments: a practical approach. New York: Springer-Verlag Publishing; 2013. p. 111–51.
42. Maciel RO, Ferreira GA, Akemy B, Cardoso F. Executive dysfunction, obsessive-compulsive symptoms, and attention deficit and hyperactivity disorder in Systemic Lupus Erythematosus: evidence for basal ganglia dysfunction? J Neurol Sci. 2016;360:94–7.
43. Kakvan M, Green R, Ruttan L, Tartaglia M, Wither J, Zandy M, et al. Performance of Montreal Cognitive Assessment (MoCA) in screening for cognitive impairment in patients with lupus compared to the neuropsychological battery [abstract]. In: Arthritis & rheumatology, vol. 71. Hoboken: Wiley; 2019.
44. Benedict RHB, Schretlen D, Groninger L, Brandt J. Hopkins verbal learning test – revised: normative data and analysis of inter-form and test-retest reliability. Clin Neuropsychol. 1998;12(1):43–55.
45. Ruff RM, Light RH, Parker SB, Levin HS. Benton controlled oral word association test: reliability and updated norms. Arch Clin Neuropsychol. 1996;11(4):329–38.
46. Panopalis P, Julian L, Yazdany J, Gillis JZ, Trupin L, Hersh A, et al. Impact of memory impairment on employment status in persons with systemic lupus erythematosus. Arthritis Rheum. 2007;57(8):1453–60.
47. Murray SG, Yazdany J, Kaiser R, Criswell LA, Trupin L, Yelin EH, et al. Cardiovascular disease and cognitive dysfunction in systemic lupus erythematosus. Arthritis Care Res. 2012;64(9):1328–33.
48. Touma Z, Moghaddam B, Su J, Katz P. Cognitive function trajectories are associated with the depressive symptoms trajectories in SLE over time. Arthritis Care Res. 2020.
49. Reeves DL, Winter KP, Bleiberg J, Kane RL. ANAM genogram: historical perspectives, description, and current endeavors. Arch Clin Neuropsychol. 2007;22(Suppl 1):S15–37.
50. Vincent AS, Roebuck-Spencer TM, Fuenzalida E, Gilliland K. Test-retest reliability and practice effects for the ANAM general neuropsychological screening battery. Clin Neuropsychol. 2018;32(3):479–94.

51. Holliday SL, Navarrete MG, Hermosillo-Romo D, Valdez CR, Saklad AR, Escalante A, et al. Validating a computerized neuropsychological test battery for mixed ethnic lupus patients. Lupus. 2003;12(9):697–703.
52. Hanly JG, Omisade A, Su L, Farewell V, Fisk JD. Assessment of cognitive function in systemic lupus erythematosus, rheumatoid arthritis, and multiple sclerosis by computerized neuropsychological tests. Arthritis Rheum. 2010;62(5):1478–86.
53. Bertsias GK, Ioannidis JP, Aringer M, Bollen E, Bombardieri S, Bruce IN, et al. EULAR recommendations for the management of systemic lupus erythematosus with neuropsychiatric manifestations: report of a task force of the EULAR standing committee for clinical affairs. Ann Rheum Dis. 2010;69(12):2074–82.
54. Bogaczewicz A, Sobow T, Kowalski J, Ząbek J, Woźniacka A, Bogaczewicz J. Cambridge Neuropsychological Test Automated Battery in assessment of cognitive parameters in patients with systemic lupus erythematosus in relation to autoantibody profile. Reumatologia. 2015;53(3):131–8.
55. Smith PJ, Need AC, Cirulli ET, Chiba-Falek O, Attix DK. A comparison of the Cambridge Automated Neuropsychological Test Battery (CANTAB) with "traditional" neuropsychological testing instruments. J Clin Exp Neuropsychol. 2013;35(3):319–28.
56. Weintraub S, Dikmen SS, Heaton RK, Tulsky DS, Zelazo PD, Bauer PJ, et al. Cognition assessment using the NIH toolbox. Neurology. 2013;80(11 Suppl 3):S54–64.
57. Weintraub S, Dikmen SS, Heaton RK, Tulsky DS, Zelazo PD, Slotkin J, et al. The cognition battery of the NIH toolbox for assessment of neurological and behavioral function: validation in an adult sample. J Int Neuropsychol Soc: JINS. 2014;20(6):567–78.
58. Gao Y, Lau EY, Wan JH, Lau CS, Mok MY. Systemic lupus erythematosus patients with past neuropsychiatric involvement are associated with worse cognitive impairment: a longitudinal study. Lupus. 2016;25(6):637–44.
59. Katz P, Julian L, Tonner MC, Yazdany J, Trupin L, Yelin E, et al. Physical activity, obesity, and cognitive impairment among women with systemic lupus erythematosus. Arthritis Care Res. 2012;64(4):502–10.
60. Coín MA, Vilar-López R, Peralta-Ramírez I, Hidalgo-Ruzzante N, Callejas-Rubio JL, Ortego-Centeno N, et al. The role of antiphospholipid autoantibodies in the cognitive deficits of patients with systemic lupus erythematosus. Lupus. 2015;24(8):875–9.
61. Correa DG, Zimmermann N, Borges RS, Pereira DB, Doring TM, Tukamoto G, et al. White-matter integrity in patients with systemic lupus erythematosus and memory deficits. Neuroradiology. 2018;31(6):587–95.
62. Harrison MJ, Ravdin LD, Lockshin MD. Relationship between serum NR2a antibodies and cognitive dysfunction in systemic lupus erythematosus. Arthritis Rheum. 2006;54(8):2515–22.
63. Sailer M, Burchert W, Ehrenheim C, Smid HGOM, Haas J, Wildhagen K, et al. Positron emission tomography and magnetic resonance imaging for cerebral involvement in patients with systemic lupus erythematosus. J Neurol. 1997;244(3):186–93.
64. Gao Y, Cheung RTF, Gao J, Lau EYY, Wan JHY, Mok MY. Electrophysiological study on cognitive function in systemic lupus erythematosus patients with previous neuropsychiatric involvement. Clin EEG Neurosci. 2017;48(4):251–8.
65. Zimmermann N, Correa DG, Kubo TA, Netto TM, Pereira DB, Fonseca RP, et al. Global cognitive impairment in systemic lupus erythematosus patients: a structural MRI study. Clin Neuroradiol. 2017;27(1):23–9.
66. Lapa AT, Pedro T, Francischinelli J, Coan AC, Costallat LT, Cendes F, et al. Abnormality in hippocampal signal intensity predicts atrophy in patients with systemic lupus erythematosus. Lupus. 2017;26(6):633–9.
67. Appenzeller S, Bonilha L, Rio PA, Min Li L, Costallat LTL, Cendes F. Longitudinal analysis of gray and white matter loss in patients with systemic lupus erythematosus. NeuroImage. 2007;34(2):694–701.
68. Appenzeller S, Cendes F, Costallat LTL. Cognitive impairment and employment status in systemic lupus erythematosus: A prospective longitudinal study. Arthritis Care Res. 2009;61(5):680–7.

69. Harboe E, Tjensvoll AB, Maroni S, Gøransson LG, Greve OJ, Beyer MK, et al. Neuropsychiatric syndromes in patients with systemic lupus erythematosus and primary Sjögren syndrome: a comparative population-based study. Ann Rheum Dis. 2009;68(10):1541.
70. Appenzeller S, Rondina JM, Li LM, Costallat LTL, Cendes F. Cerebral and corpus callosum atrophy in systemic lupus erythematosus. Arthritis Rheum. 2005;52(9):2783–9.
71. Ainiala H, Hietaharju A, Dastidar P, Loukkola J, Lehtimäki T, Peltola J, et al. Increased serum matrix metalloproteinase 9 levels in systemic lupus erythematosus patients with neuropsychiatric manifestations and brain magnetic resonance imaging abnormalities. Arthritis Rheum. 2004;50(3):858–65.
72. Hay EM, Black D, Huddy A, Creed F, Tomenson B, Bernstein RM, et al. Psychiatric disorder and cognitive impairment in systemic lupus erythematosus. Arthritis Rheum. 1992;35(4):411–6.
73. Hay EM, Huddy A, Black D, Mbaya P, Tomenson B, Bernstein RM, et al. A prospective study of psychiatric disorder and cognitive function in systemic lupus erythematosus. Ann Rheum Dis. 1994;53(5):298.
74. Carbotte RM, Denburg SD, Denburg JA. Prevalence of cognitive impairment in systemic lupus erythematosus. J Nerv Ment Dis. 1986;174(6):357–64.
75. Nishimura K, Omori M, Katsumata Y, Sato E, Gono T, Kawaguchi Y, et al. Neurocognitive impairment in corticosteroid-naive patients with active systemic lupus erythematosus: a prospective study. J Rheumatol. 2015;42(3):441.
76. Glanz BI, Slonim D, Urowitz MB, Gladman DD, Gough J, MacKinnon A. Pattern of neuropsychologic dysfunction in inactive systemic lupus erythematosus. Neuropsychiatry Neuropsychol Behav Neurol. 1997;10(4):232–8.
77. Kozora E, Arciniegas DB, Filley CM, West SG, Brown M, Miller D, et al. Cognitive and neurologic status in patients with systemic lupus erythematosus without major neuropsychiatric syndromes. Arthritis Care Res. 2008;59(11):1639–46.
78. Kozora E, Erkan D, West SG, Filley CM, Zhang L, Ramon G, et al. Site differences in mild cognitive dysfunction (MCD) among patients with systemic lupus erythematosus (SLE). Lupus. 2012;22(1):73–80.
79. Kozora E, Filley CM, Erkan D, Ulug AM, Vo A, Ramon G, et al. Longitudinal evaluation of diffusion tensor imaging and cognition in systemic lupus erythematosus. Lupus. 2018;27(11):1810–8.
80. Kozora E, Ulug AM, Erkan D, Vo A, Filley CM, Ramon G, et al. Functional magnetic resonance imaging of working memory and executive dysfunction in systemic lupus erythematosus and antiphospholipid antibody-positive patients. Arthritis Care Res. 2016;68(11):1655–63.
81. Kozora E, Erkan D, Zhang L, Zimmerman R, Ramon G, Ulug AM, et al. Cognitive dysfunction in antiphospholipid antibody (aPL)-negative systemic lupus erythematosus (SLE) versus aPL-positive non-SLE patients. Clin Exp Rheumatol. 2014;32(1):34–40.
82. Kozora E, Zell J, Swigris J, Strand M, Duggan EC, Burleson A, et al. Cardiopulmonary correlates of cognition in systemic lupus erythematosus. Lupus. 2014;24(2):164–73.
83. Brey RL, Holliday SL, Saklad AR, Navarrete MG, Hermosillo-Romo D, Stallworth CL, et al. Neuropsychiatric syndromes in lupus. Neurology. 2002;58(8):1214.
84. Tomietto P, Annese V, D'agostini S, Venturini P, La Torre G, De Vita S, et al. General and specific factors associated with severity of cognitive impairment in systemic lupus erythematosus. Arthritis Care Res. 2007;57(8):1461–72.
85. Duarte-García A, Romero-Díaz J, Juárez S, Cicero-Casarrubias A, Fragoso-Loyo H, Núñez-Alvarez C, et al. Disease activity, autoantibodies, and inflammatory molecules in serum and cerebrospinal fluid of patients with systemic lupus erythematosus and cognitive dysfunction. PLoS One. 2018;13(5):e0196487.
86. Katz PP, Andrews J, Yazdany J, Schmajuk G, Trupin L, Yelin E. Is frailty a relevant concept in SLE? Lupus Sci Med. 2017;4(1):e000186.
87. Roldan PC, Jung RE, Sibbitt WL, Qualls CR, Flores RA, Roldan CA. Correlation of neurocognitive function and brain lesion load on magnetic resonance imaging in systemic lupus erythematosus. Rheumatol Int. 2018;38(8):1539–46.

88. Magro-Checa C, Zirkzee EJ, Beaart-van de Voorde LJJ, Middelkoop HA, van der Wee NJ, Huisman MV, et al. Value of multidisciplinary reassessment in attribution of neuropsychiatric events to systemic lupus erythematosus: prospective data from the Leiden NPSLE cohort. Rheumatology (Oxford). 2017;56(10):1676–83.
89. Roebuck-Spencer TM, Yarboro C, Nowak M, Takada K, Jacobs G, Lapteva L, et al. Use of computerized assessment to predict neuropsychological functioning and emotional distress in patients with systemic lupus erythematosus. Arthritis Care Res. 2006;55(3):434–41.
90. Zirkzee EJM, Steup-Beekman GM, van der Mast RC, Bollen ELEM, van der Wee NJA, Baptist E, et al. Prospective study of clinical phenotypes in neuropsychiatric systemic lupus erythematosus; multidisciplinary approach to diagnosis and therapy. J Rheumatol. 2012;39(11):2118.
91. Hanly JG, Fisk JD, Sherwood G, Eastwood B. Clinical course of cognitive dysfunction in systemic lupus erythematosus. J Rheumatol. 1994;21(10):1825–31.
92. Hanly JG, Cassell K, Fisk JD. Cognitive function in systemic lupus erythematosus: results of a 5-year prospective study. Arthritis Rheum. 1997;40:2.
93. Carlomagno S, Migliaresi S, Ambrosone L, Sannino M, Sanges G, Di Iorio G. Cognitive impairment in systemic lupus erythematosus: a follow-up study. J Neurol. 2000;247(4):273–9.
94. Waterloo K, Omdal R, Husby G, Mellgren SI. Neuropsychological function in systemic lupus erythematosus: a five-year longitudinal study. Rheumatology (Oxford). 2002;41(4):411–5.
95. Denburg SD, Stewart KE, Hart LE, Denburg JA. How "soft" are soft neurological signs? The relationship of subjective neuropsychiatric complaints to cognitive function in systemic lupus erythematosus. J Rheumatol. 2003;30(5):1006–10.
96. Appenzeller S, Cendes F, Costallat LT. Cognitive impairment and employment status in systemic lupus erythematosus: a prospective longitudinal study. Arthritis Rheum. 2009;61(5):680–7.
97. Tayer-Shifman O, Beaton D, Green R, Ruttan L, Wither J, Tartaglia M, Kakvan M, Lombardi S, Anderson N, Su J, Bonilla D, Zandy M, Choi M, Fritzler M, Touma Z. Describing intra-individual cognitive function course over time in lupus patients: persistent and fluctuating cognitive impairment, affected cognitive domains, and severity [abstract]. Arthritis Rheumatol (Hoboken, NJ). 2019;71 (Suppl 10):1–5362.
98. Beaton D, Green R, Ruttan L, Wither J, Tayer-shifman O, Tartaglia M, Kakvan M, Anderson N, Su J, Zandy M, Choi M, Fritzler M, Touma Z. Persistent cognitive impairment in lupus patients over 1 year and associated factors [abstract]. Arthritis Rheumatol (Hoboken, NJ). 2019;71(Suppl 10):1–5362.
99. Menon S, Jameson-Shortall E, Newman SP, Hall-Craggs MR, Chinn R, Isenberg DA. A longitudinal study of anticardiolipin antibody levels and cognitive functioning in systemic lupus erythematosus. Arthritis Rheum. 1999;42(4):735–41.
100. Kwan A, Katz P, Touma Z. The assessment of anxiety and depression and its associated factors in SLE. Curr Rheumatol Rev. 2019;15(2):90–8.
101. Moustafa AT, Moazzami M, Engel L, Bangert E, Hassanein M, Marzouk S, et al. Prevalence and metric of depression and anxiety in systemic lupus erythematosus: a systematic review and meta-analysis. Semin Arthritis Rheum. 2020;50(1):84–94.
102. Ho RC, Husain SF, Ho CS. Cognitive dysfunction in patients with systemic lupus erythematosus: the challenge in diagnosis and management. Rheumatol Pract Res. 2018;3:2059902118792434.
103. Kivity S, Agmon-Levin N, Zandman-Goddard G, Chapman J, Shoenfeld Y. Neuropsychiatric lupus: a mosaic of clinical presentations. BMC Med. 2015;13(1):43.
104. Monastero R, Bettini P, Del Zotto E, Cottini E, Tincani A, Balestrieri G, et al. Prevalence and pattern of cognitive impairment in systemic lupus erythematosus patients with and without overt neuropsychiatric manifestations. J Neurol Sci. 2001;184(1):33–9.
105. Gorman JM. Comorbid depression and anxiety spectrum disorders. Depress Anxiety. 1996;4(4):160–8.
106. Petri M, Naqibuddin M, Carson KA, Wallace DJ, Weisman MH, Holliday SL, et al. Depression and cognitive impairment in newly diagnosed systemic lupus erythematosus. J Rheumatol. 2010;37(10):2032.

107. McLaurin EY, Holliday SL, Williams P, Brey RL. Predictors of cognitive dysfunction in patients with systemic lupus erythematosus. Neurology. 2005;64(2):297–303.
108. Rock PL, Roiser JP, Riedel WJ, Blackwell AD. Cognitive impairment in depression: a systematic review and meta-analysis. Psychol Med. 2014;44(10):2029–40.
109. American Psychiatric Association. Diagnostic and statistical manual of mental disorders, 5th edition: DSM-5. Arlington: American Psychiatric Association; 2013.
110. Dowlati Y, Herrmann N, Swardfager W, Thomson S, Oh PI, Van Uum S, et al. Relationship between hair cortisol concentrations and depressive symptoms in patients with coronary artery disease. Neuropsychiatr Dis Treat. 2010;6:393–400.
111. Howren MB, Lamkin DM, Suls J. Associations of depression with C-reactive protein, IL-1, and IL-6: a meta-analysis. Psychosom Med. 2009;71(2):171–86.
112. Lin T, Liu GA, Perez E, Rainer RD, Febo M, Cruz-Almeida Y, et al. Systemic inflammation mediates age-related cognitive deficits. Front Aging Neurosci. 2018;10:236.
113. Figueiredo-Braga M, Cornaby C, Cortez A, Bernardes M, Terroso G, Figueiredo M, et al. Depression and anxiety in systemic lupus erythematosus: The crosstalk between immunological, clinical, and psychosocial factors. Medicine (Baltimore). 2018;97(28):e11376-e.
114. Kozora E, Laudenslager M, Lemieux A, West SG. Inflammatory and hormonal measures predict neuropsychological functioning in systemic lupus erythematosus and rheumatoid arthritis patients. J Int Neuropsychol Soc: JINS. 2001;7(6):745–54.
115. Narushima K, Robinson RG. Stroke-related depression. Curr Atheroscler Rep. 2002;4(4):296–303.
116. Cesar B, Dwyer MG, Shucard JL, Polak P, Bergsland N, Benedict RHB, et al. Cognitive and white matter tract differences in MS and diffuse neuropsychiatric systemic lupus erythematosus. Am J Neuroradiol. 2015;36(10):1874.
117. Mak A, Ho RC, Tng HY, Koh HL, Chong JS, Zhou J. Early cerebral volume reductions and their associations with reduced lupus disease activity in patients with newly-diagnosed systemic lupus erythematosus. Sci Rep. 2016;6:22231.
118. Nave KA, Ehrenreich H. Myelination and oligodendrocyte functions in psychiatric diseases. JAMA Psychiat. 2014;71(5):582–4.
119. Tham MW, Woon PS, Sum MY, Lee TS, Sim K. White matter abnormalities in major depression: evidence from post-mortem, neuroimaging and genetic studies. J Affect Disord. 2011;132(1–2):26–36.
120. Chopra S, Shaw M, Shaw T, Sachdev PS, Anstey KJ, Cherbuin N. More highly myelinated white matter tracts are associated with faster processing speed in healthy adults. NeuroImage. 2018;171:332–40.
121. Magro-Checa C, Ercan E, Wolterbeek R, Emmer B, van der Wee NJ, Middelkoop HA, et al. Changes in white matter microstructure suggest an inflammatory origin of neuropsychiatric systemic lupus erythematosus. Arthritis Rheumatol. 2016;68(8):1945–54.
122. Ramage AE, Fox PT, Brey RL, Narayana S, Cykowski MD, Naqibuddin M, et al. Neuroimaging evidence of white matter inflammation in newly diagnosed systemic lupus erythematosus. Arthritis Rheum. 2011;63(10):3048–57.
123. Brown ES, Chandler PA. Mood and cognitive changes during systemic corticosteroid therapy. Prim Care Companion J Clin Psychiatry. 2001;3(1):17–21.
124. Zhang W, Egashira N, Masuda S. Recent topics on the mechanisms of immunosuppressive therapy-related neurotoxicities. Int J Mol Sci. 2019;20(13):3210.
125. Mackay M. Lupus brain fog: a biologic perspective on cognitive impairment, depression, and fatigue in systemic lupus erythematosus. Immunol Res. 2015;63(1–3):26–37.
126. Doria A, Rinaldi S, Ermani M, Salaffi F, Iaccarino L, Ghirardello A, et al. Health-related quality of life in Italian patients with systemic lupus erythematosus. II. Role of clinical, immunological and psychological determinants. Rheumatology (Oxford). 2004;43(12):1580–6.
127. Jolly M. How does quality of life of patients with systemic lupus erythematosus compare with that of other common chronic illnesses? J Rheumatol. 2005;32(9):1706–8.

128. Alfred S, Khoja L, Anderson M, Touma Z, Engel L. Cognitive impairments in SLE negatively related to participation and quality of life: a systematic review [abstract]. Arthritis Rheumatol (Hoboken, NJ). 2019;71.
129. Dobrowolski C, Engel L, Green R, Ruttan L, Lombardi S, Tartaglia C, et al. Cognitive impairment and health-related quality of life in a lupus cohort [abstract]. Arthritis Rheumatol (Hoboken, NJ). 2018;70.
130. Mikdashi J. Measuring and monitoring health-related quality of life responsiveness in systemic lupus erythematosus patients: current perspectives. Patient Relat Outcome Meas. 2018;9:339–43.
131. Kuriya B, Gladman DD, Ibanez D, Urowitz MB. Quality of life over time in patients with systemic lupus erythematosus. Arthritis Rheum. 2008;59(2):181–5.
132. Schmeding A, Schneider M. Fatigue, health-related quality of life and other patient-reported outcomes in systemic lupus erythematosus. Best Pract Res Clin Rheumatol. 2013;27(3):363–75.
133. Calderón J, Flores P, Aguirre JM, Valdivia G, Padilla O, Barra I, et al. Impact of cognitive impairment, depression, disease activity, and disease damage on quality of life in women with systemic lupus erythematosus. Scand J Rheumatol. 2017;46(4):273–80.
134. Tam LS, Wong A, Mok VC, Zhu YE, Kwok LW, Li TK, et al. The relationship between neuropsychiatric, clinical, and laboratory variables and quality of life of Chinese patients with systemic lupus erythematosus. J Rheumatol. 2008;35(6):1038–45.
135. Williams TS, Aranow C, Ross GS, Barsdorf A, Imundo LF, Eichenfield AH, et al. Neurocognitive impairment in childhood-onset systemic lupus erythematosus: measurement issues in diagnosis. Arthritis Care Res (Hoboken). 2011;63(8):1178–87.
136. Golder V, Ooi JJY, Antony AS, Ko T, Morton S, Kandane-Rathnayake R, et al. Discordance of patient and physician health status concerns in systemic lupus erythematosus. Lupus. 2018;27(3):501–6.
137. Mendelson C. Managing a medically and socially complex life: women living with lupus. Qual Health Res. 2006;16(7):15.
138. Gignac MA, Backman CL, Davis AM, Lacaille D, Mattison CA, Montie P, et al. Understanding social role participation: what matters to people with arthritis? J Rheumatol. 2008;35(8):1655–63.
139. Garris C, Oglesby A, Sulcs E, Lee M. Impact of systemic lupus erythematosus on burden of illness and work productivity in the United States. Lupus. 2013;22(10):1077–86.
140. Booth S, Price E, Walker E. Fluctuation, invisibility, fatigue – the barriers to maintaining employment with systemic lupus erythematosus: results of an online survey. Lupus. 2018;27(14):2284–91.
141. Drenkard C, Bao G, Dennis G, Kan HJ, Jhingran PM, Molta CT, et al. Burden of systemic lupus erythematosus on employment and work productivity: data from a large cohort in the southeastern United States. Arthritis Care Res (Hoboken). 2014;66(6):878–87.
142. Moorthy LN, Peterson MG, Hassett A, Baratelli M, Lehman TJ. Impact of lupus on school attendance and performance. Lupus. 2010;19(5):620–7.
143. Lee KKS, Chong JQ, Abu Bakar AK. School refusal in adolescents with systemic lupus erythematosus (SLE): a case series. Asian J Psychiatr. 2018;34:59–60.
144. Boomsma MM, Bijl M, Stegeman CA, Kallenberg CG, Hoffman GS, Tervaert JW. Patients' perceptions of the effects of systemic lupus erythematosus on health, function, income, and interpersonal relationships: a comparison with Wegener's granulomatosis. Arthritis Rheum. 2002;47(2):196–201.
145. Zelko F, Beebe D, Baker A, Nelson SM, Ali A, Cedeno A, et al. Academic outcomes in childhood-onset systemic lupus erythematosus. Arthritis Care Res (Hoboken). 2012;64(8):1167–74.
146. Cervera R. Antiphospholipid syndrome. Thromb Res. 2017;151(Suppl 1):S43–s7.
147. Schwartz N, Stock AD, Putterman C. Neuropsychiatric lupus: new mechanistic insights and future treatment directions. Nat Rev Rheumatol. 2019;15(3):137–52.

148. Taraborelli M, Leuenberger L, Lazzaroni MG, Martinazzi N, Zhang W, Franceschini F, et al. The contribution of antiphospholipid antibodies to organ damage in systemic lupus erythematosus. Lupus. 2016;25(12):1365–8.
149. Ho RC, Thiaghu C, Ong H, Lu Y, Ho CS, Tam WW, et al. A meta-analysis of serum and cerebrospinal fluid autoantibodies in neuropsychiatric systemic lupus erythematosus. Autoimmun Rev. 2016;15(2):124–38.
150. Yelnik CM, Kozora E, Appenzeller S. Cognitive disorders and antiphospholipid antibodies. Autoimmun Rev. 2016;15(12):1193–8.
151. Katzav A, Ben-Ziv T, Blank M, Pick CG, Shoenfeld Y, Chapman J. Antibody-specific behavioral effects: intracerebroventricular injection of antiphospholipid antibodies induces hyperactive behavior while anti-ribosomal-P antibodies induces depression and smell deficits in mice. J Neuroimmunol. 2014;272(1–2):10–5.
152. Hanly JG, Hong C, Smith S, Fisk JD. A prospective analysis of cognitive function and anticardiolipin antibodies in systemic lupus erythematosus. Arthritis Rheum. 1999;42(4):728–34.
153. Mikdashi J, Handwerger B. Predictors of neuropsychiatric damage in systemic lupus erythematosus: data from the Maryland lupus cohort. Rheumatology (Oxford). 2004;43(12):1555–60.
154. Sanna G, Bertolaccini ML, Cuadrado MJ, Laing H, Khamashta MA, Mathieu A, et al. Neuropsychiatric manifestations in systemic lupus erythematosus: prevalence and association with antiphospholipid antibodies. J Rheumatol. 2003;30(5):985–92.
155. Afeltra A, Garzia P, Mitterhofer AP, Vadacca M, Galluzzo S, Del Porto F, et al. Neuropsychiatric lupus syndromes: relationship with antiphospholipid antibodies. Neurology. 2003;61(1):108–10.
156. Moghaddam B Beaton D, Green R, Tartaglia M, Ruttan L, Kakvan M, Fritzler M, Choi M, Zandy M, Su J, Vitti M, Bonilla D, Wither J, Lombardi S, Touma Z. Prevalence of cognitive impairment in an inception lupus cohort as assessed by a comprehensive neuropsychological battery [abstract]. 2019 ACR/ARP annual meeting abstract supplement. Arthritis Rheumatol (Hoboken, NJ). 2019;71(Suppl 10):1–5362.
157. Kozora E, Filley CM, Zhang L, Brown MS, Miller DE, Arciniegas DB, et al. Immune function and brain abnormalities in patients with systemic lupus erythematosus without overt neuropsychiatric manifestations. Lupus. 2011;21(4):402–11.
158. Jacobson MW, Rapport LJ, Keenan PA, Coleman RD, Tietjen GE. Neuropsychological deficits associated with antiphospholipid antibodies. J Clin Exp Neuropsychol. 1999;21(2):251–64.
159. Tektonidou MG, Varsou N, Kotoulas G, Antoniou A, Moutsopoulos HM. Cognitive deficits in patients with antiphospholipid syndrome: association with clinical, laboratory, and brain magnetic resonance imaging findings. Arch Intern Med. 2006;166(20):2278–84.
160. Hansen KB, Yi F, Perszyk RE, Furukawa H, Wollmuth LP, Gibb AJ, et al. Structure, function, and allosteric modulation of NMDA receptors. J Gen Physiol. 2018;150(8):1081–105.
161. Kowal C, DeGiorgio LA, Nakaoka T, Hetherington H, Huerta PT, Diamond B, et al. Cognition and immunity; antibody impairs memory. Immunity. 2004;21(2):179–88.
162. Kowal C, Degiorgio LA, Lee JY, Edgar MA, Huerta PT, Volpe BT, et al. Human lupus autoantibodies against NMDA receptors mediate cognitive impairment. Proc Natl Acad Sci U S A. 2006;103(52):19854–9.
163. Khoury LE, Zarfeshani A, Diamond B. Using the mouse to model human diseases: Cognitive impairment in SLE. J Rheumatol. 2020.
164. Nestor J, Arinuma Y, Huerta TS, Kowal C, Nasiri E, Kello N, et al. Lupus antibodies induce behavioral changes mediated by microglia and blocked by ACE inhibitors. J Exp Med. 2018;215(10):2554–66.
165. Omdal R, Brokstad K, Waterloo K, Koldingsnes W, Jonsson R, Mellgren SI. Neuropsychiatric disturbances in SLE are associated with antibodies against NMDA receptors. Eur J Neurol. 2005;12(5):392–8.
166. Massardo L, Bravo-Zehnder M, Calderón J, Flores P, Padilla O, Aguirre JM, et al. Anti-N-methyl-D-aspartate receptor and anti-ribosomal-P autoantibodies contribute to cognitive dysfunction in systemic lupus erythematosus. Lupus. 2015;24(6):558–68.

167. Chang EH, Volpe BT, Mackay M, Aranow C, Watson P, Kowal C, et al. Selective impairment of spatial cognition caused by autoantibodies to the N-methyl-D-aspartate receptor. EBioMedicine. 2015;2(7):755–64.
168. Lapteva L, Nowak M, Yarboro CH, Takada K, Roebuck-Spencer T, Weickert T, et al. Anti-N-methyl-D-aspartate receptor antibodies, cognitive dysfunction, and depression in systemic lupus erythematosus. Arthritis Rheum. 2006;54(8):2505–14.
169. Hanly JG, Robichaud J, Fisk JD. Anti-NR2 glutamate receptor antibodies and cognitive function in systemic lupus erythematosus. J Rheumatol. 2006;33(8):1553–8.
170. Steup-Beekman G, Steens S, van Buchem M, Huizinga T. Anti-NMDA receptor autoantibodies in patients with systemic lupus erythematosus and their first-degree relatives. Lupus. 2007;16(5):329–34.
171. Kozora E, West SG, Maier SF, Filley CM, Arciniegas DB, Brown M, et al. Antibodies against N-methyl-D-aspartate receptors in patients with systemic lupus erythematosus without major neuropsychiatric syndromes. J Neurol Sci. 2010;295(1–2):87–91.
172. Arinuma Y, Yanagida T, Hirohata S. Association of cerebrospinal fluid anti-NR2 glutamate receptor antibodies with diffuse neuropsychiatric systemic lupus erythematosus. Arthritis Rheum. 2008;58(4):1130–5.
173. Fragoso-Loyo H, Cabiedes J, Orozco-Narváez A, Dávila-Maldonado L, Atisha-Fregoso Y, Diamond B, et al. Serum and cerebrospinal fluid autoantibodies in patients with neuropsychiatric lupus erythematosus. Implications for diagnosis and pathogenesis. PloS One. 2008;3(10):e3347-e.
174. Hirohata S, Arinuma Y, Yanagida T, Yoshio T. Blood-brain barrier damages and intrathecal synthesis of anti-N-methyl-D-aspartate receptor NR2 antibodies in diffuse psychiatric/neuropsychological syndromes in systemic lupus erythematosus. Arthritis Res Ther. 2014;16(2):R77.
175. Yoshio T, Onda K, Nara H, Minota S. Association of IgG anti-NR2 glutamate receptor antibodies in cerebrospinal fluid with neuropsychiatric systemic lupus erythematosus. Arthritis Rheum. 2006;54(2):675–8.
176. Karassa FB, Afeltra A, Ambrozic A, Chang DM, De Keyser F, Doria A, et al. Accuracy of anti-ribosomal P protein antibody testing for the diagnosis of neuropsychiatric systemic lupus erythematosus: an international meta-analysis. Arthritis Rheum. 2006;54(1):312–24.
177. Choi MY, FitzPatrick RD, Buhler K, Mahler M, Fritzler MJ. A review and meta-analysis of anti-ribosomal P autoantibodies in systemic lupus erythematosus. Autoimmun Rev. 2020;19(3):102463.
178. Gerli R, Caponi L. Anti-ribosomal P protein antibodies. Autoimmunity. 2005;38(1):85–92.
179. Nagai T, Yanagida T, Hirohata S. Anti-ribosomal P protein antibody induces Th1 responses by enhancing the production of IL-12 in activated monocytes. Mod Rheumatol. 2011;21(1):57–62.
180. Bravo-Zehnder M, Toledo EM, Segovia-Miranda F, Serrano FG, Benito MJ, Metz C, et al. Anti-ribosomal P protein autoantibodies from patients with neuropsychiatric lupus impair memory in mice. Arthritis Rheumatol (Hoboken, NJ). 2015;67(1):204–14.
181. Gerli R, Caponi L, Tincani A, Scorza R, Sabbadini MG, Danieli MG, et al. Clinical and serological associations of ribosomal P autoantibodies in systemic lupus erythematosus: prospective evaluation in a large cohort of Italian patients. Rheumatology (Oxford). 2002;41(12):1357–66.
182. Vitkovic L, Bockaert J, Jacque C. "Inflammatory" cytokines: neuromodulators in normal brain? J Neurochem. 2000;74(2):457–71.
183. Kozora E, Hanly JG, Lapteva L, Filley CM. Cognitive dysfunction in systemic lupus erythematosus: past, present, and future. Arthritis Rheum. 2008;58(11):3286–98.
184. Schaefer M, Engelbrecht MA, Gut O, Fiebich BL, Bauer J, Schmidt F, et al. Interferon alpha (IFNalpha) and psychiatric syndromes: a review. Prog Neuro-Psychopharmacol Biol Psychiatry. 2002;26(4):731–46.

185. Valentine AD. Managing the neuropsychiatric adverse effects of interferon treatment. BioDrugs. 1999;11(4):229–37.
186. Zeng J, Meng X, Zhou P, Yin Z, Xie Q, Zou H, et al. Interferon-α exacerbates neuropsychiatric phenotypes in lupus-prone mice. Arthritis Res Ther. 2019;21(1):205.
187. Huang MW, Stock AD, Mike EV, Herlitz L, Kolbeck R, Putterman C. Anti-IFNAR treatment does not reverse neuropsychiatric disease in MRL/LPR lupus mice. Lupus. 2019;28(13):1510–23.
188. Fragoso-Loyo H, Atisha-Fregoso Y, Núñez-Alvarez CA, Llorente L, Sánchez-Guerrero J. Utility of interferon-α as a biomarker in central neuropsychiatric involvement in systemic lupus erythematosus. J Rheumatol. 2012;39(3):504–9.
189. Jönsen A, Bengtsson AA, Nived O, Ryberg B, Truedsson L, Rönnblom L, et al. The heterogeneity of neuropsychiatric systemic lupus erythematosus is reflected in lack of association with cerebrospinal fluid cytokine profiles. Lupus. 2003;12(11):846–50.
190. Mooijaart SP, Sattar N, Trompet S, Lucke J, Stott DJ, Ford I, et al. Circulating interleukin-6 concentration and cognitive decline in old age: the PROSPER study. J Intern Med. 2013;274(1):77–85.
191. Fragoso-Loyo H, Richaud-Patin Y, Orozco-Narváez A, Dávila-Maldonado L, Atisha-Fregoso Y, Llorente L, et al. Interleukin-6 and chemokines in the neuropsychiatric manifestations of systemic lupus erythematosus. Arthritis Rheum. 2007;56(4):1242–50.
192. Yoshio T, Okamoto H, Kurasawa K, Dei Y, Hirohata S, Minota S. IL-6, IL-8, IP-10, MCP-1 and G-CSF are significantly increased in cerebrospinal fluid but not in sera of patients with central neuropsychiatric lupus erythematosus. Lupus. 2016;25(9):997–1003.
193. Kwieciński J, Kłak M, Trysberg E, Blennow K, Tarkowski A, Jin T. Relationship between elevated cerebrospinal fluid levels of plasminogen activator inhibitor 1 and neuronal destruction in patients with neuropsychiatric systemic lupus erythematosus. Arthritis Rheum. 2009;60(7):2094–101.
194. Wiseman SJ, Bastin ME, Hamilton IF, Hunt D, Ritchie SJ, Amft EN, et al. Fatigue and cognitive function in systemic lupus erythematosus: associations with white matter microstructural damage. A diffusion tensor MRI study and meta-analysis. Lupus. 2017;26(6):588–97.
195. Trysberg E, Carlsten H, Tarkowski A. Intrathecal cytokines in systemic lupus erythematosus with central nervous system involvement. Lupus. 2000;9(7):498–503.
196. Kello N, Anderson E, Diamond B. Cognitive dysfunction in systemic lupus erythematosus: a case for initiating trials. Arthritis Rheumatol (Hoboken, NJ). 2019;71(9):1413–25.
197. Wen J, Chen CH, Stock A, Doerner J, Gulinello M, Putterman C. Intracerebroventricular administration of TNF-like weak inducer of apoptosis induces depression-like behavior and cognitive dysfunction in non-autoimmune mice. Brain Behav Immun. 2016;54:27–37.

# Chapter 14
# Assessment of Depression and Anxiety in Lupus

**Andrew Kwan, Kathleen Bingham, Christine Peschken, Patricia P. Katz, and Zahi Touma**

## Introduction

Psychiatric manifestations are highly prevalent in patients with systemic lupus erythematosus (SLE). Among these, anxiety and depression represent the most common complaints [1], with depression occurring at four times higher prevalence when compared to a matched, non-SLE population and anxiety occurring at twice the prevalence when compared to non-SLE controls [2, 3]. Studies of depression and anxiety in SLE have shown prevalence ranging from 17% to 75% and 6% to 52%, respectively [4–6]. This range of prevalence has been attributed to varying definitions used for depression and anxiety, different study methodologies, as well as the diverse screening tools used in these studies [7–10].

In SLE, depression has been linked with increased incidence of comorbidities including cardiovascular disease [11, 12], suicidal ideation [13, 14], as well as decreased functional ability [15, 16] and adherence to treatment [10] resulting in

A. Kwan
University of Toronto, Department of Medicine, Toronto, ON, Canada

K. Bingham
Centre for Mental Health, University Health Network, Department of Psychiatry, University of Toronto, Toronto, ON, Canada

C. Peschken
University of Manitoba, Department of Medicine, Winnipeg, MB, Canada

P. P. Katz
University of California San Francisco, Department of Medicine and Institute for Health Policy Studies, San Francisco, CA, USA

Z. Touma (✉)
Centre for Prognosis in Rheumatic Disease, Toronto Lupus Clinic, Division of Rheumatology, Department of Medicine, Institute of Health Policy, Management and Evaluation, University of Toronto, Toronto, ON, Canada
e-mail: Zahi.Touma@uhn.ca



Z. Touma (ed.), *Outcome Measures and Metrics in Systemic Lupus Erythematosus*, https://doi.org/10.1007/978-3-030-73303-2_14

increased hospitalizations [17, 18] and reduced quality of life [10, 19–21]. Studies have also shown the effects of depression and anxiety on patients' ability to work [15, 22] and on increased rates of unemployment [23, 24]. As a result, it is important that anxiety and depression are promptly identified. This will highlight the need for adequate resources to manage these important comorbidities, and in turn, appropriate management may help address and improve both clinical and socioeconomic outcomes.

## Common Instruments for Assessing Anxiety and Depression in SLE

The diagnosis of anxiety and depression can often be delayed or missed in ambulatory settings. Current methods for identifying these psychiatric syndromes often require trained personnel to administer interviews, such as the Mini-International Neuropsychiatric Interview (MINI), that can be lengthy and prohibitively costly [8]. As a result, screening tools that are efficient and accurate are needed to provide early identification and management of SLE patients who may require further psychiatric assessment.

Currently, the most frequently used screening measures for anxiety and depression in patients with SLE include the Beck Depression/Anxiety Inventory (BDI/BAI) [25], the Center for Epidemiologic Studies Depression Scale (CES-D) [26], and the Hospital Anxiety and Depression Scale (HADS) [27]. These standardized instruments have been recommended by the American College of Rheumatology (ACR) as auxiliary tools for the identification of depression and anxiety in SLE patients [28] and will be described in this textbook chapter. More recent instruments, including the Patient-Reported Outcomes Measurement Information System (PROMIS) [29], the Patient Health Questionnaire-9 (PHQ-9) [30], and the Generalized Anxiety Disorder-7 (GAD-7) questionnaires, will also be briefly reviewed.

### *Beck Depression/Anxiety Inventory (BDI/BAI)*

The BDI and the BAI are self-reporting questionnaires containing 21 items that measure the severity of depression and anxiety symptoms over the past week, with an emphasis on somatic symptoms [31]. Items are scored from 0 to 3, with higher scores indicating higher levels of depression or anxiety. Patients with BDI scores >13 are considered depressed, and they are graded mild (14–19), moderate (20–28), and severe (>28). For BAI, anxiety is graded minimal (0–7), mild (8–15), moderate (16–25), and severe (>26).

The BDI and BAI have shown robust psychometric properties in studies of patients with different rheumatic diseases [32–34], though further studies are required for their validation in SLE. A recent systematic review reported the use of BDI in 14 SLE studies and BAI in only 3 SLE studies [25]. Further, this meta-analysis showed a pooled prevalence for depression and anxiety of 39.9% (95% CI: 31.1–49.1%) and 38.4% (95% CI: 34.2–42.8%) in SLE, respectively [25]. However, despite showing acceptable validity and reliability, there have been suggestions of BDI overestimating depression diagnoses in SLE, in part due to the inclusion of somatic symptoms like fatigue, which could be due to SLE rather than depression [35]. Similarly, criticisms of the BAI include its focus on the somatic aspects of anxiety – loss of appetite, sleep disturbance, nervousness, dizziness, inability to relax, etc. – which may result in the overrating of anxiety in medical or geriatric populations [36]. Further studies need to be done to validate the BAI against a non-somatic scale, such as the HADS-A, especially in rheumatologic populations.

## *Center for Epidemiologic Studies Depression Scale (CES-D)*

The CES-D is a self-reporting instruments consisting of 20 items and evaluates symptoms important in depression, including depressed mood, psychomotor retardation, loss of appetite, sleep disturbance, and feelings of helplessness, hopelessness, guilt, and worthlessness [26]. The items are scored from 0 to 3, and the total score (ranging from 0 to 60) is obtained through the sum of the 20 items; patients scoring higher than 15 are considered to be depressed [37, 38]. Compared to the BDI, items in the CES-D place less of an emphasis on somatic symptoms and primarily assess cognitive and affective (emotional) symptoms.

A meta-analysis in SLE showed the use of CES-D in 3 studies, totalling 1856 SLE patients, and demonstrated a pooled prevalence for depression of 41.5% [25]. CES-D has been studied in other rheumatic populations and has demonstrated adequate validity and reliability, especially when compared with the diagnostic Mini-International Neuropsychiatric Interview (MINI) [8]. In this study, CES-D demonstrated a sensitivity and specificity of 87% in detecting any mood disorder and correctly classified 92% of the patients diagnosed with mood disorders by the MINI [8].

## *Hospital Anxiety and Depression Scale (HADS)*

The HADS questionnaire was created to assess for depression and anxiety in hospitalized patients, though studies have also demonstrated adequate performance in ambulatory settings [39–41]. HADS consists of an anxiety (HADS-A) and depression (HADS-D) subscale, each containing seven items that are scored from 0 to 3. The items are totalled, and a score greater than 8 for either subscale classifies the patient as positive for anxiety or depression [27]. When compared with the BAI/BDI, HADS focusses predominantly on cognitive and emotional symptoms and minimizes the effects of concurrent medical illnesses by omitting items related to the somatic aspects of anxiety and depression [27].

The HADS instrument has been studied across a number of rheumatologic conditions, including Sjögren's syndrome [42], ankylosing spondylitis [43], and other forms of arthritis [44–46]. In a systematic review, HADS-D was shown to be utilized in 14 studies totalling 1238 SLE patients and HADS-A used in 12 studies totalling 1099 SLE patients. The pooled prevalences found in this study for depression and anxiety were 24.4% and 38.3%, respectively [25]. This difference in prevalence, when compared with that obtained using the BDI and CES-D, has been attributed to the different sensitivities and specificities of each tool and can also be attributed to the omission of somatic symptoms that are included in both BDI and CES-D [47].

While HADS has shown to be a reliable and valid measure for screening of anxiety and depression across different rheumatic diseases, further research needs to be performed in SLE to assess its accuracy when compared to gold standard assessment tools such as the MINI or *Diagnostic and Statistical Manual of Mental Disorders* (DSM) [48].

## *Other Screening Tools*

More recent instruments have been developed since the publication of the ACR recommended screening tools [28]. Of note, the Patient Health Questionnaire-9 (PHQ-9) [30], the Generalized Anxiety Disorder-7 (GAD-7) [49], and the Patient-Reported Outcomes Measurement Information System (PROMIS) [29] have all gained increasing attention due to their robust psychometric performances.

The anxiety and depression scales in PROMIS have demonstrated validity in general and clinical samples in the USA [29, 50, 51] and when compared with legacy measures, such as the CES-D and BDI [18, 50, 52, 53]. Similar results have been shown for PROMIS in patients across different rheumatic disease, including osteoarthritis, scleroderma, and rheumatoid arthritis [54–61], though limited studies have been performed to examine its use in SLE. Some of these studies in SLE have demonstrated good reliability [59] and responsiveness [62, 63], though further studies will have to be performed to validate its use in larger sample sizes in SLE in order to determine disease-specific cutoffs. Similarly, while there have been studies that use the PHQ-9 and GAD-7 as screening tools for depression [64, 65] and anxiety [66], their use in SLE still requires further attention. With the early promise shown by these newer instruments for screening of anxiety and depression, additional studies evaluating their use in larger sample sizes will provide further basis for their use in both clinical and research settings.

## Factors Associated with Depression and Anxiety in SLE

There have been a number of factors that have been linked with increased prevalence of depression and anxiety in patients with SLE. These can be subdivided into SLE-related factors, such as disease activity [9, 67, 68], pain [69, 70], fatigue [69, 71, 72], presence of particular antibodies [73–75], and medication use [76–78], and patient-related factors including age [68, 79], gender [21, 47, 68], ethnicity [79], and socioeconomic status [21, 80, 81].

### *SLE-Related Factors Associated with Depression*

The link between SLE disease activity and depression is one that has garnered much research attention, although the results have been inconsistent. While some studies have demonstrated higher SLE disease activity to be linked with increased risk of depression, others have reported no association between SLE disease activity and the occurrence of depressive symptoms [47, 79, 82]. The discordance in results are thought to be due to methodological limitations related to difficulties controlling for different relevant factors, e.g., cognitive dysfunction, different socioeconomic statuses, etc. [83, 84].

Furthermore, symptoms of fatigue and pain, including arthralgias, myalgias, and headache, in patients with SLE have also been shown to result in higher incidences of depression [69, 70]. Fatigue has been reported by SLE patients to be one of the most debilitating symptoms [85, 86] and has been linked with an increased risk for developing depression [69, 71, 72]. Additionally, symptoms of cognitive dysfunction in SLE are also associated with depressive symptoms – with a recent study demonstrating 60% of patients with cognitive dysfunction showing higher prevalence of depression when compared with matched controls [87]. This was also demonstrated in a recent study by Touma et al. that showed the association between cognitive impairment and depression status [88]. While fatigue and cognitive dysfunction can be symptoms of depression, they have also been shown to confer risk for depression on their own [69, 71, 72].

Treatment of SLE, especially with glucocorticoids, has been linked with neuropsychiatric manifestations of SLE. Higher doses of glucocorticoids and their chronic use have been shown to cause mood symptoms including depression [76, 89]. One proposed mechanism of glucocorticoid-related mood disturbance is via changes to brain structures related to mood and cognition, such as hippocampal atrophy [76–78, 90]. Moreover, glucocorticoids can also impact sleep and cognition and cause psychosis, as well as negatively influence body image and self-esteem, through its effects on weight gain, striae, skin atrophy, and capillary changes, which have also been associated with increased risk of depression [76–79, 91–93]. For example, in a recent paper by Eldeiry et al., they showed that younger patients with cutaneous manifestations were more likely to have depression [93], when compared to other manifestations of SLE (e.g., serositis, proteinuria, etc.) – a finding that has also been demonstrated by other studies [79].

A fairly robust literature exists linking inflammation (measured via inflammatory cytokines) to depression [94]. In patients with depression, cytokine levels have been found to be significantly elevated when compared with healthy controls [95, 96]. Further, in autoimmune diseases such as SLE, elevation in inflammatory cytokines (e.g., interleukin-6, interleukin-12, interleukin-23, etc.) has been shown to be associated with higher rates of depression [97, 98]. While the exact mechanism linking inflammation to depressive symptoms is not clear, there are a number of proposed immunologic and neurobiologic mechanisms [99] – one of which includes the effects of inflammatory damage on white matter microstructure that may impact circuits involved with mood and cognition [100]. Further investigations are required to understand this pathophysiology in order to develop therapeutic targets to prevent or reverse cytokine-induced depression [99].

Finally, autoantibodies – particularly anti-P ribosomal antibodies – have been studied for their role in the pathogenesis of depression in SLE. In studies of lupus patients, serum levels of autoantibodies have shown to correlate with severity of depressive and psychotic symptoms while showing no correlation with other manifestations of SLE [74, 101]. Further studies are required to validate these findings, as results from other reports have been inconsistent [5, 101, 102]. Other antibodies that have been studied include antineuronal and aPL, though the results of their association with depression are still inconclusive [84].

## *Patient-Related Factors Associated with Depression*

Patient-related factors, such as age, gender, ethnicity, and socioeconomic status, have also been linked with depression in SLE. Studies have shown that patients of a younger age experience higher rates of depression [68, 79, 103], with one study of pediatric inpatients with SLE showing higher rates of major depressive disorder when compared with matched controls [104]. Authors speculate that this may be a result of chronic distress on patients with early-onset SLE and the negative effects of disability and chronic illness on patients at this developmental stage [103]. In studies of gender, more severe depressive symptoms were found in female patients when compared to their male counterparts [47]. Additional studies have replicated this finding, demonstrating female gender independently associating with depression in SLE [21, 68].

Studies have also been performed to investigate the impact of ethnicity on rates of depression. In a study of SLE patients, East Asians demonstrated lower prevalence of depression when compared to other ethnicities [79]. This finding was also demonstrated in rheumatoid arthritis, where Asians had lower depressive scores when compared to patients of Latin, Caucasian, or African-American descent [105]. This has been consistent in studies of the general population, where East Asians have exhibited lower rates of depression [106, 107], and has been purported to be due to the cultural factors that may be barriers to acknowledging mood disorders [79].

Another patient-related factor associated with depression involves socioeconomic status (SES). This umbrella term includes employment status, education level, and income level, each having shown to be linked with depression [108–110]. In a study of patients with rheumatic diseases, including SLE, different levels of education were associated with increased risk of depression [81]. Further, unemployment has been shown to increase rates of depression in patients with SLE [103, 111], in patients with other rheumatic conditions [81], as well as in the general population [112]. More recent studies have shown that this effect may be more pronounced in female patients, compared with male patients [47], with factors of lower income and financial strain being additional risk factors for depression [21, 80, 113]. It is thought that risk factors associated with lower SES groups, such as increased stress exposure, weaker social supports, and poorer coping mechanisms, may all contribute to causing increased prevalence of depression [114].

Finally, obesity and physical activity have also been studied for their roles in depression. Obesity has been shown to be associated with depression in studies of the general population [115, 116], as well as in SLE [9, 117–119]. In one study by Katz et al., 716 SLE patients were studied, and higher levels of depression were found in obese women [118]. In contrast, physical activity has been shown to reduce depression across rheumatologic conditions through its effects on pain relief [120, 121], improvement of functional status [122–124], and alleviating fatigue [125–127].

## *Factors Associated with Anxiety*

Compared with depression, there have been much fewer studies focussed on anxiety in SLE and their associated factors. There are reports of links between anxiety and disease-related factors, such as disease activity [128, 129] and medication use [22, 129]. For example, studies have shown increased SLE disease activity to be predictive of severe anxiety, even after adjusting for depressive symptoms [128, 129], although these findings have not been replicated in other reports [5, 22, 130, 131]. Patient-related factors, including ethnicity [132, 133], age [132, 133], gender [131, 132], and SES [131, 133], have also been studied for their association with anxiety, with inconclusive results. Studies of gender have demonstrated lower rates of anxiety in males when compared to females, particularly in settings of unemployment, with SES showing no association with anxiety in either gender [131]. Factors such as social stress and lack of social supports have also been linked with anxiety [134]. Additional studies should be performed in SLE to understand patient- and disease-related factors that are associated with anxiety and to clarify the associations of factors that have shown conflict results as well as to investigate those that have not been studied in detail, including factors related to obesity and physical anxiety.

## Future Directions of Anxiety and Depression Screening in SLE

Anxiety and depression are significant and prevalent psychiatric manifestations affecting patients with SLE. Early screening of these symptoms may help significantly reduce the clinical impacts on this patient population. As current diagnostic tests are resource-intensive, patient-reported outcome questionnaires can be effective alternatives. ACR-recommended instruments, such as the BAI/BDI, CES-D, and HADS, are established tools that have shown robust reliability and validity in SLE patients, while newer tools such as PROMIS, PHQ-9, and GAD-7 also show promise. Further psychometric studies on these newer tools are required before they can be incorporated routinely into clinical and research settings. Similarly, additional studies should be performed in all of the aforementioned tools, specifically in SLE, to determine ideal disease-specific cutoffs specific for diagnosing depression and anxiety in this patient population. To the best of our knowledge, only two studies have been performed to compare CES-D against a gold standard diagnostic tool to derive SLE-specific thresholds for classifying depression [32, 135]. Given the plethora of available tools, it may also be advisable to develop a consensus to identify the most appropriate tool(s) to allow greater comparisons across different SLE populations, outcomes, and interventions.

As discussed in this chapter, a number of disease- and patient-related factors have been associated with depression and anxiety in SLE. While the underlying mechanisms by which they cause these psychiatric disturbances are still unclear, the results suggest that patients possessing these risk factors (e.g., female, younger age, unemployed, increased glucocorticoid use, etc.) may be targeted for screening to more readily identify depression and anxiety at an earlier stage. Moreover, patients exhibiting particular factors or clinical phenotypes of SLE may be more vulnerable to develop depression and anxiety, with cutaneous manifestations more likely to be linked with depression and anxiety, when compared to other less easily visible manifestations of SLE [79, 93]. Therefore, additional studies may also be performed to assess whether addressing these SLE-related factors decreases the severity and risk of depression and anxiety in these patients.

Further research strategies into depression and anxiety in SLE that may be of benefit, in addition to addressing limitations of previous studies, include performing longitudinal studies with larger sample sizes and assessing the effect of SLE state on depression and anxiety (e.g., determining whether depression improves with resolution of an SLE flare or discontinuation of glucocorticoids). Ultimately, randomized trials are required addressing whether screening for depression and anxiety in SLE and providing evidence-based diagnosis and intervention to those who screen positive are beneficial. Such data will allow us to move toward comprehensive and integrated mental health care for this complex patient population.

## References

1. Nikpour M, Bridge JA, Richter S. A systematic review of prevalence, disease characteristics and management of systemic lupus erythematosus in Australia: identifying areas of unmet need. Intern Med J. 2014;44(12a):1170–9.
2. Marian G, Nica EA, Ionescu BE, Carlogea DG. Depression as an initial feature of systemic lupus erythematosus? A case report. J Med Life. 2010;3(2):183–5.
3. Ainiala H, Loukkola J, Peltola J, Korpela M, Hietaharju A. The prevalence of neuropsychiatric syndromes in systemic lupus erythematosus. Neurology. 2001;57(3):496–500.
4. Afeltra A, Garzia P, Mitterhofer AP, Vadacca M, Galluzzo S, Del Porto F, et al. Neuropsychiatric lupus syndromes: relationship with antiphospholipid antibodies. Neurology. 2003;61(1):108–10.
5. Nery FG, Borba EF, Viana VS, Hatch JP, Soares JC, Bonfa E, et al. Prevalence of depressive and anxiety disorders in systemic lupus erythematosus and their association with anti-ribosomal P antibodies. Prog Neuro-Psychopharmacol Biol Psychiatry. 2008;32(3):695–700.
6. Brey RL, Holliday SL, Saklad AR, Navarrete MG, Hermosillo-Romo D, Stallworth CL, et al. Neuropsychiatric syndromes in lupus: prevalence using standardized definitions. Neurology. 2002;58(8):1214–20.
7. Matcham F, Rayner L, Steer S, Hotopf M. The prevalence of depression in rheumatoid arthritis: a systematic review and meta-analysis. Rheumatology (Oxford, England). 2013;52(12):2136–48.
8. Julian LJ, Gregorich SE, Tonner C, Yazdany J, Trupin L, Criswell LA, et al. Using the Center for Epidemiologic Studies Depression Scale to screen for depression in systemic lupus erythematosus. Arthritis Care Res. 2011;63(6):884–90.
9. Julian LJ, Tonner C, Yelin E, Yazdany J, Trupin L, Criswell LA, et al. Cardiovascular and disease related predictors of depression in SLE. Arthritis Care Res. 2011;63(4):542–9.
10. Julian LJ, Yelin E, Yazdany J, Panopalis P, Trupin L, Criswell LA, et al. Depression, medication adherence, and service utilization in systemic lupus erythematosus. Arthritis Rheum. 2009;61(2):240–6.
11. Greco CM, Li T, Sattar A, Kao AH, Danchenko N, Edmundowicz D, et al. Association between depression and vascular disease in systemic lupus erythematosus. J Rheumatol. 2012;39(2):262–8.
12. Lisitsyna TA, Vel'tishchev D, Seravina OF, Kovalevskaia OB, Marchenko AS, Novikova DS, et al. Prevalence of mental disorders in SLE patients: correlations with the disease activity and comorbid chronic conditions. Terapevticheskii arkhiv. 2009;81(6):10–6.
13. Xie LF, Chen PL, Pan HF, Tao JH, Li XP, Zhang YJ, et al. Prevalence and correlates of suicidal ideation in SLE inpatients: Chinese experience. Rheumatol Int. 2012;32(9):2707–14.
14. Zakeri Z, Shakiba M, Narouie B, Mladkova N, Ghasemi-Rad M, Khosravi A. Prevalence of depression and depressive symptoms in patients with systemic lupus erythematosus: Iranian experience. Rheumatol Int. 2012;32(5):1179–87.
15. Jonsen A, Bengtsson AA, Nived O, Ryberg B, Sturfelt G. Outcome of neuropsychiatric systemic lupus erythematosus within a defined Swedish population: increased morbidity but low mortality. Rheumatology (Oxford, England). 2002;41(11):1308–12.
16. Ward MM, Lotstein DS, Bush TM, Lambert RE, van Vollenhoven R, Neuwelt CM. Psychosocial correlates of morbidity in women with systemic lupus erythematosus. J Rheumatol. 1999;26(10):2153–8.
17. Rojas-Serrano J, Cardiel MH. Lupus patients in an emergency unit. Causes of consultation, hospitalization and outcome. A cohort study. Lupus. 2000;9(8):601–6.
18. Roy-Byrne PP, Stein MB, Russo J, Mercier E, Thomas R, McQuaid J, et al. Panic disorder in the primary care setting: comorbidity, disability, service utilization, and treatment. J Clin Psychiatry. 1999;60(7):492–9; quiz 500.

19. Pettersson S, Lovgren M, Eriksson LE, Moberg C, Svenungsson E, Gunnarsson I, et al. An exploration of patient-reported symptoms in systemic lupus erythematosus and the relationship to health-related quality of life. Scand J Rheumatol. 2012;41(5):383–90.
20. Mak A, Tang C, Ho R. Serum tumour necrosis factor-alpha is associated with poor health-related quality of life and depressive symptoms in patients with systemic lupus erythematosus. Lupus. 2013;22(3):254–61.
21. Shen B, Feng G, Tang W, Huang X, Yan H, He Y, et al. The quality of life in Chinese patients with systemic lupus erythematosus is associated with disease activity and psychiatric disorders: a path analysis. Clin Exp Rheumatol. 2014;32(1):101–7.
22. Hawro T, Krupinska-Kun M, Rabe-Jablonska J, Sysa-Jedrzejowska A, Robak E, Bogaczewicz J, et al. Psychiatric disorders in patients with systemic lupus erythematosus: association of anxiety disorder with shorter disease duration. Rheumatol Int. 2011;31(10):1387–91.
23. Appenzeller S, Cendes F, Costallat LT. Cognitive impairment and employment status in systemic lupus erythematosus: a prospective longitudinal study. Arthritis Rheum. 2009;61(5):680–7.
24. Panopalis P, Julian L, Yazdany J, Gillis JZ, Trupin L, Hersh A, et al. Impact of memory impairment on employment status in persons with systemic lupus erythematosus. Arthritis Rheum. 2007;57(8):1453–60.
25. Moustafa AH, M.; Eder, L.; Wither, J.E.; Fung, W.; Lambiris, P.; Touma, Z. Prevalence and metric of depression and anxiety in lupus: a systematic review and meta-analysis [abstract]. Arthritis Rheumatol. 2016;68
26. Radloff LS. The CES-D scale. Appl Psychol Meas. 1977;1(3):385–401.
27. Zigmond AS, Snaith RP. The hospital anxiety and depression scale. Acta Psychiatr Scand. 1983;67(6):361–70.
28. The American College of Rheumatology nomenclature and case definitions for neuropsychiatric lupus syndromes. Arthritis Rheum. 1999;42(4):599–608.
29. Cella D, Riley W, Stone A, Rothrock N, Reeve B, Yount S, et al. The Patient-Reported Outcomes Measurement Information System (PROMIS) developed and tested its first wave of adult self-reported health outcome item banks: 2005–2008. J Clin Epidemiol. 2010;63(11):1179–94.
30. Kroenke K, Spitzer RL, Williams JB. The PHQ-9: validity of a brief depression severity measure. J Gen Intern Med. 2001;16(9):606–13.
31. Beck AT, Epstein N, Brown G, Steer RA. An inventory for measuring clinical anxiety: psychometric properties. J Consult Clin Psychol. 1988;56(6):893–7.
32. Julian LJ. Measures of anxiety: State-Trait Anxiety Inventory (STAI), Beck Anxiety Inventory (BAI), and Hospital Anxiety and Depression Scale-Anxiety (HADS-A). Arthritis Care Res. 2011;63 Suppl 11:S467–72.
33. Arnold LM, Clauw D, Wang F, Ahl J, Gaynor PJ, Wohlreich MM. Flexible dosed duloxetine in the treatment of fibromyalgia: a randomized, double-blind, placebo-controlled trial. J Rheumatol. 2010;37(12):2578–86.
34. Scopaz KA, Piva SR, Wisniewski S, Fitzgerald GK. Relationships of fear, anxiety, and depression with physical function in patients with knee osteoarthritis. Arch Phys Med Rehabil. 2009;90(11):1866–73.
35. Iverson GL. Screening for depression in systemic lupus erythematosus with the British Columbia Major Depression Inventory. Psychol Rep. 2002;90(3 Pt 2):1091–6.
36. Fydrich T, Dowdall D, Chambless DL. Reliability and validity of the beck anxiety inventory. J Anxiety Disord. 1992;6(1):55–61.
37. Frerichs RR, Aneshensel CS, Clark VA. Prevalence of depression in Los Angeles County. Am J Epidemiol. 1981;113(6):691–9.
38. Harlow BL, Cohen LS, Otto MW, Spiegelman D, Cramer DW. Prevalence and predictors of depressive symptoms in older premenopausal women: the Harvard Study of Moods and Cycles. Arch Gen Psychiatry. 1999;56(5):418–24.

39. Hammerlid E, Ahlner-Elmqvist M, Bjordal K, Biorklund A, Evensen J, Boysen M, et al. A prospective multicentre study in Sweden and Norway of mental distress and psychiatric morbidity in head and neck cancer patients. Br J Cancer. 1999;80(5–6):766–74.
40. Kugaya A, Akechi T, Okuyama T, Nakano T, Mikami I, Okamura H, et al. Prevalence, predictive factors, and screening for psychologic distress in patients with newly diagnosed head and neck cancer. Cancer. 2000;88(12):2817–23.
41. Johnston M, Pollard B, Hennessey P. Construct validation of the hospital anxiety and depression scale with clinical populations. J Psychosom Res. 2000;48(6):579–84.
42. Valtysdottir ST, Gudbjornsson B, Lindqvist U, Hallgren R, Hetta J. Anxiety and depression in patients with primary Sjogren's syndrome. J Rheumatol. 2000;27(1):165–9.
43. Ertenli I, Ozer S, Kiraz S, Apras SB, Akdogan A, Karadag O, et al. Infliximab, a TNF-alpha antagonist treatment in patients with ankylosing spondylitis: the impact on depression, anxiety and quality of life level. Rheumatol Int. 2012;32(2):323–30.
44. Buszewicz M, Rait G, Griffin M, Nazareth I, Patel A, Atkinson A, et al. Self management of arthritis in primary care: randomised controlled trial. BMJ (Clin Res ed). 2006;333(7574):879.
45. Cauli A, Gladman DD, Mathieu A, Olivieri I, Porru G, Tak PP, et al. Patient global assessment in psoriatic arthritis: a multicenter GRAPPA and OMERACT study. J Rheumatol. 2011;38(5):898–903.
46. Murphy H, Dickens C, Creed F, Bernstein R. Depression, illness perception and coping in rheumatoid arthritis. J Psychosom Res. 1999;46(2):155–64.
47. Macêdo EAA, S.; Costallat, L. T. L. Depression in systemic lupus erythematosus: gender differences in the performance of the Beck Depression Inventory (BDI), Center for Epidemiologic Studies Depression Scale (CES-D), and Hospital Anxiety and Depression Scale (HADS). Lupus. 2018;27(2):179–89.
48. Diagnostic and statistical manual of mental disorders: DSM-5 (5th ed.). Arlington, VA: American Psychiatric Association, [2013]; 2013.
49. Spitzer RL, Kroenke K, Williams JB, Lowe B. A brief measure for assessing generalized anxiety disorder: the GAD-7. Arch Intern Med. 2006;166(10):1092–7.
50. Pilkonis PA, Choi SW, Reise SP, Stover AM, Riley WT, Cella D. Item banks for measuring emotional distress from the Patient-Reported Outcomes Measurement Information System (PROMIS(R)): depression, anxiety, and anger. Assessment. 2011;18(3):263–83.
51. Schalet BD, Pilkonis PA, Yu L, Dodds N, Johnston KL, Yount S, et al. Clinical validity of PROMIS Depression, Anxiety, and Anger across diverse clinical samples. J Clin Epidemiol. 2016;73:119–27.
52. Schalet BD, Cook KF, Choi SW, Cella D. Establishing a common metric for self-reported anxiety: linking the MASQ, PANAS, and GAD-7 to PROMIS Anxiety. J Anxiety Disord. 2014;28(1):88–96.
53. Choi SW, Schalet B, Cook KF, Cella D. Establishing a common metric for depressive symptoms: linking the BDI-II, CES-D, and PHQ-9 to PROMIS depression. Psychol Assess. 2014;26(2):513–27.
54. Fries JF, Cella D, Rose M, Krishnan E, Bruce B. Progress in assessing physical function in arthritis: PROMIS short forms and computerized adaptive testing. J Rheumatol. 2009;36(9):2061–6.
55. Khanna D, Maranian P, Rothrock N, Cella D, Gershon R, Khanna PP, et al. Feasibility and construct validity of PROMIS and "legacy" instruments in an academic scleroderma clinic. Value Health. 2012;15(1):128–34.
56. Jones JT, Carle AC, Wootton J, Liberio B, Lee J, Schanberg LE, et al. Validation of patient-reported outcomes measurement information system short forms for use in childhood-onset systemic lupus erythematosus. Arthritis Care Res. 2017;69(1):133–42.
57. Broderick JE, Schneider S, Junghaenel DU, Schwartz JE, Stone AA. Validity and reliability of patient-reported outcomes measurement information system instruments in osteoarthritis. Arthritis Care Res. 2013;65(10):1625–33.

58. Fung WMM, Engel L, Su J, Bonilla D, Akhavan P, Katz P, Beaton D, Touma Z. Sensitivity to Change of the Patient Reported Outcomes Measurement Information System (PROMIS) Computerized Adaptive Test (CAT) Measures in a Single Canadian Lupus Cohort [abstract]. Arthritis Rheumatol. 2019;71(suppl 10)
59. Donner A, Koval JJ. The estimation of intraclass correlation in the analysis of family data. Biometrics. 1980;36(1):19–25.
60. Hitchon CA, Zhang L, Peschken CA, Lix LM, Graff LA, Fisk JD, et al. The validity and reliability of screening measures for depression and anxiety disorders in rheumatoid arthritis. Arthritis Care Res. 2020;72(8):1130–9.
61. Bartlett SJ, Orbai A-M, Duncan T, DeLeon E, Ruffing V, Clegg-Smith K, et al. Reliability and validity of selected PROMIS measures in people with rheumatoid arthritis. PLoS ONE. 2015;10(9):e0138543-e.
62. Haringsma R, Engels GI, Beekman AT, Spinhoven P. The criterion validity of the Center for Epidemiological Studies Depression Scale (CES-D) in a sample of self-referred elders with depressive symptomatology. Int J Geriatr Psychiatry. 2004;19(6):558–63.
63. Katz P, Pedro S, Alemao E, Yazdany J, Dall'Era M, Trupin L, et al. Estimates of responsiveness, minimally important differences, and patient acceptable symptom state in five patient-reported outcomes measurement information system short forms in systemic lupus erythematosus. ACR Open Rheumatol. 2020;2(1):53–60.
64. Mitchell AJ, Yadegarfar M, Gill J, Stubbs B. Case finding and screening clinical utility of the Patient Health Questionnaire (PHQ-9 and PHQ-2) for depression in primary care: a diagnostic meta-analysis of 40 studies. BJPsych Open. 2016;2(2):127–38.
65. Manea L, Gilbody S, McMillan D. A diagnostic meta-analysis of the Patient Health Questionnaire-9 (PHQ-9) algorithm scoring method as a screen for depression. Gen Hosp Psychiatry. 2015;37(1):67–75.
66. Plummer F, Manea L, Trepel D, McMillan D. Screening for anxiety disorders with the GAD-7 and GAD-2: a systematic review and diagnostic metaanalysis. Gen Hosp Psychiatry. 2016;39:24–31.
67. Nery FG, Borba EF, Hatch JP, Soares JC, Bonfa E, Neto FL. Major depressive disorder and disease activity in systemic lupus erythematosus. Compr Psychiatry. 2007;48(1):14–9.
68. Bachen EA, Chesney MA, Criswell LA. Prevalence of mood and anxiety disorders in women with systemic lupus erythematosus. Arthritis Rheum. 2009;61(6):822–9.
69. Waldheim E, Elkan AC, Pettersson S, van Vollenhoven R, Bergman S, Frostegard J, et al. Health-related quality of life, fatigue and mood in patients with SLE and high levels of pain compared to controls and patients with low levels of pain. Lupus. 2013;22(11):1118–27.
70. Doria A, Rinaldi S, Ermani M, Salaffi F, Iaccarino L, Ghirardello A, et al. Health-related quality of life in Italian patients with systemic lupus erythematosus. II. Role of clinical, immunological and psychological determinants. Rheumatology (Oxford, England). 2004;43(12):1580–6.
71. Jump RL, Robinson ME, Armstrong AE, Barnes EV, Kilbourn KM, Richards HB. Fatigue in systemic lupus erythematosus: contributions of disease activity, pain, depression, and perceived social support. J Rheumatol. 2005;32(9):1699–705.
72. Van Exel E, Jacobs J, Korswagen LA, Voskuyl AE, Stek M, Dekker J, et al. Depression in systemic lupus erythematosus, dependent on or independent of severity of disease. Lupus. 2013;22(14):1462–9.
73. West SG, Emlen W, Wener MH, Kotzin BL. Neuropsychiatric lupus erythematosus: a 10-year prospective study on the value of diagnostic tests. Am J Med. 1995;99(2):153–63.
74. Schneebaum AB, Singleton JD, West SG, Blodgett JK, Allen LG, Cheronis JC, et al. Association of psychiatric manifestations with antibodies to ribosomal P proteins in systemic lupus erythematosus. Am J Med. 1991;90(1):54–62.
75. Jarpa E, Babul M, Calderon J, Gonzalez M, Martinez ME, Bravo-Zehnder M, et al. Common mental disorders and psychological distress in systemic lupus erythematosus are not associated with disease activity. Lupus. 2011;20(1):58–66.

76. Warrington TP, Bostwick JM. Psychiatric adverse effects of corticosteroids. Mayo Clin Proc. 2006;81(10):1361–7.
77. Mosca M, Tani C, Carli L, Bombardieri S. Glucocorticoids in systemic lupus erythematosus. Clin Exp Rheumatol. 2011;29(5 Suppl 68):S126–9.
78. Ruiz-Irastorza G, Danza A, Khamashta M. Glucocorticoid use and abuse in SLE. Rheumatology (Oxford, England). 2012;51(7):1145–53.
79. Huang X, Magder LS, Petri M. Predictors of incident depression in systemic lupus erythematosus. J Rheumatol. 2014;41(9):1823–33.
80. Trupin L, Tonner MC, Yazdany J, Julian LJ, Criswell LA, Katz PP, et al. The role of neighborhood and individual socioeconomic status in outcomes of systemic lupus erythematosus. J Rheumatol. 2008;35(9):1782–8.
81. Waheed A, Hameed K, Khan AM, Syed JA, Mirza AI. The burden of anxiety and depression among patients with chronic rheumatologic disorders at a tertiary care hospital clinic in Karachi, Pakistan. JPMA J Pak Med Assoc. 2006;56(5):243–7.
82. Hanly JG, Su L, Urowitz MB, Romero-Diaz J, Gordon C, Bae SC, et al. Mood disorders in systemic lupus erythematosus: results from an International Inception Cohort Study. Arthritis Rheumatol. 2015;67(7):1837–47.
83. Moustafa AT, Moazzami M, Engel L, Bangert E, Hassanein M, Marzouk S, et al. Prevalence and metric of depression and anxiety in systemic lupus erythematosus: a systematic review and meta-analysis. Semin Arthritis Rheum. 2020;50(1):84–94.
84. Palagini L, Mosca M, Tani C, Gemignani A, Mauri M, Bombardieri S. Depression and systemic lupus erythematosus: a systematic review. Lupus. 2013;22(5):409–16.
85. Krupp LB, LaRocca NG, Muir-Nash J, Steinberg AD. The fatigue severity scale. Application to patients with multiple sclerosis and systemic lupus erythematosus. Arch Neurol. 1989;46(10):1121–3.
86. Burgos PI, Alarcón GS, McGwin G, Crews KQ, Reveille JD, Vilá LM. Disease activity and damage are not associated with increased levels of fatigue in systemic lupus erythematosus patients from LUMINA LXVII, a Multiethnic Cohort. Arthritis Rheum. 2009;61(9):1179–86.
87. Nantes SG, Su J, Dhaliwal A, Colosimo K, Touma Z. Performance of screening tests for cognitive impairment in systemic lupus erythematosus. J Rheumatol. 2017;44(11):1583–9.
88. Touma Z, Moghaddam B, Su J, Katz P. Cognitive function trajectories are associated with the depressive symptoms trajectories in systemic lupus erythematosus over time. Arthritis Care Res. 2020;
89. Lewis DA, Smith RE. Steroid-induced psychiatric syndromes. A report of 14 cases and a review of the literature. J Affect Disord. 1983;5(4):319–32.
90. Brown ES, Woolston DJ, Frol A, Bobadilla L, Khan DA, Hanczyc M, et al. Hippocampal volume, spectroscopy, cognition, and mood in patients receiving corticosteroid therapy. Biol Psychiatry. 2004;55(5):538–45.
91. Jolly M, Pickard AS, Mikolaitis RA, Cornejo J, Sequeira W, Cash TF, et al. Body image in patients with systemic lupus erythematosus. Int J Behav Med. 2012;19(2):157–64.
92. McElhone K, Abbott J, Gray J, Williams A, Teh LS. Patient perspective of systemic lupus erythematosus in relation to health-related quality of life concepts: a qualitative study. Lupus. 2010;19(14):1640–7.
93. Eldeiry D, Zandy M, Tayer-Shifman OE, Kwan A, Marzouk S, Su J, et al. Association between depression and anxiety with skin and musculoskeletal clinical phenotypes in systemic lupus erythematosus. Rheumatology (Oxford, England). 2020;59(11):3211–20.
94. Dowlati Y, Herrmann N, Swardfager W, Liu H, Sham L, Reim EK, et al. A meta-analysis of cytokines in major depression. Biol Psychiatry. 2010;67(5):446–57.
95. Yirmiya R, Pollak Y, Morag M, Reichenberg A, Barak O, Avitsur R, et al. Illness, cytokines, and depression. Ann N Y Acad Sci. 2000;917:478–87.
96. Yirmiya R, Weidenfeld J, Pollak Y, Morag M, Morag A, Avitsur R, et al. Cytokines, "depression due to a general medical condition," and antidepressant drugs. Adv Exp Med Biol. 1999;461:283–316.

97. Fonseca R, Bernardes M, Terroso G, de Sousa M, Figueiredo-Braga M. Silent burdens in disease: fatigue and depression in SLE. Autoimmune Dis. 2014;2014:790724.
98. Braga J, Campar A. Biological causes of depression in Systemic Lupus Erythematosus. Acta Reumatol Port. 2014;39(3):218–26.
99. Felger JC, Lotrich FE. Inflammatory cytokines in depression: neurobiological mechanisms and therapeutic implications. Neuroscience. 2013;246:199–229.
100. Ramage AE, Fox PT, Brey RL, Narayana S, Cykowski MD, Naqibuddin M, et al. Neuroimaging evidence of white matter inflammation in newly diagnosed systemic lupus erythematosus. Arthritis Rheum. 2011;63(10):3048–57.
101. Nojima Y, Minota S, Yamada A, Takaku F, Aotsuka S, Yokohari R. Correlation of antibodies to ribosomal P protein with psychosis in patients with systemic lupus erythematosus. Ann Rheum Dis. 1992;51(9):1053–5.
102. Gerli R, Caponi L, Tincani A, Scorza R, Sabbadini MG, Danieli MG, et al. Clinical and serological associations of ribosomal P autoantibodies in systemic lupus erythematosus: prospective evaluation in a large cohort of Italian patients. Rheumatology. 2002;41(12):1357–66.
103. Maneeton B, Maneeton N, Louthrenoo W. Prevalence and predictors of depression in patients with systemic lupus erythematosus: a cross-sectional study. Neuropsychiatr Dis Treat. 2013;9:799–804.
104. Sibbitt WL Jr, Brandt JR, Johnson CR, Maldonado ME, Patel SR, Ford CC, et al. The incidence and prevalence of neuropsychiatric syndromes in pediatric onset systemic lupus erythematosus. J Rheumatol. 2002;29(7):1536–42.
105. Margaretten M, Yelin E, Imboden J, Graf J, Barton J, Katz P, et al. Predictors of depression in a multiethnic cohort of patients with rheumatoid arthritis. Arthritis Rheum. 2009;61(11):1586–91.
106. Andrade L, Caraveo-Anduaga JJ, Berglund P, Bijl RV, De Graaf R, Vollebergh W, et al. The epidemiology of major depressive episodes: results from the International Consortium of Psychiatric Epidemiology (ICPE) Surveys. Int J Methods Psychiatr Res. 2003;12(1):3–21.
107. Weissman MM, Bland RC, Canino GJ, Faravelli C, Greenwald S, Hwu HG, et al. Cross-national epidemiology of major depression and bipolar disorder. JAMA. 1996;276(4):293–9.
108. Stansfeld SA, Head J, Marmot MG. Explaining social class differences in depression and well-being. Soc Psychiatry Psychiatr Epidemiol. 1998;33(1):1–9.
109. Mackenbach JP, Kunst AE, Cavelaars AE, Groenhof F, Geurts JJ. Socioeconomic inequalities in morbidity and mortality in western Europe. The EU Working Group on Socioeconomic Inequalities in Health. Lancet (London, England). 1997;349(9066):1655–9.
110. Criswell LA, Katz PP. Relationship of education level to treatment received for rheumatoid arthritis. J Rheumatol. 1994;21(11):2026–33.
111. Lim SS, Agan M, Drenkard CM. Impact of systemic lupus erythematosus organ damage on unemployment or disability from a population-based cohort. Arthritis Res Ther. 2012;14(Suppl 3):A13–A.
112. Andreeva E, Magnusson Hanson LL, Westerlund H, Theorell T, Brenner MH. Depressive symptoms as a cause and effect of job loss in men and women: evidence in the context of organisational downsizing from the Swedish Longitudinal Occupational Survey of Health. BMC Public Health. 2015;15(1):1045.
113. McCormick N, Trupin L, Yelin EH, Katz PP. Socioeconomic predictors of incident depression in systemic lupus erythematosus. Arthritis Care Res. 2018;70(1):104–13.
114. Turner RJ, Lloyd DA. The stress process and the social distribution of depression. J Health Soc Behav. 1999;40(4):374–404.
115. Teychenne M, Ball K, Salmon J. Physical activity, sedentary behavior and depression among disadvantaged women. Health Educ Res. 2010;25(4):632–44.
116. Teychenne M, Ball K, Salmon J. Sedentary behavior and depression among adults: a review. Int J Behav Med. 2010;17(4):246–54.

117. Katz P, Julian L, Tonner MC, Yazdany J, Trupin L, Yelin E, et al. Physical activity, obesity, and cognitive impairment among women with systemic lupus erythematosus. Arthritis Care Res. 2012;64(4):502–10.
118. Katz P, Yazdany J, Julian L, Trupin L, Margaretten M, Yelin E, et al. Impact of obesity on functioning among women with systemic lupus erythematosus. Arthritis Care Res. 2011;63(10):1357–64.
119. Katz P, Rush S, Trupin L, Barton J, Schmaju G, Yazdany J, Tonner C, Margaretten M. Obesity is a risk factor for depression in systemic lupus erythematosus (SLE): American College of Rheumatology; 2014.
120. Baillet A, Zeboulon N, Gossec L, Combescure C, Bodin LA, Juvin R, et al. Efficacy of cardiorespiratory aerobic exercise in rheumatoid arthritis: meta-analysis of randomized controlled trials. Arthritis Care Res. 2010;62(7):984–92.
121. Conn VS, Hafdahl AR, Minor MA, Nielsen PJ. Physical activity interventions among adults with arthritis: meta-analysis of outcomes. Semin Arthritis Rheum. 2008;37(5):307–16.
122. Callahan LF, Mielenz T, Freburger J, Shreffler J, Hootman J, Brady T, et al. A randomized controlled trial of the people with arthritis can exercise program: symptoms, function, physical activity, and psychosocial outcomes. Arthritis Rheum. 2008;59(1):92–101.
123. Herring MP, Puetz TW, O'Connor PJ, Dishman RK. Effect of exercise training on depressive symptoms among patients with a chronic illness: a systematic review and meta-analysis of randomized controlled trials. Arch Intern Med. 2012;172(2):101–11.
124. Lee J, Chang RW, Ehrlich-Jones L, Kwoh CK, Nevitt M, Semanik PA, et al. Sedentary behavior and physical function: objective evidence from the Osteoarthritis Initiative. Arthritis Care Res. 2015;67(3):366–73.
125. Wolfe F, Hawley DJ, Wilson K. The prevalence and meaning of fatigue in rheumatic disease. J Rheumatol. 1996;23(8):1407–17.
126. Sterling K, Gallop K, Swinburn P, Flood E, French A, Al Sawah S, et al. Patient-reported fatigue and its impact on patients with systemic lupus erythematosus. Lupus. 2014;23(2):124–32.
127. Neill J, Belan I, Ried K. Effectiveness of non-pharmacological interventions for fatigue in adults with multiple sclerosis, rheumatoid arthritis, or systemic lupus erythematosus: a systematic review. J Adv Nurs. 2006;56(6):617–35.
128. Tay SH, Cheung PP, Mak A. Active disease is independently associated with more severe anxiety rather than depressive symptoms in patients with systemic lupus erythematosus. Lupus. 2015;24(13):1392–9.
129. Mak A, Tang CS, Chan MF, Cheak AA, Ho RC. Damage accrual, cumulative glucocorticoid dose and depression predict anxiety in patients with systemic lupus erythematosus. Clin Rheumatol. 2011;30(6):795–803.
130. Yilmaz-Oner S, Oner C, Dogukan FM, Moses TF, Demir K, Tekayev N, et al. Anxiety and depression predict quality of life in Turkish patients with systemic lupus erythematosus. Clin Exp Rheumatol. 2015;33(3):360–5.
131. Macedo EA, Appenzeller S, Costallat LT. Gender differences in systemic lupus erythematosus concerning anxiety, depression and quality of life. Lupus. 2016;25(12):1315–27.
132. Torrente-Segarra V, Carbonell-Abello J, Castro-Oreiro S, Manresa Dominguez JM. Association between fibromyalgia and psychiatric disorders in systemic lupus erythematosus. Clin Exp Rheumatol. 2010;28(6 Suppl 63):S22–6.
133. Lim LC, Lee TE, Boey ML. Psychiatric manifestation of systemic lupus erythematosus in Singapore. A cross-cultural comparison. Br J Psychiatry. 1991;159:520–3.
134. Shortall E, Isenberg D, Newman SP. Factors associated with mood and mood disorders in SLE. Lupus. 1995;4(4):272–9.
135. Kwan A, Marzouk S, Ghanean H, Kishwar A, Anderson N, Bonilla D, et al. Assessment of the psychometric properties of patient-reported outcomes of depression and anxiety in systemic lupus erythematosus. Semin Arthritis Rheum. 2019;49(2):260–6.

# Chapter 15
# Fatigue and Pain Measurements in Systemic Lupus Erythematosus

**Prabjit Ajrawat, Vibeke Strand, Mark Matsos, Lee S. Simon, and Zahi Touma**

## Introduction

Systemic lupus erythematosus (SLE) is a chronic, multisystemic, autoimmune rheumatic disease with a complex pathogenesis and diverse clinical manifestations [1]. As a result, SLE can cause substantial physical impairment, psychological disability, and reduced emotional status, which collectively impact patient-reported health-related quality of life (HRQoL) [2–4]. With the increased survival rate and life expectancy of individuals with SLE, and the recommendations made by the Outcome Measures in Rheumatology (OMERACT) group, it is important to measure patient-reported outcomes (PROs) that reflect the impact of disease on HRQoL [2]. Fatigue and pain are two frequently encountered physical health complaints that can substantially compromise HRQoL of individuals with SLE by impacting family and social life, work, emotional well-being, and cognition [1, 5, 6]. Both fatigue and

P. Ajrawat
University of Toronto, Division of Rheumatology, Department of Medicine, Toronto, ON, Canada

V. Strand
Division of Immunology & Rheumatology, Department of Medicine, Stanford University School of Medicine, Palo Alto, CA, USA

M. Matsos
McMaster University, Division of Rheumatology, Department of Medicine, Hamilton, ON, Canada

L. S. Simon
SDG, LLC, Cambridge, MA, USA

Z. Touma (✉)
Centre for Prognosis in Rheumatic Disease, Toronto Lupus Clinic, Division of Rheumatology, Department of Medicine, Institute of Health Policy, Management and Evaluation, University of Toronto, Toronto, ON, Canada
e-mail: Zahi.Touma@uhn.ca



Z. Touma (ed.), *Outcome Measures and Metrics in Systemic Lupus Erythematosus*, https://doi.org/10.1007/978-3-030-73303-2_15

pain have been correlated with declining HRQoL in patients with SLE and are major determinants of morbidity [7–10]. Studies have demonstrated that approximately 53–90% and up to 71–90% of SLE patients present with fatigue and pain as primary complaints during the course of their disease, respectively [5, 11]. Fatigue- and pain-related symptoms occurring in SLE can substantially increase direct, indirect, and intangible healthcare costs and resource utilization [12, 13].

## Clinical Impacts, Prevalence, and Association of Fatigue and Pain in SLE

### *Fatigue*

Chronic fatigue is the most frequent and disabling manifestation with multiple adverse consequences for individuals with SLE. Fatigue in SLE remains an elusive symptom that is poorly understood by healthcare providers [14, 15]. Patients often describe fatigue as unforeseeable, paralyzing, insurmountable, dominating, and a controlling symptom [6]. A large proportion of patients living with SLE report that debilitating fatigue limits their activities of daily living (ADL), reduces their participation in physical activity, and forces early resignation from work [5, 16–18]. One study that evaluated the perceived unmet needs of 386 SLE patients from attaining optimal health and HRQoL found that fatigue was recorded as a perceived area of unmet need by 81% [19]. The association of fatigue intensification with disease activity in SLE remains controversial with some studies exhibiting a positive correlation, while other studies demonstrating no significant correlation [11, 14, 20–23].

Clinically, self-reported fatigue in SLE has been directly correlated with reduced sleep quality and insomnia, increased disease activity, pain exacerbations, diminished functionality, and heightened states of anxiety and depression [5, 6, 14]. Importantly, fibromyalgia (FM) often congruently presents with fatigue in SLE patients, which may intensify fatigue. In fact, approximately 10–30% of SLE patients reporting fatigue fulfill the American College of Rheumatology (ACR) criteria for FM [24, 25]. Accordingly, it is crucial for physicians to screen for FM in SLE patients complaining of fatigue. These fatigue-induced clinical complications play an important role in severely decreasing SLE patients' HRQoL. Disease-specific HRQoL tools have indicated that fatigue was the most affected domain with the greatest impairment to HRQoL [26].

### *Pain*

Patients with SLE often describe their pain sensations as tender, aching, and/or burning [15, 27]. Of the patients with higher levels of pain, 70% reported their present pain as distressing and negatively impacting their HRQoL [27]. SLE-related pain often presents in the early stages of the disease and before diagnosis. When comparing SLE patients against healthy controls, SLE patients reported significantly worse pain [9]. One study demonstrated that approximately one quarter of SLE patients reported a high degree of pain on the visual analogue scale (i.e., ≥ 40 mm) [27]. The chronic nature of SLE-related pain often manifests in the musculoskeletal system as arthralgias, arthritis, or myalgias but can also present as headaches, abdominal pain, pain related to avascular necrosis of joints, chest pains (from serositis, myositis, costochondritis), generalized body pain, or pain caused by Raynaud's phenomenon. These SLE-pain related symptoms are similar to FM, which may coexist with SLE [28]. Despite the symptomatic burden of SLE-related pain, studies from Australia and the United States have shown that 73–80% of SLE patients rated their pain needs as being highly unmet [19, 29].

Similar to fatigue, SLE-related pain significantly limits the ability to perform ADL, reduces compliance with physical activity/rehabilitation programs, and can significantly impair physical function [9, 30, 31]. Furthermore, SLE-related pain is associated with higher levels of anxiety and depression, self-reported cognitive problems, increasing incidence of sleep disorders, and greater fatigue [27, 32–34]. Collectively, these SLE-related pain consequences negatively impact HRQoL and lead to a significant economic burden on the society as a whole [9, 10, 12, 27].

## Common Metrics for Assessing Fatigue and Pain in SLE

Fatigue and pain are frequent and disabling issues in SLE; however, both complications are difficult to quantify. In addition, significant heterogeneity exists among clinical studies with the utilization of different metrics for measuring fatigue and pain in SLE (Tables 15.1 and 15.2) [35–37]. For instance, in 2007, the Ad Hoc Committee on SLE Response Criteria for Fatigue conducted a systematic review of fatigue instruments used in SLE studies. Among the 34 SLE-included studies, 15 different instruments were used to measure fatigue; however, the study recommended using the Fatigue Severity Scale (FSS) for evaluating fatigue in SLE patients [38]. More recently, in 2020, a new systematic review confirmed the measurement properties (validity, reliability, and responsiveness) of the Functional Assessment of Chronic Illness Therapy-Fatigue Scale (FACIT-F) based on data from SLE randomized clinical trials and observational studies and recommended FACIT-F for clinical trials and observational SLE studies [37].

### *Fatigue Metrics*

1. *Functional Assessment of Chronic Illness Therapy-Fatigue Scale (FACIT-F)*

The FACIT-F is a self-reported inventory consisting of 13 items measuring various aspects of fatigue (i.e., physical, functional, emotional, and social) within the

**Table 15.1** Measurement properties and summary of fatigue instruments

| Reference | Population | Validity | | | | | Reliability | | Responsiveness | |
|---|---|---|---|---|---|---|---|---|---|---|
| | | *Face/ content* | *Construct* | *Convergent* | *Divergent* | *Known groups* | *Internal consistency* | *Test-retest* | *Ability to detect change* | *MCID/ MID* |
| FACIT-F | | | | | | | | | | |
| Strand 2014 [45] | SLE | | ✔ | | | | | | | |
| Kosinski 2013 [42] | SLE | ✔ | ✔ | | | | | | | ✔ |
| Lai 2011 [44] | SLE | | ✔ | | | ✔ | ✔ | ✔ | ✔ | ✔ |
| Goligher 2008 [43] | SLE | | ✔ | | | | ✔ | ✔ | ✔ | ✔ |
| Chandran 2007 [46] | PsA | | ✔ | | | | ✔ | ✔ | | |
| FSS | | | | | | | | | | |
| Goligher 2008 [43] | SLE | | | | | | | | | ✔ |
| Mattsson 2008 [49] | SLE | ✔ | ✔ | | | | ✔ | ✔ | | |
| AHCSLERCF 2007 [38] | SLE | | ✔ | | | | ✔ | | ✔ | |
| Austin 1996 [50] | SLE | | ✔ | | | | | | | |
| Krupp 1989 [47] | SLE | | ✔ | ✔ | ✔ | ✔ | ✔ | ✔ | | |
| SF-36 VT | | | | | | | | | | |
| Baba 2018 [69] | SLE | | ✔ | | | | ✔ | ✔ | ✔ | |
| Nantes 2018 [67] | SLE | | ✔ | | | | | | | |
| McElhone 2016 [66] | SLE | | ✔ | | | | | | ✔ | ✔ |
| Devilliers 2015 [65] | SLE | | | | | | | | ✔ | ✔ |
| Touma 2011 [68] | SLE | | ✔ | | | | | | ✔ | |
| Colangelo 2009 [64] | SLE | | | | | | | | | ✔ |
| Linde 2008 [63] | RA | | | ✔ | ✔ | ✔ | ✔ | | ✔ | |
| Goligher 2008 [43] | SLE | | | | | | | | | ✔ |

| | | | | | | | | | | |
|---|---|---|---|---|---|---|---|---|---|---|
| AHCSLERCF 2007 [38] | SLE | | ✔ | | | | ✔ | | | |
| Strand 2005 [51] | SLE | | | | | | | | | ✔ |
| Cella 2005 [39] | RA | | | ✔ | | | ✔ | | ✔ | ✔ |
| Strombeck 2005 [61] | SS | | ✔ | | | | | | | |
| Wolfe 2004 [60] | RA | | | | | | | | ✔ | |
| Wanders 2004 [59] | AS | | | | | | | | ✔ | |
| Thumboo 2000 [70] | SLE | | ✔ | | | | ✔ | ✔ | | |
| Soderman 2000 [58] | OA | ✔ | ✔ | | | | ✔ | ✔ | | |
| Thumboo 1999 [71] | SLE | | ✔ | | | | ✔ | ✔ | | |
| VAS | | | | | | | | | | |
| Rohekar 2009 [73] | RA | | | | | | | ✔ | | |
| Colangelo 2009 [64] | SLE | | | | | | | | | ✔ |
| d'Elia 2008 [74] | SS | ✔ | ✔ | ✔ | | | | ✔ | | |
| AHCSLERCF 2007 [38] | SLE | | ✔ | | | | | | | |
| LupusQoL fatigue domain | | | | | | | | | | |
| Meseguer 2017 [90] | SLE | ✔ | ✔ | | | | ✔ | | | |
| McElhone 2016 [66] | SLE | | | | | | | | ✔ | ✔ |
| Anindito 2016 [88] | SLE | | ✔ | | | | ✔ | ✔ | | |
| Devilliers 2015 [65] | SLE | | | | | | | | ✔ | ✔ |
| Touma 2011 [68] | SLE | | ✔ | | | ✔ | | | ✔ | |
| Jolly 2010 [89] | SLE | ✔ | ✔ | ✔ | ✔ | | ✔ | ✔ | | |
| McElhone 2007 [75] | SLE | | ✔ | | | ✔ | | ✔ | | |

*Abbreviations: SLE* Systemic lupus erythematosus, *RA* Rheumatoid arthritis, *SS* Sjögren's syndrome, *PsA* Psoriatic arthritis, *OA* Osteoarthritis, *MCID* Minimal clinically important difference, *MID* Minimal important difference, *AHCSLERCF* Ad Hoc Committee on Systemic Lupus Erythematosus Response Criteria for Fatigue

**Table 15.2** Measurement properties and summary of pain instruments

| Reference | Population | Validity | | | | | Reliability | | Responsiveness | |
|---|---|---|---|---|---|---|---|---|---|---|
| | | *Face/ content* | *Construct* | *Convergent* | *Divergent* | *Known groups* | *Internal consistency* | *Test-retest* | *Ability to detect change* | *MCID/ MID* |
| VAS | | | | | | | | | | |
| Hawker 2011 [52] | Various patients | | ✔ | | | | | ✔ | ✔ | |
| Wollaston 2004 [78] | SLE | | | | | | | | ✔ | |
| Ferraz 1990 [77] | RA | | | | | | | ✔ | | |
| Downie 1978 [76] | Various RD | ✔ | | | | | | | ✔ | |
| Joyce 1975 [79] | CP | | | | | | | ✔ | | |
| SF-36 BPS | | | | | | | | | | |
| Nantes 2018 [67] | SLE | | ✔ | | | | | | | |
| Hawker 2011 [52] | Various patients | | ✔ | | | | ✔ | ✔ | ✔ | ✔ |
| Escobar 2007 [82] | Orthopedic | | | | | | ✔ | | ✔ | ✔ |
| Koh 2006 [83] | RA | | ✔ | | | | ✔ | ✔ | ✔ | |
| Strand 2005 [51] | SLE | | | | | | | | | ✔ |
| Quintana 2005 [81] | Orthopedic | | | | | | ✔ | | ✔ | ✔ |
| Salaffi 2003 [85] | OA | | ✔ | ✔ | ✔ | | | | | |
| Bombardier 1995 [84] | Orthopedic | | | ✔ | ✔ | | | | | |
| Brazier 1992 [80] | General Patients | | ✔ | ✔ | ✔ | ✔ | ✔ | ✔ | | |

| LupusQoL pain domain | | | | | | | | | | |
|---|---|---|---|---|---|---|---|---|---|---|
| Nantes 2018 [67] | SLE | | ✔ | | | | | | | |
| Meseguer 2017 [90] | SLE | | ✔ | | | | ✔ | | | |
| McElhone 2016 [66] | SLE | | | | | | | | ✔ | ✔ |
| Anindito 2016 [88] | SLE | | ✔ | | | | ✔ | ✔ | | |
| Pamuk 2015 [92] | SLE | | | ✔ | ✔ | ✔ | ✔ | ✔ | | |
| Devilliers 2015 [65] | SLE | | | | | | | | ✔ | ✔ |
| Wang 2013 [91] | SLE | ✔ | ✔ | ✔ | ✔ | ✔ | ✔ | ✔ | | |
| Devilliers 2012 [87] | SLE | ✔ | ✔ | ✔ | ✔ | ✔ | ✔ | ✔ | | |
| Touma 2011 [68] | SLE | | ✔ | | | ✔ | | | ✔ | |
| Jolly 2010 [89] | SLE | ✔ | ✔ | ✔ | ✔ | | ✔ | ✔ | | |
| McElhone 2007 [75] | SLE | | ✔ | | | ✔ | | ✔ | | |

*Abbreviations*: *SLE* Systemic lupus erythematosus, *RA* Rheumatoid arthritis, *RD* Rheumatic diseases, *CP* Chronic pain, *OA* Osteoarthritis, *MCID* Minimal clinically important difference, *MI*, Minimal important difference past 7 days [39–41]. Originally, the FACIT-F was developed in 1997 for the assessment of fatigue in oncology patients with anemia demonstrating good reliability and validity [39–41]. Items are scored from 0 to 4 on a 5-point Likert scale ranging from "Not at all" to "Very much so." FACIT-F score is summed to provide a final score that can range from 0 to 52, with higher scores reflecting less fatigue and scores <30 suggesting severe fatigue [40, 41]. More recently, the FACIT-F has been utilized in various chronic and rheumatic conditions including SLE, in which the content validity was confirmed (Table 15.1) [37, 39, 41, 42]. The construct validity of the FACIT-F has been assessed in three RCTs, which have shown moderate-to-high correlations ($r$ = 0.49–0.87) between FACIT-F and other established legacy instruments, including the SF-36 vitality domain and Physical Component Summary (PCS) and Mental Component Summary (MCS) scores, Systemic Lupus Activity Questionnaire (SLAQ – PROs to assess disease activity based on Systemic Lupus Activity Measure [SLAM]), and patient global assessment scores [37, 43–45]. The internal consistency of the FACIT-F was demonstrated with a Cronbach's alpha of >0.95 [44]. Although the test-retest reliability of the FACIT-F is currently unknown in SLE patients, the FACIT-F test-retest reliability has been shown in psoriatic arthritis [46]. In the SLE population, FACIT-F ability to detect meaningful change over time has been consistently demonstrated. In one study [44], authors concluded that the minimal clinically important difference (MCID) of the FACIT-F in SLE responders ranged from 3 to 4 points. Another study [43] used an unpaired linear regression analysis after paired interviews and estimated that MCID of FACIT-F in SLE patients to be −5.9 points using the original FACIT-F scaling. Overall, the FACIT-F is a well-established instrument with good psychometric properties and sensitivity to change for measuring fatigue in SLE patients [37]. It covers a range of fatigue concepts in easy to understand language and is timely (<5 min) to administer in clinical and research settings where a global fatigue score is required [41].

2. *Fatigue Severity Scale (FSS)*

The FSS is a self-reported questionnaire initially developed to assess the impact of fatigue in multiple sclerosis and SLE patients [47]. Precisely, the FSS is a nine-item questionnaire designed to evaluate the impact of fatigue on specific types of physical, social, and cognitive functioning during the preceding 2 weeks [41]. Each item is scored from 1 to 7 ranging from "Strongly disagree" to "Strongly agree," and the global score is calculated as the sum and average of the 9 scores with higher scores reflecting greater fatigue [41]. The maximum score is 7, and any score ≥4 is considered a clinically relevant level of fatigue [41]. The 2007 Ad Hoc Committee on SLE Response Criteria for Fatigue recommended using the FSS in assessing SLE-related fatigue [38]. As a result, from 2007 to 2018, the FSS continues to be, along with FACIT-F, one of the most frequently used instruments in measuring fatigue in the SLE population [48].

The FSS has appropriate psychometric properties for measuring fatigue in SLE [41] (Table 15.1). The reliability of the FSS has been evaluated in SLE patients indicating an internal consistency of a Cronbach's alpha of 0.89–0.94 with no significant difference observed in the FSS in clinically stable SLE patients over 1 week

[47, 49]. With regard to the construct discriminative validity, one study indicated that the FSS accurately discriminated 90% of 29 SLE patients from healthy controls [47]. Moreover, FSS construct validity was established, and in one review, the results indicated a range of correlations with the FSS and various domains including disease activity (0.16–0.53), depression (0.22–0.59), and pain (0.35–0.54) [38]. Another study with 22 SLE patients demonstrated moderate-to-strong correlations with the FSS and pain, general health, and physical and social roles (0.59–0.60) and moderate correlations with function, emotional role, and mental health (0.41–0.44) [49]. The construct validity of the FSS was also assessed in 29 SLE patients suggesting strong correlations with visual analogue scale (VAS) of fatigue (0.81) and SF-36 vitality domain (0.56–0.63) [47, 49]. However, the content validity of the FSS in SLE has yet to be evaluated. Using the FSS in 58 SLE patients who underwent two telephone counseling interventions for improving functional status, effect sizes of 0.55 and 0.44 were specified for fatigue [50]. A further study using a linear regression analysis indicated that the effect size required to shift to a different fatigue category was 0.41 (95% CI 0.2–0.57) and concluded the MCID to be 0.6 (95% CI 0.3–0.9) [43]. A systematic review of earlier SLE studies recommended that ≤15% decreases in FSS were clinically relevant [38]. In summary, FSS is a short, timely (2–3 minutes), easy to interpret, and validated instrument with good internal consistency, reliability, responsiveness, construct validity, and sensitivity to change in SLE [41]. It has been translated, adapted, and validated from English into several other languages [41].

3. *Short Form-36 Vitality Domain (SF-36 VT)*

The SF-36 is a generic self-reported questionnaire that measures HRQOL and has been validated in multiple languages and various populations, including SLE [41]. It consists of 36 questions that assesses eight domains related to HRQOL, including physical functioning, physical role, bodily pain, general health, vitality, social functioning, emotional role, and mental health. Domain scores are measured on a scale of 0 (worst) to 100 (best) [51]. Patients with higher scores represent greater mental and/or physical health. The SF-36 is available in two versions (classic and acute) that measure different recall periods of pain (i.e., 4 weeks or 1 week) [52]. The SF-36 has been extensively studied and validated in various rheumatic populations, including SLE, and has been shown to reflect SLE-related impact on all domains [37] including the vitality domain (Table 15.1). The SF-36 vitality domain assesses energy levels (e.g., vitality and fatigue) and contains four items, each with 6 possible responses ranging from "all of the time" to "none of the time" pertaining to the previous 4 weeks to yield a single score on a 0–100 numeric scale, with higher scores representing less fatigue [41]. Studies have reported mean SF-36 vitality scores for healthy controls ranging between 57.4 and 62.2 points and an average of approximately 36 points for SLE patients [53–55]. In SLE patients, changes of 5–10 points in domain scores (including vitality domain) and 2.5–5 points in PCS an MCS scores represent MCID [51, 56]. The SF-36 vitality domain displays good internal consistency, reliability, construct and convergent validity, and appropriate ability to detect change in various rheumatic populations [37, 39, 41, 43, 57–63]. More specifically in the SLE literature, several studies have assessed the various SF-36 domains and concluded it to be a valid, reliable, and responsive questionnaire for assessing HRQOL in SLE patients [37, 64–71]. The SF-36 must be used in its entirety, and the SF-36 vitality domain should not be administered separate from SF-36.

4. *Visual Analogue Scale (VAS)*

The VAS is a self-reported, unidimensional instrument that measures the severity and intensity of mental and physical fatigue [41]. It generally comprises of a 0–100 mm horizontal line per an item (the number of items is decided upon the investigators), where respondents are instructed to indicate a marking between two anchored statements usually ranging from "not at all tired" to "very tired" that reflects their fatigue status within the previous week [41]. However, researchers often develop their own anchoring statements that often best reflect their patient population. Typically, higher scores represent greater fatigue [41]. VAS scores for healthy controls and SLE patients have been reported in previous studies as 20.5 ± 0.02 and 50.4 ± 30.6, respectively [64, 72]. Assessment of the test-retest reliability of fatigue VAS indicated intra-class correlations (ICC) ranging from 0.66 to 0.74 in various rheumatic disease populations [73, 74]. Patients have reported VAS as a relevant, easy to understand and complete tool that can accurately reflected their fatigue VAS strongly correlated with the FSS ($r = 0.6$) and the Chalder Fatigue Scale (ChFS) ($r = 0.6$) [38] (Table 15.1). An improvement of 10 points on the VAS (0–100 mm) when assessing fatigue is considered to be MCID [56]. The fatigue VAS is quick (<1 min), simple to administer and score, and easy to interpret with minimal respondent burden [41]. It is suitable and easy to implement in clinical practice and is frequently used in rheumatology research where a rapid global fatigue assessment is needed [41]. However, the fatigue VAS yields limited information on fatigue, and the inability to administer it online or by phone limits its usability, but it can be changed to a numerical rating scale [41]. In summary, the fatigue VAS is a valid instrument for assessing fatigue in SLE patients with good reliability and construct validity but with limited information on the construct being measured.

5. *Lupus Quality of Life Questionnaire Fatigue Domain (LupusQoL)*

The LupusQoL is a multidimensional, patient-derived, disease-specific tool that was developed in 2007 to evaluate the HRQoL in patients with SLE [75]. It includes 34 items that are grouped into 8 domains, which include physical health, pain, planning, intimate relationships, burden to others, emotional health, body image, and fatigue [75]. The LupusQoL includes questions measured on a 5-point Likert scale from 0 to 100, where higher scores indicate less impact in the past 4 weeks [75]. With regard to its psychometric properties, the LupusQoL has been shown to be a valid and reliable tool measuring HRQOL in SLE patients and is widely accepted and responsive in SLE patients in different languages and geographic locations [37, 65] (Table 15.1). All LupusQoL domains, including fatigue, are sensitive to change with improvements and worsening. A study by Touma and colleagues that used SLEDAI-2 K as an anchor showed that the LupusQoL displayed responsiveness

[68]. Specifically, among patients who improved, moderate effects were reported in the pain, fatigue, and physical health domains, while there were only small effects in emotional health, body image, burden to others, and planning domains. The study also demonstrated that patients with worsening disease activity reported moderate effects in the fatigue domain and a small effect in the burden to others domain [68]. The responsiveness of LupusQoL domains using a 100-mm VAS indicated that clinically improved patients reported significant improvements in LupusQoL physical health, pain, emotional health, and fatigue [65]. The physical health, planning, and fatigue domain scores declined significantly in patients with worsening disease activity [65]. The MCIDs for the LupusQoL domains have been established [37]. MCID estimates for deterioration and improvement ranged from −2.4 (body image domain) to −8.7 (intimate relationships domain) and 3.5 (body image domain) to 7.3 (burden to others domain), respectively [66]. Furthermore, the LupusQoL domain MCIDs ranged from 12.9 (emotional health) to 16.7 (intimate relationships) [66]. MCID for the LupusQoL has been derived using an anchor-based approach, which ranged from 1.1 to 9.2 for improvements and from −0.5 to −6.4 for deteriorations [65]. Studies have also indicated that LupusQoL is responsive to changes in QoL in SLE patients over 3-month to 1-year time intervals [65, 68]. Overall, evidence has indicated that the LupusQoL is a valid, reliable, and responsive questionnaire among SLE patients [37]. The LupusQoL must be used in its entirety, and the fatigue domain should not be administered separate from LupusQoL.

## *Pain Metrics*

1. *Visual Analogue Scale (VAS)*

The VAS is a unidimensional, single item, self-completed pain intensity measure and is often administered in rheumatic disease patients, including SLE [52]. Specifically, it comprises of a continuous horizontal or vertical line that tends to range from tends 0 to 100 mm in length, and completing the VAS for respondents takes less than 1 minute [52]. Respondents are asked to place a perpendicular mark to the VAS line at a point that most accurately represents their pain intensity. To avoid confusion among respondents, the line usually only consists of two anchored statements for each symptom extreme that reflects the respondents pain intensity within the previous week, such as "no pain" (score of 0) to "worst imaginable pain" (score of 100) [52]. While various anchor statements are used in research, there appears to be no benefit in selecting one set of anchor statements over another. Therefore, researchers often develop their own anchoring statements that often best reflect their patient population symptoms. Scoring is determined by placing a ruler and measuring the distance (mm) from 0 ("no pain" anchor) to the patient's perpendicular mark on the line. Typically, higher scores (i.e., closer to 100) obtained represent greater pain intensity [52].

Previous research has reported the VAS-pain for rheumatic patients as valid and reliable instrument [52] (Table 15.2). The test-retest reliability has been shown to be good ($r = 0.71–0.94$), and the VAS-pain has demonstrated good construct validity as it is highly correlated with a 5-point Likert scale (0.71–0.78) and the numerical rating scale (NRS) (0.62–0.91) among rheumatology patients [76, 77]. Another study with 80 SLE patients demonstrated that the pain VAS correlated well with both the SLEDAI and BILAG scores [78]. The pain VAS has demonstrated the ability to detect changes in pain intensity among patients with chronic inflammatory conditions, when assessed every hour until 4 hours and upward until 4 weeks following pain management therapy [52, 79]. Although the VAS-pain MCID for SLE patients has yet to be established, in general a 10-point change on the VAS (0–100 mm) when assessing pain is considered to be MCID [56]. Overall, the VAS-pain is a simple and adaptable measure that is easily administered to SLE patients in clinical settings; however, patients with cognitive and motor skill impairments may require additional assistance [52].

2. *Short Form-36 Bodily Pain Domain (SF-36 BP)*

The two-item SF-36 bodily pain domain is one of the eight domains of the SF-36 HRQOL questionnaire, which specifically measures the bodily pain intensity and pain interference with activities of daily living and work [52]. The bodily pain intensity portion is assessed using a 6-point scale that ranges from "none" to "very severe," while the pain interference portion is measured using a 5-point scale that ranges from "not at all" to "extremely" [52]. Scoring the SF-36 bodily pain domain requires both the bodily pain intensity and pain interference portions to be completed. Scoring and interpretation require minimal effort and training [52]. The SF-36 bodily pain domain is generally accepted among patients with a high response and completion rate as it is easy to administer taking roughly 2 minutes to complete [80]. With regard to its psychometric properties, the SF-36 bodily pain domain is considered to be a valid and reliable domain of SF-36 in assessing pain among diverse patient populations [52, 80] (Table 15.2). In terms of reliability and the internal consistency for the SF-36 bodily pain domain, the Cronbach's α among osteoarthritic, chronic musculoskeletal, and RA patients was 0.72–0.77, 0.91, and 0.59, respectively [81–83]. The test-retest reliability for the SF-36 bodily pain domain over a 2-week time interval ranged from 0.78 to 0.82 in various patient populations, including RA [80, 83]. The construct validity has been examined in arthroplasty patients with the SF-36 bodily pain domain against the WOMAC, which indicated moderate correlations (0.55) with no pain reporting of 13.6% and 32.2%, respectively [84]. In lower extremity osteoarthritic patients, the SF-36 bodily pain domain and WOMAC pain scale correlations ranged from 0.6 to 0.7 [80, 85, 86]. The SF-36 bodily pain domain has shown to be responsive in detecting improvements in pain [52]. One study that included SLE patients with active disease showed that the SF-36 was sensitive to change, which reflected both worsening and improvement [67]. Studies including SLE have indicated that a 5–10 point improvement in individual domain scores of the SF-36 and a 2.5–5 point improvement in the physical and mental components' summary scores of the SF-36 are representative of MCID [51]. Overall, the SF-36 bodily pain domain is a simple, easy, and useful tool in measuring general bodily pain in a research setting in diverse patient populations, including SLE patients [37, 52]. The SF-36 must be used in its entirety, and the SF-36 bodily pain domain should not be administered separate from SF-36.

3. *Lupus Quality of Life Questionnaire Pain Domain (LupusQoL)*

The LupusQoL pain domain is a self-reported measure that can be utilized to evaluate pain in SLE patients [75]. The LupusQoL pain domain uses a 5-point Likert scale (0 = "all the time," 1 = "most of the time," 2 = "a good bit of time," 3 = "occasionally," 4 = "never") to assess pain intensity within the previous 4 weeks [75]. As each domain in the LupusQoL is scored separately, scoring for the LupusQoL pain domain is obtained by dividing the mean raw score by 4 and then multiplying it by 100; scores range 0 (worst pain, worst HRQoL) to 100 (no pain, best HRQoL) [75]. In particular, the floor and ceiling effects of the LupusQoL pain domains are 2.6 and 18.1, respectively [67]. The LupusQoL pain domain also demonstrated construct validity when compared to the equivalent domains of SF-36 ($r$ = 0.38–0.83), the EQ5D analogic scale ($r$ = 0.76–0.80), EQ5D domains ($r$ = 0.50–0.68), and the SLAQ symptom scale ($r$ = −0.70 to −0.76) [68] (Table 15.2). Another study indicated good external convergent validity ($r$ = 0.59–0.78) with SF-36 and satisfactory divergent validity with SLEDAI [68, 87]. Another study showed that the associations between LupusQoL and SLEDAI scores were small ($r$ = −0.02 to 0.25), which confirmed divergent validity with SLE disease activity [68]. With respect to reliability, studies have shown that the LupusQoL has good internal consistency reliability (ICR) with a Cronbach's α ranging from 0.85 to 0.95 [87–90]. Studies have also shown the LupusQoL to have good test-retest reliability ($r$ = 0.68–0.93) [75, 88, 89]. Another study indicated that the ICR of the LupusQoL pain domain was 0.91 [91]. The LupusQoL pain domain was also able to discriminate between active and inactive SLE Turkish-speaking and Chinese patients [91, 92]. Another study examining known-groups' validity suggested that mean LupusQoL domain scores, with exception of intimate relationships, did not significantly differ between improved and same/worsened groups on SLEDAI-2 K ($p$ >0.05 for all domains) [68]. Overall, the LupusQoL including the pain domain is a valid and reliable SLE-specific instrument that can adequately capture SLE-related pain characteristics and intensity. The LupusQoL must be used in its entirety, and the pain domain should not be administered separate from LupusQoL.

## Factors Associated with Fatigue and Pain in SLE

### *Fatigue: Association with patient-reported and disease specific factors*

Fatigue is often one of the first symptoms that is consistently experienced by SLE patients. The etiology of fatigue in the SLE population is multifactorial and associated with a plethora of disease-specific and patient-reported factors including physical activity, obesity, sleep quality, comorbidities, SLE disease activity, vitamin D deficiency/insufficiency, and/or medications used (Fig. 15.1).

1. *Fatigue in the Context of Active Disease*
   1. *Disease Activity*
      All inflammatory autoimmune diseases are associated with fatigue, ranging from mild to profound manifestations. Although SLE disease activity contributes to fatigue, there are conflicting results in the literature indicating both positive and weak or no correlations between SLE disease activity and fatigue, conflicting results in studies indicate both positive and others exhibiting weak or no correlations [11, 47, 93–96]. In particular, one study reported no significant correlations with fatigue as measured by the FSS and disease activity measured by the SLEDAI [23]. In contrast, another study revealed that SLE-related fatigue was not associated with serologic markers but did correlate with physician's rating of disease activity [97]. Likewise, a longitudinal study using multiple regression analyses concluded that SLE disease activity predicted fatigue at two-time intervals [95].
   2. Medications
      Studies have indicated that the adverse effects associated with certain medications utilized to treat SLE may contribute to SLE-related fatigue. In one study, SLE patients administered with corticosteroids did not report increased fatigue scores; however, patients receiving NSAIDs indicated greater fatigue than NSAID-naïve SLE patients [94]. In addition, methotrexate is a common therapy used to treat SLE joint pain; however, patients frequently report associated fatigue. Although fatigue is a common side effect of various antide-

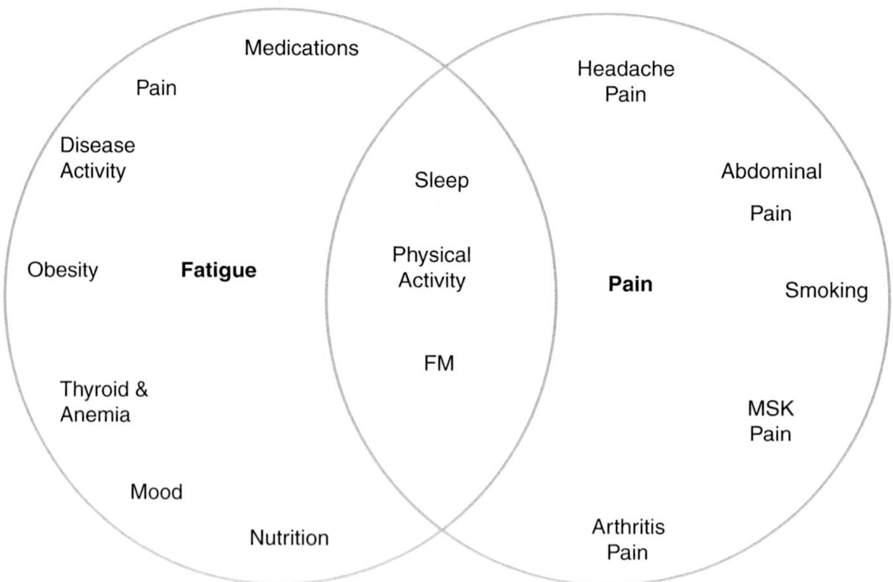


**Fig. 15.1** Factors associated with fatigue and pain in the context of SLE. FM fibromyalgia, MSK musculoskeletal

pressants or anxiolytic medications, reports showed that these medications did not significantly induce fatigue in SLE patients [94].

2. *Fatigue in the Context of Comorbidities*
   1. *Fibromyalgia*
   Fibromyalgia (FM) refers to the disruption of the central pain processing system, commonly referred to as central sensitization [98]. It is estimated that approximately 10–30% of SLE patients have clinically evident fibromyalgia [24, 25, 28, 99]. The high prevalence of FM in SLE patients suggests common mechanisms related to pain and distress in both conditions [98]. Although the prevalence of concomitant FM in SLE is common, it varies depending on geographical regions. For instance, in a Mexican cohort of SLE patients, there was a 10% prevalence rate of FM in comparison to a 22% among a US cohort of SLE patients [28, 100]. Patients with SLE and FM are often highly symptomatic and display poor physical function [98]. Changes to the central nervous system and sensory input processing caused by FM can lead to cognitive dysfunction, fatigue, poor sleep, and depression commonly seen in patients with SLE [98]. FM-induced fatigue is often reported as moderate to severe and is chronic. One study indicated that SLE patients with more fatigue also had more tender points ($p = 0.014$, $r = 0.34$) [24]. This study also showed that the number of tender points was significantly higher in SLE patients with secondary FM than in patients with primary Sjögren's syndrome with FM [24]. However, another study indicated that while 50% of SLE patients complained of fatigue, only 10% met the clinical criteria for FM [25]. Symptoms manifesting from SLE can be divided into two types (i.e., type 1 and 2) [101]. Type 1 manifestations represent the classic inflammatory symptoms of SLE (e.g., arthritis and vasculitis). Type 2 manifestations represent chronic, noninflammatory symptoms such as fatigue, widespread body pain, depression, anxiety, cognitive dysfunction, and sleep disturbance, which often resemble that of FM [101]. Since FM may coexist with SLE, it should be considered in causing fatigue, and a differential diagnosis should be made.
   2. *Thyroid Disease and Anemia*
   Studies have implicated that anemia- and thyroid-related complications may heighten fatigue in SLE patients. Research has shown that hematological abnormalities are frequent in SLE, with approximately 50% of SLE patients having anemia [102]. Anemia of chronic disease (ACD) is the most common form of anemia in SLE patients as well as iron deficiency as a result of menorrhagia and increased gastrointestinal blood loss caused by various medications [102, 103]. Fatigue is the most common symptom associated with anemia in SLE patients. Functional iron deficiency has been shown to be associated with fatigue in SLE patients [104].

   Thyroid disease has been associated with SLE with hypothyroidism being the most common, occurring in 15–19% of SLE patients [105–107]. Hyperthyroidism occurs less often in SLE patients when compared to hypothyroidism at a prevalence rate of 3–9% [105, 106]. A previous study showed that 45% of SLE patients had elevated levels of thyroid-stimulating hormone,

34% had low T3 levels, and 18% had high anti-microsomal antibody titers [108]. One study has shown a significant correlation between SLE disease activity and clinical symptoms of hyperthyroidism ($r = 0.4$, $P = 0.004$) [109]. In a study of 100 Brazilian SLE patients, 76% of SLE patients had symptoms associated with thyroid dysfunction, of which 36% had symptoms of fatigue [110]. Given that thyroid disease and SLE have overlapping symptoms, including fatigue, clinicians may mistakenly attribute these symptoms to SLE alone rather than the co-existent thyroid disease [108].

3. *Depression and Anxiety*
   Mood disorders, including depression and anxiety, are common in SLE patients with a prevalence of 28% and 24%, respectively [111]. Various studies have consistently indicated that both anxiety and depression are factors that contribute to heighten fatigue in SLE patients [11, 22, 97, 112]. For instance, one study indicated that SLE patients had higher depression scores than the general population and their depression scores correlated with higher fatigue scores [97]. More specifically, using the Hospital Anxiety and Depression (HAD) scale, one study indicated that in approximately one third of SLE patients, HAD scores suggested a mood disorder and roughly 13% of these patients were taking antidepressant medications and reported a moderate correlation between HAD depression scores and fatigue [11]. Overall, current evidence suggests that depression and anxiety both contribute to increasing fatigue experienced by SLE patients.
4. *Cognitive Dysfunction*
   Cognitive dysfunction is a common complaint in the SLE population with a prevalence ranging from 27% to 61% [113–117]. In a recent study and meta-analysis that included nine studies, SLE patients had more microstructural brain white matter damage and elevated IL-6 levels, which may contribute to the fatigue issues experienced in SLE [118]. Despite this finding, there is limited evidence on the mechanisms of cognitive dysfunction and its relation to fatigue in SLE patients, and this relationship should be explored in larger datasets.
5. *Pain*
   Pain along with other psychosocial factors is associated with elevated levels of fatigue in SLE patients. Specifically, arthralgias and arthritis occur in the SLE populations with a prevalence of roughly 95% [5]. In one study, significant correlations were noted between self-reported increases in pain and elevated levels of fatigue [119]. Another study that included 127 SLE patients and utilized a correlational analysis found that fatigue was moderately related to greater pain intensity measured by a VAS ($r = 0.43$; $p < 0.001$) [94]. Studies have demonstrated a higher prevalence of fatigue in SLE patients who report higher pain levels [11, 24]. Evidence suggests a direct relationship between heightened self-reported pain intensity and increasing sensations of fatigue in SLE patients.

3. *Fatigue in the Context of Lifestyle Factors*
   1. *Physical Activity*
      Optimal aerobic capacity, exercise tolerance, and muscular strength are required to perform essential activities of daily living and can improve health outcomes, limit the incidence of chronic conditions, and increase HRQoL [120–123]. One study assessed the physical activity capacity in SLE patients, reflecting reduced levels of aerobic fitness, exercise capacity, muscle strength, and resting lung function [124]. Studies comparing aerobic capacity in women with SLE to sedentary women and healthy controls demonstrated that SLE women had lower aerobic capacity measured by peak oxygen consumption (i.e., $VO_2$ max) than non-SLE counterparts [125, 126]. Low physical activity levels in SLE patients also increase the risk of cardiovascular disease through amplified pro-inflammatory biomarkers and carotid plaque solidification [127, 128]. Interestingly, emerging evidence has suggested that SLE patients who are physically inactive and thereby more unfit in terms of aerobic and/or muscular endurance and strength have significantly higher levels of fatigue [129–132]. Using a linear regression model, research has shown a correlation between physical disability due to poor exercise capacity and higher levels of fatigue in SLE patients [124]. A further study indicated that physiologic deconditioning was highly correlated with the perception of severe, activity-limiting fatigue in SLE patients [126]. Several RCTs have demonstrated that exercise can be well-tolerated and significantly reduce fatigue in SLE patients compared with controls [62, 133–135]. However, research has shown there to be a lack of enthusiasm to participate in exercise training as only 24% of SLE patients continued to exercise regularly [62, 136].
   2. *Obesity and Body Mass Index*
      Research estimates that approximately 30–50% of SLE patients are classified as clinically obese [137–139]. SLE and obesity are both considered to be chronic systematic inflammatory conditions as reflected by increases in inflammatory biomarkers TNF-α, CRP, and IL-6 [140]. Obese SLE patients are more likely to experience higher levels of fatigue. Although direct studies examining the relationship between obesity and fatigue in SLE are scare, data from the LUMINA cohort documented that 28% of SLE patients were obese (BMI >30 kg/m$^2$) and associated with greater fatigue [141]. Likewise, another clinical cohort study indicated that 39% of SLE patients were clinically obese and demonstrated a positive correlation between obesity and increased fatigue [142]. One study indicated that diets can induce weight loss and correspondingly reduce fatigue in SLE [136, 143]. However, these mean reductions assessed by the FSS were not ≥ MCID [136, 143].
   3. *Sleep*
      It is estimated that nearly 92% of SLE patients experience some form of sleep disorder including sleep-wake disturbances and non-restorative sleep, which can lead to poor sleep quality and intensify disease-specific symptoms such as fatigue [11, 144–146]. Sleep disturbances and difficulties in SLE may be

attributed to pain severity, functional impairment, mood disorders, certain medications (i.e., prednisone), physical inactivity, stress, and cumulative damage and/or heightened disease activity [5, 130, 147]. Studies have indicated that SLE participants indicated greater fatigue with more sleep-related issues and non-restorative sleep such as deficits in slow-wave sleep, low sleep efficiency, and high levels of α-EEG sleep activity compared to healthy controls [148]. The authors concluded that sleep-related issues in SLE may be related to patients' experience of fatigue. In addition, studies have also found a higher prevalence of sleep fragmentation, sleep apnea, and abnormal limb movement in SLE patients, possibly leading to increased daytime sleepiness [25, 149]. Finally, another study in 100 SLE female patients indicated that 56% of the cohort reported moderate-to-severe sleep impairments [145].

4. *Nutrition and Supplementation*
   Nutritional deficiency in various vitamins and minerals is common in SLE patients. Vitamin D insufficiency and deficiency in SLE patients are suggested to be multifactorial, which may be specifically related to sunlight avoidance, use of sunscreen, renal insufficiency, and SLE itself [5, 150]. For instance, SLE patients are generally advised to avoid sun exposure [5, 150], and medication usage (i.e., chloroquine and prednisone) may interfere with vitamin D metabolism [150]. In particular, vitamin D deficiency (25[OH]D below 10 ng/ml) and insufficiency (25[OH]D below 30 ng/ml) have been reported based on serum levels in SLE patients [150–153]. Although the role of vitamin D in the SLE pathogenesis remains unknown, lower vitamin D levels may be associated with fatigue in SLE [154, 155]. One study reported that SLE patients were 75% and 15% vitamin D insufficient and deficient, respectively [154]. From this study, researchers identified lower serum vitamin D levels as an independent predictor of increased and exacerbated fatigue levels reported by VAS. The same research group administered oral vitamin D supplementation to vitamin D-deficient SLE patients and observed reduction in VAS fatigue levels, which were not ≥ MCID [155]. Findings from these preliminary studies support routine vitamin D supplementation for improvement of fatigue [150, 156–158].

## *Pain: Association with patient-reported and disease specific factors*

1. *Pain in the Context of Active Lupus Disease*
   1. Arthritis and Musculoskeletal Complications
      Inflammatory musculoskeletal (MSK) manifestations, including arthralgia, myalgia, arthritis, and occasionally tenosynovitis, are among the most commonly reported pain-related symptoms, affecting approximately 50–95% of SLE patients [159]. Importantly, inflammatory MSK pain symptoms have

been shown to strongly correlate with reduced HRQOL, morbidity, and work disability [159]. Although clinical assessments may underestimate joint and tendon inflammation in SLE patients, ultrasonography and MRI have demonstrated synovitis in affected joints [159, 160]. Similar to other inflammatory diseases, musculoskeletal pain in SLE reflects production of pro-inflammatory cytokines and mediators, including IL-6, IL-17, interferon-α, IL-18, and TNF-α [161–163].

2. *Headache Pain*
   Headache-related pain is a common source of pain and discomfort associated with SLE. Headache pain in SLE may be described as severe, persistent, intermittent, migrainous, and non-migrainous [164]. Numerous studies have indicated varying prevalence rates ranging from 10% to 62% [165–167]. Migraine headaches have been reported in 10–39% of SLE patients and may be as common as tension headaches [165–167]. Although the clinical relationship between SLE disease activity and headaches frequently remains unclear, some of the causes include neuropsychiatric SLE, vascular injury, circulating pro-inflammatory cytokines, central nervous system disorder, and neuropathic pain [164]. Studies have also suggested that headaches associated with SLE may be attributed to antiphospholipid antibodies (aPL) [168, 169]. However, one prospective study in 103 SLE patients with SLE and 58 patients with migraine without SLE found a high frequency of headache in SLE patients without an association with aPL [170].
3. *Abdominal Pain*
   Abdominal pain in SLE is often a complex diagnosis and is reported by approximately 8–40% of SLE patients [171, 172]. The occurrence of SLE-related abdominal pain is due to a variety of causes, including peritonitis, mesenteric vasculitis, pancreatitis, ulcers, and lupus enteritis [172, 173]. One previous study identified 38/175 (22%) of SLE patients who presented with acute abdominal pain with the most common cause being lupus enteritis [174]. Abdominal pain in SLE may also be attributed to drug-induced adverse effects.

2. *Pain in the Context of Comorbidities*
   1. *Fibromyalgia*
      It is well established that SLE patients with concomitant FMS have significantly more frequent and severe pain-related symptoms, including muscle soreness and tenderness, widespread pain, headaches, menstrual pains, chest pains, stiffness, myalgias, and arthralgia [98].
3. *Pain in the Context of Lifestyle*
   1. *Sleep*
      A systematic review comprising of nine studies indicated that the prevalence of sleep disorders in SLE ranged from 55% to 85%; however, authors noted that significant variability existed in assessment techniques among studies [34]. From this review, the majority of included studies also displayed an association between sleep disorders and pain in SLE patients [34]. Polysomnographic data shows that SLE patients' sleep is often characterized

by respiratory (sleep apnea or abnormal respiration) or movement disorders [175]. A key predictor of poor sleep quality in SLE patients is pain [11, 145, 175–178]. One study [146] indicated that pain severity was one of the factors correlated with poor sleep quality in SLE patients. Another study showed that SLE patients reported more pain when trying to fall asleep and during the night compared with healthy controls [179]. Additionally, in the German LuLa cohort, one of the predictors of severe sleep disorders was pain. Pain attributed to arthralgias, arthritis, and FM commonly seen in SLE patients cause significant sleep disruption [146]. Theoretically, sleep disorders and pain associated with SLE can alter inflammatory markers and cytokine regulation, both of which are hypothesized as possible factors that impact pain intensification in SLE [34].

2. *Smoking*
   Tobacco or cigarette smoking has been identified as an environmental risk factor for increasing the incidence of developing autoimmune diseases, including SLE [1, 180–182]. In fact, there is a dose-response association between the number of cigarettes smoked per year and the development of SLE [1]. The toxins from tobacco smoking can directly damage endogenous proteins and DNA leading to genetic mutations and influence both cell-mediated and humoral immune responses, which could be involved in the development of SLE [183]. Elevated titers of anti-dsDNA antibodies have also been reported in current or past smokers with SLE [184]. SLE patients who smoke may increase their risk of heightened pain severity as smoking can lead to increased oxidative stress and activate cytokine-driven pathways of systemic inflammation [170, 182], and patients with FM who smoke reported significantly more pain than nonsmokers [185]. Within the SLE literature, several studies have shown increased disease activity among SLE smokers compared with nonsmokers [186–188]. One study with 181 SLE women showed that smokers reported increased bodily pain [189]. Another study indicated that smoking exposure is associated with cumulative chronic damage in Brazilian SLE patients [190].

   Our findings indicate that smoking exposure is associated with cumulative chronic damage, as determined by the SDI score, in patients with SLE. Smoking exposure may have deleterious effects on lupus morbidity, and more detailed studies of this association are needed.
3. *Physical Activity*
   Physical activity has emerged as an adjuvant therapy in the treatment of SLE patients for mitigating various symptoms, such as pain. The accumulation of fatigue, depressed mood, and disability associated with SLE can drive patients toward a physically inactive lifestyle, thus fostering a sedentary state, leading to further fatigue and exacerbated pain [130]. However, physical exercise could be a treatment to break this vicious sedentary cycle [191]. It is well established that long-term exercise and physical activity provide anti-inflammatory effects that can theoretically reduce pain severity and increase pain tolerance [192–194], as well as immunomodulatory effects and downregula-

tion of inflammatory gene expression [192, 194, 195]. Several studies have shown that various forms of exercise, such as stretching, Wii Fit programming, aquatic exercise, and aerobic exercise, can reduce pain and suggest a beneficial effect of exercise in SLE patients [194, 196–198]. Exercise can also promote higher sleep quality and increase weight loss, which can further limit the occurrence of pain in SLE patients [199]. However, one study reported an improvement in the exercise group when compared to the control group in all SF-36 domains except for the pain domain. The exercise group also did not report statistically significant improvements in pain by VAS (MD −1.31 [95% CI −3.06 to 0.44]) [200]. Despite exercise interventions being safe, tolerable, and not adversely affecting SLE disease activity, there is a possibility of transient joint pain among SLE patients when exercising [131, 201]. This temporary joint pain may make SLE patients reluctant to exercise and more likely to become sedentary.

## Conclusions

Fatigue and pain are primary complaints of patients with SLE. The dynamic interplay between various disease-specific and lifestyle factors may contribute to heighted fatigue and pain experienced by SLE patients. As such, it is of clinical importance to accurately and consistently monitor patient-reported fatigue and pain in routine practice and in clinical trials in order to ensure the highest quality of care. Evidence from this chapter supports the measurement properties of the SF-36, LupusQoL, FSS, VAS, and FACIT-F in their entirety for assessing pain and fatigue in SLE patients. From these instruments, recent research has suggested the utilization of the FACIT-F in RCTs and longitudinal observational studies when assessing SLE-related fatigue based on its validated psychometric properties [37]. Although other instruments for measuring pain do exist, including the McGill Pain Questionnaire, Brief Pain Inventory, and numerical rating scale, further research of the psychometric properties of these instruments within the context of SLE is required.

## References

1. Kaul A, Gordon C, Crow MK, Touma Z, Urowitz MB, van Vollenhoven R, et al. Systemic lupus erythematosus. Nat Rev Dis Primers. 2016;2:16039. Epub 2016/06/17
2. Strand V, Gladman D, Isenberg D, Petri M, Smolen J, Tugwell P. Endpoints: consensus recommendations from OMERACT IV. Outcome measures in rheumatology. Lupus. 2000;9(5):322–7. Epub 2000/07/06
3. Archenholtz B, Burckhardt CS, Segesten K. Quality of life of women with systemic lupus erythematosus or rheumatoid arthritis: domains of importance and dissatisfaction. Qual Life Res. 1999;8(5):411–6. Epub 1999/09/04

4. Strand V, Galateanu C, Pushparajah DS, Nikai E, Sayers J, Wood R, et al. Limitations of current treatments for systemic lupus erythematosus: a patient and physician survey. Lupus. 2013;22(8):819–26. Epub 2013/07/03
5. Ahn GE, Ramsey-Goldman R. Fatigue in systemic lupus erythematosus. Int J Clin Rheumtol. 2012;7(2):217–27. Epub 2012/06/28
6. Olesinska M, Saletra A. Quality of life in systemic lupus erythematosus and its measurement. Reumatologia. 2018;56(1):45–54. Epub 2018/04/25
7. Du X, Zhao Q, Zhuang Y, Chen H, Shen B. Fatigue of systemic lupus erythematosus in China: contributors and effects on the quality of life. Patient Prefer Adherence. 2018;12:1729–35. Epub 2018/09/21
8. Holloway L, Humphrey L, Heron L, Pilling C, Kitchen H, Hojbjerre L, et al. Patient-reported outcome measures for systemic lupus erythematosus clinical trials: a review of content validity, face validity and psychometric performance. Health Qual Life Outcomes. 2014;12:116. Epub 2014/07/23
9. Waldheim E, Ajeganova S, Bergman S, Frostegard J, Welin E. Variation in pain related to systemic lupus erythematosus (SLE): a 7-year follow-up study. Clin Rheumatol. 2018;37(7):1825–34. Epub 2018/04/15
10. Waldheim E, Elkan AC, Pettersson S, van Vollenhoven R, Bergman S, Frostegard J, et al. Health-related quality of life, fatigue and mood in patients with SLE and high levels of pain compared to controls and patients with low levels of pain. Lupus. 2013;22(11):1118–27. Epub 2013/08/31
11. Tench CM, McCurdie I, White PD, D'Cruz DP. The prevalence and associations of fatigue in systemic lupus erythematosus. Rheumatology (Oxford). 2000;39(11):1249–54. Epub 2000/11/21
12. Sutcliffe N, Clarke AE, Taylor R, Frost C, Isenberg DA. Total costs and predictors of costs in patients with systemic lupus erythematosus. Rheumatology (Oxford). 2001;40(1):37–47. Epub 2001/02/07
13. Tanaka Y, Mizukami A, Kobayashi A, Ito C, Matsuki T. Disease severity and economic burden in Japanese patients with systemic lupus erythematosus: a retrospective, observational study. Int J Rheum Dis. 2018;21(8):1609–18. Epub 2018/08/28
14. Cleanthous S, Tyagi M, Isenberg DA, Newman SP. What do we know about self-reported fatigue in systemic lupus erythematosus? Lupus. 2012;21(5):465–76. Epub 2012/02/22
15. Mattsson M, Moller B, Stamm T, Gard G, Bostrom C. Uncertainty and opportunities in patients with established systemic lupus erythematosus: a qualitative study. Musculoskeletal Care. 2012;10(1):1–12. Epub 2011/10/20
16. Benitha R, Tikly M. Functional disability and health-related quality of life in south Africans with rheumatoid arthritis and systemic lupus erythematosus. Clin Rheumatol. 2007;26(1):24–9. Epub 2006/03/16
17. Pettersson S, Bostrom C, Eriksson K, Svenungsson E, Gunnarsson I, Henriksson EW. Lifestyle habits and fatigue among people with systemic lupus erythematosus and matched population controls. Lupus. 2015;24(9):955–65. Epub 2015/02/24
18. Robinson D Jr, Aguilar D, Schoenwetter M, Dubois R, Russak S, Ramsey-Goldman R, et al. Impact of systemic lupus erythematosus on health, family, and work: the patient perspective. Arthritis Care Res (Hoboken). 2010;62(2):266–73. Epub 2010/03/02
19. Moses N, Wiggers J, Nicholas C, Cockburn J. Prevalence and correlates of perceived unmet needs of people with systemic lupus erythematosus. Patient Educ Couns. 2005;57(1):30–8. Epub 2005/03/31
20. Azizoddin DR, Gandhi N, Weinberg S, Sengupta M, Nicassio PM, Jolly M. Fatigue in systemic lupus: the role of disease activity and its correlates. Lupus. 2019;28(2):163–73. Epub 2018/12/26
21. McElhone K, Abbott J, Teh LS. A review of health related quality of life in systemic lupus erythematosus. Lupus. 2006;15(10):633–43. Epub 2006/11/24

22. McKinley PS, Ouellette SC, Winkel GH. The contributions of disease activity, sleep patterns, and depression to fatigue in systemic lupus erythematosus. A proposed model. Arthritis Rheum. 1995;38(6):826–34. Epub 1995/06/01
23. Wang B, Gladman DD, Urowitz MB. Fatigue in lupus is not correlated with disease activity. J Rheumatol. 1998;25(5):892–5. Epub 1998/05/23
24. Iannuccelli C, Spinelli FR, Guzzo MP, Priori R, Conti F, Ceccarelli F, et al. Fatigue and widespread pain in systemic lupus erythematosus and Sjogren's syndrome: symptoms of the inflammatory disease or associated fibromyalgia? Clin Exp Rheumatol. 2012;30(6 Suppl 74):117–21. Epub 2013/02/27
25. Taylor J, Skan J, Erb N, Carruthers D, Bowman S, Gordon C, et al. Lupus patients with fatigue-is there a link with fibromyalgia syndrome? Rheumatology (Oxford). 2000;39(6):620–3. Epub 2000/07/11
26. Gordon C, Isenberg D, Lerstrom K, Norton Y, Nikai E, Pushparajah DS, et al. The substantial burden of systemic lupus erythematosus on the productivity and careers of patients: a European patient-driven online survey. Rheumatology (Oxford). 2013;52(12):2292–301. Epub 2013/09/21
27. Waldheim E, Elkan AC, Bergman S, Frostegard J, van Vollenhoven R, Henriksson EW. Extent and characteristics of self-reported pain in patients with systemic lupus erythematosus. Lupus. 2013;22(2):136–43. Epub 2012/11/30
28. Wolfe F, Petri M, Alarcon GS, Goldman J, Chakravarty EF, Katz RS, et al. Fibromyalgia, systemic lupus erythematosus (SLE), and evaluation of SLE activity. J Rheumatol. 2009;36(1):82–8. Epub 2008/11/13
29. Danoff-Burg S, Friedberg F. Unmet needs of patients with systemic lupus erythematosus. Behav Med. 2009;35(1):5–13. Epub 2009/03/20
30. Greco CM, Rudy TE, Manzi S. Effects of disease activity, pain, and distress on activity limitations in patients with systemic lupus erythematosus. J Rheumatol. 2004;31(2):260–7. Epub 2004/02/05
31. McElhone K, Abbott J, Gray J, Williams A, Teh LS. Patient perspective of systemic lupus erythematosus in relation to health-related quality of life concepts: a qualitative study. Lupus. 2010;19(14):1640–7. Epub 2010/08/17
32. Figueiredo-Braga M, Cornaby C, Cortez A, Bernardes M, Terroso G, Figueiredo M, et al. Depression and anxiety in systemic lupus erythematosus: the crosstalk between immunological, clinical, and psychosocial factors. Medicine (Baltimore). 2018;97(28):e11376. Epub 2018/07/12
33. Kozora E, Ellison MC, West S. Depression, fatigue, and pain in systemic lupus erythematosus (SLE): relationship to the American College of Rheumatology SLE neuropsychological battery. Arthritis Rheum. 2006;55(4):628–35. Epub 2006/07/29
34. Palagini L, Tani C, Mauri M, Carli L, Vagnani S, Bombardieri S, et al. Sleep disorders and systemic lupus erythematosus. Lupus. 2014;23(2):115–23. Epub 2014/01/15
35. Izadi Z, Gandrup J, Katz PP, Yazdany J. Patient-reported outcome measures for use in clinical trials of SLE: a review. Lupus Sci Med. 2018;5(1):e000279. Epub 2018/09/01
36. Strand V, Gladman D, Isenberg D, Petri M, Smolen J, Tugwell P. Outcome measures to be used in clinical trials in systemic lupus erythematosus. J Rheumatol. 1999;26(2):490–7. Epub 1999/02/11
37. Strand V, Simon LS, Meara AS, Touma Z. Measurement properties of selected patient-reported outcome measures for use in randomised controlled trials in patients with systemic lupus erythematosus: a systematic review. Lupus Sci Med. 2020;7(1) Epub 2020/06/28
38. Ad Hoc Committee on Systemic Lupus Erythematosus Response Criteria for F. Measurement of fatigue in systemic lupus erythematosus: a systematic review. Arthritis Rheum. 2007;57(8):1348–57. Epub 2007/12/01
39. Cella D, Yount S, Sorensen M, Chartash E, Sengupta N, Grober J. Validation of the Functional Assessment of Chronic Illness Therapy Fatigue Scale relative to other instrumentation in patients with rheumatoid arthritis. J Rheumatol. 2005;32(5):811–9.

40. Yellen SB, Cella DF, Webster K, Blendowski C, Kaplan E. Measuring fatigue and other anemia-related symptoms with the Functional Assessment of Cancer Therapy (FACT) measurement system. J Pain Symptom Manag. 1997;13(2):63–74. Epub 1997/02/01
41. Hewlett S, Dures E, Almeida C. Measures of fatigue: Bristol Rheumatoid Arthritis Fatigue Multi-Dimensional Questionnaire (BRAF MDQ), Bristol Rheumatoid Arthritis Fatigue Numerical Rating Scales (BRAF NRS) for severity, effect, and coping, Chalder Fatigue Questionnaire (CFQ), Checklist Individual Strength (CIS20R and CIS8R), Fatigue Severity Scale (FSS), Functional Assessment Chronic Illness Therapy (Fatigue) (FACIT-F), Multi-Dimensional Assessment of Fatigue (MAF), Multi-Dimensional Fatigue Inventory (MFI), Pediatric Quality Of Life (PedsQL) Multi-Dimensional Fatigue Scale, Profile of Fatigue (ProF), Short Form 36 Vitality Subscale (SF-36 VT), and Visual Analog Scales (VAS). Arthritis Care Res (Hoboken). 2011;63 Suppl 11:S263–86. Epub 2012/05/25
42. Kosinski M, Gajria K, Fernandes AW, Cella D. Qualitative validation of the FACIT-fatigue scale in systemic lupus erythematosus. Lupus. 2013;22(5):422–30. Epub 2013/02/21
43. Goligher EC, Pouchot J, Brant R, Kherani RB, Avina-Zubieta JA, Lacaille D, et al. Minimal clinically important difference for 7 measures of fatigue in patients with systemic lupus erythematosus. J Rheumatol. 2008;35(4):635–42. Epub 2008/03/07
44. Lai JS, Beaumont JL, Ogale S, Brunetta P, Cella D. Validation of the functional assessment of chronic illness therapy-fatigue scale in patients with moderately to severely active systemic lupus erythematosus, participating in a clinical trial. J Rheumatol. 2011;38(4):672–9. Epub 2011/01/18
45. Strand V, Levy RA, Cervera R, Petri MA, Birch H, Freimuth WW, et al. Improvements in health-related quality of life with belimumab, a B-lymphocyte stimulator-specific inhibitor, in patients with autoantibody-positive systemic lupus erythematosus from the randomised controlled BLISS trials. Ann Rheum Dis. 2014;73(5):838–44. Epub 2013/03/26
46. Chandran V, Bhella S, Schentag C, Gladman DD. Functional assessment of chronic illness therapy-fatigue scale is valid in patients with psoriatic arthritis. Ann Rheum Dis. 2007;66(7):936–9. Epub 2007/02/28
47. Krupp LB, LaRocca NG, Muir-Nash J, Steinberg AD. The fatigue severity scale. Application to patients with multiple sclerosis and systemic lupus erythematosus. Arch Neurol. 1989;46(10):1121–3. Epub 1989/10/01
48. Barbacki A, Petri M, Avina-Zubieta A, Alarcon GS, Bernatsky S. Fatigue measurements in systemic lupus erythematosus. J Rheumatol. 2019;46(11):1470–7. Epub 2019/02/03
49. Mattsson M, Moller B, Lundberg I, Gard G, Bostrom C. Reliability and validity of the Fatigue Severity Scale in Swedish for patients with systemic lupus erythematosus. Scand J Rheumatol. 2008;37(4):269–77. Epub 2008/07/10
50. Austin JS, Maisiak RS, Macrina DM, Heck LW. Health outcome improvements in patients with systemic lupus erythematosus using two telephone counseling interventions. Arthritis Care Res. 1996;9(5):391–9. Epub 1996/10/01
51. Strand V, Crawford B. Improvement in health-related quality of life in patients with SLE following sustained reductions in anti-dsDNA antibodies. Expert Rev Pharmacoecon Outcomes Res. 2005;5(3):317–26. Epub 2005/06/01
52. Hawker GA, Mian S, Kendzerska T, French M. Measures of adult pain: Visual Analog Scale for Pain (VAS Pain), Numeric Rating Scale for Pain (NRS Pain), McGill Pain Questionnaire (MPQ), Short-Form McGill Pain Questionnaire (SF-MPQ), Chronic Pain Grade Scale (CPGS), Short Form-36 Bodily Pain Scale (SF-36 BPS), and Measure of Intermittent and Constant Osteoarthritis Pain (ICOAP). Arthritis Care Res (Hoboken). 2011;63 Suppl 11:S240–52. Epub 2012/05/25
53. Gilboe IM, Kvien TK, Husby G. Disease course in systemic lupus erythematosus: changes in health status, disease activity, and organ damage after 2 years. J Rheumatol. 2001;28(2):266–74. Epub 2001/03/15

54. Segal B, Bowman SJ, Fox PC, Vivino FB, Murukutla N, Brodscholl J, et al. Primary Sjogren's Syndrome: health experiences and predictors of health quality among patients in the United States. Health Qual Life Outcomes. 2009;7:46. Epub 2009/05/29
55. Wolfe F, Michaud K, Li T, Katz RS. EQ-5D and SF-36 quality of life measures in systemic lupus erythematosus: comparisons with rheumatoid arthritis, noninflammatory rheumatic disorders, and fibromyalgia. J Rheumatol. 2010;37(2):296–304. Epub 2009/12/25
56. Strand V, Boers M, Idzerda L, Kirwan JR, Kvien TK, Tugwell PS, et al. It's good to feel better but it's better to feel good and even better to feel good as soon as possible for as long as possible. Response criteria and the importance of change at OMERACT 10. J Rheumatol. 2011;38(8):1720–7. Epub 2011/08/03
57. Busija L, Osborne RH, Nilsdotter A, Buchbinder R, Roos EM. Magnitude and meaningfulness of change in SF-36 scores in four types of orthopedic surgery. Health Qual Life Outcomes. 2008;6:55. Epub 2008/08/01
58. Soderman P, Malchau H. Validity and reliability of Swedish WOMAC osteoarthritis index: a self-administered disease-specific questionnaire (WOMAC) versus generic instruments (SF-36 and NHP). Acta Orthop Scand. 2000;71(1):39–46. Epub 2000/04/01
59. Wanders AJ, Gorman JD, Davis JC, Landewe RB, van der Heijde DM. Responsiveness and discriminative capacity of the assessments in ankylosing spondylitis disease-controlling antirheumatic therapy core set and other outcome measures in a trial of etanercept in ankylosing spondylitis. Arthritis Rheum. 2004;51(1):1–8. Epub 2004/02/12
60. Wolfe F. Fatigue assessments in rheumatoid arthritis: comparative performance of visual analog scales and longer fatigue questionnaires in 7760 patients. J Rheumatol. 2004;31(10):1896–902. Epub 2004/10/07
61. Strombeck B, Theander E, Jacobsson LT. Assessment of fatigue in primary Sjogren's syndrome: the Swedish version of the Profile of Fatigue. Scand J Rheumatol. 2005;34(6):455–9. Epub 2006/01/06
62. Tench CM, McCarthy J, McCurdie I, White PD, D'Cruz DP. Fatigue in systemic lupus erythematosus: a randomized controlled trial of exercise. Rheumatology (Oxford). 2003;42(9):1050–4. Epub 2003/05/06
63. Linde L, Sorensen J, Ostergaard M, Horslev-Petersen K, Hetland ML. Health-related quality of life: validity, reliability, and responsiveness of SF-36, 15D, EQ-5D [corrected] RAQoL, and HAQ in patients with rheumatoid arthritis. J Rheumatol. 2008;35(8):1528–37. Epub 2008/05/20
64. Colangelo KJ, Pope JE, Peschken C. The minimally important difference for patient reported outcomes in systemic lupus erythematosus including the HAQ-DI, pain, fatigue, and SF-36. J Rheumatol. 2009;36(10):2231–7. Epub 2009/09/03
65. Devilliers H, Amoura Z, Besancenot JF, Bonnotte B, Pasquali JL, Wahl D, et al. Responsiveness of the 36-item Short Form Health Survey and the Lupus Quality of Life questionnaire in SLE. Rheumatology (Oxford). 2015;54(5):940–9. Epub 2014/11/02
66. McElhone K, Abbott J, Sutton C, Mullen M, Lanyon P, Rahman A, et al. Sensitivity to change and minimal important differences of the LupusQoL in patients with systemic lupus erythematosus. Arthritis Care Res (Hoboken). 2016;68(10):1505–13. Epub 2016/01/28
67. Nantes SG, Strand V, Su J, Touma Z. Comparison of the sensitivity to change of the 36-item short form health survey and the lupus quality of life measure using various definitions of minimum clinically important differences in patients with active systemic lupus erythematosus. Arthritis Care Res (Hoboken). 2018;70(1):125–33. Epub 2017/03/21
68. Touma Z, Gladman DD, Ibanez D, Urowitz MB. Is there an advantage over SF-36 with a quality of life measure that is specific to systemic lupus erythematosus? J Rheumatol. 2011;38(9):1898–905. Epub 2011/07/05
69. Baba S, Katsumata Y, Okamoto Y, Kawaguchi Y, Hanaoka M, Kawasumi H, et al. Reliability of the SF-36 in Japanese patients with systemic lupus erythematosus and its associations with disease activity and damage: a two-consecutive year prospective study. Lupus. 2018;27(3):407–16. Epub 2017/08/11

70. Thumboo J, Feng PH, Boey ML, Soh CH, Thio S, Fong KY. Validation of the Chinese SF-36 for quality of life assessment in patients with systemic lupus erythematosus. Lupus. 2000;9(9):708–12. Epub 2001/02/24
71. Thumboo J, Fong KY, Ng TP, Leong KH, Feng PH, Thio ST, et al. Validation of the MOS SF-36 for quality of life assessment of patients with systemic lupus erythematosus in Singapore. J Rheumatol. 1999;26(1):97–102. Epub 1999/01/26
72. Slatkowsky-Christensen B, Mowinckel P, Loge JH, Kvien TK. Health-related quality of life in women with symptomatic hand osteoarthritis: a comparison with rheumatoid arthritis patients, healthy controls, and normative data. Arthritis Rheum. 2007;57(8):1404–9. Epub 2007/12/01
73. Rohekar G, Pope J. Test-retest reliability of patient global assessment and physician global assessment in rheumatoid arthritis. J Rheumatol. 2009;36(10):2178–82. Epub 2009/09/17
74. d'Elia HF, Rehnberg E, Kvist G, Ericsson A, Konttinen Y, Mannerkorpi K. Fatigue and blood pressure in primary Sjogren's syndrome. Scand J Rheumatol. 2008;37(4):284–92. Epub 2008/07/10
75. McElhone K, Abbott J, Shelmerdine J, Bruce IN, Ahmad Y, Gordon C, et al. Development and validation of a disease-specific health-related quality of life measure, the LupusQol, for adults with systemic lupus erythematosus. Arthritis Rheum. 2007;57(6):972–9. Epub 2007/08/01
76. Downie WW, Leatham PA, Rhind VM, Wright V, Branco JA, Anderson JA. Studies with pain rating scales. Ann Rheum Dis. 1978;37(4):378–81. Epub 1978/08/01
77. Ferraz MB, Quaresma MR, Aquino LR, Atra E, Tugwell P, Goldsmith CH. Reliability of pain scales in the assessment of literate and illiterate patients with rheumatoid arthritis. J Rheumatol. 1990;17(8):1022–4. Epub 1990/08/01
78. Wollaston SJ, Farewell VT, Isenberg DA, Gordon C, Merrill JT, Petri MA, et al. Defining response in systemic lupus erythematosus: a study by the Systemic Lupus International Collaborating Clinics group. J Rheumatol. 2004;31(12):2390–4. Epub 2004/12/01
79. Joyce CR, Zutshi DW, Hrubes V, Mason RM. Comparison of fixed interval and visual analogue scales for rating chronic pain. Eur J Clin Pharmacol. 1975;8(6):415–20. Epub 1975/08/14
80. Brazier JE, Harper R, Jones NM, O'Cathain A, Thomas KJ, Usherwood T, et al. Validating the SF-36 health survey questionnaire: new outcome measure for primary care. BMJ. 1992;305(6846):160–4. Epub 1992/07/18
81. Quintana JM, Escobar A, Bilbao A, Arostegui I, Lafuente I, Vidaurreta I. Responsiveness and clinically important differences for the WOMAC and SF-36 after hip joint replacement. Osteoarthr Cartil. 2005;13(12):1076–83. Epub 2005/09/13
82. Escobar A, Quintana JM, Bilbao A, Arostegui I, Lafuente I, Vidaurreta I. Responsiveness and clinically important differences for the WOMAC and SF-36 after total knee replacement. Osteoarthr Cartil. 2007;15(3):273–80. Epub 2006/10/21
83. Koh ET, Leong KP, Tsou IY, Lim VH, Pong LY, Chong SY, et al. The reliability, validity and sensitivity to change of the Chinese version of SF-36 in oriental patients with rheumatoid arthritis. Rheumatology (Oxford). 2006;45(8):1023–8. Epub 2006/02/24
84. Bombardier C, Melfi CA, Paul J, Green R, Hawker G, Wright J, et al. Comparison of a generic and a disease-specific measure of pain and physical function after knee replacement surgery. Med Care. 1995;33(4 Suppl):AS131–44. Epub 1995/04/01
85. Salaffi F, Leardini G, Canesi B, Mannoni A, Fioravanti A, Caporali R, et al. Reliability and validity of the Western Ontario and McMaster Universities (WOMAC) Osteoarthritis Index in Italian patients with osteoarthritis of the knee. Osteoarthr Cartil. 2003;11(8):551–60. Epub 2003/07/26
86. Gandhi R, Tsvetkov D, Dhottar H, Davey JR, Mahomed NN. Quantifying the pain experience in hip and knee osteoarthritis. Pain Res Manag. 2010;15(4):224–8. Epub 2010/09/03

87. Devilliers H, Amoura Z, Besancenot JF, Bonnotte B, Pasquali JL, Wahl D, et al. LupusQoL-FR is valid to assess quality of life in patients with systemic lupus erythematosus. Rheumatology (Oxford). 2012;51(10):1906–15. Epub 2012/07/25
88. Anindito B, Hidayat R, Koesnoe S, Dewiasty E. Validity and reliability of lupus quality of life questionnaire in patients with systemic lupus erythematosus in Indonesia. Indones J Rheumatol. 2016;8(2)
89. Jolly M, Pickard AS, Wilke C, Mikolaitis RA, Teh LS, McElhone K, et al. Lupus-specific health outcome measure for US patients: the LupusQoL-US version. Ann Rheum Dis. 2010;69(1):29–33. Epub 2009/01/08
90. Meseguer-Henarejos AB, Gascon-Canovas JJ, Lopez-Pina JA. Components of quality of life in a sample of patients with lupus: a confirmatory factor analysis and Rasch modeling of the LupusQoL. Clin Rheumatol. 2017;36(8):1789–95. Epub 2017/05/04
91. Wang SL, Wu B, Leng L, Bucala R, Lu LJ. Validity of LupusQoL-China for the assessment of health related quality of life in Chinese patients with systemic lupus erythematosus. PLoS One. 2013;8(5):e63795. Epub 2013/05/30
92. Pamuk ON, Onat AM, Donmez S, Mengus C, Kisacik B. Validity and reliability of the Lupus QoL index in Turkish systemic lupus erythematosus patients. Lupus. 2015;24(8):816–21. Epub 2014/12/30
93. Bruce IN, Mak VC, Hallett DC, Gladman DD, Urowitz MB. Factors associated with fatigue in patients with systemic lupus erythematosus. Ann Rheum Dis. 1999;58(6):379–81. Epub 1999/05/26
94. Jump RL, Robinson ME, Armstrong AE, Barnes EV, Kilbourn KM, Richards HB. Fatigue in systemic lupus erythematosus: contributions of disease activity, pain, depression, and perceived social support. J Rheumatol. 2005;32(9):1699–705. Epub 2005/09/06
95. Tayer WG, Nicassio PM, Weisman MH, Schuman C, Daly J. Disease status predicts fatigue in systemic lupus erythematosus. J Rheumatol. 2001;28(9):1999–2007. Epub 2001/09/12
96. Wysenbeek AJ, Leibovici L, Weinberger A, Guedj D. Fatigue in systemic lupus erythematosus. Prevalence and relation to disease expression. Br J Rheumatol. 1993;32(7):633–5. Epub 1993/07/01
97. Krupp LB, LaRocca NG, Muir J, Steinberg AD. A study of fatigue in systemic lupus erythematosus. J Rheumatol. 1990;17(11):1450–2. Epub 1990/11/01
98. Staud R. Are patients with systemic lupus erythematosus at increased risk for fibromyalgia? Curr Rheumatol Rep. 2006;8(6):430–5. Epub 2006/11/10
99. Fung W, Lim LSH, Tomlinson G, Engel L, Su J, Diaz-Martinez JP, et al. Joint trajectories of disease activity, and physical and mental health-related quality of life in an inception lupus cohort. Rheumatology (Oxford). 2020;59:3032–41.
100. Valencia-Flores M, Cardiel MH, Santiago V, Resendiz M, Castano VA, Negrete O, et al. Prevalence and factors associated with fibromyalgia in Mexican patients with systemic lupus erythematosus. Lupus. 2004;13(1):4–10. Epub 2004/02/12
101. Pisetsky DS, Clowse MEB, Criscione-Schreiber LG, Rogers JL. A novel system to categorize the symptoms of systemic lupus erythematosus. Arthritis Care Res (Hoboken). 2019;71(6):735–41. Epub 2018/10/26
102. Giannouli S, Voulgarelis M, Ziakas PD, Tzioufas AG. Anaemia in systemic lupus erythematosus: from pathophysiology to clinical assessment. Ann Rheum Dis. 2006;65(2):144–8. Epub 2005/08/05
103. Voulgarelis M, Kokori SI, Ioannidis JP, Tzioufas AG, Kyriaki D, Moutsopoulos HM. Anaemia in systemic lupus erythematosus: aetiological profile and the role of erythropoietin. Ann Rheum Dis. 2000;59(3):217–22. Epub 2000/03/04
104. Wincup CR. A. Evaluating the prevalence of iron deficiency and anaemia in systemic lupus erythematosus. Rheumatology (Oxford). 2018;57
105. Domingues SL, Goncalves FT, Jorge M, Limongi JE, Ranza R, Jorge PT. High prevalence of hypothyroidism in systemic lupus erythematosus patients without an increase in circulating anti-thyroid antibodies. Endocr Pract. 2017;23(11):1304–10. Epub 2017/08/18

106. Klionsky Y, Antonelli M. Thyroid disease in lupus: an updated review. ACR Open Rheumatol. 2020;2(2):74–8. Epub 2020/02/12
107. Luo W, Mao P, Zhang L, Yang Z. Association between systemic lupus erythematosus and thyroid dysfunction: a meta-analysis. Lupus. 2018;27(13):2120–8. Epub 2018/10/31
108. Miller FW, Moore GF, Weintraub BD, Steinberg AD. Prevalence of thyroid disease and abnormal thyroid function test results in patients with systemic lupus erythematosus. Arthritis Rheum. 1987;30(10):1124–31. Epub 1987/10/01
109. Appenzeller S, Pallone AT, Natalin RA, Costallat LT. Prevalence of thyroid dysfunction in systemic lupus erythematosus. J Clin Rheumatol. 2009;15(3):117–9. Epub 2009/03/21
110. KakehasiI M, Dias V, Duarte J II, et al. Thyroid abnormalities in systemic lupus erythematosus: a study in 100 Brazilian patients. Rev Bras Reumatol. 2006;46(6)
111. Brey RL, Holliday SL, Saklad AR, Navarrete MG, Hermosillo-Romo D, Stallworth CL, et al. Neuropsychiatric syndromes in lupus: prevalence using standardized definitions. Neurology. 2002;58(8):1214–20. Epub 2002/04/24
112. Wang C, Mayo NE, Fortin PR. The relationship between health related quality of life and disease activity and damage in systemic lupus erythematosus. J Rheumatol. 2001;28(3):525–32. Epub 2001/04/12
113. Denburg SD, Carbotte RM, Denburg JA. Cognitive impairment in systemic lupus erythematosus: a neuropsychological study of individual and group deficits. J Clin Exp Neuropsychol. 1987;9(4):323–39. Epub 1987/08/01
114. Denburg SD, Carbotte RM, Ginsberg JS, Denburg JA. The relationship of antiphospholipid antibodies to cognitive function in patients with systemic lupus erythematosus. J Int Neuropsychol Soc. 1997;3(4):377–86. Epub 1997/07/01
115. Kozora E, West SG, Kotzin BL, Julian L, Porter S, Bigler E. Magnetic resonance imaging abnormalities and cognitive deficits in systemic lupus erythematosus patients without overt central nervous system disease. Arthritis Rheum. 1998;41(1):41–7. Epub 1998/01/20
116. Touma Z, Moghaddam B, Su J, Katz P. Cognitive function trajectories are associated with the depressive symptoms trajectories in systemic lupus erythematosus over time. Arthritis Care Res (Hoboken). 2020;
117. Rayes HA, Tani C, Kwan A, Marzouk S, Colosimo K, Medina-Rosas J, et al. What is the prevalence of cognitive impairment in lupus and which instruments are used to measure it? A systematic review and meta-analysis. Semin Arthritis Rheum. 2018;48(2):240–55.
118. Wiseman SJ, Bastin ME, Hamilton IF, Hunt D, Ritchie SJ, Amft EN, et al. Fatigue and cognitive function in systemic lupus erythematosus: associations with white matter microstructural damage. A diffusion tensor MRI study and meta-analysis. Lupus. 2017;26(6):588–97. Epub 2016/10/01
119. Zonana-Nacach A, Roseman JM, McGwin G Jr, Friedman AW, Baethge BA, Reveille JD, et al. Systemic lupus erythematosus in three ethnic groups. VI: Factors associated with fatigue within 5 years of criteria diagnosis. LUMINA Study Group. LUpus in MInority populations: NAture vs Nurture. Lupus. 2000;9(2):101–9. Epub 2000/04/29
120. Febbraio MA. Exercise metabolism in 2016: health benefits of exercise - more than meets the eye! Nat Rev Endocrinol. 2017;13(2):72–4. Epub 2017/01/05
121. Fiuza-Luces C, Santos-Lozano A, Joyner M, Carrera-Bastos P, Picazo O, Zugaza JL, et al. Exercise benefits in cardiovascular disease: beyond attenuation of traditional risk factors. Nat Rev Cardiol. 2018;15(12):731–43. Epub 2018/08/18
122. Gill DL, Hammond CC, Reifsteck EJ, Jehu CM, Williams RA, Adams MM, et al. Physical activity and quality of life. J Prev Med Public Health. 2013;46 Suppl 1:S28–34. Epub 2013/02/21
123. Warburton DER, Bredin SSD. Health benefits of physical activity: a systematic review of current systematic reviews. Curr Opin Cardiol. 2017;32(5):541–56. Epub 2017/07/15
124. Tench C, Bentley D, Vleck V, McCurdie I, White P, D'Cruz D. Aerobic fitness, fatigue, and physical disability in systemic lupus erythematosus. J Rheumatol. 2002;29(3):474–81. Epub 2002/03/23

125. Bostrom C, Dupre B, Tengvar P, Jansson E, Opava CH, Lundberg IE. Aerobic capacity correlates to self-assessed physical function but not to overall disease activity or organ damage in women with systemic lupus erythematosus with low-to-moderate disease activity and organ damage. Lupus. 2008;17(2):100–4. Epub 2008/02/06
126. Keyser RE, Rus V, Cade WT, Kalappa N, Flores RH, Handwerger BS. Evidence for aerobic insufficiency in women with systemic lupus erythematosus. Arthritis Rheum. 2003;49(1):16–22. Epub 2003/02/13
127. McMahon M, Grossman J, Skaggs B, Fitzgerald J, Sahakian L, Ragavendra N, et al. Dysfunctional proinflammatory high-density lipoproteins confer increased risk of atherosclerosis in women with systemic lupus erythematosus. Arthritis Rheum. 2009;60(8):2428–37. Epub 2009/08/01
128. Volkmann ER, Grossman JM, Sahakian LJ, Skaggs BJ, FitzGerald J, Ragavendra N, et al. Low physical activity is associated with proinflammatory high-density lipoprotein and increased subclinical atherosclerosis in women with systemic lupus erythematosus. Arthritis Care Res (Hoboken). 2010;62(2):258–65. Epub 2010/03/02
129. Mancuso CA, Perna M, Sargent AB, Salmon JE. Perceptions and measurements of physical activity in patients with systemic lupus erythematosus. Lupus. 2011;20(3):231–42. Epub 2010/12/25
130. Margiotta DPE, Basta F, Dolcini G, Batani V, Lo Vullo M, Vernuccio A, et al. Physical activity and sedentary behavior in patients with Systemic Lupus Erythematosus. PLoS One. 2018;13(3):e0193728. Epub 2018/03/06
131. O'Dwyer T, Durcan L, Wilson F. Exercise and physical activity in systemic lupus erythematosus: a systematic review with meta-analyses. Semin Arthritis Rheum. 2017;47(2):204–15. Epub 2017/05/10
132. Lipovskiy LBC, Seifert O. Reasons for deficiency of physical inactivity in patients with systemic lupus erythematosus. Ann Rheum Dis. 2017;76:308–9.
133. Robb-Nicholson LC, Daltroy L, Eaton H, Gall V, Wright E, Hartley LH, et al. Effects of aerobic conditioning in lupus fatigue: a pilot study. Br J Rheumatol. 1989;28(6):500–5. Epub 1989/12/01
134. Daltroy LH, Robb-Nicholson C, Iversen MD, Wright EA, Liang MH. Effectiveness of minimally supervised home aerobic training in patients with systemic rheumatic disease. Br J Rheumatol. 1995;34(11):1064–9. Epub 1995/11/01
135. Ramsey-Goldman R, Schilling EM, Dunlop D, Langman C, Greenland P, Thomas RJ, et al. A pilot study on the effects of exercise in patients with systemic lupus erythematosus. Arthritis Care Res. 2000;13(5):262–9. Epub 2003/11/26
136. Yuen HK, Cunningham MA. Optimal management of fatigue in patients with systemic lupus erythematosus: a systematic review. Ther Clin Risk Manag. 2014;10:775–86. Epub 2014/10/21
137. Katz P, Gregorich S, Yazdany J, Trupin L, Julian L, Yelin E, et al. Obesity and its measurement in a community-based sample of women with systemic lupus erythematosus. Arthritis Care Res (Hoboken). 2011;63(2):261–8. Epub 2010/09/09
138. Katz P, Yazdany J, Julian L, Trupin L, Margaretten M, Yelin E, et al. Impact of obesity on functioning among women with systemic lupus erythematosus. Arthritis Care Res (Hoboken). 2011;63(10):1357–64. Epub 2011/06/28
139. Petri M. Detection of coronary artery disease and the role of traditional risk factors in the Hopkins lupus cohort. Lupus. 2000;9(3):170–5. Epub 2000/05/11
140. Ellulu MS, Patimah I, Khaza'ai H, Rahmat A, Abed Y. Obesity and inflammation: the linking mechanism and the complications. Arch Med Sci. 2017;13(4):851–63. Epub 2017/07/20
141. Chaiamnuay S, Bertoli AM, Fernandez M, Apte M, Vila LM, Reveille JD, et al. The impact of increased body mass index on systemic lupus erythematosus: data from LUMINA, a multiethnic cohort (LUMINA XLVI) [corrected]. J Clin Rheumatol. 2007;13(3):128–33. Epub 2007/06/07

142. Oeser A, Chung CP, Asanuma Y, Avalos I, Stein CM. Obesity is an independent contributor to functional capacity and inflammation in systemic lupus erythematosus. Arthritis Rheum. 2005;52(11):3651–9. Epub 2005/11/01
143. Davies RJ, Lomer MC, Yeo SI, Avloniti K, Sangle SR, D'Cruz DP. Weight loss and improvements in fatigue in systemic lupus erythematosus: a controlled trial of a low glycaemic index diet versus a calorie restricted diet in patients treated with corticosteroids. Lupus. 2012;21(6):649–55. Epub 2012/02/09
144. Greenwood KM, Lederman L, Lindner HD. Self-reported sleep in systemic lupus erythematosus. Clin Rheumatol. 2008;27(9):1147–51. Epub 2008/04/15
145. Da Costa D, Bernatsky S, Dritsa M, Clarke AE, Dasgupta K, Keshani A, et al. Determinants of sleep quality in women with systemic lupus erythematosus. Arthritis Rheum. 2005;53(2):272–8. Epub 2005/04/09
146. Chandrasekhara PK, Jayachandran NV, Rajasekhar L, Thomas J, Narsimulu G. The prevalence and associations of sleep disturbances in patients with systemic lupus erythematosus. Mod Rheumatol. 2009;19(4):407–15. Epub 2009/06/13
147. D.D. C. Sleep and systemic lupus erythematosus. In: Verster JC, P-PSR, Streiner DL, editors. Sleep and quality of life in clinical medicine: Humana Press; 2008.
148. Iaboni A, Ibanez D, Gladman DD, Urowitz MB, Moldofsky H. Fatigue in systemic lupus erythematosus: contributions of disordered sleep, sleepiness, and depression. J Rheumatol. 2006;33(12):2453–7. Epub 2006/12/05
149. Valencia-Flores M, Resendiz M, Castano VA, Santiago V, Campos RM, Sandino S, et al. Objective and subjective sleep disturbances in patients with systemic lupus erythematosus. Arthritis Rheum. 1999;42(10):2189–93. Epub 1999/10/19
150. Hassanalilou T, Khalili L, Ghavamzadeh S, Shokri A, Payahoo L, Bishak YK. Role of vitamin D deficiency in systemic lupus erythematosus incidence and aggravation. Auto Immun Highlights. 2017;9(1):1. Epub 2017/12/28
151. Huisman AM, White KP, Algra A, Harth M, Vieth R, Jacobs JW, et al. Vitamin D levels in women with systemic lupus erythematosus and fibromyalgia. J Rheumatol. 2001;28(11):2535–9. Epub 2001/11/16
152. Kamen DL, Cooper GS, Bouali H, Shaftman SR, Hollis BW, Gilkeson GS. Vitamin D deficiency in systemic lupus erythematosus. Autoimmun Rev. 2006;5(2):114–7. Epub 2006/01/25
153. Muller K, Kriegbaum NJ, Baslund B, Sorensen OH, Thymann M, Bentzen K. Vitamin D3 metabolism in patients with rheumatic diseases: low serum levels of 25-hydroxyvitamin D3 in patients with systemic lupus erythematosus. Clin Rheumatol. 1995;14(4):397–400. Epub 1995/07/01
154. Ruiz-Irastorza G, Egurbide MV, Olivares N, Martinez-Berriotxoa A, Aguirre C. Vitamin D deficiency in systemic lupus erythematosus: prevalence, predictors and clinical consequences. Rheumatology (Oxford). 2008;47(6):920–3. Epub 2008/04/16
155. Ruiz-Irastorza G, Gordo S, Olivares N, Egurbide MV, Aguirre C. Changes in vitamin D levels in patients with systemic lupus erythematosus: effects on fatigue, disease activity, and damage. Arthritis Care Res (Hoboken). 2010;62(8):1160–5. Epub 2010/03/18
156. Nguyen MH, Bryant K, O'Neill SG. Vitamin D in SLE: a role in pathogenesis and fatigue? A review of the literature. Lupus. 2018;27(13):2003–11. Epub 2018/08/31
157. Karimzadeh H, Shirzadi M, Karimifar M. The effect of Vitamin D supplementation in disease activity of systemic lupus erythematosus patients with Vitamin D deficiency: a randomized clinical trial. J Res Med Sci. 2017;22:4. Epub 2017/04/13
158. Sousa JR, Rosa EPC, Nunes I, Carvalho C. Effect of vitamin D supplementation on patients with systemic lupus erythematosus: a systematic review. Rev Bras Reumatol Engl Ed. 2017;57(5):466–71. Epub 2017/10/19
159. Torrente-Segarra V, Monte TCS, Corominas H. Musculoskeletal involvement and ultrasonography update in systemic lupus erythematosus: new insights and review. Eur J Rheumatol. 2018;5(2):127–30. Epub 2018/09/06

160. Zayat AS, Md Yusof MY, Wakefield RJ, Conaghan PG, Emery P, Vital EM. The role of ultrasound in assessing musculoskeletal symptoms of systemic lupus erythematosus: a systematic literature review. Rheumatology (Oxford). 2016;55(3):485–94. Epub 2015/10/09
161. Umare V, Pradhan V, Nadkar M, Rajadhyaksha A, Patwardhan M, Ghosh KK, et al. Effect of proinflammatory cytokines (IL-6, TNF-alpha, and IL-1beta) on clinical manifestations in Indian SLE patients. Mediat Inflamm. 2014;2014:385297. Epub 2014/12/31
162. Ohl K, Tenbrock K. Inflammatory cytokines in systemic lupus erythematosus. J Biomed Biotechnol. 2011;2011:432595. Epub 2011/10/27
163. Eilertsen GO, Nikolaisen C, Becker-Merok A, Nossent JC. Interleukin-6 promotes arthritis and joint deformation in patients with systemic lupus erythematosus. Lupus. 2011;20(6):607–13. Epub 2011/03/23
164. Cuadrado MJ, Sanna G. Headache and systemic lupus erythematosus. Lupus. 2003;12(12):943–6. Epub 2004/01/13
165. Glanz BI, Venkatesan A, Schur PH, Lew RA, Khoshbin S. Prevalence of migraine in patients with systemic lupus erythematosus. Headache. 2001;41(3):285–9. Epub 2001/03/27
166. Sfikakis PP, Mitsikostas DD, Manoussakis MN, Foukaneli D, Moutsopoulos HM. Headache in systemic lupus erythematosus: a controlled study. Br J Rheumatol. 1998;37(3):300–3. Epub 1998/05/05
167. Mitsikostas DD, Sfikakis PP, Goadsby PJ. A meta-analysis for headache in systemic lupus erythematosus: the evidence and the myth. Brain. 2004;127(Pt 5):1200–9. Epub 2004/03/30
168. Sanna G, Bertolaccini ML, Cuadrado MJ, Khamashta MA, Hughes GR. Central nervous system involvement in the antiphospholipid (Hughes) syndrome. Rheumatology (Oxford). 2003;42(2):200–13. Epub 2003/02/22
169. Tanasescu R, Nicolau A, Caraiola S, Ticmeanu M, Cojocaru IM, Frasineanu A, et al. Antiphospholipid antibodies and migraine: a retrospective study of 428 patients with inflammatory connective tissue diseases. Rom J Intern Med. 2007;45(4):355–63. Epub 2008/09/05
170. Pryor WA, Stone K. Oxidants in cigarette smoke. Radicals, hydrogen peroxide, peroxynitrate, and peroxynitrite. Ann N Y Acad Sci. 1993;686:12–27; discussion -8. Epub 1993/05/28
171. Prouse PJ, Thompson EM, Gumpel JM. Systemic lupus erythematosus and abdominal pain. Br J Rheumatol. 1983;22(3):172–5. Epub 1983/08/01
172. Tian XP, Zhang X. Gastrointestinal involvement in systemic lupus erythematosus: insight into pathogenesis, diagnosis and treatment. World J Gastroenterol. 2010;16(24):2971–7. Epub 2010/06/24
173. Kirby JM, Jhaveri KS, Maizlin ZV, Midia M, Haider E, Khalili K. Abdominal manifestations of systemic lupus erythematosus: spectrum of imaging findings. Can Assoc Radiol J. 2009;60(3):121–32. Epub 2009/07/14
174. Lee CK, Ahn MS, Lee EY, Shin JH, Cho YS, Ha HK, et al. Acute abdominal pain in systemic lupus erythematosus: focus on lupus enteritis (gastrointestinal vasculitis). Ann Rheum Dis. 2002;61(6):547–50. Epub 2002/05/15
175. Chehab G, Carnarius H, Schneider M. What matters for lupus patients? Presse Med. 2014;43(6 Pt 2):e197–207. Epub 2014/05/06
176. Inoue M, Shiozawa K, Yoshihara R, Yamane T, Shima Y, Hirano T, et al. Predictors of poor sleep quality in patients with systemic lupus erythematosus. Clin Rheumatol. 2017;36(5):1053–62. Epub 2017/02/01
177. Vina ER, Green SL, Trivedi T, Kwoh CK, Utset TO. Correlates of sleep abnormalities in systemic lupus: a cross-sectional survey in an urban, academic center. J Clin Rheumatol. 2013;19(1):7–13. Epub 2013/01/16
178. Kasitanon N, Achsavalertsak U, Maneeton B, Wangkaew S, Puntana S, Sukitawut W, et al. Associated factors and psychotherapy on sleep disturbances in systemic lupus erythematosus. Lupus. 2013;22(13):1353–60. Epub 2013/10/02
179. Gudbjornsson B, Hetta J. Sleep disturbances in patients with systemic lupus erythematosus: a questionnaire-based study. Clin Exp Rheumatol. 2001;19(5):509–14. Epub 2001/10/03

180. Ekblom-Kullberg S, Kautiainen H, Alha P, Leirisalo-Repo M, Julkunen H. Smoking and the risk of systemic lupus erythematosus. Clin Rheumatol. 2013;32(8):1219–22. Epub 2013/03/22
181. Ghaussy NO, Sibbitt WL Jr, Qualls CR. Cigarette smoking, alcohol consumption, and the risk of systemic lupus erythematosus: a case-control study. J Rheumatol. 2001;28(11):2449–53. Epub 2001/11/16
182. Speyer CB, Costenbader KH. Cigarette smoking and the pathogenesis of systemic lupus erythematosus. Expert Rev Clin Immunol. 2018;14(6):481–7. Epub 2018/05/05
183. Arnson Y, Shoenfeld Y, Amital H. Effects of tobacco smoke on immunity, inflammation and autoimmunity. J Autoimmun. 2010;34(3):J258–65. Epub 2010/01/01
184. Freemer MM, King TE Jr, Criswell LA. Association of smoking with dsDNA autoantibody production in systemic lupus erythematosus. Ann Rheum Dis. 2006;65(5):581–4. Epub 2005/09/10
185. Yunus MB, Arslan S, Aldag JC. Relationship between fibromyalgia features and smoking. Scand J Rheumatol. 2002;31(5):301–5. Epub 2002/11/29
186. Bourre-Tessier J, Peschken CA, Bernatsky S, Joseph L, Clarke AE, Fortin PR, et al. Association of smoking with cutaneous manifestations in systemic lupus erythematosus. Arthritis Care Res (Hoboken). 2013;65(8):1275–80. Epub 2013/02/13
187. Turchin I, Bernatsky S, Clarke AE, St-Pierre Y, Pineau CA. Cigarette smoking and cutaneous damage in systemic lupus erythematosus. J Rheumatol. 2009;36(12):2691–3. Epub 2009/11/04
188. Ghaussy NO, Sibbitt W Jr, Bankhurst AD, Qualls CR. Cigarette smoking and disease activity in systemic lupus erythematosus. J Rheumatol. 2003;30(6):1215–21. Epub 2003/06/05
189. Barta Z, Harrison MJ, Wangrangsimakul T, Shelmerdine J, Teh LS, Pattrick M, et al. Health-related quality of life, smoking and carotid atherosclerosis in white British women with systemic lupus erythematosus. Lupus. 2010;19(3):231–8. Epub 2009/12/17
190. Montes RA, Mocarzel LO, Lanzieri PG, Lopes LM, Carvalho A, Almeida JR. Smoking and its Association with Morbidity in Systemic Lupus Erythematosus Evaluated by the Systemic Lupus International Collaborating Clinics/American College of Rheumatology Damage Index: Preliminary Data and Systematic Review. Arthritis Rheumatol. 2016;68(2):441–8. Epub 2015/09/12
191. Gualano B, Bonfa E, Pereira RMR, Silva CA. Physical activity for paediatric rheumatic diseases: standing up against old paradigms. Nat Rev Rheumatol. 2017;13(6):368–79. Epub 2017/05/24
192. Sharif K, Watad A, Bragazzi NL, Lichtbroun M, Amital H, Shoenfeld Y. Physical activity and autoimmune diseases: get moving and manage the disease. Autoimmun Rev. 2018;17(1):53–72. Epub 2017/11/08
193. Beavers KM, Brinkley TE, Nicklas BJ. Effect of exercise training on chronic inflammation. Clin Chim Acta. 2010;411(11–12):785–93. Epub 2010/03/02
194. Barnes JN, Tanaka H. Cardiovascular benefits of habitual exercise in systemic lupus erythematosus: a review. Phys Sportsmed. 2012;40(3):43–8. Epub 2013/03/27
195. Perandini LA, Sales-de-Oliveira D, Mello SB, Camara NO, Benatti FB, Lima FR, et al. Exercise training can attenuate the inflammatory milieu in women with systemic lupus erythematosus. J Appl Physiol (1985). 2014;117(6):639–47. Epub 2014/07/20
196. Yuen HK, Holthaus K, Kamen DL, Sword DO, Breland HL. Using Wii Fit to reduce fatigue among African American women with systemic lupus erythematosus: a pilot study. Lupus. 2011;20(12):1293–9. Epub 2011/06/28
197. Bogdanovic G, Stojanovich L, Djokovic A, Stanisavljevic N. Physical activity program is helpful for improving quality of life in patients with systemic lupus erythematosus. Tohoku J Exp Med. 2015;237(3):193–9. Epub 2015/10/23
198. An MP, IH. Effect of stretching exercise on depression, pain, and fatigue in patients with systemic lupus erythematosus. J Muscle Joint Health. 2006;13(1):43–52.

199. Ayan C, Martin V. Systemic lupus erythematosus and exercise. Lupus. 2007;16(1):5–9. Epub 2007/02/08
200. Carvalho MR, Sato EI, Tebexreni AS, Heidecher RT, Schenkman S, Neto TL. Effects of supervised cardiovascular training program on exercise tolerance, aerobic capacity, and quality of life in patients with systemic lupus erythematosus. Arthritis Rheum. 2005;53(6):838–44. Epub 2005/12/13
201. Clarke-Jenssen AC, Fredriksen PM, Lilleby V, Mengshoel AM. Effects of supervised aerobic exercise in patients with systemic lupus erythematosus: a pilot study. Arthritis Rheum. 2005;53(2):308–12. Epub 2005/04/09

# Chapter 16
# Frailty: An Emerging Concept in Lupus

**John G. Hanly and Alexandra Legge**

## The Concept of Frailty

Individuals of the same chronological age vary considerably in terms of their health status and life expectancy. Similar observations have been made in nonhuman species, whereby same-strain animals raised in controlled environments will develop age-related diseases and die at variable rates [1]. This unmeasured variability in the risk of death among people of the same age gave rise to the term "frailty" [2]. The concept has since been generalized to describe the propensity for certain individuals to experience greater susceptibility to adverse health outcomes than others despite comparable exposures [3].

While the concept of frailty initially emerged through the study of community-dwelling older adults [4], frailty has since become a topic of interest across a wide range of medical disciplines [5–8]. A more recent area of inquiry has been the evaluation of frailty in populations where accelerated aging is commonly observed, such as disease-specific cohorts of patients with hematologic malignancies or individuals living with HIV infection [5, 8]. Frailty may be particularly relevant in a complex, multisystem disease like systemic lupus erythematosus (SLE), where the risk of morbidity and mortality is increased compared with similarly aged individuals without SLE and where significant unexplained heterogeneity in health outcomes exists between patients.

J. G. Hanly (✉)
Division of Rheumatology, Department of Medicine, and Department of Pathology, Dalhousie University and Queen Elizabeth II Health Sciences Centre, Halifax, NS, Canada
e-mail: john.hanly@nshealth.ca

A. Legge
Division of Rheumatology, Department of Medicine, Dalhousie University and Queen Elizabeth II Health Sciences Centre, Halifax, NS, Canada
e-mail: alex.legge@dal.ca

 
Z. Touma (ed.), *Outcome Measures and Metrics in Systemic Lupus Erythematosus*, https://doi.org/10.1007/978-3-030-73303-2_16

There is also biological plausibility for the hypothesis that frailty may play a significant role in the disproportionately poor outcomes observed among individuals with SLE. The link between chronic inflammation and frailty is well recognized. Elevated levels of systemic inflammatory markers have been observed among frail, older adults when compared to those who are not frail [9]. Furthermore, specific pro-inflammatory cytokines, such as interleukin-6, have been implicated in the pathogenesis of both frailty and SLE [9, 10]. While the role of immune dysregulation in the development of frailty has yet to be fully elucidated, this represents a potential mechanism for accelerated aging among individuals with SLE.

Conceptually, frailty can be defined as a diminished capacity to withstand and recover from stressors due to a loss of physiologic reserve [3]. Thus, a definitive diagnosis of frailty can only be made retrospectively by observing a disproportionately poor response to a stressful event, such as a critical illness or major surgery. However, in order for frailty to be useful clinically, it must be identified prior to an inciting event to allow opportunity for intervention. Therefore, alternative strategies are required to estimate the probability of frailty prospectively, using the gold standard definition of frailty as a reference.

While the conceptual definition of frailty is generally accepted, there is debate regarding how best to measure frailty in clinical settings, and various types of instruments have been developed [11, 12]. The two main approaches for operationalizing frailty are (1) the phenotypic approach and (2) the deficit accumulation approach [13]. These two approaches have different strengths and limitations, and together they provide valuable and complementary information [13]. Both approaches have been successfully applied to measure frailty among individuals with SLE [14, 15].

## The Phenotypic Approach to Frailty

The phenotypic approach views frailty as a clinical syndrome characterized by a cluster of physiologic signs and symptoms commonly observed in vulnerable older adults. The frailty phenotype arises through the progressive age-related loss of muscle mass and strength known as sarcopenia, which is accelerated in frail individuals [16]. The phenotypic approach views sarcopenia as the biological substrate and key pathophysiologic mechanism leading to physical frailty [17, 18], which is characterized clinically by a cycle of decline with concurrent reductions in physical activity, gait speed, muscle strength, energy level, and nutritional status [16]. Thus, in this operational definition, frailty is a biological syndrome of aging that is multifactorial in etiology but leads to the common pathway of sarcopenia, manifested clinically via the five phenotypic criteria listed above.

## *The Fried Frailty Phenotype*

The original frailty phenotype (Table 16.1), published in 2001 by Fried and colleagues [16], determined the presence or absence of frailty based on five clinical criteria: weight loss (≥10 pounds or ≥5% unintentional weight loss over the prior year), exhaustion (based on self-report), physical inactivity (lowest quintile based on the Minnesota Leisure Time Activities Questionnaire), slow walking speed (lowest quintile based on a timed 15 meter walk), and reduced grip strength (lowest quintile based on dynamometric measurement) [16]. Individuals meeting three or more of these criteria were classified as frail, those with one or two criteria were said to be pre-frail, and those meeting none of the criteria were considered non-frail or robust [16].

The Fried frailty phenotype was first evaluated using observational data from the Cardiovascular Health Study, which included over 5000 community-dwelling adults aged 65 years or older in the United States. Seven percent of participants were classified as frail at baseline [16]. Construct validity was assessed by measuring self-reported disability and chronic disease concurrently [16]. While significant overlap was observed between disability, chronic illness, and frailty, many frail participants neither were disabled nor did they have comorbid medical illness [16]. This supports the hypothesis that phenotypic frailty is a distinct biological entity independent of disability and chronic disease.

Predictive validity analyses from the Cardiovascular Health Study demonstrated that individuals meeting the phenotypic criteria for frailty were at significantly higher risk for incident falls, worsening mobility, functional disability, hospitalization, and mortality [16]. Pre-frailty status showed intermediate risk for these

**Table 16.1** Phenotypic criteria for frailty

| The following five criteria are used to define phenotypic frailty: |
|---|
| 1. Weight loss (≥10 pounds or ≥5% unintentional weight loss over the past year) |
| 2. Exhaustion (based on self-report) |
| 3. Physical inactivity (lowest quintile on the Minnesota Leisure Time Activities Questionnaire) |
| 4. Slow gait speed (lowest quintile based on a timed 15 meter walk) |
| 5. Reduced grip strength (lowest quintile based on dynamometric measurement) |
| Based on the presence or absence of these five criteria, individuals are classified as follows: |
| Non-frail: None of the above criteria met |
| Pre-frail: One or two criteria met |
| Frail: Three or more criteria met |

Adapted from the criteria originally described by Fried et al. [16]

outcomes [16], demonstrating a dose-response relationship. Pre-frailty was also associated with increased risk of fulfilling the criteria for phenotypic frailty over time [16]. These results have subsequently been confirmed in several large cohort studies of older adults [19, 20], as well as in multiple systematic reviews and meta-analyses [21–24].

Since its initial publication, the Fried phenotype has become a popular clinical and research tool for identifying frailty in older adults [11]. However, strategies for identifying phenotypic criteria have varied across studies, and a recent systematic review identified 262 modifications to the original Fried phenotype [25]. Physical inactivity and weight loss are the most frequently modified criteria [25]. Such modifications result in significant variability in estimates of the prevalence of frailty, as well as differences in the predictive validity of the frailty phenotype for mortality risk [25]. Therefore, the comparability of studies using different modifications of the original Fried criteria for frailty is very limited. Furthermore, many of these modified definitions of phenotypic frailty have not been adequately validated.

## *Advantages of the Phenotypic Approach*

As phenotypic frailty arises as a consequence of underlying sarcopenia, a major strength of this approach is its physiologic basis [17, 18], which contributes to its content validity. This positions frailty as a separate biological entity distinct from other concepts such as disability and comorbidity [26]. As a result, the evaluation of phenotypic frailty is a novel addition to clinical assessment that lacks redundancy with other measures. Thus, the frailty phenotype facilitates evaluation of the specific impact of sarcopenia and resultant physical frailty on health outcomes, independent of other prognostic factors. Finally, with only five criteria, phenotypic frailty can be assessed in less than 10 minutes, allowing it to be incorporated into clinical practice with relative ease [12].

Another advantage of operationalizing frailty using a sarcopenic phenotype is that it allows clinicians to address frailty using therapeutic interventions that specifically target sarcopenia [26]. Individuals with sarcopenia benefit from interventions such as physical activity programs and nutritional supplementation that help increase muscle mass and improve strength [17]. A randomized trial of community-dwelling older adults confirmed that physical activity, nutritional, cognitive, and combined interventions are capable of significantly reducing the prevalence of phenotypic frailty when compared to usual care [27]. Thus, defining frailty as a clinical syndrome driven by sarcopenia not only facilitates its identification but also its treatment.

## *Disadvantages of the Phenotypic Approach*

One limitation of the Fried frailty phenotype is its lack of granularity, as it only identifies three risk categories – frail, pre-frail, and non-frail. In some populations, such as community-dwelling older adults, there is a possible floor effect, with the majority of individuals being classified as non-frail [28]. This issue may be less problematic in chronic disease populations, where the proportion of individuals who are either frail or pre-frail is expected to be higher. Still, this characterization of frailty as an all-or-none phenomenon does not account for differences in susceptibility to adverse outcomes between individuals with varying degrees of frailty, which may necessitate different treatment approaches.

From a practical standpoint, evaluation of the Fried phenotype includes physical performance measures that require specialized equipment and trained assessors, which may be barriers to implementation in certain settings [12]. Furthermore, data regarding some components of the phenotype, such as grip strength and gait speed, are less likely to be available in pre-existing health datasets, limiting the feasibility of evaluating phenotypic frailty using secondary data sources. Finally, this approach does not capture psychosocial and cognitive factors that may also contribute to vulnerability and lead to disproportionately poor health outcomes in certain individuals. To address this shortcoming, separate assessments of other domains such as disability, comorbidity, and cognition [26] are required.

## *Phenotypic Frailty in Chronic Disease Populations*

The Fried frailty phenotype has been applied to study unexplained variability in health outcomes in specific chronic disease populations. Chronic medical conditions are associated with many of the underpinnings of sarcopenia, including mitochondrial dysfunction, inadequate nutrition, malabsorption, disuse atrophy, and elevated levels of pro-inflammatory cytokines [17]. Thus, the prevalence of phenotypic frailty is expected to be increased among patients with chronic diseases compared to the general population. Indeed, up to 54% of patients with congestive heart failure [29] and up to 73% of patients on chronic hemodialysis [30] meet the phenotypic criteria for frailty. In these populations, the prevalence of frailty tends to increase with increasing disease severity [29–31]. The Fried phenotype also consistently predicts adverse health outcomes such as hospitalizations and mortality in chronic disease populations, including among individuals with chronic kidney disease [30], congestive heart failure [29], and chronic obstructive pulmonary disease [31, 32].

## *Phenotypic Frailty in SLE*

Several of the individual elements comprising the frailty phenotype have been observed with increased frequency among SLE patients, including muscle weakness [33, 34], fatigue [33, 35, 36], and physical inactivity [37, 38]. Furthermore, higher rates of objectively measured sarcopenia have been noted among SLE patients compared to healthy controls [39], with increased risk of sarcopenia among SLE patients with more active disease and higher levels of systemic inflammation [39]. Based on these findings, it is hypothesized that the prevalence of phenotypic frailty may be increased among SLE patients, which may contribute to the increased risk of adverse health outcomes that is observed in this population.

In 2017, Katz and colleagues evaluated the frailty phenotype in a prevalent cohort of 152 women with SLE [14]. This study used the original Fried criteria for phenotypic frailty with slight variations in the definitions of weight loss and physical inactivity. Overall, 20.4% of SLE patients were classified as frail and 50.7% as pre-frail [14], which is a substantially higher prevalence of frailty when compared to similarly aged women in the general population, where the prevalence of frailty is typically reported to be less than 10% [40]. This is perhaps unsurprising when one considers the many factors that could potentially contribute to the accelerated development of sarcopenia in patients with SLE.

Among the 152 women with SLE in the study by Katz et al., the presence of frailty at baseline was associated with greater functional disability and higher rates of cognitive impairment [14]. Each of the five individual frailty criteria was also significantly associated with concurrent physical function, demonstrating internal consistency. However, the association between phenotypic frailty and physical function was not fully explained by the individual effects of the five frailty components alone, highlighting the importance of the cumulative effect of these variables.

In the same study by Katz et al., predictive validity analyses showed that women with SLE who were classified as frail at baseline were at increased risk of experiencing functional decline and cognitive impairment during follow-up [14]. Furthermore, during a mean follow-up time of 7.2 years, the risk of death among frail women with SLE was nearly six times higher than the mortality risk among robust women, even after adjusting for age, SLE disease duration, and baseline organ damage [14]. Overall, these results suggest that the frailty phenotype is relevant in SLE and warrants further study in this population.

## The Deficit Accumulation Approach to Frailty

The deficit accumulation approach views frailty as a multidimensional risk state that can be measured by counting an individual's health problems [41, 42]. In this model, frailty reflects a stochastic dynamic process in a system with high redundancy of multiple interdependent items. As deficits accumulate, they impair the ability of the system to recover from their impact and withstand future insults [41, 42]. In other words, this approach suggests that frailty is a loss of physiologic reserve that arises from the accumulation of health deficits over time. As health deficits accumulate with increasing age, they impair the ability of the individual to respond to and recover from future health challenges (Fig. 16.1). Individuals with few deficits are relatively fit, while those with an increasing number of health deficits are considered increasingly frail and therefore at greater risk for future adverse health outcomes. Because individuals may accrue health deficits at different rates, the deficit accumulation approach aids in our understanding of the differential vulnerability to adverse outcomes observed between individuals of the same chronological age.

That many small effects can aggregate to produce larger ones is well recognized in other disciplines, such as computer science. Applying this principle in medicine allows us to capture the cumulative effect of numerous small deficits, which individually may lack statistical significance but, once combined, will have clinically meaningful impact. In this approach to operationalizing frailty, it is the number of health deficits that is felt to be important, with less emphasis placed on the presence or absence of specific, individual risk factors.

With aging, individual health deficits may accumulate in varying patterns, from increasing slowly at a near-constant rate to either negative or upward curvature. However, when considered as a group, these varying health deficits will demonstrate a typical pattern of slow, gradual accumulation across the lifespan. As health deficits accumulate and individuals become more frail, alterations in disease risk and expression occur, which can have important implications for both prognostication and management. Thus, measuring frailty in clinical settings via the quantification of health deficits may allow for more personalized and patient-centered care.

## *Quantifying Deficit Accumulation Using a Frailty Index*

The deficit accumulation approach to frailty can be operationalized using the frailty index (FI) [13]. An FI can be developed from any existing health dataset using a standard procedure (Table 16.2) previously outlined by Searle and colleagues [43]. In brief, a frailty index is constructed using a set of health deficits, where a single health deficit can be any symptom, physical sign, disease process, functional impairment, or laboratory abnormality meeting the criteria of being acquired, associated with adverse health outcomes, and associated with increasing chronological age [43]. Importantly, there is no requirement for each individual health deficit to have a statistically significant association with either age or adverse outcomes. Instead, the FI combines many small pieces of information from different health domains into a single variable that represents their cumulative effect on an individual's health.

If deficits are either too infrequent (prevalence <1%) or too common (prevalence >80%) in the dataset, they are unlikely to help differentiate between individuals with respect to their risk of adverse outcomes and thus should be excluded [43].

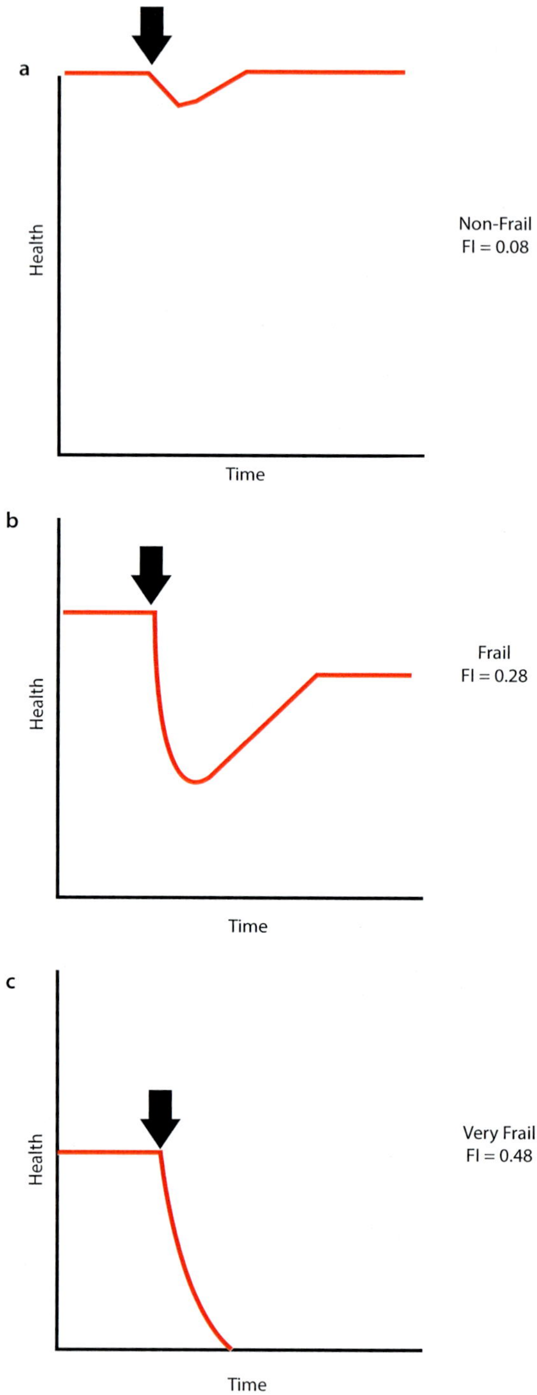


**Fig. 16.1** The impact of deficit accumulation on recovery from health challenges, using a hypothetical frailty index (FI) comprised of 50 health deficits. The black arrows represent the occurrence of an inciting health event (e.g., a critical illness or major surgery). (**a**) This individual possesses only 4 of the 50 health deficits, resulting in an FI score of 0.08. With this FI score, they are considered non-frail or robust. A new insult may only result in a minor disruption in their overall health status, with rapid recovery back to their previous baseline. (**b**) With 14 of the 50 total deficits and a resulting FI score of 0.28, this individual would be considered frail. A new health challenge may cause them to become more unwell. Recovery will be slower, and they may never fully recover back to their previous baseline. (**c**) An individual with 24 of the 50 health deficits would be considered severely frail, based on an FI score of 0.48. They may not have enough physiologic reserve to withstand an additional health insult and may die as a result. (Modified from Legge et al. *Curr Treat Options Rheumatol* (2020). https://doi.org/10.1007/s40674-020-00150-1)

**Table 16.2** Selection of health deficits for inclusion in a frailty index

| *Definition of a health deficit:* |
|---|
| Any health variable, such as a symptom, physical sign, disease process, functional impairment, or laboratory/radiographic abnormality |
| *Criteria to be met by each individual health deficit:* |
| 1. Must be acquired, as opposed to innate |
| 2. Must be associated with adverse health outcomes |
| 3. Prevalence typically increases with increasing chronological age |
| 4. Must be present in at least 1%, but no more than 80% of the sample |
| 5. Must have non-missing values for at least 95% of the sample |
| *Criteria to be met by the overall set of health deficits:* |
| 1. Must cover a range of physiologic organ systems |
| 2. Must include variables indicative of repair potential, such as measures of functional status, resiliency, and other health protective factors |
| 3. Must include at least 30–40 health deficits in total |
| *An individual's frailty index score should only be calculated if there are non-missing values for at least 80% of included health deficits.* |

Adapted from the process for constructing a frailty index outlined by Searle et al. [43]

Likewise, if a single item is missing values for >5% of the sample, it should not be included as a health deficit in an FI [43]. Finally, an individual's FI score should only be calculated if there are non-missing values for at least 80% of the included health deficits.

As a whole, the health deficits included in an FI must cover several organ systems. Furthermore, frailty not only is a measure of cumulative organ damage but also quantifies an individual's potential for recovery or repair. Therefore, in addition to disease manifestations and comorbidities, a frailty index must also include other variables that can impact repair potential, including measures of function, mobility, resiliency, and other health protective factors [43]. As a result, FI scores have the potential to fluctuate up and down over time, thereby reflecting dynamic changes in health status throughout the life course.

Once identified, each health deficit in the FI is assigned a scoring system from 0 to 1, with a score of 0 representing complete absence of the deficit, a score of 1 representing the deficit fully expressed, and intermediate scores indicating partial expression [43]. Finally, individual deficits are combined to produce an FI score, which is a proportion, between 0 and 1, calculated from the sum of individual health deficit scores divided by the total number of deficits that were considered [43]. For example, using an FI consisting of 40 deficits, an individual in whom ten of the health deficits are fully expressed would have an FI score of 10/40 = 0.25. As individuals may become frail via multiple different pathways, a large number of variables are typically required in order to capture all aspects of frailty. Prior studies suggest that at least 30–40 health deficits should be included in an FI in order to achieve stable and precise estimates of frailty [44].

## *Properties of the Frailty Index*

Previous work in community-dwelling older adults has demonstrated remarkably consistent properties for the FI across a wide range of study designs and settings. In general, FI scores in these population samples of older adults tend to approximate a gamma distribution [43, 45]. The majority of people exhibit relatively low FI scores resulting in positive skew, while a small number of more frail individuals are represented by the long, right-sided tail of the distribution. The nonlinear rate of deficit accumulation with increasing age has also remained stable across different cohorts, with individuals accumulating deficits at an average rate of 3% per year on a logarithmic scale after the age of 70 [43, 45–48]. Women consistently accumulate more deficits than men of similar age, yielding higher FI scores [44, 45]. In addition, there appears to be a biological limit to the number of health deficits an individual can accumulate, beyond which any further deficit accumulation is incompatible with life. FI measures have consistently demonstrated a 99% submaximal limit of approximately 0.70, or 70% of the total deficits considered [43, 45, 48, 49]. Depending on the prevalence and information value of the health deficits included in a particular FI, a slightly lower submaximal limit may be observed. Finally, across all studies, the FI has shown predictive validity for future adverse health outcomes. Higher FI values have been consistently associated with increased risk of falls, fractures, hospitalization, institutionalization, and mortality [24, 43, 45, 50, 51].

The reproducibility of the above findings is impressive, given that these studies utilized separate datasets and incorporated different types and numbers of health deficits, based on data availability. To further illustrate the construct validity of the FI approach, one study re-calculated FI scores using 80% of its total health deficits, randomly selected [43]. In 1000 iterations to this procedure, the properties of the FI remained unchanged, suggesting that it is the cumulative effect of deficit accumulation, and not the isolated effects of specific health deficits, that is important [43]. Remarkably, with respect to the FI, it is not necessary to measure the same items, or even the same number of items, in order to achieve similar results.

In studies comparing the phenotypic and deficit accumulation approaches to identify frailty in older adults, FI scores greater than 0.21–0.25 have been consistently associated with phenotypic frailty [48]. Therefore, FI scores in this range have been utilized as cutoff values to identify frail individuals [40]. Studies evaluating minimally important differences in FI scores have suggested that changes in the FI by more than 0.03 are clinically meaningful.

## *Advantages of the Deficit Accumulation Approach*

The generalizability of the FI approach is seen as one of its major strengths. The validity of the FI has been demonstrated not only in older adults but also in a variety of disease-specific clinical cohorts [52–54], among younger adults [40], and even in animal studies [1, 42]. It has also been successfully applied across different cultural contexts [50, 51]. The flexibility afforded by the FI approach with respect to the number and type of included health deficits also means that an FI can be constructed from nearly any existing health dataset without the need for additional data collection, making this a suitable approach for evaluating frailty using secondary health data sources.

The granularity of the deficit accumulation approach is another advantage, as it allows for the identification of varying levels of frailty across a broad spectrum. The degree of frailty present in a given individual is critically important in both determining their risk of adverse health outcomes and for planning future care. Furthermore, as subclinical health deficits, such as laboratory abnormalities, can be included in the FI, there is less risk of a floor effect, as well as greater potential for the early detection of individuals who are at risk for becoming frail.

## *Disadvantages of the Deficit Accumulation Approach*

In contrast to the phenotypic approach, the FI may include health deficits that overlap considerably with other constructs such as comorbidity and functional disability. This is a potential limitation of the FI approach, as it introduces redundancy that may be problematic when incorporating the FI into clinical prediction models [26, 55]. Alternatively, the holistic nature of the FI may be advantageous for prognostication, as this approach incorporates information from many different domains into a stand-alone measure of overall health status that can accurately predict susceptibility to adverse health outcomes. One challenge of such an all-encompassing measure may be providing targeted therapeutic interventions to individuals who are identified as frail using the FI, as the underlying factors driving frailty may differ between individuals, necessitating different treatment approaches [26, 55].

Unlike phenotypic frailty, which has a strong biological foundation with its pathophysiologic link to sarcopenia, the deficit accumulation approach lacks a physiologic basis. However, the remarkably consistent properties of the FI across contexts and even across different species would suggest that it does have some innate biological meaning. Finally, a practical limitation of the FI approach is the large number of included health deficits, which makes the FI approach very challenging and time-consuming to administer in clinical settings. Moving forward, electronic health records could be used to improve the clinical feasibility of the FI approach [56].

## *Deficit Accumulation in Chronic Disease Populations*

In individuals with chronic medical conditions, deficit accumulation may be accelerated, as physiologic stressors are more frequent and recovery is slower when compared to healthy individuals. The FI approach has been applied to several disease-specific clinical cohorts, including patients with chronic kidney disease [54], human immunodeficiency virus [53], and systemic sclerosis [52]. It appears that many of the properties of the FI described in older adults are also valid in these disease-specific patient populations. For example, in disease-specific cohorts, FI scores have demonstrated similar submaximal limits of no more than 0.7 [52, 53]. Women still tend to exhibit higher FI scores than men at a given age. Most importantly, higher FI values continue to consistently predict the occurrence of future adverse health outcomes, including mortality [52, 53].

There are also a few notable differences when the FI is applied to disease-specific cohorts as opposed to population-based samples of community-dwelling older adults. First, in some clinical samples, FI scores have been found to be normally distributed [53]. Second, mean FI scores in chronic disease cohorts tend to be higher than expected for similarly aged healthy individuals [52–54], confirming that deficit accumulation is likely accelerated in this population. Last, the relationship between chronological age and FI scores tends to be less pronounced in disease-specific clinical cohorts when compared to population-based samples [52, 53]. This may reflect the potential for individuals with chronic illnesses to demonstrate considerable frailty even at relatively young ages.

## *Deficit Accumulation in SLE*

Health issues rarely occur in isolation, and this is particularly true for a complex, multisystem disease like SLE. The deficit accumulation approach provides an opportunity to incorporate health deficits across organ systems into a single outcome measure, regardless of whether the deficits represent manifestations of SLE, complications of its treatment, or unrelated comorbidities. Some SLE patients will accumulate health deficits more rapidly than others, leading to disproportionately poor health outcomes. Indeed, the clinical course of SLE is highly variable and challenging to predict, ranging from a relatively benign illness to gradually progressive organ damage or even fulminant organ failure. The FI approach may aid in our understanding of this unexplained heterogeneity in health outcomes among SLE patients.

Legge and colleagues [15] have employed the deficit accumulation approach to construct a frailty index specifically for patients with SLE using data from the Systemic Lupus International Collaborating Clinics (SLICC) Inception Cohort. This is an international, multicenter, prospective observational study of 1826 SLE patients enrolled within 15 months of SLE diagnosis and followed with annual clinical and laboratory assessments. There were 222 variables identified as potential health deficits from the SLICC database. The majority of these variables were derived from existing, well-validated SLE instruments, including the SLE Disease Activity Index 2000 (SLEDAI-2K), SLICC/American College of Rheumatology (ACR) Damage Index (SDI), and the Medical Outcomes Survey Short Form 36 (SF-36). The use of a well-established, standard procedure to identify health deficits further enhanced content validity [43].

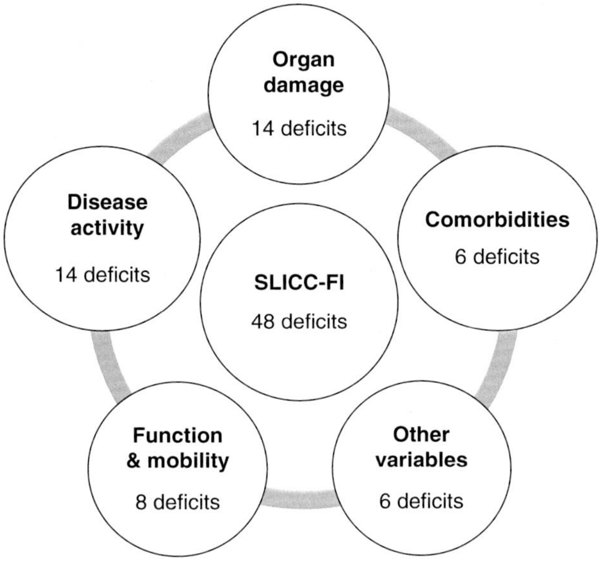


**Fig. 16.2** Health deficits included in the Systemic Lupus International Collaborating Clinics Frailty Index (SLICC-FI). The 48 health deficits included 14 items related to organ damage (e.g., congestive heart failure and chronic kidney disease), 14 items reflecting active inflammatory disease (e.g., serositis and inflammatory arthritis), 6 items representing comorbid conditions (e.g., hypertension and obesity), 8 variables related to functional impairment and mobility, and 6 other variables including self-reported health status and other health protective factors. (Based on original data from Legge et al. [15])

Of the 222 candidate variables, there were 48 items that met the required criteria for inclusion as health deficits in the SLICC-FI (Fig. 16.2). The properties of the SLICC-FI were initially evaluated in a baseline dataset of 1683 SLICC Inception Cohort patients who were mostly female (89%) with a mean age of 35.7 years and mean SLE disease duration of 18.8 months [57]. Baseline SLICC-FI scores ranged from 0 to 0.51 with a mean score of 0.17 [57]. There were 27.1% of SLE patients who were classified as frail [15], which is substantially higher than the prevalence of frailty observed among similarly aged individuals in general population samples, where the prevalence of frailty is typically less than 10% [40]. The prevalence of frailty among SLE patients in the SLICC Inception Cohort was low compared to other disease-specific clinical cohorts [52, 53], which may be partly explained by higher mean age in these other samples, as deficits tend to accumulate with increasing age.

The measurement properties of the SLICC-FI in the SLICC Inception Cohort were similar to those consistently demonstrated by other frailty indices in non-SLE populations. First, women demonstrated higher mean SLICC-FI scores compared to men at a given age [57]. Second, similar to other clinical cohorts, there was a weak, positive correlation between chronological age and SLICC-FI values [57]. Third, the distribution of baseline SLICC-FI scores was similar to the distribution of FI scores described in previous disease-specific cohorts and most closely approximated a beta distribution [57]. Fourth, the upper limit of SLICC-FI scores was in keeping with the submaximal limit for FI values reported in prior studies [57]. Last, in terms of concurrent validity, baseline SLICC-FI values demonstrated weak, positive associations with SLEDAI-2K and SDI scores from the same time point, which persisted even when overlapping items were omitted from the SLICC-FI [57].

Importantly, the SLICC-FI demonstrates predictive validity for future adverse health outcomes among SLE patients in the SLICC Inception Cohort. Higher baseline SLICC-FI values predicted increased risk of mortality [57] and organ damage accrual [58] during follow-up, and these associations persisted after adjusting for other important prognostic factors. In sensitivity analyses, the associations of baseline SLICC-FI values with adverse health outcomes remained unchanged when items related to organ damage were omitted from the SLICC-FI and when patients without baseline organ damage were considered [57, 58], suggesting that the predictive validity of the SLICC-FI was not dependent on the impact of organ damage alone. Furthermore, when the SLICC-FI and the SDI were included as independent variables in the same models, both measures were independent predictors of mortality risk and organ damage accrual during follow-up. Similar findings have been reported in other disease-specific cohort studies, whereby both the FI and existing measures of disease severity maintain independent associations with the risk of adverse health outcomes.

Similar measurement properties were observed for SLICC-FI scores at last follow-up in the SLICC Inception Cohort, again demonstrating the construct validity of this instrument. Interestingly, mean SLICC-FI scores remained unchanged during an average follow-up period of 7.2 years, which is uncommon in FI studies with such prolonged follow-up. When changes in SLICC-FI values during follow-up were evaluated, approximately two-thirds of patients had clinically meaningful changes in their SLICC-FI scores over time, with 26% of patients having an increase in SLICC-FI score, while 42% had a decrease in their SLICC-FI score during follow-up [57]. These results may reflect the impact of treatment, or a trade-off of deficits related to active SLE early in disease with later deficits due to irreversible organ damage. Regardless, these findings provide important insights into the attenuated relationship between chronological age and frailty in chronic disease populations. The potential for SLICC-FI scores to decrease over time reinforces the notion that frailty is a reversible process that is potentially treatable. To this end, frailty could be a novel therapeutic target in SLE, and the SLICC-FI may warrant investigation as a possible outcome measure for future intervention studies. Of note, the SLICC-FI has only been evaluated in a cohort of relatively young SLE patients early in their disease course. External validation of the SLICC-FI is required to determine its generalizability to other SLE populations, including among older patients with long-standing SLE.

## Other Approaches to Measuring Frailty

While phenotypic frailty and deficit accumulation have been the most frequently used approaches, numerous other operational definitions for frailty have been proposed [12]. A 2016 systematic review identified 67 instruments for the measurement of frailty in the medical literature [11]. Many of these frailty scales have been developed for use in specific research settings and have not been externally validated in other populations. The systematic review identified nine frailty instruments that had been frequently cited (>200 citations) in the medical literature [11]. While the frailty phenotype and the frailty index were the most commonly used approaches, other frequently cited instruments include the Clinical Frailty Scale [59] and the Vulnerable Elders Survey [60]. To date, none of these other frailty scales have been applied to patients with SLE.

Many studies have attempted to directly compare different instruments for the measurement of frailty. In a study by Theou and colleagues [61], eight different frailty scales were applied to a representative sample of middle-aged and older Europeans in the Survey of Health, Ageing, and Retirement in Europe (SHARE). While all eight scales identified frail individuals and predicted all-cause mortality, they varied in the accuracy of their mortality prediction, and each instrument was noted to capture slightly different domains of frailty [61]. Several factors should be considered when selecting an instrument to measure frailty, including its intended purpose, the domains of frailty captured, its measurement properties in prior studies, and its feasibility in a particular setting [11]. Although there is ongoing debate regarding the best approach for measuring frailty, it seems that different frailty instruments may be better suited for different clinical and research settings, depending upon the above factors.

## Research Agenda

While early research suggests that frailty may be a helpful concept for better understanding the health of SLE patients, several unanswered questions remain. Many important areas for future research have been identified and are outlined below.

### *Phenotypic Frailty in SLE: Areas for Future Research*

Among SLE patients, the prevalence of certain components of the original Fried frailty phenotype is very different from previous observations in community-dwelling older adults. While exhaustion was found to be much more common in

SLE, slow gait speed was rarely observed [14]. This suggests that certain components of the frailty phenotype, as defined in geriatric medicine, may have limited utility in SLE, and perhaps a lupus-specific phenotype would more accurately identify frail SLE patients. This reflects the broader debate regarding the generalizability of the frailty phenotype to diverse populations where the phenotypic expression of frailty may differ significantly from community-dwelling older adults. Another important area for future work will be to explore whether targeted interventions, such as physical activity programs, can prevent and treat phenotypic frailty in SLE and whether this will translate into improved clinical outcomes for this patient population.

## *Deficit Accumulation in SLE: Areas for Future Research*

First, it must be acknowledged that the SLICC-FI has been developed and evaluated in a single cohort of relatively young SLE patients early in their disease course. External validation of the SLICC-FI is required to determine its generalizability to other SLE populations, including among older patients with longer-standing SLE. Future work should also aim to compare the SLICC-FI to general population FI measures for the prediction of adverse health outcomes among individuals with SLE, in order to determine the extent to which a disease-specific FI provides additional prognostic value.

Recent reports suggest that rapidly increasing frailty is associated with worse health outcomes when compared to arriving at the same level of frailty more slowly [62]. Therefore, in addition to examining absolute SLICC-FI values, how the past trajectory of SLICC-FI scores influences its future predictive value is of great interest. Future work should aim to better understand the trajectories of SLICC-FI scores over time and how these trajectories relate to the risk of adverse health outcomes among SLE patients.

While the FI has been consistently shown to be a strong predictor of future health risks, significant unexplained variability in outcomes is still observed among individuals with the same FI score. Recent work suggests that differences in social vulnerability, as well as in health protective factors such as resiliency, may account for some of this heterogeneity. Undoubtedly, these factors should be taken into consideration when determining the risk of adverse outcomes. However, whether social factors should be incorporated as health deficits in the FI itself versus adjusted for at the level of the model remains unclear [42]. This is a critical area for future study, given the abundance of evidence demonstrating the important role of social factors in determining health outcomes in SLE.

## Conclusions

Frailty is a useful concept for understanding the unexplained variability in health outcomes that is observed among individuals with SLE. While many different instruments have been developed to measure frailty, two main approaches for operationalizing frailty have emerged – the phenotypic approach and the deficit accumulation approach. Each of these approaches has strengths and limitations, and the optimal method for measuring frailty may differ depending on the context. Both approaches have been shown to be relevant among individuals with SLE.

The SLICC-FI embraces the heterogeneity and complexity of SLE, by placing less emphasis on specific, individual risk factors and instead focusing on the cumulative impact of multiple interrelated health issues. Following additional validation studies, the SLICC-FI may be a useful prognostic tool for identifying high-risk SLE patients who may warrant closer monitoring or changes in therapy to reduce the risk of adverse health outcomes. Given that frailty is potentially reversible, the SLICC-FI may also be useful as an outcome measure for future intervention studies. Meanwhile, the Fried frailty phenotype is useful for understanding the specific impact of sarcopenia and physical frailty in SLE and will play an important role in the design and evaluation of interventions for the prevention and treatment of physical frailty among SLE patients.

## References

1. Rockwood K, Blodgett JM, Theou O, Sun MH, Feridooni HA, Mitnitski A, et al. A frailty index based on deficit accumulation quantifies mortality risk in humans and in mice. Sci Rep. 2017;7:43068.
2. Vaupel JW, Manton KG, Stallard E. The impact of heterogeneity in individual frailty on the dynamics of mortality. Demography. 1979;16:439–54.
3. Fulop T, Larbi A, Witkowski JM, McElhaney J, Loeb M, Mitnitski A, et al. Aging, frailty and age-related diseases. Biogerontology. 2010;11:547–63.
4. Clegg A, Young J, Iliffe S, Rikkert MO, Rockwood K. Frailty in elderly people. Lancet. 2013;381:752–62.
5. Abel GA, Klepin HD. Frailty and the management of hematologic malignancies. Blood. 2018;131:515–24.
6. Partridge JSL, Harari D, Dhesi JK. Frailty in the older surgical patient: a review. Age Ageing. 2012;41:142–7.
7. Ness KK, Armstrong GT, Kundu M, Wilson CL, Tchkonia T, Kirkland JL. Frailty in childhood cancer survivors. Cancer. 2015;121:1540–7.
8. Brothers TD, Kirkland S, Guaraldi G, Falutz J, Theou O, Johnston BL, et al. Frailty in people aging with human immunodeficiency virus (HIV) infection. J Infect Dis. 2014;210:1170–9.

9. Soysal P, Stubbs B, Lucato P, Luchini C, Solmi M, Peluso R, et al. Inflammation and frailty in the elderly: a systematic review and meta-analysis. Ageing Res Rev. 2016;31:1–8.
10. Jacob N, Stohl W. Cytokine disturbances in systemic lupus erythematosus. Arthritis Res Ther. 2011;13:228.
11. Buta BJ, Walston JD, Godino JG, Park M, Kalyani RR, Xue Q-L, et al. Frailty assessment instruments: systematic characterization of the uses and contexts of highly-cited instruments. Ageing Res Rev. 2016;26:53–61.
12. de Vries NM, Staal JB, van Ravensberg CD, Hobbelen JSM, Rikkert MGMO, Nijhuis-Van der Sanden MW. Outcome instruments to measure frailty: a systematic review. Ageing Res Rev. 2011;10:104–14.
13. Theou O, Walston J, Rockwood K. Operationalizing frailty using the frailty phenotype and deficit accumulation approaches. Interdiscip Top Gerontol. 2015;41:66–73.
14. Katz PP, Andrews J, Yazdany J, Schmajuk G, Trupin L, Yelin E. Is frailty a relevant concept in SLE? Lupus Sci Med. 2017;4:e000186.
15. Legge A, Kirkland S, Rockwood K, Andreou P, Bae S-C, Gordon C, et al. Construction of a frailty index as a novel health measure in systemic lupus erythematosus. J Rheumatol. 2019;47:72–81.
16. Fried LP, Tangen CM, Walston J, Newman AB, Hirsch C, Gottdiener J, et al. Frailty in older adults: evidence for a phenotype. J Gerontol A Biol Sci Med Sci. 2001;56A:M146–56.
17. Walrand S, Guillet C, Salles J, Cano N, Boirie Y. Physiopathological mechanism of sarcopenia. Clin Geriatr Med. 2011;27:365–85.
18. Landi F, Calvani R, Cesari M, Tosato M, Martone AM, Bernabei R, et al. Sarcopenia as the biological substrate of physical frailty. Clin Geriatr Med. 2015;31:367–74.
19. Bandeen-Roche K, Seplaki CL, Huang J, Buta B, Kalyani RR, Varadhan R, et al. Frailty in older adults: a nationally representative profile in the United States. J Gerontol A Biol Sci Med Sci. 2015;70:1427–34.
20. Zaslavsky O, Zelber-Sagi S, Gray SL, LaCroix AZ, Brunner RL, Wallace RB, et al. Comparison of frailty phenotypes for prediction of mortality, incident falls, and hip fracture in older women. J Am Geriatr Soc. 2016;64:1858–62.
21. Kojima G. Frailty as a predictor of fractures among community-dwelling older people: a systematic review and meta-analysis. Bone. 2016;90:116–22.
22. Kojima G. Frailty as a predictor of nursing home placement among community-dwelling older adults: a systematic review and meta-analysis. J Geriatr Phys Ther. 2018;41:42–8.
23. Shamliyan T, Talley KMC, Ramakrishnan R, Kane RL. Association of frailty with survival: a systematic literature review. Ageing Res Rev. 2013;12:719–36.
24. Kojima G, Iliffe S, Walters K. Frailty index as a predictor of mortality: a systematic review and meta-analysis. Age Ageing. 2018;47:193–200.
25. Theou O, Cann L, Blodgett J, Wallace LMK, Brothers TD, Rockwood K. Modifications to the frailty phenotype criteria: systematic review of the current literature and investigation of 262 frailty phenotypes in the Survey of Health, Ageing, and Retirement in Europe. Ageing Res Rev. 2015;21:78–94.
26. Fried LP, Ferrucci L, Darer J, Williamson JD, Anderson G. Untangling the concepts of disability, frailty, and comorbidity: implications for improved targeting and care. J Gerontol A Biol Sci Med Sci. 2004;59:255–63.
27. Fairhall N. Physical, nutritional, cognitive and combination interventions reduce frailty in community-dwelling prefrail and frail older people. Evid Based Med. 2016;21:142.
28. Kulminski AM, Ukraintseva SV, Kulminskaya IV, Arbeev KG, Land K, Yashin AI. Cumulative deficits better characterize susceptibility to death in elderly people than phenotypic frailty: lessons from the Cardiovascular Health Study. J Am Geriatr Soc. 2008;56:898–903.
29. Jha SR, Ha HSK, Hickman LD, Hannu M, Davidson PM, Macdonald PS, et al. Frailty in advanced heart failure: a systematic review. Heart Fail Rev. 2015;20:553–60.
30. Chowdhury R, Peel NM, Krosch M, Hubbard RE. Frailty and chronic kidney disease: a systematic review. Arch Gerontol Geriatr. 2017;68:135–42.

31. Kennedy CC, Novotny PJ, LeBrasseur NK, Wise RA, Sciurba FC, Benzo RP. Frailty and clinical outcomes in chronic obstructive pulmonary disease. Ann Am Thorac Soc. 2019;16:217–24.
32. Maddocks M, Kon SSC, Canavan JL, Jones SE, Nolan CM, Labey A, et al. Physical frailty and pulmonary rehabilitation in COPD: a prospective cohort study. Thorax. 2016;71:988–95.
33. Stockton KA, Kandiah DA, Paratz JD, Bennell KL. Fatigue, muscle strength and vitamin D status in women with systemic lupus erythematosus compared with healthy controls. Lupus. 2012;21:271–8.
34. Andrews JS, Trupin L, Schmajuk G, Barton J, Margaretten M, Yazdany J, et al. Muscle strength, muscle mass, and physical disability in women with systemic lupus erythematosus. Arthritis Care Res. 2015;67:120–7.
35. Sterling K, Gallop K, Swinburn P, Flood E, French A, Sawah Al S, et al. Patient-reported fatigue and its impact on patients with systemic lupus erythematosus. Lupus. 2014;23:124–32.
36. Mahieu MA, Ahn GE, Chmiel JS, Dunlop DD, Helenowski IB, Semanik P, et al. Fatigue, patient reported outcomes, and objective measurement of physical activity in systemic lupus erythematosus. Lupus. 2016;25:1190–9.
37. Ahn GE, Chmiel JS, Dunlop DD, Helenowski IB, Semanik PA, Song J, et al. Self-reported and objectively measured physical activity in adults with systemic lupus erythematosus. Arthritis Care Res. 2015;67:701–7.
38. Legge A, Blanchard C, Hanly JG. Physical activity, sedentary behaviour and their associations with cardiovascular risk in systemic lupus erythematosus. Rheumatology (Oxford). 2020;59:1128–36.
39. Santos MJ, Vinagre F, Canas da Silva J, Gil V, Fonseca JE. Body composition phenotypes in systemic lupus erythematosus and rheumatoid arthritis: a comparative study of Caucasian female patients. Clin Exp Rheumatol. 2011;29:470–6.
40. Rockwood K, Song X, Mitnitski A. Changes in relative fitness and frailty across the adult lifespan: evidence from the Canadian National Population Health Survey. Can Med Assoc J. 2011;183:E487–94.
41. Mitnitski A, Rockwood K. Aging as a process of deficit accumulation: its utility and origin. Interdiscip Top Gerontol. 2015;40:85–98.
42. Rockwood K, Howlett SE. Age-related deficit accumulation and the diseases of ageing. Mech Ageing Dev. 2019;180:107–16.
43. Searle SD, Mitnitski A, Gahbauer EA, Gill TM, Rockwood K. A standard procedure for creating a frailty index. BMC Geriatr. 2008;8:731–10.
44. Rockwood K, Mitnitski A. Frailty defined by deficit accumulation and geriatric medicine defined by frailty. Clin Geriatr Med. 2011;27:17–26.
45. Mitnitski A, Song X, Skoog I, Broe GA, Cox JL, Grunfeld E, et al. Relative fitness and frailty of elderly men and women in developed countries and their relationship with mortality. J Am Geriatr Soc. 2005;53:2184–9.
46. Mitnitski A, Rockwood K. The rate of aging: the rate of deficit accumulation does not change over the adult life span. Biogerontology. 2016;17:199–204.
47. Goggins WB, Woo J, Sham A, Ho SC. Frailty index as a measure of biological age in a Chinese population. J Gerontol A Biol Sci Med Sci. 2005;60:1046–51.
48. Rockwood K, Andrew M, Mitnitski A. A comparison of two approaches to measuring frailty in elderly people. J Gerontol A Biol Sci Med Sci. 2007;62:738–43.
49. Rockwood K, Mitnitski A. Limits to deficit accumulation in elderly people. Mech Ageing Dev. 2006;127:494–6.
50. Fang X, Shi J, Song X, Mitnitski A, Tang Z, Wang C, et al. Frailty in relation to the risk of falls, fractures, and mortality in older Chinese adults: results from the Beijing longitudinal study of aging. J Nutr Health Aging. 2012;16:903–7.
51. Song X, Mitnitski A, Rockwood K. Prevalence and 10-year outcomes of frailty in older adults in relation to deficit accumulation. J Am Geriatr Soc. 2010;58:681–7.
52. Rockwood MR, MacDonald E, Sutton E, Rockwood K, Scleroderma Research Group, Baron M. Frailty index to measure health status in people with systemic sclerosis. J Rheumatol. 2014;41:698–705.

53. Guaraldi G, Brothers TD, Zona S, Stentarelli C, Carli F, Malagoli A, et al. A frailty index predicts survival and incident multimorbidity independent of markers of HIV disease severity. AIDS. 2015;29:1633–41.
54. Hubbard RE, Peel NM, Smith M, Dawson B, Lambat Z, Bak M, et al. Feasibility and construct validity of a frailty index for patients with chronic kidney disease. Australas J Ageing. 2015;34:E9–12.
55. Afilalo J. Conceptual models of frailty: the sarcopenia phenotype. Can J Cardiol. 2016;32:1051–5.
56. Clegg A, Bates C, Young J, Ryan R, Nichols L, Ann Teale E, et al. Development and validation of an electronic frailty index using routine primary care electronic health record data. Age Ageing. 2016;45:353–60.
57. Legge A, Kirkland S, Rockwood K, Andreou P, Bae S-C, Gordon C, et al. Evaluating the properties of a frailty index and its association with mortality risk among patients with systemic lupus erythematosus. Arthritis Rheumatol. 2019;11:455–11.
58. Legge A, Kirkland S, Rockwood K, Andreou P, Bae S-C, Gordon C, et al. Prediction of damage accrual in systemic lupus erythematosus using the Systemic Lupus International Collaborating Clinics Frailty Index (SLICC-FI). Arthritis Rheumatol. 2020;72:658–66.
59. Rockwood K, Song X, MacKnight C, Bergman H, Hogan DB, McDowell I, et al. A global clinical measure of fitness and frailty in elderly people. Can Med Assoc J. 2005;173:489–95.
60. Saliba D, Elliott M, Rubenstein LZ, Solomon DH, Young RT, Kamberg CJ, et al. The Vulnerable Elders Survey: a tool for identifying vulnerable older people in the community. J Am Geriatr Soc. 2001;49:1691–9.
61. Theou O, Brothers TD, Mitnitski A, Rockwood K. Operationalization of frailty using eight commonly used scales and comparison of their ability to predict all-cause mortality. J Am Geriatr Soc. 2013;61:1537–51.
62. Stow D, Matthews FE, Hanratty B. Frailty trajectories to identify end of life: a longitudinal population-based study. BMC Med. 2018;16:171–7.

# Chapter 17
# Work Disability and Prevention in SLE: A Focus on Assessment and Function

**Behdin Nowrouzi-Kia and Zahi Touma**

## Introduction

Systemic lupus erythematosus (SLE) is a chronic relapsing-remitting autoimmune disease that attacks different organ systems and results in substantial disability and mortality [1]. Exacerbating matters is that medical status is not always congruent with functional and disability status. Within the biopsychosocial model, work disability (WD) is conceptualized as a complex relationship between physical, psychosocial, and cultural factors [2]. For instance, some patients successfully return to work even before their symptoms completely resolve. Conversely, other patients with comparable injuries indicate long-term work incapacity. The heterogeneity of clinical presentations provides numerous compelling arguments to develop and distribute measures of work disability outcomes.

This chapter describes issues and measures related to work disability prevention in SLE. The chapter provides an overview of the importance of addressing work disability and ways to measure its impact on patients' functioning and associated disability. Participation in work is a significant component of a patient's life. When a patient experiences limitations of employment activities, these should be examined rigorously to mitigate their impact on work participation.

B. Nowrouzi-Kia (✉)
Department of Occupational Science and Occupational Therapy, Temerty Faculty of Medicine, University of Toronto, Toronto, ON, Canada
e-mail: behdin.nowrouzi.kia@utoronto.ca

Z. Touma
Centre for Prognosis in Rheumatic Disease, Toronto Lupus Clinic, Division of Rheumatology, Department of Medicine, Institute of Health Policy, Management and Evaluation, University of Toronto, Toronto, ON, Canada
e-mail: Zahi.Touma@uhn.ca



Z. Touma (ed.), *Outcome Measures and Metrics in Systemic Lupus Erythematosus*, https://doi.org/10.1007/978-3-030-73303-2_17

## Overview of SLE and Impact on Work (Focus on Prevention)

Work participation or employment is a major area of people's lives [3]. However, when a patient becomes affected with a health condition, illness, or disease, work disability may result and prevent the patient from working. For SLE patients, work disability is related with personal challenges, including limitations in functioning, decreased income [4], restrictions in activity participation [5, 6], and diminished health-related quality of life [7, 8]. SLE is a chief cause of work limitation [5, 6], and it equates to lost productivity costs (C$4494/patient/year) [4], and in Canadian cohorts, mean lost productivity costs were $55,827 over 4 years [9]. In addition, work disability may lead to diminished productivity and increased societal costs. Work disability poses a great burden and challenge to both developing [10] and developed nations [11–13] as indirect costs make up the bulk of the burden in industrialized countries, approximately 80% [14, 15]. The challenge is to mitigate WD-related burden and sustain optimal work participation.

Increased WD rates have been reported in many studies and range from 20% to 50% and vary drastically between SLE populations reported in the literature [9, 16–19]. The examination of WD and function in SLE requires the recognition of the complexity, multidimensionality, temporal dimensions of SLE, and its relationship to work and warrants a multidisciplinary perspective. There is a dearth of evidence regarding the use of a multidisciplinary team approach in improving WD and functional outcomes in SLE, in particular pertaining to the assessment of WD. A meta-analysis of 26 studies ($n = 9886$ patients) estimated that 46% (confidence intervals 40–52%) of patients were employed, and 34% experienced WD [20]. Moreover, evidence suggests that SLE may diminish a patient's ability to work and results in elevated rates of WD [18, 21] and lower productivity by 43% [22]. Observational studies have reported that SLE has impacted patient's employment, career choices, and productivity. One study reported that 28% of patients had altered careers within the first year after their diagnosis [6]. Sixty percent had lowered the number of hours worked, and 70% indicated that SLE had impacted their career, in such ways as selecting to work flexible hours, requesting disability benefits (e.g., short- and long-term disability), using sick leaves, and changing careers [6]. The impact of SLE on career development is significant and presents challenges at work [23]. For some patients, they may need to revaluate their career due to the disability and periods of exacerbation and remission caused by SLE and its impact on work [24].

The inability to participate in paid employment has been associated with a variety of psychosocial and disease outcomes including age, race, sex and gender, socioeconomic status, education attainment, disease activity, duration of pain, fatigue anxiety, and cognitive development [18].

In the labor force, patients with SLE have experienced deleterious occupational outcomes, including their ability to do paid work early in life [25–28], early retirement [29], increased work absenteeism rates [25, 28], lower productivity [27], and high direct costs (e.g., lost values for paid or unpaid labor) [26]. One study reported a mean average work absenteeism rate of 14–16 days per year in patients with SLE

[26]; another study found that 21% of patients with SLE were absent from work due to health issues for more than 15 days per year when compared to with 11% in matched controls [16]. One of the challenges that persists is the heterogeneity of the data sources (e.g., secondary data vs cohort/population based, varying countries of origin), study criteria, and outcome measures used to evaluate WD. To address this challenge, WD in patients with SLE should be evaluated through a biopsychosocial framework that is patient-centric and grounded in disability management.

## *Conceptual View and Framework for Measuring Work Disability Prevention*

### International Classification of Functioning (ICF), Work Disability, and Health

Approximately 20 years ago, the World Health Assembly approved the International Classification of Functioning (ICF) as the conceptual model and terminology to define human functioning and disability's totality [30]. The ICF is a biopsychosocial framework and also a classification system with applications to health service delivery, research, occupational health, and clinical services, including rheumatology. Furthermore, the conceptual model may be used to determine health and health-related domains, as a universal language of work disability, and as a foundation to compare assessment information across geographical settings. Another strength of the ICF is that it may be used across work settings, culture, and context. As a conceptual model, the ICF demonstrates the relationship between SLE and its ramifications on a patient's functioning (as demonstrated by the model's activities and participation aspects). These different aspects represent work disability in SLE patients and may be under the influence of contextual factors (e.g., environmental, personal). As a framework, the ICF demonstrates the interrelationship between SLE and its impact on the person's body and participation in work (see Fig. 17.1).

### Work Disability Prevention (WDP) Framework

Preventing WD allows patients to have fewer lost time injuries and improve their participation in the labor force in several ways. The work disability framework presented by Loisel et al. (2001) recognizes that disability in the workplace is not only due to the patients' characteristics but also due to environmental factors. The WDP framework is framed in disability management and is patient centered. The framework indicates the patient, the workplace, the healthcare system, and the compensation system to be influential stakeholders in regard to WD [31]. The patient interacts with all four systems depending on the context of the interaction. Figure 17.2 provides the model with its four systems, including the person (physical and psychosocial), the workplace, the healthcare system, and the compensation system.

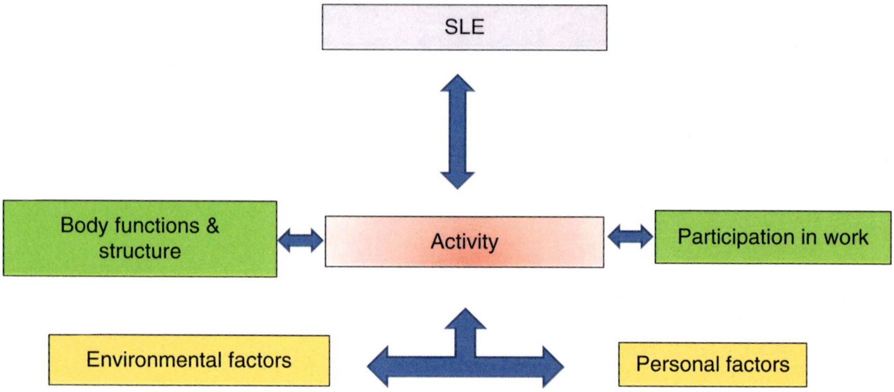


**Fig. 17.1** The ICF is a biopsychosocial framework that defines human functioning and disability. The figure depicts the interaction between body functions and structure, activity, environmental and personal factors, and participation in work with activity and its relationship with SLE. (Adapted from The International Classification of Functioning, Disability and Health (ICF) [30])

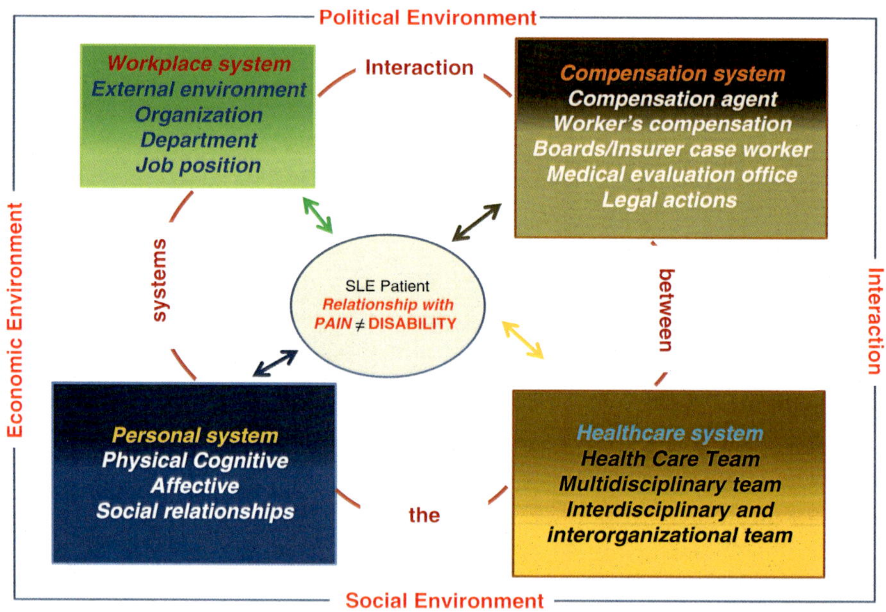


**Fig. 17.2** Work Disability Prevention Framework represents the interactions with and between the workplace, compensation, personal and healthcare systems, and the SLE patient at the center of the model. The patient-centric model emphasizes a biopsychosocial and preventive approach to work disability. (Adapted from the Work Disability Prevention Framework [31])

## *Work Disability and SLE: The Potential in Using a Preventative Approach*

A general understanding of work disability is vital to improve research utilization and to promote unified approaches to prevent work disability [32, 33]. Figure 17.2 represents a conceptual model of "Work Disability Prevention" based and inspired by the work of Loisel et al. (2001) and underpinned by the biopsychosocial model [34]. The model about "WDP" is anchored by the patient. The central location of the patient emphasizes the importance of his/her place within the WDP paradigm. Loisel et al. proposed a WDP intervention [31], known as the Sherbrooke model of management of subacute occupational back pain and functioning, which combines occupational and clinical interventions. Researchers analyzed the cost-benefit and cost-effectiveness for each experimental arm (Sherbrooke model, standard care, occupational intervention, and clinical intervention) to decide which approach is the most productive at preventing occupational back pain and work disability [31]. The highest experimental intervention costs were in the Sherbrooke model arm, but after a 1-year follow-up, the consequence of disease costs was highest in the standard care [31]. Following up about 6 years later, the Sherbrooke model had moderately higher savings than the other groups. The Sherbrooke group also had the lowest absenteeism 6 years later compared to the other experimental arms. Although the Sherbrooke model was the most cost-beneficial, the WDP framework states that it was not statistically significant compared to the other arms, which may be caused by the skewed distributions of costs on a few cases [31].

The WDP provides a roadmap for the patient with SLE to follow in the context of WD through its biopsychosocial underpinnings. For instance, the patient may interact with their healthcare team regarding the medical management of SLE. Once their symptoms are controlled, the focus may shift toward addressing the wide range of functional limitations that are dependent upon the body system or organs that have been affected. Next, the patient will connect with the workplace system and work with a healthcare professional such as an occupational therapist to maximize work functioning and return to work in a timely and safe manner. The patient may also interact with the worker's compensation system to establish a return-to-work plan that is supported by their employer and effectively communicated by a designed case manager or adjudicator. The patient may also use social supports systems and build networks at work to support their transition to paid employment.

The conceptual model emphasizes the different facets and their various levels, from the person (physical and psychosocial), the workplace, the compensation system, and the healthcare system that may influence WDP [31]. Additionally, the model demonstrates the challenges and opportunities of the return-to-work process in the workplace, from the patient's job position to the whole workplace organization and even possibly to the external environment in which the firm functions [31].

In Canada and the United States, chronic pain is a leading cause of healthcare utilization and disability. Statistics suggest that approximately 60 million people in the United States and 7 million people in Canada live with devastating chronic pain [35–37]. As well, the diagram (Fig. 17.2) depicts the psychological factors involved in the transition from acute to chronic pain through biopsychosocial lens [38]. Also noteworthy is that a disability framework takes into account the rehabilitation services provided to the patient by different stakeholders in the healthcare system (e.g., attending physician, other members of the multidisciplinary team, the patients' compensation, personal supports). Three RCTs have provided evidence of relatively large reductions in time lost from work because of widely differing interventions for patients still off work 6–8 weeks after the onset of low back pain symptoms [39–41]. Patients with SLE with WD have higher pain, fatigue, and depressive symptoms and have poorer cognitive functioning [6, 9, 17–19, 42, 43]. However, the evidence regarding the relationship between pain and subsequent risk of WD in SLE has not been explored, for example, how may pain influence a patient's perception of WD and work participation. A few studies have reported that the majority of work loss was due to WD rather than decreased labor force participation (e.g., fewer hours worked) [44].

In further understanding work disability and its relationship on work, the diagram depicts the relationship between the physical and mental characteristics of the work and the patient's social connections [31]. The model also examines the disability paradigm and the various stakeholder interactions that exist between the patient and the public or private compensation system.

## *Work Disability and Disability Management in SLE*

A work disability paradigm should incorporate the medical and rehabilitation services provided to the patient by different healthcare management.For a patient with SLE to participate in work, an analysis of personal, occupational and environmental must be considered, and personal factors. A work disability framework (e.g., WDP) allows for a patient-centric approach that is biopsychosocial (e.g., ICF) in nature and recognizes the complexity involved in mitigating WD and in promoting work participation. This framework is particularly important given the episodic nature of flare-ups in patients with SLE and given that it is grounded in disability management. Disability management uses a proactive approach and assumes joint responsibility in decision-making related to employment-based interventions of services for patients with SLE. Through a multidisciplinary approach that is framed in disability management principles, a patient with SLE may return to work or participate in work.

Work disability management is a workplace-based process that requires the integration of complex issues related to WD, intervention, rehabilitation, and management participation. Health professionals provide expertise, though it is necessary for organizations to work as a team and assist co-workers in making a successful transition back to work for a patient with SLE or to promote work participation. Disability management includes the education and involvement of patients with SLE and employers working together as a team, the use of prevention strategies, and many more factors. Furthermore, disability management will also address strategies to lower work absenteeism rates, fatigue, and pain through assessment and intervention in the workplace. Vital factors involved in facilitating return to work and work participation for patients with SLE include employer participation, a supportive work environment, and cooperation between labor and management [45–47]. Patient expectations regarding their SLE diagnosis, communication, and involvement in decision-making should be considered to an extent [48]. Numerous factors are recommended to be considered when conducting applied research in WDP with a patient with SLE; barriers and facilitators of returning to work should be identified, finding effective ways to reassure patients with work disability, investigating modified work that is effective to improve return to regular work, and finding a system that enhances stakeholders' collaboration [49].

## *Patient-Reported Outcomes of Work Disability and Functioning*

Patient-reported outcomes (PROs) provide crucial knowledge about a patient's health, functional status, symptoms, treatment preferences, satisfaction, and quality of life from their perspective [50]. PROs provide the patient's perspective and facilitate a richer understanding of the effects of SLE and treatment on symptoms, functioning, and other outcomes [51, 52]. For many chronic diseases, including SLE, PROs provide crucial health information in evaluating functioning and work disability. The application of relevant and psychometrically sound PROs helps patients and clinicians understand the comprehensive impact of interventions on patients' functioning and work disability.

### Health Assessment Questionnaire (HAQ)

The HAQ is a widely used self-reported functional status and work disability measure. It contains eight domains, including dressing, arising, eating, walking, hygiene, reach, grip, and activities. There are two or three questions per domain. The measure is widely used to assess and monitor patients with rheumatic diseases [53] including SLE [54–56]. Scoring for each domain is from 0 (without any difficulty) to 3 (unable to do). The eight scores of the eight domains are summed and divided by nine and generate a functional disability index score [57].

## The World Health Organization-Disability Assessment Schedule 2.0 (WHO-DAS 2.0)

The WHO-DAS 2.0 measures 6 domains related to work disability and functioning. The *WHO-DAS 2.0* definition of disability [58, 59] and grounded in the ICF framework [59] and the Diagnostic and Statistical Manual of Mental Disorders (fifth edition) [60, 61]. The WHO-DAS 2.0 theoretical construct is based on the International Classification of Functioning. This definition takes into account multiple levels of difficulty for each *WHODAS 2.0* item across the six domains, and it is available as 12-item version and 36-item version. Scores on the 12-item version account for 85% of the variance in scores on the full 36-item version [59]. The six domains include cognition, mobility, self-care, getting along, life activities, and participation. Item response options are "none," "mild," "moderate," "severe," and "extreme" separately. The aggregate score is calculated by differentially weighting the items and the levels of severity [58]. Higher scores indicate severe disability.

## Work Ability Index

The Work Ability Index (WAI) is developed by the Finnish Institute of Occupational Health [62]. Work ability is operationalized as the ability of a patient to perform their job duties, based on specific physical and mental health demands of the job. The WAI uses point scales between one and five and contains seven subscales [63]. The seven subscales include as follows: (1) current work ability compared with lifetime best, (2) work ability to the demands of the job, (3) the number of current diseases diagnosed by a physician, (4) estimated work impairment due to diseases, (5) sick leave during the past year, (6) the patient's prognosis of work ability 2 years from now, and (7) mental resources. A psychometric evaluation for internal reliability on data from ten European countries found that the Cronbach's alpha for total sample amounted to 0.72 (0.54 to 0.79) [64]. Overall, the internal reliability for nine out of ten countries was deemed satisfactory with the exception of one country (Slovakia) which had a sample that deviated from the other national samples. A patient's responses may range from 0 to 10 with possible scores ranging from 7 to 49. Scores are categorized as "poor work ability" (7–27), "moderate work ability" (28–36), "good work ability" (37–43), and "excellent work ability" (44–49).

## Work Role Functioning Questionnaire v2.0

The *Work Role Functioning Questionnaire v2.0* is an outcome measure related to a person's health and their ability to meet work demands given a particular state of health. The measure contains 27 items across 4 subscales on a 5-point scale (0–4). Subscale scores are tabulated as the mean of item scores multiplied by 25 to obtain scores between 0 and 100. Higher scores indicate better work role functioning. The second version consists of 27 items and is divided into five subscales. The subscales include work scheduling and output demands, physical demands, mental and social demands, and flexibility demands [62]. The measure has shown consistent structural validity across samples, and its subscale scores are recommended to compare across different clinical and working samples [62].

### Work Limitation Questionnaire

The Work Limitation Questionnaire is used to evaluate the impact of chronic health conditions such as SLE on work performance [65]. The instrument contains 25 items and 4 subscales: time, physical demands, mental-interpersonal, and output demand. Each item is scored on a five-point Likert scale, with higher values indicating more severe work limitation. The Work Limitation Questionnaire has been validated with numerous populations, including those with back pain [65], cancer [66], obstructive sleep apnea [67], rheumatoid arthritis [68], insomnia [69], and depression [70].

## *Clinician-Administered Evaluations*

### Functional Capacity Evaluations

Functional capacity evaluations (FCEs) are a comprehensive, systematic, and objective assessment of a patient's ability to perform work-related activity [71–73]. FCEs are considered the gold standard of functional assessment [74]. For over 40 years, FCEs have been used to support and assist healthcare professionals in making return-to-work decisions and were primarily performed by occupational therapists and other healthcare professionals [75]. Currently, the findings of FAEs may be used in numerous ways to inform the functional status of a patient, including those with SLE. For example, FAEs may be used to assess and provide a determination about a timely and safe return to work for patients with SLE. A typical assessment includes an examination of their medical records, social history and interview, a physical examination including a functional screening of their physical capabilities and performance, and the production of a report [73]. The components of a FCE include data gathering (e.g., patient's medical, social, and work history). This information helps with determining the patient's abilities. Some FCE will include a physical (musculoskeletal) examination, physiological measurement (e.g., muscular endurance), functional performance (e.g., physical demands of work), and an evaluation of the patient's capabilities as compared to the job requirements [73]. FCE should be used as part of an overall assessment of work disability and functioning.

### Vocational Evaluations

Vocational evaluations are a comprehensive procedure that systematically evaluates work, in real or simulated environments for the purpose of vocational assessment and in supporting patients in their vocational rehabilitation and return to work [76]. Vocational evaluations consider both the physical (e.g., strength, positioning) and mental components (e.g., cognitive, emotional, attitude) of the job and fit with the patient. These assessments may last between 3 and 10 consecutive days and vary by the goal of the assessment [77].

### Job Demand Analysis

The job demand analysis seeks to understand the actual cognitive and physical demands of the job and is performed by regulated health professionals. Assessing the job demands of a job using a job demand analysis provides objective information about the patient's work ability and their fit with the job. The job demand evaluation includes essential job duties, cognitive (e.g., attention, concentration, mental fatigue) and physical requirements (e.g., kneeling, pushing, pulling) (see Fig. 17.3), educational requirements, use of equipment, the work environment including exposure to occupational hazards, and recommendations to support return to work. Data is collected by using questionnaires, observing the patient perform the job, interviewing co-workers and supervisors, and formal measurement (e.g., measuring strength, range of motion) [79].

## *Return to Work*

Supporting return to work provides patients purpose, financial security, opportunity to advance their careers and better quality of life, purpose, opportunity to advance their careers and in their health. The WDP framework provides a patient-centric approach to supporting their return-to-work journey. The unpredictable nature of

| Physical demands requirements for disability case manager | | | |
|---|---|---|---|
| Physical demand | Occasional | Frequent | Constant |
| Level | 0–33% | 33–66% | 66–100% |
| Sedentary | 1–10 lbs | Negligible | Negligible |
| Light | 11–20 lbs | 1–10 lbs | Negligible |
| Medium | 21–50 lbs | 11–25 lbs | 1–10 lbs |
| Heavy | 51–100 lbs | 26–50 lbs | 11–20 lbs |
| Very heavy | Over 100 lbs | Over 50 lbs | Over 20 lbs |

**Fig. 17.3** Physical demand characteristics of work using a job demand analysis approach. (Adapted from the Dictionary of Occupational Titles-Volume II, Fourth Edition, Revised 1991 [78])

SLE leads to a decline in function and, ultimately, a decrease in quality of life and absence from the workplace. Supporting a patient's return to work or work participation should include a multidisciplinary approach. This approach espouses the complexity of the return-to-work process and values the contributions of many disciplines including health and human resources. For example, the patient's treating physician can support their medical recovery and control symptoms of the disease (healthcare system). The patient's family may contribute to augmenting their mental and physical health through social support that can include assisting the patients when they are fatigued and providing encouragement. In the workplace, the supervisor or human resources professionals can create and foster an environment of inclusion where a patient that returns to work feels welcome.

Furthermore, this work environment should provide accommodations that support the chronic nature of SLE. For example, a patient may be allowed to take multiple breaks or have paid time off work to attend medical appointments. In the worker's compensation system, healthcare providers such as occupational therapists can work closely with the patient and various other stakeholders from the other systems to promote maximal functioning and reduce work disability. The case management of SLE patients requires precise and timely communication to encourage a timely and safe return to work.

## *Conclusion and Future Direction*

Work disability impedes functioning and impacts quality of life in a patient with SLE functioning and impacts the quality of life and health. The use of a holistic approach that is grounded in a patient-centered approach that uses the ICF or WDP framework will permit for improvements in the patient's health and well-being. This biopsychosocial perspective also recognizes the use of a multidisciplinary team that brings collective expertise to support return to work and functioning. Together, healthcare providers can encapsulate and measure the complex functioning aspects of SLE and improve patients' health.

## References

1. Scofield L, Reinlib L, Alarcón GS, Cooper GS. Employment and disability issues in systemic lupus erythematosus: a review. Arthritis Care Res. 2008;59:1475–9.
2. Schultz IZ, Stowell AW, Feuerstein M, Gatchel RJ. Models of return to work for musculoskeletal disorders. J Occup Rehabil. 2007;17:327–52.
3. Waddell G, Burton AK, Kendall NA. Vocational rehabilitation–what works, for whom, and when? (Report for the Vocational Rehabilitation Task Group): TSO; 2008.
4. McCormick N, Marra CA, Sadatsafavi M, Kopec JA, Aviña-Zubieta JA. Excess productivity costs of systemic lupus erythematosus, systemic sclerosis, and Sjögren's syndrome: a general population–based study. Arthritis Care Res. 2019;71:142–54.

5. Rapoza KA, Kenney-Riley K, Berkowitz SS, Lewis AN, Rosen RM. Lupus in culturally diverse populations: a transdisciplinary model for vocational rehabilitation counseling. J Appl Rehabil Couns. 2017;48:18–27.
6. Gordon C, et al. The substantial burden of systemic lupus erythematosus on the productivity and careers of patients: a European patient-driven online survey. Rheumatology. 2013;52:2292–301.
7. Katz P, Morris A, Trupin L, Yazdany J, Yelin E. Disability in valued life activities among individuals with systemic lupus erythematosus. Arthritis Care Res. 2008;59:465–73.
8. Yazdany J, et al. Quality of care in systemic lupus erythematosus: application of quality measures to understand gaps in care. J Gen Intern Med. 2012;27:1326–33.
9. Panopalis P, et al. The systemic lupus erythematosus tri-nation study: cumulative indirect costs. Arthritis Care Res. 2007;57:64–70.
10. Chan CC, Zhuo, D.-h. Occupational rehabilitation in twenty-first century Asia Pacific: facilitating health and work: an introduction. J Occup Rehabil. 2011;21:1–4.
11. Stubbs J, Deaner G. When considering vocational rehabilitation: describing and comparing the Swedish and American systems and professions. Work. 2005;24:239–49.
12. Burkhauser RV, Daly MC, McVicar D, Wilkins R. Disability benefit growth and disability reform in the US: lessons from other OECD nations. IZA J Labor Pol. 2014;3:4.
13. Nowrouzi B, et al. Workplace system factors of obstetric nurses in Northeastern Ontario, Canada: using a work disability prevention approach. Saf Health Work. 2015;6:305–11.
14. Shuey KM, Willson AE. Trajectories of work disability and economic insecurity approaching retirement. J Gerontol Ser B. 2019;74:1200–10.
15. Dagenais S, Caro J, Haldeman S. A systematic review of low back pain cost of illness studies in the United States and internationally. Spine J. 2008;8:8–20.
16. Campbell R, Cooper GS, Gilkeson GS. The impact of systemic lupus erythematosus on employment. J Rheumatol. 2009;36:2470–5.
17. Appenzeller S, Cendes F, Costallat LT. Cognitive impairment and employment status in systemic lupus erythematosus: a prospective longitudinal study. Arthritis Care Res. 2009;61:680–7.
18. Baker K, Pope J. Employment and work disability in systemic lupus erythematosus: a systematic review. Rheumatology. 2009;48:281–4.
19. Baker K, et al. Work disability in systemic lupus erythematosus is prevalent and associated with socio-demographic and disease related factors. Lupus. 2009;18:1281–8.
20. Bachen EA, Chesney MA, Criswell LA. Prevalence of mood and anxiety disorders in women with systemic lupus erythematosus. Arthritis Rheum. 2009;61:822–9.
21. Yelin E, et al. Work dynamics among persons with systemic lupus erythematosus. Arthritis Care Res. 2007;57:56–63.
22. Agarwal N, Yasui NY, Kumar V. Lupus: vocational aspects and the best rehabilitation practices. J Vocat Rehabil. 2015;43:83–90.
23. Dhanhani AA. (2010). The workplace challenges of lupus patients (Master's dissertation). https://central.bac-lac.gc.ca/.item?id=MR72493&op=pdf&app=Library&oclc_number=1019482792.
24. Garris C, Oglesby A, Sulcs E, Lee M. Impact of systemic lupus erythematosus on burden of illness and work productivity in the United States. Lupus. 2013;22:1077–86.
25. Carls G, et al. Direct and indirect costs to employers of patients with systemic lupus erythematosus with and without nephritis. J Occup Environ Med. 2009;51:66–79.
26. Clarke AE, et al. Underestimating the value of women: assessing the indirect costs of women with systemic lupus erythematosus. J Rheumatol. 2000;27:2597–604.
27. Panopalis P, et al. Health care costs and costs associated with changes in work productivity among persons with systemic lupus erythematosus. Arthritis Care Res. 2008;59:1788–95.
28. Pelletier EM, Ogale S, Yu E, Brunetta P, Garg J. Economic outcomes in patients diagnosed with systemic lupus erythematosus with versus without nephritis: results from an analysis of data from a US claims database. Clin Ther. 2009;31:2653–64.
29. Kozora E, Ellison MC, West S. Depression, fatigue, and pain in systemic lupus erythematosus (SLE): relationship to the American College of Rheumatology SLE neuropsychological battery. Arthritis Care Res. 2006;55:628–35.

30. World Health Organization. ICF: international classification of functioning, disability and health. Geneva, Switzerland: World Health Organization; 2001.
31. Loisel P, et al. Disability prevention. Dis Manag Health Out. 2001;9:351–60.
32. Black K, Feuerstein M, Loisel P. Models in WDP. In: Loisel P, Anema H, editors. Handbook of work disability: prevention and management. New York: Springer Science+Business Media; 2013.
33. Nowrouzi B, et al. Lost-time illness, injury and disability and its relationship with obesity in the workplace: a comprehensive literature review. Int J Occup Med Environ Health. 2016;29:749–66.
34. Waddell G, Main CJ, Morris EW, Di Paola M, Gray IC. Chronic low-back pain, psychologic distress, and illness behavior. Spine. 1984;9:209–13.
35. Moulin DE, Clark AJ, Speechley M, Morley-Forster PK. Chronic pain in Canada–prevalence, treatment, impact and the role of opioid analgesia. Pain Res Manag. 2002;
36. Arden N, Nevitt MC. Osteoarthritis: epidemiology. Best Pract Res Clin Rheumatol. 2006;20:3–25.
37. Kopec JA, et al. Descriptive epidemiology of osteoarthritis in British Columbia, Canada. J Rheumatol. 2007;34:386–93.
38. Sullivan M, Martel M, Trost Z. Pain, chronicity, and disability. In: Loisel P, Anema H, editors. Handbook of work disability: prevention and management. New York: Springer Science+Business Media; 2013.
39. Loisel P, et al. A population-based, randomized clinical trial on back pain management. Spine. 1997;22:2911–8.
40. Lindström I, et al. The effect of graded activity on patients with subacute low back pain: a randomized prospective clinical study with an operant-conditioning behavioral approach. Phys Ther. 1992;72:279–90.
41. Indahl A, Velund L, Reikeraas O. Good prognosis for low back pain when left untampered: a randomized clinical trial. Spine. 1995;20:473–7.
42. Yelin E, et al. Work loss and work entry among persons with systemic lupus erythematosus: comparisons with a national matched sample. Arthritis Care Res. 2009;61:247–58.
43. Almehed K, Carlsten H, Forsblad-d'Elia H. Health-related quality of life in systemic lupus erythematosus and its association with disease and work disability. Scand J Rheumatol. 2010;39:58–62.
44. Faurschou M, Dreyer L, Kamper AL, Starklint H, Jacobsen S. Long-term mortality and renal outcome in a cohort of 100 patients with lupus nephritis. Arthritis Care Res. 2010;62:873–80.
45. Jetha A, Pransky G, Hettinger LJ. Capturing complexity in work disability research: application of system dynamics modeling methodology. Disabil Rehabil. 2016;38:189–94.
46. Breslin FC, Lay AM, Jetha A, Smith P. Examining occupational health and safety vulnerability among Canadian workers with disabilities. Disabil Rehabil. 2018;40:2138–43.
47. Williams RM, Westmorland M. Perspectives on workplace disability management: a review of the literature. Work. 2002;19:87–93.
48. Verbeek J, Sengers M-J, Riemens L, Haafkens J. Patient expectations of treatment for back pain: a systematic review of qualitative and quantitative studies. Spine. 2004;29:2309–18.
49. Loisel P, et al. Prevention of work disability due to musculoskeletal disorders: the challenge of implementing evidence. J Occup Rehabil. 2005;15:507–24.
50. Bruce B, Fries JF. The health assessment questionnaire (HAQ). Clin Exp Rheumatol. 2005;23:S14.
51. Leidy NK, Revicki DA, Genesté B. Recommendations for evaluating the validity of quality of life claims for labeling and promotion. Value Health. 1999;2:113–27.
52. Revicki DA, et al. Recommendations on health-related quality of life research to support labeling and promotional claims in the United States. Qual Life Res. 2000;9:887–900.
53. Wolfe F, Pincus T. Listening to the patient: a practical guide to self-report questionnaires in clinical care. Arthritis Rheum. 1999;42:1797–808.
54. Parodis I, et al. The impact of belimumab and rituximab on health-related quality of life in patients with systemic lupus erythematosus. Arthritis Care Res. 2019;71:811–21.

55. Duruöz M, et al. The validity and reliability of Systemic Lupus Erythematosus Quality of Life Questionnaire (L-QoL) in a Turkish population. Lupus. 2017;26:1528–33.
56. Milligan S, et al. An assessment of the Health Assessment Questionnaire functional ability index among women with systemic lupus erythematosus. J Rheumatol. 1993;20:972–6.
57. Wolfe F. Data collection and utilization: a methodology for clinical practice and clinical research. In: Wolfe F, Pincus T, Dekker M, editors. Rheumatoid arthritis: pathogenesis, assessment, outcome and treatment. New York: Marcel Dekker; 1994. p. 463–514.
58. World Health Organization. WHO disability assessment schedule 2.0 WHODAS 2.0, vol. 2020. Geneva, Switzerland: World Health Organization; 2020.
59. Federici S, Bracalenti M, Meloni F, Luciano JV. World Health Organization disability assessment schedule 2.0: an international systematic review. Disabil Rehabil. 2017;39:2347–80.
60. Association, A.P. Diagnostic and statistical manual of mental disorders (DSM-5®): American Psychiatric Pub; 2013.
61. Migone P. Presentazione del DSM-5. Psicoterapia e Scienze Umane; 2013.
62. Abma FI, et al. The work role functioning questionnaire v2. 0 showed consistent factor structure across six working samples. J Occup Rehabil. 2018;28:465–74.
63. Ilmarinen J. The work ability index (WAI). Occup Med. 2007;57:160.
64. Radkiewicz P, Widerszal-Bazyl M, Group, N.-S. Psychometric properties of Work Ability Index in the light of comparative survey study. In: International congress series, vol. 1280: Elsevier; 2005. p. 304–9.
65. Lerner D, et al. The work limitations questionnaire. Med Care. 2001:72–85.
66. Peugeot M Relation of cognitive measures to perceived work limitations in cancer survivors. (Uniformed Services University of the Health Sciences Bethesda MD F Edward Hebert …; 2009.
67. Nena E, Steiropoulos P, Constantinidis TC, Perantoni E, Tsara V. Work productivity in obstructive sleep apnea patients. J Occup Environ Med. 2010;52:622–5.
68. Zhang W, et al. Validity of the work productivity and activity impairment questionnaire-general health version in patients with rheumatoid arthritis. Arthritis Res Ther. 2010;12:R177.
69. Yang M, Morin CM, Schaefer K, Wallenstein GV. Interpreting score differences in the Insomnia Severity Index: using health-related outcomes to define the minimally important difference. Curr Med Res Opin. 2009;25:2487–94.
70. Montgomery SA, Nielsen RZ, Poulsen LH, Häggström L. A randomised, double-blind study in adults with major depressive disorder with an inadequate response to a single course of selective serotonin reuptake inhibitor or serotonin–noradrenaline reuptake inhibitor treatment switched to vortioxetine or agomelatine. Hum Psychopharmacol Clin Exp. 2014;29:470–82.
71. Gibson L, Strong J. A conceptual framework of functional capacity evaluation for occupational therapy in work rehabilitation. Aust Occup Ther J. 2003;50:64–71.
72. Hart DL, Isernhagen SJ, Matheson LN. Guidelines for functional capacity evaluation of people with medical conditions. J Orthop Sports Phys Ther. 1993;18:682–6.
73. King PM, Tuckwell N, Barrett TE. A critical review of functional capacity evaluations. Phys Ther. 1998;78:852–66.
74. McFadden S, MacDonald A, Fogarty A, Le S, Merritt BK. Vocational assessment: a review of the literature from an occupation-based perspective. Scand J Occup Ther. 2010;17:43–8.
75. Isernhagen S. Advancements in functional capacity evaluation. Back Pain Rehabil. 1993:180–204.
76. Eser G. Overview of vocational evaluation. Las Vegas, NV: Workshop, S.U.T.; 1983.
77. Holmes D. The role of the occupational therapist–work evaluator. Am J Occup Ther. 1985;39:308–13.
78. United States Department of Labor. United States Employment, S. & the North Carolina Occupational Analysis Field, C. Dictionary of Occupational Titles (DOT): Revised Fourth Edition, 1991. ([distributor], 2006).
79. Baum CM, Law M. Occupational therapy practice: focusing on occupational performance. Am J Occup Ther. 1997;51:277–88.

# Chapter 18
# Metrics and Outcomes of SLE Clinical Trials

**Shereen Oon and Mandana Nikpour**

## Introduction

The systemic lupus erythematosus (SLE) clinical trial landscape has been marred by the failure of multiple mechanistically promising drugs to meet their primary endpoints at the final hurdle of a phase III clinical trial. Although a number of factors have contributed to these failures, the choice of primary endpoint can be a critical determinant of trial success or failure. Developing a robust and clinically relevant trial outcome measure in SLE is challenging, given the heterogeneity and fluctuating nature of the disease and the lack of consensus regarding a definition of remission in the disease. In 1987, members of the Systemic Lupus International Collaborating Clinics (SLICC) began to develop a consensus for disease activity indices and outcome measures for SLE randomized clinical trials (RCTs) [1]. A variety of outcome measures have subsequently been employed in SLE clinical trials. This chapter discusses these different SLE outcome measures and their advantages and limitations when used in the clinical trial setting (Table 18.1).

---

S. Oon
Department of Medicine at St Vincent's Hospital, The University of Melbourne, Parkville, VIC, Australia

Department of Rheumatology, St Vincent's Hospital, Fitzroy, VIC, Australia

Department of Rheumatology, The Royal Melbourne Hospital, Parkville, VIC, Australia

M. Nikpour (✉)
Department of Medicine at St Vincent's Hospital, The University of Melbourne, Parkville, VIC, Australia

Department of Rheumatology, St Vincent's Hospital, Fitzroy, VIC, Australia
e-mail: m.nikpour@unimelb.edu.au



Z. Touma (ed.), *Outcome Measures and Metrics in Systemic Lupus Erythematosus*, https://doi.org/10.1007/978-3-030-73303-2_18

**Table 18.1** Outcome measures in SLE clinical trials: advantages and disadvantages

| Outcome measure | Definition | Advantages | Disadvantages | Trials utilized in |
|---|---|---|---|---|
| **SRI-X** (Systemic Lupus Erythematosus Responder Index) | 1. ≥X reduction in SELENA-SLEDAI score<br>2. No new BILAG A or <1 new BILAG B domain scores<br>3. No deterioration from baseline in PGA ≥0.3 points | Composite index<br>Better at capturing disease activity globally and within organ systems than single indices | Greater complexity<br>Time-consuming<br>Requires training to complete<br>SLEDAI-based measure – may be less sensitive than BILAG-based composite measures in detecting changes in disease activity within organ systems. | * *SRI-4:* Belimumab phase III trials – BLISS-52 [5], BLISS-76 [4], BLISS-SC [6][a,b]<br>* *SRI-4:* Anifrolumab phase III TULIP-1 trial [10][a]<br>* *SRI-5*: Tabalumab phase III trials – ILLUMINATE-1 [7][a], ILLUMINATE-2 [8][a,b]<br>* *SRI-6*: Blisibimod phase III trial [9] |
| **BICLA** (BILAG-Based Composite Lupus Assessment) | 1. Improvement in moderate-severe BILAG-2004 activity<br>2. No worsening in global and organ-specific disease activity (no new BILAG-2004 A or ≤1 new BILAG B score, no worsening of SLEDAI-2K score from baseline to endpoint and no worsening in PGA (<10%))<br>3. No treatment failure (addition of non-protocol SLE treatments) | Composite index<br>Better at capturing disease activity globally and within organ systems than single indices<br>May be more sensitive than SLEDAI-based composite indices in detecting changes in disease activity within individual organ systems<br>Stringent endpoint | Greater complexity<br>Time-consuming<br>Requires training to complete | * Epratuzumab phase IIb trial – EMBLEM [12][a]<br>* Epratuzumab phase III trials – EMBODY-1 and EMBODY-2 [13][a]<br>* Anifrolumab phase III TULIP-2 trial [11][a,b] |

| | | | | |
|---|---|---|---|---|
| **LDAS** (Lupus Low Disease Activity State) | 1. SLEDAI-2K ≤4, with no activity in major organ systems, no haemolytic anaemia or gastrointestinal activity<br>2. No new features of lupus disease activity compared with previous assessment<br>3. PGA score ≤1<br>4. Current prednisolone-equivalent dose ≤7.5 mg/day<br>5. Standard maintenance doses of immunosuppressive drugs and approved biologics allowed | Composite index<br>Stringent measure – fewer patients attain LLDAS compared to SRI<br>Clinically relevant – LLDAS attainment associated with reduced damage accrual and better health-related quality of life | Greater complexity<br>More time-consuming to complete | * Belimumab phase III intravenous trials – BLISS-52 and BLISS-76 [21][b,c])<br>* Anifrolumab phase II trial – MUSE [19][b,c]<br>* Atacicept phase II trial – ADDRESS [20][b,c]<br>* Baricitinib phase II trial [18][b,c] |
| **SLEDAI** (Systemic Lupus Erythematosus Disease Activity Index) | Sum of scores across 24 weighted items | Relatively simple to complete | May lack accuracy in assessing global disease activity, due to limited items included, and relies on presence rather than severity of organ activity item | * Belimumab phase II trial [2][a] |
| **BILAG** (British Isles Lupus Assessment Group Index) | Includes 97 items across 9 organ system domains<br>Complex algorithm required to score | Better captures changes in disease activity within organs as it measures severity of manifestations rather than presence, as compared to the SLEDAI | Greater complexity and time required to complete<br>BILAG-2004 greater sensitivity than earlier BILAG version | * Rituximab phase III non renal trial – EXPLORER [36][a]<br>* Atacicept phase II/III trial [37][a]<br>* Abatacept phase IIb trial [35][a]<br>* Rontalizumab phase II trial – ROSE [38][a] |

(continued)

**Table 18.1** (continued)

| Outcome measure | Definition | Advantages | Disadvantages | Trials utilized in |
|---|---|---|---|---|
| **CLASI** (Cutaneous Lupus Erythematosus Disease Area and Severity Index) | Single-page tool assessing both disease activity and damage; accounts for presence of skin lesions, mucous membrane disease and alopecia | Relatively simple and quick to complete<br>Provides comprehensive information on both activity and damage<br>High intra- and inter-rater reliability (both dermatologists and rheumatologists) | Affected body parts weighted equally regardless of surface area or number of lesions present. | * Anifrolumab phase III TULIP-1 trial [10][b,d]<br>* Baricitinib phase II trial [18][d] |
| **Joint indices** | SLEDAI-2K improvement in joint count<br>28 tender and swollen joint counts<br>LARI (Lupus Arthritis Responder Index) – (a) ≥50% decrease in combined tender and swollen joint count compared to baseline, (b) ≥1 letter improvement in BILAG musculoskeletal system score compared to baseline, (c) specified steroid reduction compared to baseline | 28 joint count: relatively simple to complete but provides comprehensive information | 28 joint count: excludes certain joints such as hips, ankles and feet | * *SLEDAI-2K improvement in joint count:* Baricitinib phase II trial [18][a,b] – combined endpoint with SLEDAI-2K improvement in rash<br>* *28 tender and swollen joint counts:* Baricitinib phase II trial [18][b,d] |
| **Renal indices** | Complete and partial responses dependent upon specified improvement in proteinuria, urinary sediment and renal function<br>Definitions of renal 'flare' | | No agreement as to cut-offs for complete and partial response across studies | * *Renal flare* – abetimus sodium phase III trial [49][a]<br>*Complete/partial response*<br>* Rituximab phase III in renal lupus (LUNAR) trial [51][a] |

[a]primary endpoint
[b]positive result
[c]applied post hoc
[d]secondary or exploratory endpoint

## Composite Outcome Measures in SLE Clinical Trials

The majority of recent phase II and III trials in SLE have utilized a composite outcome measure as their primary outcome measure. These composite measures usually comprise a SLEDAI (Systemic Lupus Erythematosus Disease Activity Index), BILAG (British Isles Lupus Assessment Group Index)-based component and the PGA (Physician Global Assessment). The most commonly utilized composite measure has been the SLEDAI-based Systemic Lupus Erythematosus Responder Index (SRI); the BILAG-based BICLA (BILAG-Based Composite Lupus Assessment) has been used in more recent trials. These composite measures generally have better sensitivity in capturing subtle changes in disease activity, as opposed to single indices, at the expense of requiring greater expertise and time to score, with the attendant associated increased costs, for example, to employ adjudication committees to verify scoring during trial data collection.

### *Systemic Lupus Erythematosus Responder Index (SRI)*

#### Definition

The Systemic Lupus Erythematosus Responder Index (SRI) was developed following the large phase II trial of intravenous belimumab (an anti-B-cell-activating factor (BAFF) monoclonal antibody) for non-renal SLE [2], and its utility was first demonstrated in a post hoc analysis of a subpopulation of patients from that study [1]. The study had not met its co-primary endpoints of a percentage change in SELENA-SLEDAI score from baseline to week 24 and time to first mild/moderate or severe flare as defined by the SFI (SELENA-SLEDAI Flare Index) during 52 weeks. However, a subset of serologically active patients (ANA $\geq$1:80 and/or anti-dsDNA $\geq$30 IU/mL) were seen to respond better to belimumab than placebo, and it was to this population of patients that the SRI was first applied. To overcome the potential limitations of using single disease measures, the SRI was formulated to measure global improvement using the SELENA-SLEDAI, ensure no worsening in organ systems with the BILAG and capture potential worsening of overall disease activity missed by the SELENA-SLEDAI or BILAG, with the PGA. In the analysis for this study, the SRI was defined as meeting three criteria: (1) a $\geq$X reduction in SELENA-SLEDAI score (e.g. a $\geq$4 point reduction in SELENA-SLEDAI score is termed as SRI-4 and a $\geq$5 point reduction as SRI-5; a cut-off of $\geq$4 is generally used based on the established minimally clinically important difference for the SLEDAI [3]); (2) no new BILAG A or $\leq$1 new BILAG B domain scores; and (3) no deterioration from baseline in the PGA by $\geq$0.3 points on a 0 to 3 scale, where 0 is no disease activity and 3 is maximum possible disease activity. A significant difference at week 52 was seen in attainment of an SRI-4 between belimumab-treated patients and placebo (46% versus 29%, $p = 0.006$); a significant difference in attainment of an

SRI-5 was also seen (35.9% vs 22.5%, $p = 0.034$). A trend to a greater percentage of patients receiving belimumab attaining an SRI-6 or SRI-7 was also evident. Moreover, analysis of the entire trial population, regardless of baseline autoantibody status, showed a significantly higher week 52 SRI-4 response in the belimumab compared to placebo group (45.9% vs 35.4%, $p = 0.045$). These responses remained in spite of removal of anti-dsDNA and complement values from the SELENA-SLEDAI.

## Performance

Since its development, the SRI has been utilized as the primary outcome measure in a number of clinical trials, most notably the phase III intravenous (BLISS-52 and BLISS-76) [4, 5] and subcutaneous (BLISS-SC) [6] belimumab trials, in which the primary endpoint of an SRI-4 was met in all three trials. Modest but significant differences in the percentage of patients (all of whom were seropositive) attaining a week 52 SRI-4 response were seen in the belimumab 10 mg/kg group compared to placebo for both intravenous studies (58% versus 44%, $p = 0.013$ for the BLISS-52 trial and 43.2% versus 33.5%, $p = 0.017$ for the BLISS-76 trial); however the difference between belimumab and placebo at week 76 in the BLISS-76 trial was not statistically significant. A similarly modest but significant difference in SRI-4 attainment was demonstrated in the BLISS-SC trial (61.4% versus 48.4%, $p = 0.0006$).

The SRI was also utilized in the two phase III trials of another anti-BAFF monoclonal antibody (mAb), tabalumab (ILLUMINATE 1 [7] and ILLUMINATE 2 [8]). In these trials, the primary endpoint of an SRI-5 at week 52 was met only for the higher dose of 120 mg subcutaneously 2 weekly (compared to 120 mg 4 weekly) in the ILLUMINATE-2 trial; in this group, SRI-4, SRI-6, SRI-7, SRI-9 and SRI-10 were also obtained. Higher SRIs (i.e. those that require a greater improvement in SLEDAI) may be a more stringent discriminator between drug and placebo, although they may be harder to achieve. Key secondary endpoints were also not met; however, biological activity was seen, with significant reductions in antibody levels and increases in complement. An SRI-6 at week 52 was chosen as the primary endpoint in the phase III trial of blisibimod, another anti-BAFF mAb [9]. The primary endpoint was not met (46.9% with blisibimod compared to 42.3% with placebo, $p = 0.352$); however the result may have been confounded by higher steroid doses throughout the trial in the standard of care group; in this trial, biological activity was also seen with reduction in autoantibodies and B cells and increases in complement levels.

Recently, the SRI-4 was used as the primary endpoint in the TULIP-1 trial of intravenous anifrolumab (an anti-type I interferon receptor monoclonal antibody), which was a negative study [10]. Interestingly, a different, BILAG-based primary endpoint (the BICLA) was chosen as the primary endpoint for the parallel phase III TULIP-2 trial [11], which was a positive study (attained by 47.8% in the anifrolumab group compared to 31.5% in the placebo group, $p = 0.001$). The differences in attainment of primary endpoint may have been because the BICLA is based on the BILAG-2004, which can register both partial and complete improvement within an organ system, whereas the SRI (a SLEDAI-based measure) requires complete resolution within a particular item to register change.

### Advantages and Disadvantages

The SRI better captures changes in disease activity, compared to solitary disease activity indices, by incorporating global measures of disease activity and the ability to measure change within individual organ systems, and has been used successfully in several phase III clinical trials. However, being a primarily SLEDAI-based measure, the SRI may not be as sensitive a measure of change compared to BILAG-based composite measures such as the BICLA, which can capture partial improvement in addition to complete resolution of activity within an organ system, as seen in the phase III anifrolumab trials.

## *BILAG-Based Combined Lupus Assessment (BICLA)*

### Definition

The BICLA (BILAG-Based Composite Lupus Assessment) was first used as a primary endpoint in the phase IIb trial of epratuzumab, a mAb that binds CD22, a cell surface marker present on mature B cells (EMBLEM) [12]. Similar to the SRI, the BICLA requires improvement in baseline disease activity and no worsening (global or organ specific) of disease; in addition, there can be no 'treatment failure'. The criteria for the BICLA response require as follows: (1) improvement in moderate-severe BILAG-2004 activity (all A scores at study entry improved to B/C/D, and all B scores improved to C/D); (2) no worsening in global and organ-specific disease activity (no new BILAG-2004 A or $\leq 1$ new BILAG B scores, no worsening of SLEDAI-2K score from baseline to endpoint, and no worsening in PGA (<10% worsening)); and (3) no treatment failure (addition of non-protocol SLE treatments, such as new/increased immunosuppressants or antimalarials, increased or parenteral corticosteroids or premature discontinuation from study treatment). A primary endpoint of a week 12 BICLA was utilized for this study, which examined epratuzumab at 5 doses (cumulative dose per month ranging from 200 to 3600 mg, dosed at weekly or fortnightly intervals). A statistically significant overall treatment effect of epratuzumab was not seen for the primary endpoint; however the placebo effect was low at 21.1%, potentially reflecting the stringent nature of the endpoint, and a benefit for the 2400 mg dose, compared to placebo, was shown (43.2%, $p = 0.02$), as early as week 8 of the study.

## Performance

The BICLA was subsequently employed in the phase III trials of epratuzumab (EMBODY-1 and EMBODY-2 [13]), with the primary endpoint defined at week 48. In these trials, there was no statistically significance difference seen in the primary endpoint between treatment groups (600 mg weekly and 1200 mg every other week, given for the first 4 weeks in a 12-week repeating cycle) compared to placebo, with response rates ranging between 33.5% and 39.8%. This result was consistent across multiple outcome measures including various sensitivity analyses and a post hoc analysis using an adjusted BICLA definition of response, which omitted the 'treatment' failure portion of the criteria. Similarly, key secondary endpoints, various exploratory endpoints, and a post hoc analysis using a modified SRI response at an SRI-4, SRI-6 or SRI-8 showed no difference between treatment and placebo groups.

As mentioned previously, the BICLA at week 52 was utilized as the primary outcome measure in the recently published second phase III trial of anifrolumab, TULIP-2 [11]. The earlier published trial, TULIP-1 [10], had utilized the SRI-4 at week 52 as its primary outcome measure, based on its successful use in the belimumab trials, but had returned a negative result. However, benefit in pre-specified secondary endpoints, including the BICLA, was seen. Informed by these results, the primary endpoint for TULIP-2 was changed in a protocol amendment before unblinding of the TULIP-2 trial data, from an SRI-4, to the BICLA [11]. A significant difference in week 52 BICLA was seen (47.8% responders in the anifrolumab group compared to 31.5% in the placebo group, $p = 0.001$); additionally, a difference in SRI-4 across multiple timepoints was seen; however it was not formally assessed for statistical significance.

## Advantages and Disadvantages

Like the SRI, the BICLA, as a composite outcome measure, more comprehensively captures changes in disease activity compared to single indices such as the SLEDAI or BILAG. In contrast to the SRI, the BICLA may better capture subtle changes in disease activity, as the SRI relies on the *presence* of disease activity (as required in the SLEDAI) as opposed to reflecting a change in *severity* of disease (as captured by the BILAG), a phenomenon that may have contributed to the differential results of the two anifrolumab phase III trials. Interestingly though, the BICLA has been found to be less sensitive than the SRI in determining clinically significant improvement (as determined by the treating physician), potentially due to the BICLA requiring at minimum partial improvement in organ systems [14].

## *Low Disease Activity and Remission States*

### Definition

In recent years, there has been increasing interest in utilizing various treat-to-target measures as clinical trial endpoints. These include measures of low disease activity such as the Lupus Low Disease Activity State (LLDAS) and states of 'remission'. The LLDAS was conceptually defined as 'a state which, if sustained, is associated with a low likelihood of adverse outcome, considering disease activity and medication safety' and has been found to correlate with reduced damage accrual in SLE in both retrospective and prospective studies [15, 16] and with improved health-related quality of life [17]. It is defined as being attained if all of the following criteria are met: (1) a SLEDAI-2K score ≤4, with no activity in major organ systems (renal, central nervous system, cardiopulmonary, vasculitis and fever) and no haemolytic anaemia or gastrointestinal activity; (2) no new features of lupus disease activity compared with the previous assessment; (3) a PGA score ≤1; 4) current prednisolone-equivalent dosage ≤7.5 mg/day; and (5) standard maintenance dosages of immunosuppressive drugs and approved biologics allowed.

### Performance

To date, these treat-to-target measures have not been utilized as the primary endpoint in SLE clinical trials; however the LLDAS has been employed as an exploratory endpoint in the phase II baricitinib trial [18] and examined in post hoc analyses of various phase II and III clinical trials, including the phase II trial of anifrolumab (MUSE) [19] and atacicept (ADDRESS II) [20] and the phase III trials of intravenous belimumab [21]. In these trials, the LLDAS has been seen to be able to discriminate responders (to drug) from non-responders and to be a potentially more stringent measure than the SRI-4 and BICLA, with fewer patients overall, and very few patients on placebo, attaining LLDAS than both of these measures. In a post hoc analysis of the phase III intravenous belimumab trials [21], significantly more patients attained LLDAS on belimumab 10 mg/kg compared to placebo, although the rates of attainment compared to the SRI-4 were much lower (12.5% vs 5.8%, OR 2.32, $p = 0.02$ for BLISS-52; 14.4% vs 7.8%, OR 1.98, $p = 0.04$ for BLISS-76). However, at week 52, for belimumab 10 mg/kg, only 17.0% and 19.3% of patients who achieved an SRI-4 also attained LLDAS in the BLISS-52 and BLISS-76 trials, respectively. A post hoc analysis of the phase IIb trial of anifrolumab (MUSE) [19] showed that the LLDAS was positively associated but more stringent than the SRI-4 and BICLA – 87% and 74% of LLDAS responders were SRI-4 and BICLA responders, respectively (both nominal $p < 0.001$); only 47% of SRI-4 and 51% of BICLA responders reached LLDAS.

In a post hoc analysis of the phase IIb atacicept trial (ADDRESS II) [20], both low disease activity and remission were seen to be more stringent than SRI-4 (and SRI-6) responses at week 24. In this analysis, both the LLDAS and LDA (low disease activity) were used as low disease activity outcome measures, with the LDA being simply defined as a SLEDAI-2K $\leq 2$. The remission state was defined using the Definitions of Remission in SLE (DORIS) criteria (clinical SLEDAI-2K = 0; prednisolone-equivalent dosage $\leq$5 mg/day; PGA < 0.5). In this study, it was also shown that the low disease activity and remission states were able to be obtained from a high initial disease activity state (SLEDAI-2K $\leq 10$).

### Advantages and Disadvantages

These data indicate that low disease activity and remission states represent clinically relevant and robust outcome measures when applied in the clinical trial setting, with the ability to discriminate responders, whilst being more stringent than accepted composite primary outcome measures such as the SRI and the BICLA.

## Single Outcome Measures in SLE Clinical Trials

Single disease indices such as the SLEDAI and BILAG (and their various iterations) have been shown to correlate with each other [22–24] and have been validated in long-term observational studies and utilized reliably in this context, although baseline scores did not always predict subsequent damage or other outcomes [25, 26]. Use in RCTs indicates that these indices correlate with response rates, disease remission and flare prevention [27]. These single disease indices generally fall into two groups – the first, measuring changes in global disease activity, such as the SLEDAI, and the second, reflecting changes in disease activity within organ systems, such as the BILAG. Single disease indices were used as the primary outcome measures in early SLE RCTs; later trials utilize these measures largely as secondary endpoints.

## *Global Disease Indices (e.g. SLEDAI, SFI)*

### SLEDAI

The SLEDAI (Systemic Lupus Erythematosus Disease Activity Index) is discussed in further detail in other chapters; however, in brief, there have been several versions of the SLEDAI – the original [28], the SELENA-SLEDAI [29] and the SLEDAI-2K [30], of which the SLEDAI-2K is now most frequently utilized in clinical trials. The SLEDAI comprises the sum of the score of 24 items present (generally in the last

10 days, with SLEDAI-2K capturing activity in the last 30 days), weighted for severity (e.g. vasculitis scores 8, alopecia 2). The different versions include the same items for scoring; however some items have different definitions (largely relating to proteinuria, rash, ulcers and alopecia).

An advantage of the SLEDAI is its simplicity of use; however, it may lack accuracy in judging global disease activity, because it reflects only the presence of an item, rather than its magnitude of severity. The included disease manifestations are also limited, with severe manifestations such as gastrointestinal inflammation not being included. Neuropsychiatric manifestations are given a slight overemphasis, each being assigned a weighted score of 8, whereas thrombocytopenia is only scored as 1, regardless of severity.

### SLEDAI Flare Index (SFI)

The SELENA-SLEDAI Flare Index (SFI) is another commonly employed secondary endpoint commonly employed secondary endpoint in SLE RCTs. It represents a composite outcome of SELENA-SLEDAI score, the PGA, a change in treatment decision and the presence of different disease manifestations of varying severity, which allows classification into mild/moderate or severe flares [31].

Both the SELENA-SLEDAI and SFI were used as co-primary endpoints in the phase II intravenous belimumab trial [2], an outcome which was not met and the limitations of which led to the development of the composite indices used in more recent trials.

## *Organ-Specific Disease Indices (e.g. BILAG, CLASI, Renal Indices)*

### BILAG

Similar to the SLEDAI, the original BILAG [32] has been revised a number of times, with the BILAG-2004 [33] (revised also in 2009 [34]) currently utilized in SLE clinical trials. Unlike the SLEDAI, the BILAG reflects the *severity* and *change over time* of disease activity within organ systems, however, with the trade-off of greater complexity, requiring increased time and training to evaluate. The BILAG comprises 97 items across 9 organ system domains (e.g. mucocutaneous, musculoskeletal) which are scored as 0 (not present), 1 (improving), 2 (same), 3 (worse) or 4 (new), comparing activity in the last 4 weeks to the previous 4 weeks. An A (severe), B (moderate), C (mild), D (no activity) or E (no history) score is then assigned to each domain, utilizing a complicated determination algorithm. It is in theory possible to reflect global disease activity with the BILAG by adding the scores of each domain together; however this is not usually done.

Earlier RCTs such as the phase IIb abatacept in non-renal SLE [35], the phase III rituximab in non-renal SLE [36] and phase II/III atacicept trial in SLE [37] had utilized the original BILAG, whereas more recent trials such as the phase II rontalizumab (anti-IFNα mAb) trial employed the BILAG-2004 [38]. As the latest version of the BILAG is generally more sensitive in reflecting disease activity, reporting less false positive disease activity than the original [39], the difference in versions may explain variances in trial outcomes to some degree. BILAG-related endpoints are generally expressed either as an improvement in BILAG domains (BILAG response) or as a flare (BILAG flares) or a combination thereof. For example, in the phase III rituximab in non-renal lupus (EXPLORER) [36] trial, a major clinical response was defined as an improvement to BILAG C scores or better in all organ systems at week 24, without experiencing a severe flare (defined as 1 new BILAG A score or 2 new BILAG B scores), maintained without a moderate or severe flare (≥1 new BILAG A or B score) to week 52 of the trial. The definition of BILAG-based endpoints varies between different studies, which makes comparison between study outcomes difficult.

## Cutaneous Lupus (CLASI) Index

Although the SLEDAI and BILAG include some cutaneous disease items, neither of these comprehensively track cutaneous lupus erythematosus (CLE) disease activity [40, 41]. The Cutaneous Lupus Erythematosus Disease Area and Severity Index (CLASI) was therefore developed in 2005 [42, 43], in order to provide a quantitative measure of the burden of cutaneous disease *activity* and *damage*, thereby allowing standardized assessments of disease progression [44]. Recently, an international group of dermatologists agreed unanimously that the CLASI be used in clinical trials as a measure of skin activity [45, 46].

The CLASI is a single-page tool, which assigns activity scores to each part of the body, based on the presence of erythema, scale, mucous membrane lesions and alopecia, with points weighted for severity. The presence of dyspigmentation, scarring and scarring alopecia contributes to the damage score. Scores for each area are based on the worst lesion in the assigned area, and affected body parts are weighted equally regardless of surface area or number of lesions present; higher weighting of visible areas reflects greater patient impairment. The total score for activity and damage is calculated by the addition of the individual component scores. The CLASI is relatively simple and quick to complete whilst providing comprehensive information regarding current CLE activity (average time to completion 5.25 minutes, ranging from 1 to 11 minutes [42]). The CLASI has been found to have high intra- and inter-rater reliability with both dermatologists and rheumatologists [42] and clinical responsiveness [47].

The CLASI has been used as an endpoint in a number of clinical trials including the TULIP-1 phase III trial of anifrolumab [10] and the phase II trial of baricitinib in SLE [18]. In the TULIP-1 trial, although the primary endpoint of an SRI-4 was not met, benefit for skin disease was suggested by an improvement of at least 50%

by week 12 in those with a CLASI score of at least 10 at baseline (42% in the anifrolumab 300 mg group as compared with 25% in the placebo group).

## Arthritis Indices in Lupus

Similar to cutaneous lupus, items capturing activity of lupus arthritis are included in both the SLEDAI and the BILAG; however these do not provide as complete an assessment as specific arthritis outcome measures (e.g. the SLEDAI-2K defines arthritis simply as ≥2 joints with pain and signs of inflammation, i.e. tenderness, swelling or effusion). In recent SLE trials, arthritis is often captured as an exploratory or secondary endpoint in a 28 tender and swollen joint count, such as that validated for use in rheumatoid arthritis. This tool includes the shoulders, elbows, wrist, metacarpophalangeal joints, interphalangeal joints and knees but does not include other joints such as the hips, ankle and feet. In the phase Ib trial of AMG 557 (an anti-ICOSL monoclonal antibody), the LARI (Lupus Arthritis Responder Index), a novel composite endpoint focussing on arthritis activity, was used as the primary endpoint. This was defined as a ≥50% decrease in the combined tender and swollen joint counts on day 169 compared with baseline, ≥1 letter improvement in the BILAG musculoskeletal system score on day 169 compared with baseline and a reduction in and maintenance of the dosage of prednisone (or its equivalent) to ≤50% of baseline or ≤7.5 mg/day, whichever was lower, from day 85 to day 169 in patients not treated with immunosuppressants at baseline; and ≤7.5 mg/day of prednisolone from day 85 to day 169 and discontinuation of immunosuppressants by day 29 in patients treated with immunosuppressants at baseline [48]. Although numbers were small in this pilot study, there was a trend to greater LARI response in AMG 557-treated patients, as compared to placebo.

The primary outcome in the phase II trial of baricitinib in SLE [18] was determined as the resolution of SLEDAI-2K arthritis *or* rash. This endpoint was met for the 4 mg dose at week 24; however analysis of the CLASI and 28 tender and swollen joint count showed that a significant difference was seen in the 28 tender joint count, rather than CLASI, indicating that organ-specific disease indices can assist in determining specific organ systems that may benefit from particular therapies, which is not easily appreciated in complex composite indices.

## Renal Indices

Various outcome measures have been used to gauge lupus nephritis disease activity, including a change in, or specific level of, proteinuria, urinary sediment and/or renal function. Some earlier trials used renal flare as an outcome measure [49]. Composite endpoints designated as 'complete' or 'partial' response, defined as improvements to pre-specified levels in these renal outcome measures, have been used in more recent clinical trials, although the precise definition of response varies between studies. This lack of consensus in renal response endpoints can drastically alter trial results, as shown in a study [50] analysing the data of the IM101075 trial (phase II/III trial of abatacept in lupus nephritis) with endpoints from a number of other lupus nephritis trials, the LUNAR (phase III rituximab) [51], ALMS (mycophenolate mofetil) [52] and ACCESS (abatacept and cyclophosphamide combination) [53] trials. The definitions of complete response differed in terms of urine protein/creatinine ratio required to be reached (between ≤0.20 and 0.50 g/g), level of improvement in creatinine or estimated glomerular filtration rate reached (normal, or within 10–25% of screening or baseline value), the presence of urinalysis cells or cast (normal, or not assessed), steroid taper required (none, not included or required) and whether the complete response criteria was required to be met over two consecutive visits. Analysed with their pre-specified complete response criteria, there was no difference among treatment groups in the IM101075 trial; however, when analysed with the criteria from the other three trials, a difference in response was seen, which was highest when the most lenient criteria were applied.

## Patient-Reported Outcomes (PROs) in SLE Clinical Trials

Patient-reported outcomes represent an important adjunct to assessing the global health of a lupus patient, as there is a well-known disparity between physician and patient assessment of SLE activity [54]. PROs are routinely included in most recent SLE clinical trials as secondary endpoints and enable the systematic collection of data concerning the patient's experience of disease, which is not readily captured in traditional disease activity indices. A detailed discussion of lupus PROs is included in a separate chapter; however in the clinical trials, the most frequently used PRO measure is the Short Form 36 (SF-36) [55, 56]. The FACIT-Fatigue (Functional Assessment of Chronic Illness Therapy-Fatigue) score [57] and EQ-5D (EuroQoL) [58] are also commonly included. Although there has been discordance between PROs and disease activity indices [55], trials that have met their primary endpoint have also found improvements in PRO outcomes, such as in the belimumab phase III trials [59].

## Other Measures

### *Physician Global Assessment (PGA)*

In SLE clinical trials, the PGA comprises a component of the composite outcome measures or at times is used alone as a secondary endpoint. Compared to the other (single) outcome measures, it perhaps best reflects a global state of disease activity, being able to take into account items that are not formally scored in the SLEDAI or

BILAG (e.g. fatigue). A recent case-based survey of lupus experts [60] found that whilst there was excellent inter-rater reliability of the PGA when applied to a set of real-life-based clinical scenarios, knowledge of laboratory indicators of SLE disease activity affected the PGA score. Therefore, scoring the PGA on the day of a study visit, as is often mandated in SLE trials, may undermine the accuracy of the PGA as laboratory tests are not available at the time of scoring. Additionally, the study found that clinicians were differentially influenced by various factors in determining the PGA score (e.g. medication use and patient-reported outcomes), indicating that further work in standardizing the scoring of the PGA may be required for its optimal application in the trial setting.

## *Corticosteroid Reduction*

Corticosteroid reduction is often included as a secondary endpoint in SLE clinical trials. However, given the importance of steroids as a risk factor for cumulative organ damage in SLE [61, 62], and the potential masking of drug efficacy by high-dose corticosteroid use (which may be partly mitigated in some studies by mandated steroid tapering regimens), routinely incorporating steroid reduction into a composite primary endpoint, or even utilizing it alone as a primary outcome measure, has been suggested [63].

A meta-analysis of steroid-sparing effect in recent phase III trials [64] found that the different trials reported similar, but slightly different corticosteroid reduction endpoints:

- ≤7.5 mg/day and by ≥25% from baseline between weeks 40 and 52 (belimumab, BLISS-52 [5], BLISS-76 [4], BLISS-SC [6]; blisibimod, CHABLIS-SC [9])
- ≤7.5 mg/day, between weeks 24 and 52 for ≥3 consecutive months, without increase in antimalarials/immunosuppressants (tabalumab, ILLUMINATE-1 [7], ILLUMINATE-2 [8])
- ≤10 mg/day or ≤7.5 mg/day by week 24 (epratuzumab – ALLEVIATE-1 and ALLEVIATE-2, respectively [65])
- <10 mg/day between weeks 24 and 52, with a major clinical response (rituximab – EXPLORER [36])

The results of the meta-analysis showed that despite many of these trials having failed to meet their (mostly composite) primary endpoints, almost all (apart from the EXPLORER trial of rituximab in SLE [36] and the lower dose of tabalumab in the ILLUMINATE-1 trial [7]) showed a steroid-sparing effect. These data suggest that the inclusion of steroid-sparing effect in the composite endpoints utilized in SLE clinical trials may be of benefit. This could be captured as a specified dose reduction or dose reached or potentially incorporated into existing disease activity measures, such as in the SLEDAI-2KG [66], a version of the SLEDAI-2 K which includes a steroid reduction item.

## Discussion and Conclusion

SLE clinical trials have employed a wide variety of outcome measures, with most recent trials choosing complex composite indices as their primary endpoints, with single or organ-specific indices and patient-reported outcomes included as secondary or exploratory endpoints. The composite indices have the advantage of being able to better capture global changes in disease activity, in addition to changes in activity within individual organ systems, compared to single indices. However, this comes at the expense of far greater complexity and time and training required to complete them. It should be noted also that these indices have been applied to trials which have mostly excluded more severe lupus manifestations such as severe active lupus nephritis and severe active central nervous system disease. There is a lack of consistency in endpoints chosen between trials, a phenomenon which has been shown to drastically affect the outcome of the trial and also makes results difficult to compare across trials. A minimally clinically important difference is also rarely stated for these outcome measures. Given the frequent failure of promising therapeutics to meet their primary endpoints in recent phase III clinical trials, an urgent review of the use of lupus outcome measures in SLE RCTs is required.

## References

1. Furie R, Petri M, Wallace D, Ginzler E, Merrill J, Stohl W, et al. Novel evidence-based systemic lupus erythematosus responder index. Arthritis Rheum. 2009;61:1143–51.
2. Wallace DJ, Stohl W, Furie RA, Lisse JR, McKay JD, Merrill JT, et al. A phase II, randomized, double-blind, placebo-controlled, dose-ranging study of belimumab in patients with active systemic lupus erythematosus. Arthritis Rheum. 2009;61:1168–78.
3. Gladman DD, Urowitz MB, Kagl A, Hallett D. Accurately describing changes in disease activity in systemic lupus erythematosus. J Rheumatol. 2000;27(2):377–9.
4. Furie R, Petri M, Zamani O, Cervera R, Wallace DJ, Tegzová D, et al. A phase III, randomized, placebo-controlled study of belimumab, a monoclonal antibody that inhibits B lymphocyte stimulator, in patients with systemic lupus erythematosus. Arthritis Rheum. 2011;63(12):3912–30.
5. Navarra S, Guzmán R, Gallacher A, Hall S, Levy R, Jimenez RE, et al. Efficacy and safety of belimumab in patients with active systemic lupus erythematosus: a randomised, placebo-controlled, phase 3 trial. Lancet. 2011;377:721–31.
6. Stohl W, Schwarting A, Okada M, Scheinberg M, Doria A, Hammer AE, et al. Efficacy and safety of subcutaneous belimumab in systemic lupus erythematosus: a fifty-two-week randomized, double-blind, placebo-controlled study. Arthritis Rheumatol. 2017;69(5):1016–27.
7. Isenberg DA, Petri M, Kalunian K, Tanaka Y, Urowitz MB, Hoffman RW, et al. Efficacy and safety of subcutaneous tabalumab in patients with systemic lupus erythematosus: results from ILLUMINATE-1, a 52-week, phase III, multicentre, randomised, double-blind, placebo-controlled study. Ann Rheum Dis. 2016;75:323–31.
8. Merrill JT, van Vollenhoven RF, Buyon JP, Furie RA, Stohl W, Morgan-Cox M, et al. Efficacy and safety of subcutaneous tabalumab, a monoclonal antibody to B-cell activating factor, in patients with systemic lupus erythematosus: results from ILLUMINATE-2, a 52-week,

phase III, multicentre, randomised, double-blind, placebo-controlled study. Ann Rheum Dis. 2016;75:332–40.
9. Merrill JT, Shanahan WR, Scheinberg M, Kalunian KC, Wofsy D, Martin RS. Phase III trial results with blisibimod, a selective inhibitor of B-cell activating factor, in subjects with systemic lupus erythematosus (SLE): results from a randomised, double-blind, placebo-controlled trial. Ann Rheum Dis. 2018;77:883–9.
10. Furie RA, Morand EF, Bruce IN, Manzi S, Kalunian K, Vital E, et al. Type 1 interferon inhibitor anifrolumab in active systemic lupus erythematosus (TULIP-1): a randomised, controlled, phase 3 trial. Lancet Rheumatol. 2019;1:e208–19.
11. Morand EF, Furie R, Tanaka Y, Bruce IN, Askanase AD, Richez C, et al. Trial of anifrolumab in active systemic lupus erythematosus. NEJM. 2020;382:211–21.
12. Wallace DJ, Kalunian K, Petri A, Strand V, Houssiau F, Pike M, et al. Efficacy and safety of epratuzumab in patients with moderate/severe active systemic lupus erythematosus: results from EMBLEM, a phase IIb, randomised, double-blind, placebo-controlled, multicentre study. Ann Rheum Dis. 2014;73:183–90.
13. Clowse MEB, Wallace D, Furie R, Petri M, Pike M, Leszczyński P, et al. Efficacy and safety of epratuzumab in moderately to severely active systemic lupus erythematosus. Arthritis Rheumatol. 2017;69:362–75.
14. Thanou A, Chakravarty E, James J, Merrill JT. Which outcome measures in SLE clinical trials best reflect medical judgement? Lupus Sci Med. 2014;1:e000005. https://doi.org/10.1136/lupus-2013-000005.
15. Franklyn K, Lau CS, Navarra SV, Louthrenoo W, Lateef A, Hamijoyo L, et al. Definition and initial validation of a Lupus Low Disease Activity State (LLDAS). Ann Rheum Dis. 2016;75:1615–21.
16. Golder V, Kandane-Rathnayake R, Huq M, Louthrenoo W, Luo SF, Wu YJJ, et al. Evaluation of remission definitions for systemic lupus erythematosus: a prospective cohort study. Lancet Rheumatol. 2019;1:E103–10.
17. Golder V, Kandane-Rathnayake R, Hoi A, Huq M, Louthrenoo W, An Y, et al. Association of the Lupus Low Disease Activity State (LLDAS) with health-related quality of life in a multinational prospective study. Arthritis Res Ther. 2017;19:62.
18. Wallace DJ, Furie RA, Tanaka Y, Kalunian K, Mosca M, Petri MA, et al. Baricitinib for systemic lupus erythematosus: a double-blind, randomised, placebo-controlled, phase 2 trial. Lancet. 2018;392:222–31.
19. Morand EF, Trasieva T, Berglind A, Illei GG, Tummala R. Lupus Low Disease Activity State (LLDAS) attainment discriminates responders in a systemic lupus erythematosus trial: post-hoc analysis of the phase IIb MUSE trial of anifrolumab. Ann Rheum Dis. 2018;77:706–13.
20. Morand EF, Isenberg D, Wallace DJ, Kao AH, Vazquez-Mateo C, Chang P, et al. Attainment of treat-to-target endpoints in SLE patients with high disease activity in the atacicept phase 2b ADDRESS II study. Rheumatology. 2020:1–9.
21. Oon S, Huq M, Golder M, Ong PX, Morand EF, Nikpour M. Lupus Low Disease Activity State (LLDAS) discriminates responders in the BLISS-52 and BLISS-76 phase III trials of belimumab in systemic lupus erythematosus. Ann Rheum Dis. 2019;78:629–33.
22. Griffiths B, Mosca M, Gordon C. Assessment of patients with systemic lupus erythematous and the use of lupus disease activity indices. Best Pract Res Clin Rheumatol. 2005;19:685–708.
23. Gladman DD, Goldsmith CH, Urowitz MB, Bacon P, Bombardier C, Isenberg D, et al. Cross-cultural validation and reliability of 3 disease activity indices in systemic lupus erythematosus. J Rheumatol. 1992;19:608–11.
24. Ward MM, Marx AS, Barry NN. Comparison of the validity and sensitivity to change of 5 activity indices in systemic lupus erythematosus. J Rheumatol. 2000;27:664–70.
25. Rahman P, Gladman DD, Urowitz MB, Hallett D, Tam LS. Early damage as measured by the SLICC/ACR Damage Index is a predictor of mortality in systemic lupus erythematosus. Lupus. 2001;10:93–6.

26. Stoll T, Sutcliffe N, Mach J, Klaghofer R, Isenberg DA. Analysis of the relationship between disease activity and damage in patients with systemic lupus erythematosus: a 5-year prospective study. Rheumatology (Oxford). 2004;43:1039–44.
27. Romero-Diaz J, Isenberg D, Ramsey-Goldman R. Measures of adult systemic lupus erythematosus: updated version of British Isles Lupus Assessment Group (BILAG 2004), European Consensus Lupus Activity Measurements (ECLAM), Systemic Lupus Activity Measure, Revised (SLAM-R), Systemic Lupus Activity Questionnaire for Population Studies (SLAQ), Systemic Lupus Erythematosus Disease Activity Index 2000 (SELDAI-2K), and Systemic Lupus International Collaborating Clinics/American College of Rheumatology Damage Index (SDI). Arthritis Care Res. 2011;63:0–11.
28. Bombardier C, Gladman DD, Urowitz MB, Caron D, Chang CH. Derivation of the SLEDAI. A disease activity index for lupus patients. The Committee on Prognosis Studies in SLE. Arthritis Rheum. 1992;35:630–40.
29. Petri M, Kim MY, Kalunian KC, Grossman J, Hanh BH, Sammaritano LR, et al. OC-SELENA Trial. Combined oral contraceptives in women with systemic lupus erythematosus. N Engl J Med. 2005;353:2550–8.
30. Gladman DD, Ibanez D, Urowitz MB. Systemic lupus erythematosus disease activity index 2000. J Rheumatol. 2002;29:288–91.
31. Buyon JP, Petric MA, Kim MY, Kalunian KC, Grossman J, Hanh BH, et al. The effect of combined estrogen and progesterone hormone replacement therapy on disease activity in systemic lupus erythematosus: a randomized trial. Ann Intern Med. 2005;142:953–62.
32. Hay EM, Bacon PA, Gordon C, Isenberg DA, Maddison P, Snaith ML, et al. The BILAG index: a reliable and valid instrument for measuring clinical disease activity in systemic lupus erythematosus. Q J Med. 1993;86:447–58.
33. Isenberg DA, Rahman A, Allen E, Farewell V, Akil M, Bruce IN, et al. BILAG 2004. Development and initial validation of an updated version of the British Isles Lupus Assessment Group's disease activity index for patients with systemic lupus erythematosus. Rheumatology (Oxford). 2005;44:902–6.
34. Yee CS, Farewell V, Isenberg DA, Griffiths B, The LS, Bruce IN, et al. The BILAG-2004 index is sensitive to change for assessment of SLE disease activity. Rheumatology (Oxford). 2009;48:691–5.
35. Merrill JT, Burgos-Vargas R, Westhovens R, Chalmers A, D'Cruz D, Wallace DJ, et al. The efficacy and safety of abatacept in patients in non-life threatening manifestations of systemic lupus erythematosus: results of a twelve-month, multicentre, exploratory, phase IIb, randomized, double-blind, placebo-controlled trial. Arthritis Rheum. 2010;62:3077–87.
36. Merrill JT, Neuwelt CM, Wallace DJ, Shanahan JC, Latinis KM, Oates JC, et al. Efficacy and safety of rituximab in moderately-to-severely active systemic lupus erythematosus: the randomized, double-blind, phase II/III systemic lupus erythematosus evaluation of rituximab trial. Arthritis Rheum. 2010;62:222–33.
37. Isenberg D, Gordon C, LIcu D, Copt S, Rossi CP, Wofsy D. Efficacy and safety of atacicept for prevention of flares in patients with moderate-to-severe systemic lupus erythematosus (SLE): 52-week data (APRIL-SLE randomised trial). Ann Rheum Dis. 2015;74:2006–15.
38. Kalunian KC, Merrill JT, Maciuca R, McBride JM, Townsend MJ, Wei X, et al. A phase II study of the efficacy and safety of rontalizumab (rhuMAb interferon-α) in patients with systemic lupus erythematosus (ROSE). Ann Rheum Dis. 2016;75:196–202.
39. Ohmura K. Which is the best SLE activity index for clinical trials? Mod Rheumatol. 2020;16:1–9.
40. Parodi A, Massone C, Cacciapuoti M, Aragone MG, Bondavalli P, Cattarini G, et al. Measuring the activity of the disease in patients with cutaneous lupus erythematosus. Br J Dermatol. 2000;142:457–60.
41. Merrill JT. Measuring disease activity in systemic lupus: progress and problems. J Rheumatol. 2002;29:2256–7.

42. Albrecht J, Taylor L, Berlin JA, Dulay S, Ang G, Fakharzadeh S, et al. The CLASI (Cutaneous Lupus Erythematosus Disease Area and Severity Index): an outcome instrument for cutaneous lupus erythematosus. J Invest Dermatol. 2005;125:889–94.
43. Albrecht J, Werth VP. Development of the CLASI as an outcome instrument for cutaneous lupus erythematosus. Dermatol Ther. 2007;20:93–101.
44. Klein RS, Morganroth PA, Werth VP. Cutaneous lupus and CLASI instrument. Rheum Dis Clin N Am. 2010;36:33–51.
45. Concha JS, Patsatsi A, Marshak-Rothstine A, Liu ML, Sinha AA, Lee LA, et al. Advances in cutaneous lupus erythematosus and dermatomyositis: a report from the 4th international conference on cutaneous lupus erythematosus – an ongoing need for international consensus and collaborations. J Invest Dermatol. 2019;139:270–6.
46. Chen KL, Krain RL, Werth VP. Advancing understanding, diagnosis, and therapies for cutaneous lupus erythematosus within the broader context of systemic lupus erythematosus. F1000Res. 2019;8:F1000 Faculty Rev-332.
47. Bonilla-Martinez ZL, Albrecht J, Troxel AB, Taylor L, Okawa J, Dulay S, et al. The cutaneous lupus erythematosus disease area and severity index: a responsive instrument to measure activity and damage in patients with cutaneous lupus erythematosus. Arch Dermatol. 2008;144:173–80.
48. Cheng L, Amoura Z, Cheah B, Hiepe F, Sullivan B, Zhou L, et al. A randomized, double-blind, parallel-group, placebo-controlled, multiple-dose study to evaluate AMG 557 in patients with systemic lupus erythematosus and active lupus arthritis. Arthritis Rheumatol. 2018;70:1071–6.
49. Cardiel MH, Tumlin JA, Furie RA, Wallace DJ, Joh T, Linnik MD, et al. Abetimus sodium for renal flare in systemic lupus erythematosus: results of a randomized, controlled phase III trial. Arthritis Rheum. 2008;58:2470–80.
50. Wofsy D, Hillson JL, Diamond B. Abatacept for lupus nephritis. Alternative definitions of complete response support conflicting conclusions. Arthritis Rheum. 2012;64:3660–5.
51. Rovin BH, Furie R, Latinis K, Looney RJ, Fervenza FC, Sanchez-Guerrero J, et al., for the LUNAR Investigator Group. Efficacy and safety of rituximab in patients with active proliferative lupus nephritis: the Lupus Nephritis Assessment with Rituximab study. Arthritis Rheum. 2012;64:1215–26.
52. Appel GB, Contreras G, Dooley MA, Ginzler EM, Isenberg D, Jayne D, et al. Mycophenolate mofetil versus cyclophosphamide for induction treatment of lupus nephritis. J Am Soc Nephrol. 2009;20:1103–12.
53. Askanase A, Byron M, Keyes-Elstein L, Cagnoli P, McCune J, Chatham W, et al. Treatment of lupus nephritis with abatacept: the abatacept and cyclophosphamide combination efficacy and safety study. Arthritis Rheumatol. 2014;66:3096–104.
54. Alarcón GS, McGwin G, Brooks K, Roseman JM, Fessler BJ, Sanchez ML, et al. Systemic lupus erythematosus in three ethnic groups. XI. Source of discrepancy in perception of disease activity: a comparison of physician and patient visual analog scale scores. Arthritis Rheum. 2002;47:408–13.
55. Annapureddy N, Devilliers H, Jolly M. Patient-reported outcomes in lupus clinical trials with biologics. Lupus. 2016;25:1111–21.
56. Ware JEJ, Sherbourne CD. The MOS 36-item Short Form health survey (SF-36). I. Conceptual framework and item selection. Med Care. 1992;30:473–83.
57. Yellen SB, Cella D, Webster K, Blendowski C, Kaplan E. Measuring fatigue and other anemia-related symptoms with the Functional Assessment of Cancer Therapy (FACT) measurement system. J Pain Symptom Manag. 1997;13:67–74.
58. Aggarwal R, Wilke CT, Pickard AS, Vats V, Mikolaitis R, Fogg L, et al. Psychometric properties of the EuroQol-5D and Short Form-6D in patients with systemic lupus erythematosus. J Rheumatol. 2009;36:1209–16.
59. Furie R, Petri MA, Strand V, Gladman DD, Zhong J, Freimuth WW, and the BLISS-52 and BLISS-76 study groups. Clinical, laboratory and health-related quality of life correlates of

Systemic Lupus Erythematosus Responder Index response: a post hoc analysis of the phase 3 belimumab trials. Lupus Sci Med. 2014;1:e000031.

60. Aranow C*, Askanase A*, Oon S, Huq M, Calderone A, Morand EF, Nikpour M (* equal contributors). Laboratory investigation results influence Physician's Global Assessment (PGA) of Disease Activity in SLE. Ann Rheum Dis. 2020;79:787–92.
61. Al Sawah S, Zhang X, Zhu B, Magder L, Foster S, Iikuni N, et al. Effect of corticosteroid use by dose on the risk of developing organ damage over time in systemic lupus erythematosus – the Hopkins Lupus Cohort. Lupus Sci Med. 2015;2:e000066.
62. Apostopoulos D, Kandane-Rathnayake R, Raghunath S, Hoi A, Nikpour M, Morand EF. Independent association of glucocorticoids with damage accrual in SLE. Lupus Sci Med. 2016;3:e000157.
63. Houssiau FA. Time to change the primary outcome of lupus trials. Ann Rheum Dis. 2019;78:581–2.
64. Oon S, Huq M, Nikpour M. Steroid sparing effect: an essential element in assessing therapeutic efficacy in SLE: response to 'time to change the primary outcome of lupus trials' by Houssiau. Ann Rheum Dis. 2019. https://doi.org/10.1136/annrheumdis-2019-216113. Online ahead of print.
65. Strand V, Petri M, Kalunian K, Gordon C, Wallace DJ, Hobbs K, et al. Epratuzumab for patients with moderate to severe flaring SLE: health related quality of life outcomes and corticosteroid use in the randomized controlled ALLEVIATE trials and extension study SL0006. Rheumatology (Oxford). 2014;53:502–11.
66. Touma Z, Gladman DD, Zandy M, Su J, Anderson N, Urowitz M. Identifying a response for the systemic lupus erythematosus disease activity glucocorticoid index (SLEDAI-2KG). Arthritis Care Res. 2020. https://doi.org/10.1002/acr.24261. Online ahead of print.

# Chapter 19
# Metrics and Outcomes of Systemic Lupus Erythematosus in Clinical Practice

**Ambika Gupta, Janet Pope, Zahi Touma, and Stephanie Keeling**

## Introduction

Systemic lupus erythematosus (SLE) is a heterogeneous, complex, chronic, multi-system autoimmune disease. There are targeted autoantibody production and variable manifestations between patients. For this reason, careful assessment is necessary to determine if the disease is active or in remission and to include all potential organ involvement. Disease damage (the burden of irreversible damage since the diagnosis of SLE whether directly from lupus or not) is also important to distinguish from disease activity when assessing SLE patients, as it has implications for immunosuppressive therapy escalation and glucocorticoids use.

Disease activity and outcome metrics were originally developed for clinical research purposes and have since been incorporated into randomized controlled trials in SLE. While many tools have been developed since the late 1980s, no one standardized metric for a particular domain (e.g., disease activity, damage) has been consistently used in these studies. Moreover, these tools have evolved due to

A. Gupta (✉)
Division of Rheumatology, Department of Medicine, University of Toronto, Toronto, ON, Canada
e-mail: ambika.gupta@uhnresearch.ca

J. Pope
Division of Rheumatology, Department of Medicine, University of Western Ontario, London, ON, Canada

Z. Touma
Centre for Prognosis in Rheumatic Disease, Toronto Lupus Clinic, Division of Rheumatology, Department of Medicine, Institute of Health Policy, Management and Evaluation, University of Toronto, Toronto, ON, Canada

S. Keeling
Division of Rheumatology, Department of Medicine, University of Alberta, Edmonton, AB, Canada



Z. Touma (ed.), *Outcome Measures and Metrics in Systemic Lupus Erythematosus*, https://doi.org/10.1007/978-3-030-73303-2_19

studying the results of trials and using them in subsequent trials. For example, the SLE Responder Index (SRI) encompasses several disease activity metrics, particularly the SLE Disease Activity Index (SLEDAI), British Isles Lupus Assessment Group Disease Activity Index (BILAG), and physician-rated disease activity (PGA). Some of these metrics may have applicability in day-to-day clinical practice, and we have tried to outline instruments that are more likely to be used in clinical practice when assessing SLE patients in this chapter. The important consideration would be to apply a tool early in disease and to be consistent in using the same tool in future clinical visits to allow for accurate comparisons. It can be considered advantageous to have several tools to choose from when it comes to assessing disease activity and damage as each has its respective advantages and disadvantages. Some may be more helpful than others when looking at specific manifestations.

## Advantages of Using Validated Metrics for SLE Assessment in Clinical Practice

Validated disease activity metrics allow the clinician to be comprehensive and to assess each organ system thoroughly. They can serve as a memory aid to do so. For example, the SLEDAI assesses seven manifestations of neurologic involvement and ensures that the clinician asks about each of these areas separately. Using these tools can also allow for more objective assessments from visit to visit as well.

Validated disease activity metrics can provide insight into future risk of morbidity and mortality as recently reviewed in a systematic review used to inform Canadian SLE recommendations for monitoring SLE patients [1]. This group evaluated four different disease activity metrics including the BILAG and the SLEDAI and its derivations in 30 studies. They reported that higher mortality was found in six studies with higher SLEDAI scores at baseline or over time (weight-adjusted hazard ratio [HR] 1.14, 95% confidence interval [CI] 1.06–1.22) and a greater risk of mortality in those with more than 10 years of follow-up (HR 1.13, 95% CI 1.06–1.21). They found three studies that demonstrated higher SLEDAI scores in those that were dead compared to alive. Moreover, they found that higher disease activity scores were associated with greater damage. There was greater damage in patients with higher SLEDAI scores at baseline in three studies (odd ratio [OR] 1.08 (95% CI 1.03–1.12). An increase in the BILAG scores was also been shown to be predictive of damage and mortality [2].

## Challenges of Using Validated Metrics

Often in clinical practice, disease activity metrics are not completed due to lack of familiarity or perception that these metrics are time-intensive which is something that many clinicians do not have. A recent survey of 175 Canadian rheumatologists revealed that validated metrics of SLE disease activity and damage were not commonly used with only 16% of respondents using the SLEDAI (Table 19.1) [3].

**Table 19.1** Use of validated disease activity and damage measures by academic and nonacademic Canadian centers

| Index | Group | | Survey | Responses, *n* (%) | | |
|---|---|---|---|---|---|---|
| | | Always | Sometimes | Never | Would like to | *P** |
| SLEDAI,<br>$n = 145$ | Academic, $n = 96$<br>Nonacademic,<br>$n = 49$ | 24 (25)<br>2 (4) | 29 (30)<br>17 (35) | 31 (32)<br>26 (53) | 12 (13)<br>4 (8) | 0.002 |
| BILAG,<br>$n = 150$ | Academic, $n = 101$<br>Nonacademic,<br>$n = 49$ | 1 (1)<br>0 (0) | 20 (20)<br>3 (6) | 70 (69)<br>42 (86) | 10 (10)<br>4 (8) | 0.02 |
| SLAM,<br>$n = 149$ | Academic, $n = 101$<br>Nonacademic,<br>$n = 48$ | 3 (3)<br>0 (0) | 16 (16)<br>2 (6) | 78 (77)<br>42 (88) | 4 (4)<br>4 (8) | 0.03 |
| SLICC,<br>$n = 150$ | Academic, $n = 101$<br>Nonacademic,<br>$n = 49$ | 2 (2)<br>0 (0) | 22 (22)<br>4 (8) | 67 (66)<br>41 (84) | 10 (10)<br>4 (8) | 0.02 |

Table adapted from Keeling et al. [3]

Interestingly, the individual items on disease activity and damage metrics such as the SLEDAI or SLICC/ACR DI (SLE International Collaborating Clinics/ACR Damage Index) are likely captured in a thorough history of a lupus patient, which is standard of care for the assessment of lupus patients overall. This implies that the additional use of these metrics would likely not add significant time while providing a useful metric per visit for the same patient.

Significant heterogeneity exists when comparing the results on the use of validated metrics between academic and nonacademic centers. This may be explained on the basis that academic centers are interested in research and, as such, would often use validated tools. Furthermore, reimbursement of medications is not tied to performance metrics as it is for other diseases such as rheumatoid arthritis. As such, physicians are not required to use these validated metrics, even though it would be recommended as per current guidelines (see below). However, even academics always used the SLEDAI in a quarter of physicians, and the other metrics were far less often used.

Mikdashi et al. discuss some of the challenges in choosing disease activity metrics in SLE. These difficulties include the absence of a gold standard instrument. Some tools impose an administrative burden including having a knowledge of the instruments, the time to complete the instrument, the complexity in scoring, and sometimes the cost associated with the use of a specific instrument [4].

## Current Guidelines

The Canadian Rheumatology Association (CRA) recommends that disease activity be assessed with a validated instrument of disease activity during baseline and follow-up visits; however, the recommendations do not specify which instrument should be used on purpose due to a lack of a gold standard disease activity tool [5].

They also recommend assessing disease damage annually with a validated metric, and currently there is one main physician-reported metric, the SDI.

The EULAR (European League Against Rheumatism) guidelines recommend monitoring SLE through validated disease activity and chronicity (damage) indices, which include physician global assessment [6]. The decision is left to the rheumatologist in regard to which tool to choose. The choice should incorporate knowledge on the specific test, the administrative burden, and any associated cost.

## Instruments of Disease Activity/Damage That Can Be Used in Clinics

### *Systemic Lupus Erythematosus Disease Activity Index (SLEDAI)*

The SLEDAI is a validated clinical global assessment of disease activity in SLE [7]. Chapter 6 outlines full scoring details of this metric. It assesses nine organ systems using 24 descriptors of disease activity using both clinical and laboratory/imaging variables. Manifestations are weighted depending on their severity. For example, vasculitis and neurological symptoms are given a higher weight. Furthermore, manifestations of proteinuria, alopecia, rash, and mucous membrane lesions were considered active at their first occurrence or at a recurrence. As such, chronic manifestations and persistent disease activity were not included in the original SLEDAI. The SLEDAI 2000 (SLEDAI-2K) modified the SLEDAI to include chronic active manifestations [8]. The SLEDAI-2K was validated against the SLEDAI and was also found to be a predictor of mortality and disease activity [8]. Further studies confirmed the validity of SLEDAI-2K 30 days against SLEDAI-2K 10 days [9].

The SELENA (Safety of Estrogens in Lupus Erythematosus National Assessment) studies, which assessed oral contraception or hormone replacement therapy in patients with SLE, modified the scoring of SLEDAI to capture new or worsening disease activity (e.g., new or worsening proteinuria but not ongoing proteinuria) and developed the SELENA-SLEDAI Flare Index (SFI) which gathers information on medication changes, hospitalizations, and physician global score to grade different levels of flares [10, 11]. The differences in scoring between the SLEDAI and its derivatives are highlighted in Chap. 6.

Although these metrics are generally easy to use, criticisms of these disease activity metrics are that they assessed disease activity only in the preceding 30 days and the scoring was binary with either a "yes" or "no" response to each disease manifestation. For this reason, the SLEDAI-2K Responder Index-50 (S2K RI-50) was developed and validated. It could document a minimum 50% improvement in disease manifestations and assess disease activity in the preceding 30 days [12]. S2K RI-50 describes the disease activity overall; however, the details regarding specific organ systems can easily be seen on the data form. S2K RI-50 has also been assessed in longitudinal research studies and RCTs.

## Systemic Lupus Erythematosus Activity Measure (SLAM)

The SLAM assesses symptoms that occurred during the previous month and includes 30 clinical manifestations and 8 laboratory parameters to assess organs that cannot otherwise be measured [13]. Both disease activity and severity are incorporated into the scales. Symptoms are determined to be active or inactive. The severity is additionally assessed based on treatment needed, need to follow the patient more closely, or prognostic consequences. The SLAM was found to be a reliable and valid index [13]. The SLAM-revised (SLAM-R) further clarified some of the manifestations and included 23 clinical manifestations and 7 laboratory parameters. Reliability and validity were also established for the SLAM-R [14]. A disadvantage of the SLAM is that many of the items are subjective and rely on reporting by the patient [4]. However, physicians are often criticized for not taking patient opinion and concerns into account when making their judgments. These tools allow physicians to do so. Additionally, another disadvantage is that all manifestations are given an equal weight. For example, neurological symptoms are graded similar in severity to oral ulcers even though these manifestations imply differing treatment strategies with differing degrees of potency and side effects. Full scoring details are outlined in Chap. 6.

## SLE Disease Activity Score (SLE-DAS)

The SLE-DAS is a continuous global disease activity metric which encompasses 17 of the 24 items of SLEDAI-2K in the previous 30 days. The SLE-DAS was modeled on the PGA to reflect the opinion of an expert clinician in the management of SLE. In this new metric, four items are scored as continuous variables to reflect on the severity of the manifestation within each item (arthritis, proteinuria, leukopenia, and thrombocytopenia), and new weighted scores, different from the original scores of SLEDAI-2K, were derived to all items. In the original publication by the developers of this instrument, the SLE-DAS was found to have good validity and was better at identifying clinically significant changes in disease activity and in predicting damage accrual than the SLEDAI-2K [15].

## British Isles Lupus Assessment Group Disease Activity Index (BILAG)

The BILAG measures organ-specific scores for eight organ systems with an alphabetical grading system, and a total score is not calculated. It assesses both newly presenting manifestations and changes in previous disease manifestations [16]. It has high reliability and has been validated [13, 16]. The BILAG grading system was modified to derive the BILAG-2004 index [17]. The BILAG tests are more comprehensive and allow clinicians to compare changes in organ systems across various domains.

Disadvantages of the indices include that formal training is required to administer a BILAG and BILAG-2004, laboratory results are needed, and the instrument can take up to 50 minutes to administer and complete, while scoring is generated by the BILAG computerized software [4]. This makes this test less realistic to use in clinical settings. Physicians would need ample time and would have needed to have laboratory test results available in advance. Often, blood work is ordered after the visit depending on the clinical need.

## *Cutaneous Lupus Erythematosus Disease Area and Severity Index (CLASI)*

The CLASI is an organ-specific metric and composed of two scores: there is a score for activity of the disease, and the second is a score for damage done by the disease. The disease activity is scored based on erythema, scale/hyperkeratosis, mucous membrane involvement, acute hair loss, and nonscarring alopecia. The disease damage is scored based on dyspigmentation and scarring, including scarring alopecia. The extent of the disease is also taken into account. Visual analog scales separately report associated symptoms of pruritus, pain, and fatigue. Studies confirmed the inter-rater reliability and validity of disease activity and damage scales [18]. This index would be difficult to administer in a general rheumatology setting, as all rheumatologists would not have this degree of dermatology knowledge, but it is not difficult to get a training on this instrument.

## *SLE Responder Index (SRI)*

The SRI is a composite index to evaluate changes in disease activity, and it utilizes the SELENA-SLEDAI, BILAG, and a 3 cm visual analog scale of physician-rated disease activity (PGA). It evaluates response to therapy by looking at reductions in the SELENA-SLEDAI, no worsening in organ systems in BILAG, and minimal change in the PGA (no worsening) to ensure that the patient's overall condition is not compromised at the expense of improvements in disease activity [19]. As with the SLEDAI, partial improvements are not captured in this index. Training on all components (SELENA-SLEDAI, BILAG, and PGA) of SRI is also required for optimal performance [4]. Although developed for research, this index would be difficult to apply in clinical practice due to the multiple components required for assessment and the training required for administration.

## BILAG-Based Composite Lupus Assessment (BICLA)

The BICLA is a composite index to assess response to treatment in RCTs. It assesses improvement in the BILAG-2004 and requires no worsening in disease activity, no worsening of the total SLEDAI-2K score, no significant deterioration in PGA, and no treatment failure. This responder index requires a more stringent response with improvement in all active organ systems and no worsening of any individual organ system [4]. Thanou et al. compared the SRI with the BICLA and found that the BICLA may be less sensitive in detecting improvement, especially in patients with multiple organs involved [20]. As with the SRI, this index is not realistic to be used in clinical practice due to the various components required for assessment and the training required.

## Systemic Lupus International Collaborating Clinics/American College of Rheumatology Damage Index (SDI)

The SDI was developed to assess damage in patients with SLE from any cause. The manifestation must be present and irreversible for at least 6 months to differentiate from active inflammation. The damage could be a result of previously active disease, from medication, or from a comorbidity [21]. Petri et al. found that age, hypertension, and corticosteroid use were important predictors of damage accrual [22]. This tool is easy to use and does not require any formal training. This would be helpful to assess irreversible damage in patients with SLE and could be done annually as recommended by the CRA.

## The Brief Index of Lupus Damage (BILD)

The BILD is a patient-reported metric of disease in SLE. It was designed for telephone or interviewer administration [23]. It was found to have predictive validity and ability to detect change in damage over time [24].

This is a forest plot in Fig. 19.1 from a recent systematic review used to inform Canadian SLE recommendations for monitoring SLE patients which demonstrates that there is an increased risk of mortality seen with higher SLEDAI scores [1]. The forest plots in Fig. 19.2 demonstrate an increased risk of damage accrual and neuropsychiatric damage with higher SLEDAI scores and higher damage accrual with higher SLAM scores. The researchers also found that there was a higher risk of damage with higher BILAG scores. The forest plots in Fig. 19.3 demonstrate an increased risk of mortality with higher SRI scores as well. There was also a trend toward a risk of damage based on past damage as depicted in the forest plot in Fig. 19.4.

*Hazard Ratios for risk of mortality with higher scores at baseline and over time*

| Study or Subgroup | log[Risk Ratio] | SE | Weight | Risk Ratio IV, Random, 95% CI |
|---|---|---|---|---|
| Becker-Merok 2006 | 0.8883768 | 0.362087 | 1.0% | 2.42 [1.19, 4.92] |
| Ibanez 2007 | 0.14842 | 0.022006 | 34.5% | 1.16 [1.11, 1.21] |
| Liang 2010 | 0.09531 | 0.111053 | 8.2% | 1.10 [0.88, 1.37] |
| Telles 2013 | 0.113329 | 0.054387 | 20.7% | 1.12 [1.01, 1.25] |
| Wu (2) 2014 | 1.4884 | 0.565716 | 0.4% | 4.43 [1.46, 13.43] |
| Wu 2014 | 0.09 | 0.02 | 35.3% | 1.09 [1.05, 1.14] |
| **Total (95% CI)** | | | **100.0%** | **1.14 [1.06, 1.22]** |

Heterogeneity: $Tau^2 = 0.00$; $Chi^2 = 14.26$, $df = 5$ ($P = 0.01$); $I^2 = 65\%$
Test for overall effect: $Z = 3.59$ ($P = 0.0003$)

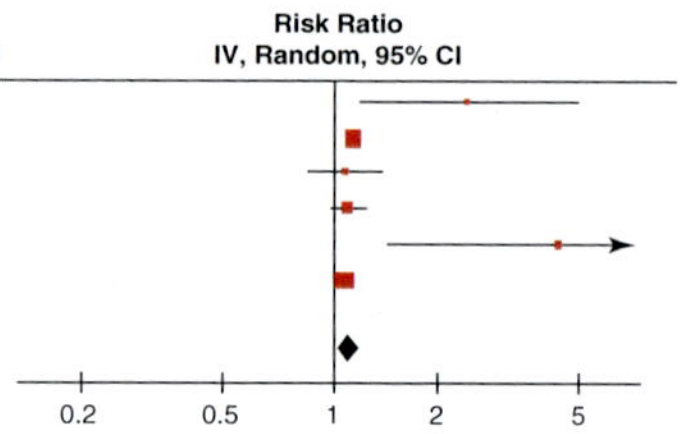


*Mean Difference between dead and alive SLE patients with higher SLEDAI scores*

| Study or Subgroup | Dead Mean | Dead SD | Dead Total | Alive Mean | Alive SD | Alive Total | Weight | Mean Difference IV, Random, 95% CI |
|---|---|---|---|---|---|---|---|---|
| Nossent 1993 | 15 | 9 | 22 | 8 | 9 | 46 | 40.3% | 7.00 [2.43, 11.57] |
| Pons-Estel 2004 | 19.6 | 13.3 | 34 | 13 | 8.1 | 1180 | 41.7% | 6.60 [2.11, 11.09] |
| Zonana-Nacach 2007 | 23 | 12 | 16 | 15 | 9 | 25 | 17.9% | 8.00 [1.14, 14.86] |
| **Total (95% CI)** | | | **72** | | | **1251** | **100.0%** | **7.01 [4.11, 9.92]** |

Heterogeneity: $Tau^2 = 0.00$; $Chi^2 = 0.11$, $df = 2$ ($P = 0.95$); $I^2 = 0\%$
Test for overall effect: $Z = 4.73$ ($P < 0.00001$)

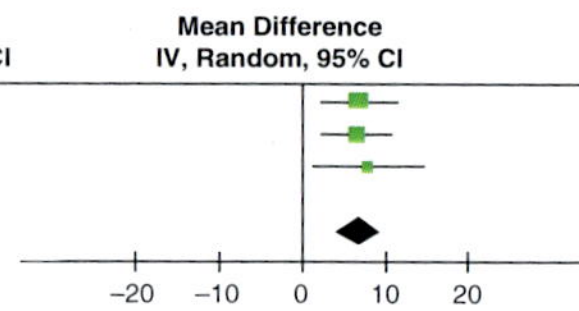


**Fig. 19.1** Forest plots on the risk of mortality associated with higher disease activity measured by SLEDAI

## Is It Time to Talk About Treat-to-Target (T2T): How Can We Do It?

There has been interest in using treat-to-target strategies to achieve low disease activity or remission in SLE, like other rheumatic diseases such as rheumatoid arthritis. Although this has not been adopted in clinical practice, it is being used as exploratory endpoint in clinical trials as outlined in more detail in Chap. 18. An example of this is the Lupus Low Disease Activity State (LLDAS) which has been defined as attaining all of the following criteria: (1) a SLEDAI-2K score ≤4 with no activity in major organ systems (renal, central nervous system, cardiopulmonary, vasculitis, and fever) and no hemolytic anemia or gastrointestinal activity; (2) no new features of lupus disease activity compared with the previous assessment; (3) a PGA score ≤1; (4) current prednisolone-equivalent dosage ≤7.5 mg/day; and (5) standard maintenance dosages of immunosuppressive drugs and approved biologics allowed. Remission has also been defined using the Definitions of Remission in SLE (DORIS) criteria (clinical SLEDAI-2K = 0; prednisolone-equivalent dosage ≤5 mg/day; PGA <0.5).

## Conclusion

For a general rheumatology practice, the SLEDAI and its derivatives, or the SLAM, are reasonable and easy to use validated tools that can be used to assess SLE disease activity although all of the validated metrics mentioned can be used and have their own advantages and disadvantages. It is helpful to use these validated metrics early

*Odds ratio for accruing damage based on the SLEDAI at baseline*

| Study or Subgroup | log[Odds Ratio] | SE | Weight | Odds Ratio IV, Random, 95% CI |
|---|---|---|---|---|
| Gilboe 2001 | 0.131028 | 0.062976 | 10.6% | 1.14 [1.01 1.29] |
| Lilleby 2005 | 0.057 | 0.0245 | 69.8% | 1.06 [1.01 1.11] |
| Lin 2012 | 0.098034 | 0.046174 | 19.6% | 1.10 [1.01, 1.21] |
| **Total (95% CI)** | | | **100.0%** | **1.08 [1.03, 1.12]** |

Heterogeneity: Tau$^2$ = 0.00; Chi$^2$ = 1.57, df = 2 (P = 0.46); I$^2$ = 0%
Test for overall effect: Z = 3.56 (P = 0.0004)

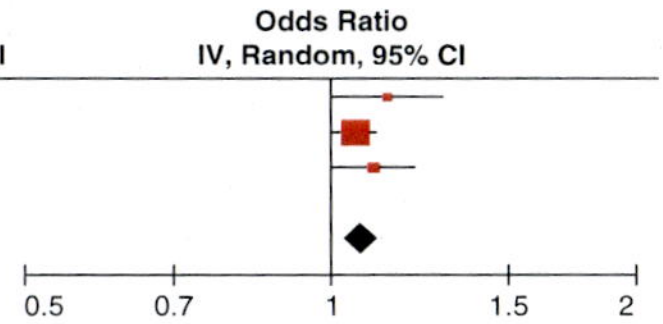


*Hazard ratio measuring the impact of the SLEDAI over time on the outcome of damage accrual*

| Study or Subgroup | log[Odds Ratio] | SE | Weight | Odds Ratio IV, Random, 95% CI |
|---|---|---|---|---|
| Becker-Merok 2006 | 0.850151 | 0.369517 | 3.6% | 2.34 [1.13, 4.83] |
| Bruce 2015 | 0.223144 | 0.040904 | 32.3% | 1.25 [1.15, 1.35] |
| Ibanez 2005 | 0.039221 | 0.012326 | 35.4% | 1.04 [1.02, 1.07] |
| Nossent 2010 | 0.182322 | 0.061522 | 28.7% | 1.20 [1.06, 1.35] |
| **Total (95% CI)** | | | **100.0%** | **1.18 [1.02, 1.37]** |

Heterogeneity: Tau$^2$ = 0.02; Chi$^2$ = 27.28, df = 3 (P < 0.00001); I$^2$ = 89%
Test for overall effect: Z = 2.28 (P = 0.02)

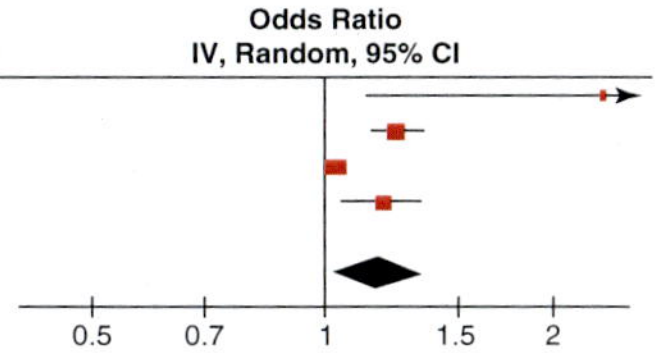


*Odds Ratio for Neuropsychiatric Damage based on the SLEDAI score*

| Study or Subgroup | Damage Mean | Damage SD | Damage Total | No Damage Mean | No Damage SD | No Damage Total | Weight | Mean Difference IV, Random, 95% CI |
|---|---|---|---|---|---|---|---|---|
| Mikdashi 2004 | 15.4 | 2.55 | 66 | 4.8 | 1.28 | 64 | 51.2% | 10.60 [9.91, 11.29] |
| Mok 2006 | 15.3 | 6.9 | 50 | 11 | 5.5 | 232 | 48.8% | 4.30 [2.26, 6.34] |
| **Total (95% CI)** | | | **116** | | | **296** | **100.0%** | **7.53 [1.35, 13.70]** |

Heterogeneity: Tau$^2$ = 0.19.24; Chi$^2$ = 32.89, df = 1 (P < 0.00001); I$^2$ = 97%
Test for overall effect: Z = 2.39 (P = 0.02)

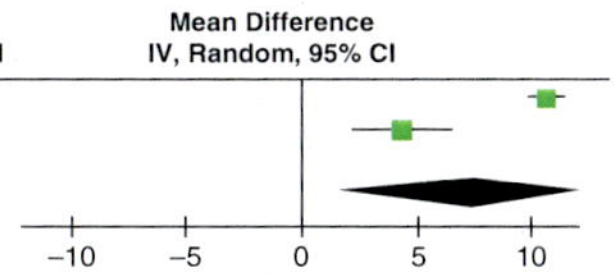


*Odds ratio for damage accrual based on the SLAM score*

| Study or Subgroup | log[Odds Ratio] | SE | Weight | Odds Ratio IV, Random, 95% CI |
|---|---|---|---|---|
| Alarcon 2003 | 0.0705 | 0.0129 | 44.6% | 1.07 [1.05, 1.10] |
| Karlson 1997 | 0.05 | 0.0182 | 22.4% | 1.05 [1.01, 1.09] |
| Peschken 2009 | 0.049 | 0.015 | 33.0% | 1.05 [1.02, 1.08] |
| **Total (95% CI)** | | | **100.0%** | **1.06 [1.04, 1.08]** |

Heterogeneity: Tau$^2$ = 0.00; Chi$^2$ = 1.48, df = 2 (P = 0.48); I$^2$ = 0%
Test for overall effect: Z = 6.83 (P = 0.00001)

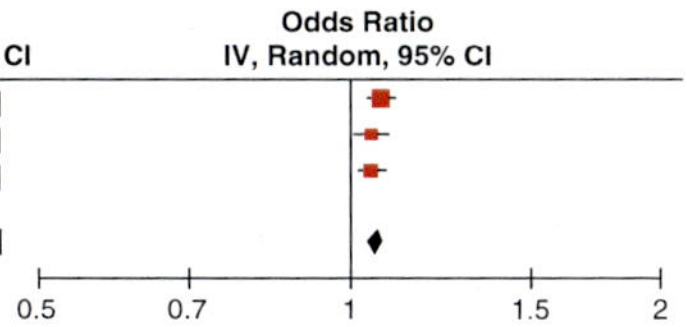


**Fig. 19.2** Forest plots depicting risk of damage accrual (measured by the SDI) with higher SLEDAI, BILAG, and SLAM scores

in the diagnosis of a patient with SLE and to continue using the same validated tool in subsequent follow-up visits.

For patients with more severe organ manifestations, a clinician may prefer to use the SLEDAI and its derivatives as different organs are weighted differently depending on their severity. The SLAM can be considered for the clinician who would like to incorporate patient-reported manifestations into their assessment since this is imbedded in this metric. The CLASI is likely a tool most useful in specialized SLE clinics or for skin experts (e.g., dermatologists) as dermatology knowledge including morphology is required. The BILAG and the responder indices, SRI and BICLA, are very comprehensive and useful over time; their application may seem too onerous for daily clinical practice although with increased use, they can be performed relatively more quickly and are endorsed by many lupus experts internationally.

The SDI is a reasonably easy to use metric of damage that can be completed annually by the physician. While the tool may seem long, it is performed relatively

*Risk of mortality (hazard ratio) with higher damage scores as measured by the SDI*

| Study or Subgroup | log[Risk Ratio] | SE | Weight | Risk Ratio IV, Random, 95% CI |
|---|---|---|---|---|
| Bruce 2015 | 0.378436 | 0.109136 | 14.7% | 1.46 [1.18, 1.81] |
| Cardoso 2008 | 0.29267 | 0.083266 | 19.1% | 1.34 [1.14, 1.58] |
| Chambers 2009 | 0.277632 | 0.097917 | 16.5% | 1.32 [1.09, 1.60] |
| Lopez 2012 | 0.530628 | 0.165 | 8.6% | 1.70 [1.23, 2.35] |
| Mok 2014 | 0.270027 | 0.050798 | 25.8% | 1.31 [1.19, 1.45] |
| Rahman 2001 | 1.229641 | 0.33 | 2.7% | 3.42 [1.79, 6.53] |
| Telles 2013 | 0.451076 | 0.125288 | 12.5% | 1.57 [1.23, 2.01] |
| **Total (95% CI)** | | | **100.0%** | **1.44 [1.29, 1.61]** |

Heterogeneity: $Tau^2 = 0.01$; $Chi^2 = 11.87$, df = 6 (P = 0.06); $I^2 = 49\%$
Test for overall effect: Z = 6.41 (P < 0.00001)

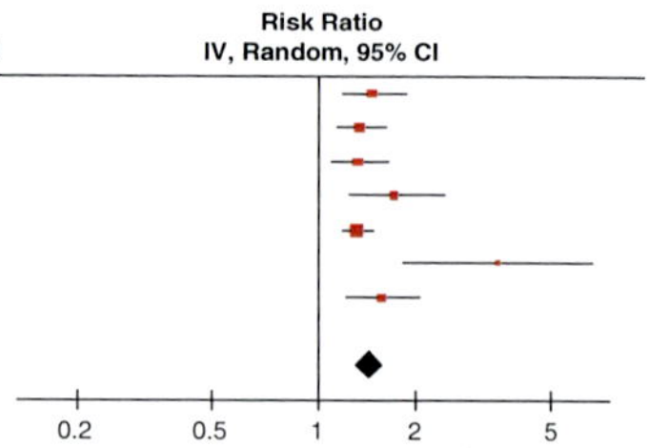


*Difference of past damage (measured by the SDI) between dead and alive SLE patients*

| Study or Subgroup | Dead Mean | Dead SD | Dead Total | Alive Mean | Alive SD | Alive Total | Weight | Mean Difference IV, Random, 95% CI |
|---|---|---|---|---|---|---|---|---|
| Gladman 2000 | 1.56 | 1.5 | 99 | 0.99 | 1.5 | 1198 | 48.6% | 0.57 [0.26, 0.88] |
| Liang 2010 | 4.63 | 2.07 | 8 | 4.04 | 1.37 | 30 | 11.2% | 0.59 [−0.93, 2.11] |
| Pons-Estel 2004 | 2.1 | 2.6 | 34 | 0.54 | 1 | 1180 | 24.0% | 1.56 [0.68, 2.44] |
| Zonana-Nacach 2007 | 2.9 | 2.1 | 16 | 1.6 | 1.5 | 25 | 16.2% | 1.30 [1.11, 2.49] |
| **Total (95% CI)** | | | **157** | | | **2433** | **100.0%** | **0.93 [0.36, 1.49]** |

Heterogeneity: $Tau^2 = 0.15$; $Chi^2 = 5.39$, df = 3 (P = 0.15); $I^2 = 44\%$
Test for overall effect: Z = 3.22 (P = 0.001)

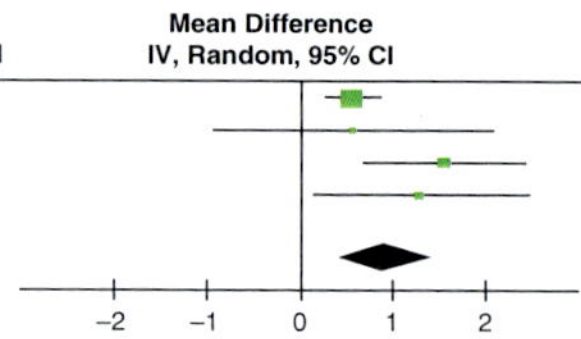


**Fig. 19.3** Forest plots associating damage with mortality in patients with SLE

*Risk of damage from early damage*

| Study or Subgroup | log[Odds Ratio] | SE | Weight | Odds Ratio IV, Random, 95% CI |
|---|---|---|---|---|
| Alarcon 2003 | 0.0687 | 0.01428 | 66.9% | 1.07 [1.04, 1.10] |
| Gilboe 2001 | 0.41871 | 0.20408 | 33.1% | 1.52 [1.02, 2.27] |
| **Total (95% CI)** | | | **100.0%** | **1.20 [1.87, 1.66]** |

Heterogeneity: $Tau^2 = 0.04$; $Chi^2 = 2.93$, df = 1 (P = 0.09); $I^2 = 66\%$
Test for overall effect: Z = 1.12 (P = 0.26)

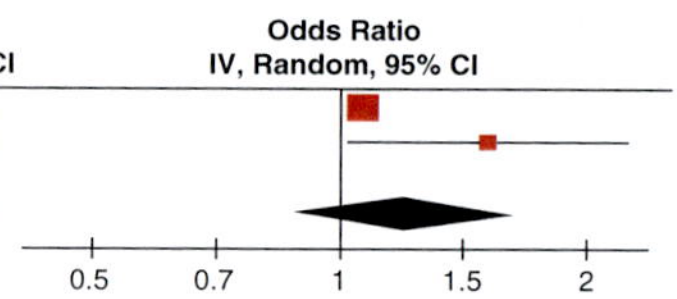


**Fig. 19.4** Forest plots depicting risk of damage (SDI) from past damage

infrequently and does supply helpful clinical information over time while following a lupus patient. The use of patient-reported damage indices such as BILD may be useful but has had less uptake clinically to date.

Beyond the use in clinical trials, these tools provide a metric in clinic which allows for comparisons for that patient over time. As newer treatments arise for lupus, reimbursement criteria by government and private payers, respectively, will likely require that patients be assessed by valid and reliable metrics in a standardized way and meet particular disease activity cutoffs to be eligible for a particular medication. This has already been seen worldwide in other diseases such as rheumatoid arthritis and spondyloarthritis. Moreover, in various countries, reimbursement of belimumab for lupus often requires a disease activity score suggesting moderate to severe disease activity using either the SLEDAI or BILAG. In a heterogenous disease such as lupus, the regular use of these tools in clinic will therefore allow better understanding of each person's disease severity to stratify them along certain treatment algorithms. In the end, this is important as it is clear that greater disease activity and damage lead to more damage and death.

## References

1. Keeling SO, Vandermeer B, Medina J, Chatterley T, Nevskaya T, Pope J, et al. Measuring disease activity and damage with validated metrics: a systematic review on mortality and damage in systemic lupus erythematosus. J Rheumatol. 2018;45(10):1448–61.
2. Nuttall A, Isenberg DA. Assessment of disease activity, damage and quality of life in systemic lupus erythematosus: new aspects. Best Pract Res Clin Rheumatol. 2013;27(3):309–18.
3. Keeling SO, Bissonauth A, Bernatsky S, Vandermeer B, Fortin PR, Gladman DD, et al. Practice variations in the diagnosis, monitoring, and treatment of systemic lupus erythematosus in Canada. J Rheumatol. 2018;45(10):1440–7.
4. Mikdashi J, Nived O. Measuring disease activity in adults with systemic lupus erythematosus: the challenges of administrative burden and responsiveness to patient concerns in clinical research. Arthritis Res Ther. 2015;17:183.
5. Keeling SO, Alabdurubalnabi Z, Avina-Zubieta A, Barr S, Bergeron L, Bernatsky S, et al. Canadian Rheumatology Association recommendations for the assessment and monitoring of systemic lupus erythematosus. J Rheumatol. 2018;45(10):1426–39.
6. Fanouriakis A, Kostopoulou M, Alunno A, Aringer M, Bajema I, Boletis JN, et al. 2019 update of the EULAR recommendations for the management of systemic lupus erythematosus. Ann Rheum Dis. 2019;78(6):736–45.
7. Bombardier C, Gladman DD, Urowitz MB, Caron D, Chang CH. Derivation of the SLEDAI. A disease activity index for lupus patients. The Committee on Prognosis Studies in SLE. Arthritis Rheum. 1992;35(6):630–40.
8. Gladman DD, Ibañez D, Urowitz MB. Systemic lupus erythematosus disease activity index 2000. J Rheumatol. 2002;29(2):288–91.
9. Touma Z, Urowitz MB, Ibañez D, Gladman DD. SLEDAI-2K 10 days versus SLEDAI-2K 30 days in a longitudinal evaluation. Lupus. 2011;20(1):67–70.
10. Petri M, Kim MY, Kalunian KC, Grossman J, Hahn BH, Sammaritano LR, et al. Combined oral contraceptives in women with systemic lupus erythematosus. N Engl J Med. 2005;353(24):2550–8.
11. Buyon JP, Petri MA, Kim MY, Kalunian KC, Grossman J, Hahn BH, et al. The effect of combined estrogen and progesterone hormone replacement therapy on disease activity in systemic lupus erythematosus: a randomized trial. Ann Intern Med. 2005;142(12 Pt 1):953–62.
12. Touma Z, Gladman DD, Ibañez D, Urowitz MB. Development and initial validation of the systemic lupus erythematosus disease activity index 2000 responder index 50. J Rheumatol. 2011;38(2):275–84.
13. Liang MH, Socher SA, Larson MG, Schur PH. Reliability and validity of six systems for the clinical assessment of disease activity in systemic lupus erythematosus. Arthritis Rheum. 1989;32(9):1107–18.
14. Bae SC, Koh HK, Chang DK, Kim MH, Park JK, Kim SY. Reliability and validity of systemic lupus activity measure-revised (SLAM-R) for measuring clinical disease activity in systemic lupus erythematosus. Lupus. 2001;10(6):405–9.
15. Jesus D, Matos A, Henriques C, Zen M, Larosa M, Iaccarino L, et al. Derivation and validation of the SLE Disease Activity Score (SLE-DAS): a new SLE continuous measure with high sensitivity for changes in disease activity. Ann Rheum Dis. 2019;78(3):365–71.
16. Hay EM, Bacon PA, Gordon C, Isenberg DA, Maddison P, Snaith ML, et al. The BILAG index: a reliable and valid instrument for measuring clinical disease activity in systemic lupus erythematosus. Q J Med. 1993;86(7):447–58.
17. Yee CS, Cresswell L, Farewell V, Rahman A, Teh LS, Griffiths B, et al. Numerical scoring for the BILAG-2004 index. Rheumatology (Oxford). 2010;49(9):1665–9.
18. Albrecht J, Taylor L, Berlin JA, Dulay S, Ang G, Fakharzadeh S, et al. The CLASI (Cutaneous Lupus Erythematosus Disease Area and Severity Index): an outcome instrument for cutaneous lupus erythematosus. J Invest Dermatol. 2005;125(5):889–94.

19. Furie RA, Petri MA, Wallace DJ, Ginzler EM, Merrill JT, Stohl W, et al. Novel evidence-based systemic lupus erythematosus responder index. Arthritis Rheum. 2009;61(9):1143–51.
20. Thanou A, Chakravarty E, James JA, Merrill JT. Which outcome measures in SLE clinical trials best reflect medical judgment? Lupus Sci Med. 2014;1(1):e000005.
21. Gladman D, Ginzler E, Goldsmith C, Fortin P, Liang M, Urowitz M, et al. The development and initial validation of the Systemic Lupus International Collaborating Clinics/American College of Rheumatology damage index for systemic lupus erythematosus. Arthritis Rheum. 1996;39(3):363–9.
22. Petri M, Purvey S, Fang H, Magder LS. Predictors of organ damage in systemic lupus erythematosus: the Hopkins Lupus Cohort. Arthritis Rheum. 2012;64(12):4021–8.
23. Yazdany J, Trupin L, Gansky SA, Dall'era M, Yelin EH, Criswell LA, et al. Brief index of lupus damage: a patient-reported measure of damage in systemic lupus erythematosus. Arthritis Care Res (Hoboken). 2011;63(8):1170–7.
24. Katz P, Trupin L, Rush S, Yazdany J. Longitudinal validation of the Brief Index of Lupus Damage. Arthritis Care Res (Hoboken). 2014;66(7):1057–62.

# Chapter 20
# Socioeconomic Impact of SLE: Metrics Utilized in the Determination of Direct and Indirect Costs and Future Directions

**Megan R. W. Barber and Ann E. Clarke**

## Introduction

A comprehensive economic assessment includes direct, indirect, and intangible components. Direct costs are those generated by SLE diagnosis and management. Lupus often presents insidiously, with diverse manifestations. Consequently, a formal diagnosis is often delayed, with an average time from first seeking medical attention to diagnosis of 3.5 years [1]. Even during this pre-diagnostic period, healthcare costs accumulate. In the year prior to diagnosis, adjusted incremental direct costs are $3473 (2013 Canadian dollars) compared to the age-, sex- and calendar year-matched general population [2]. Direct costs in the first year after SLE diagnosis average $12,019 (2013 Canadian dollars), about fivefold the cost of the matched general population [2]. Across international studies, annual direct cost estimates range between $13,494 and $55,344 (2015 US dollars) [3]. This wide variation in reported costs is not just due to geographic region but to differences in study methodology. One of the most costly and dreaded SLE complication is lupus nephritis, with predicted 10-year cumulative direct costs in those with lupus nephritis and an estimated glomerular filtration rate (GFR) <30 ml/minute of $310,579 (2015 Canadian dollars) versus $19,987 in patients with no nephritis and normal renal function [4]. As organ damage increases over time, direct costs also accumulate. Predicted 10-year cumulative direct costs are almost ninefold higher for those with the highest Systemic Lupus International Collaborating Clinics/American College of Rheumatology (SLICC/ACR) Damage Index (SDI) scores compared to those with the lowest SDIs [5]. Other well-established direct cost predictors include age, disease activity and severity, and flares (reviewed in [3, 6, 7]). Lupus

M. R. W. Barber · A. E. Clarke (✉)
Division of Rheumatology, Department of Medicine, Cumming School of Medicine, University of Calgary, Calgary, AB, Canada
e-mail: aeclarke@ucalgary.ca





Z. Touma (ed.), *Outcome Measures and Metrics in Systemic Lupus Erythematosus*, https://doi.org/10.1007/978-3-030-73303-2_20

disproportionately affects marginalized patients, who suffer increased disease activity, damage, and mortality [3]. Costs are also higher in those with low socioeconomic status. In the US, costs are higher in Medicaid-insured versus commercially insured patients [8]. Even in publicly funded healthcare systems, low socioeconomic status is associated with increased costs [2, 9].

Lupus patients often develop severe disease which may require inpatient care. More than 174,000 SLE-related hospital admissions were identified in the United States in 2016 alone [10]. Many studies report hospitalization as the largest single driver of direct costs [6], representing close to 60% of costs in the first year after diagnosis [2]. Almost one quarter of SLE patients in a large American cohort required admission on an annual basis [11], with mean annual hospitalization costs per patient of $42,253 (2015 US dollars) [11].

Indirect costs capture the economic impact of diminished engagement in paid and unpaid work, such as childcare and housework. These costs include both absenteeism (or time away from work) and presenteeism, which refers to decreased work productivity. Relatively few studies report indirect costs in SLE, as they are difficult to calculate. Yet, because SLE predominantly affects young woman at the height of their working and reproductive years, indirect costs actually exceed direct costs [12, 13]. Of more than 1200 patients in the University of California, San Francisco, Lupus Outcomes Study, 42% of patients with increased disease activity stopped paid employment by 4 years of follow-up [14]. More than 40% of surveyed SLE patients in the United Kingdom reported having left work due to their disease [15]. Employment rates were only 36–55% across 11 SLE cost-of-illness studies [6]. Work disability is independently associated with higher disease activity and damage, lower education, and lupus nephritis [16]. Indirect costs are also incurred by caregivers, with a 13% decrease in paid work time and a 34% reduction in work productivity [17]. Economic studies that do not include indirect costs may underestimate the cost-effectiveness of treatments, particularly those that allow patients to return to work or reduce their dependence on caregivers.

Intangible costs refer to the psychosocial impact of illness and cannot easily be valued. Typically, they are represented as health-related quality of life. Further discussion regarding the assessment of health-related quality of life is included in Chap. 12.

The remainder of this chapter provides an overview of economic evaluation in SLE and the means by which direct and indirect costs are determined. Thoughtful design of economic studies will help capture more complete and reliable economic data, crucial information for resource allocation.

## Economic Evaluation Design

Cost of illness studies are the most common economic study design in SLE. They describe both direct and indirect expenditures but without respect to the effect on health. Other types of evaluation include cost minimization studies, which compare the cost of different interventions that are assumed to have equivalent health outcomes. Cost-effectiveness analysis compares the cost and health outcomes of different interventions. Cost-utility analysis is a variant of cost-effectiveness analysis which values health outcomes in health measures such as quality-adjusted life years (QALY), whereas cost-benefit analysis values outcomes with monetary units [18].

Sources of health service utilization data include insurance claims databases and clinic-based cohorts. Although studies based on insurance claims databases may benefit from a larger and more representative patient population and are generally less costly to conduct, a major disadvantage is diagnostic uncertainty, as the diagnosis is typically confirmed with International Classification of Diseases (ICD) codes and is subject to misdiagnosis or miscoding [19]. Further, disease characteristics such as specific organ involvement, activity, and damage are unknown, which means it is difficult to stratify costs, an important consideration in a disease as heterogenous as SLE. Claims-based studies also do not include the costs of noninsured services or indirect costs. The results may also not apply to uninsured populations. Clinic-based cohorts have the advantages of a physician-confirmed diagnosis and the ability to stratify costs according to disease characteristics. However, these cohorts may be biased to more severe cases, and thus results may not be applicable to the general SLE population [19].

Given the complexity of SLE and its myriad manifestations, it is not possible to confidently identify whether costs are attributable to the disease, rather than treatment-related complications or patient comorbidities. Hence, total costs are typically reported, irrespective of the cause [19]. However, incremental costs can be determined through comparison with the general population.

A further consideration in study design is the perspective, which determines the relevancy of costs. The most comprehensive and least biased perspective is societal, which includes all direct and indirect costs [6, 20, 21]. The other perspective includes only costs that are relevant to the payer, such as the government, healthcare system, insurance corporation, or patient.

Other methodological considerations include the use of discounting, which is a method that expresses future costs in their present value [6]. A sensitivity analysis should also be performed to account for any uncertainty in cost estimates [6, 22]. Finally, the time horizon of the study should be sufficiently long as to appreciate all relevant costs [23].

## Metrics for the Determination of Direct Costs

Efforts have been made to standardize the cost domains that are included in economic evaluations of rheumatic diseases [24]. The two major direct cost domains are healthcare costs and other disease-related costs [24]. Healthcare costs include outpatient costs (visits to physicians, emergency room visits, nonphysician services, outpatient surgery, medications, diagnostic and therapeutic procedures and tests, and devices and aids) and inpatient costs. The other disease-related cost category includes transportation associated with obtaining medical care, home healthcare, home remodeling, medical equipment, alternative therapy, and patient time associated with receiving medical care.

In clinic-based cohorts, direct cost assessment is often based on patient self-report of health services utilized [25–27] and can be supplemented by medical chart audit, provider utilization databases, and payer claims data. Self-report questionnaires have been validated for use in SLE [28] and allow for evaluation of all goods and services utilized by the patient, including those that are not reimbursed by insurers, although they may be subject to recall bias [19].

Direct costs are valued by assigning a dollar value to each service used. Detailed recommendations outline how to properly measure and value healthcare resources within local settings. For instance, the Canadian Agency for Drugs and Technologies in Health (CADTH) has published a guidance document for the costing of healthcare resources in the Canadian setting [23].

## Metrics for the Determination of Indirect Costs

Indirect costs include impaired patient and caregiver engagement in paid work through time away from work (absenteeism) and decreased productivity (presenteeism), as well as reduced unpaid labor.

Patient-reported outcomes (PROs) are the most common method of measuring indirect costs. Examples include the Work Productivity and Activity Impairment (WPAI) Questionnaire-Lupus [29], which assesses absenteeism, presenteeism, overall work impairment, and activity impairment over the previous 7 days. The Valuation of Lost Productivity (VOLP) questionnaire assesses employment status, absenteeism, work performance, working environment and characteristics, and unpaid work. It was initially validated in patients with rheumatoid arthritis [30] but has been used in SLE research [31]. Other methods of indirect cost calculation include review of insurance data or employer records.

Once productivity losses are quantified, they are valued with either the human capital approach or friction cost method [20, 32, 33]. Most studies use the human capital approach, which adopts the patient's perspective by using age- and sex-matched wages to value the entire duration of a patient's work absence, up to retirement age [20]. This approach assumes that the patient would remain employed if it were not for their illness [34]. Unpaid work can be valued as either equivalent to time in the labor market (opportunity cost) or the market value of the unpaid work (replacement cost). The friction cost method values lost time from the employer's perspective, by only calculating the cost to replace an employee, up to 3 months [20]. This assumes that each employee's absence can be replaced by an unemployed individual [34]. The friction period refers to the period of the time that it takes to identify and train a replacement worker, after which point it is assumed that there is no longer lost productivity. Unpaid work is not considered in the friction cost method. Over the long term, the human capital approach results in higher cost estimates [20].

## Future Directions

Lupus principally affects young women, often in the midst of demanding professional and child-rearing years, leading to substantial economic impact. Extrapolation of annual direct costs from US insurance databases estimates the annual direct cost burden of insured SLE patients to be between 1.4 and 3.2 billion 2016 US dollars [35].

Many economic studies only consider direct costs, although indirect costs generally exceed direct costs by several folds [6]. Indirect costs should be included to appreciate the cost-effectiveness of interventions that allow patients to continue employment, as well as to inform policy around work accommodations. Other cost components that are typically less well studied but important contributors to total illness costs include the pre-diagnosis period [2] and cost borne by caregivers [17]. Future studies should also include the cost of nontraditional therapies, as most SLE patients use complementary and alternative medicine [36].

Mean costs exceed median costs in most studies, suggesting that a subset of severe patients drive the majority of costs [21]. However, relatively few economic studies have assessed cost stratified by disease activity, damage, or specific organ involvement. Future economic studies should consider subpopulations of SLE, as therapies may be cost-effective for segments of the SLE population, but not others.

Consistent methodology should be applied to studies and used for their appraisal. Turchetti et al. performed a systematic review of SLE cost studies from 2002 to 2012. Out of 26 publications that met inclusion criteria, none provided cost-effectiveness analysis, cost-utility analysis, or cost-benefit analysis. The target population, disease manifestations and severity, design, perspective, methodology, and time horizon varied considerably [37]. The Consolidated Health Economic Evaluation Reporting Standards (CHEERS) statement was published in 2013 to optimize reporting of health economic evaluations [38]. It contains a 24-item checklist of items to include when reporting health intervention evaluations. A recent systematic review identified six decision-analytic model-based cost-effectiveness analyses that have been performed in SLE [39]. None of these studies completely adhered to CHEERS reporting criteria. Using standardized reporting can ensure that resource allocation decisions are based on complete data.

Controlling disease activity such that at least half of a patient's disease course is spent in a Lupus Low Disease Activity State (LLDAS) results in a 26% reduction in annual direct costs [40]. Conventional immunosuppressants have been the cornerstone of SLE treatment for several decades, with belimumab, a humanized monoclonal antibody against B-lymphocyte stimulator, currently the only approved biologic [41]. Patients on belimumab have reduced damage accumulation compared to those on standard of care [42], and over time this may translate into reduced expenditures. Additional effective targeted therapies for SLE are rapidly being developed, including anifrolumab [43] and baricitinib [44]. For these and other treatments to become routinely available, their cost will need to be justified by rigorous cost analyses. In many cases, the upfront investment in treatment will be high. However, therapeutics that control disease activity and damage accumulation may result in long-term direct and indirect cost savings, in addition to an improved quality of life.

## References

1. Sawah S, Daly RP, Foster S, Naegeli A, Katay B, Doll H, Bong G, Moshkovich O, Alarcón G. SAT0423 understanding delay in diagnosis, access to care and satisfaction with care in lupus: findings from a cross-sectional online survey in the United States. Ann Rheum Dis. 2015;74:812.
2. McCormick N, Marra CA, Sadatsafavi M, Avina-Zubieta JA. Incremental direct medical costs of systemic lupus erythematosus patients in the years preceding diagnosis: a general population-based study. Lupus. 2018;27(8):1247–58.
3. Carter EE, Barr SG, Clarke AE. The global burden of SLE: prevalence, health disparities and socioeconomic impact. Nat Rev Rheumatol. 2016;12(10):605–20.
4. Barber MRW, Hanly JG, Su L, Urowitz MB, St Pierre Y, Romero-Diaz J, et al. Economic evaluation of lupus nephritis in the systemic lupus international collaborating clinics inception cohort using a multistate model approach. Arthritis Care Res (Hoboken). 2018;70(9):1294–302.
5. Barber MRW, Hanly JG, Su L, Urowitz MB, St Pierre Y, Romero-Diaz J, et al. Economic evaluation of damage accrual in an international SLE inception cohort using a multi-state model approach. Arthritis Care Res (Hoboken). 2020;72:1800–8.
6. Zhu TY, Tam LS, Li EK. Cost-of-illness studies in systemic lupus erythematosus: a systematic review. Arthritis Care Res (Hoboken). 2011;63(5):751–60.
7. Slawsky KA, Fernandes AW, Fusfeld L, Manzi S, Goss TF. A structured literature review of the direct costs of adult systemic lupus erythematosus in the US. Arthritis Care Res (Hoboken). 2011;63(9):1224–32.
8. Clarke AE, Yazdany J, Kabadi SM, Durden E, Winer I, Griffing K, et al. The economic burden of systemic lupus erythematosus in commercially- and medicaid-insured populations in the United States. Semin Arthritis Rheum. 2020;50(4):759–68.
9. McCormick N, Marra CA, Sadatsafavi M, Avina-Zubieta JA. Socioeconomic status at diagnosis influences the incremental direct medical costs of systemic lupus erythematosus: a longitudinal population-based study. Semin Arthritis Rheum. 2020;50(1):77–83.
10. Dhital R, Pandey RK, Poudel DR, Oladunjoye O, Paudel P, Karmacharya P. All-cause hospitalizations and mortality in systemic lupus erythematosus in the US: results from a national inpatient database. Rheumatol Int. 2020;40(3):393–7.
11. Anandarajah AP, Luc M, Ritchlin CT. Hospitalization of patients with systemic lupus erythematosus is a major cause of direct and indirect healthcare costs. Lupus. 2017;26(7):756–61.
12. Jönsen A, Bengtsson AA, Hjalte F, Petersson IF, Willim M, Nived O. Total cost and cost predictors in systemic lupus erythematosus – 8-years follow-up of a Swedish inception cohort. Lupus. 2015;24(12):1248–56.
13. Sutcliffe N, Clarke AE, Taylor R, Frost C, Isenberg DA. Total costs and predictors of costs in patients with systemic lupus erythematosus. Rheumatology (Oxford). 2001;40(1):37–47.

14. Yelin E, Tonner C, Trupin L, Gansky SA, Julian L, Katz P, et al. Longitudinal study of the impact of incident organ manifestations and increased disease activity on work loss among persons with systemic lupus erythematosus. Arthritis Care Res (Hoboken). 2012;64(2):169–75.
15. Booth S, Price E, Walker E. Fluctuation, invisibility, fatigue - the barriers to maintaining employment with systemic lupus erythematosus: results of an online survey. Lupus. 2018;27(14):2284–91.
16. Abu Bakar F, Shaharir SS, Mohd R, Kamaruzaman L, Mohamed Said MS. Work disability in a multi-ethnic Malaysian systemic lupus erythematosus cohort: a cross-sectional study. Int J Rheum Dis. 2019;22(6):1002–7.
17. Al Sawah S, Daly RP, Foster SA, Naegeli AN, Benjamin K, Doll H, et al. The caregiver burden in lupus: findings from UNVEIL, a national online lupus survey in the United States. Lupus. 2017;26(1):54–61.
18. Husereau D, Drummond M, Petrou S, Carswell C, Moher D, Greenberg D, et al. Consolidated health economic evaluation reporting standards (CHEERS) statement. Int J Technol Assess Health Care. 2013;29(2):117–22.
19. Gordon C, Clarke A. Quality of life and economic evaluation in SLE clinical trials. Lupus. 1999;8:645–54.
20. van den Hout WB. The value of productivity: human-capital versus friction-cost method. Ann Rheum Dis. 2010;69(Suppl 1):i89–91.
21. Zhu TY, Tam LS, Li EK. The socioeconomic burden of systemic lupus erythematosus: state-of-the-art and prospects. Expert Rev Pharmacoecon Outcomes Res. 2012;12(1):53–69.
22. Hodgson TA, Meiners MR. Cost-of-illness methodology: a guide to current practices and procedures. Milbank Mem Fund Q Health Soc. 1982;60(3):429–62.
23. Jacobs P, Budden A, Lee K. Guidance document for the costing of health care resources in the Canadian setting | CADTH.ca 2020. Available from: https://www.cadth.ca/dv/guidance-document-costing-health-care-resources-canadian-setting.
24. Merkesdal S, Ruof J, Huelsemann JL, Schoeffski O, Maetzel A, Mau W, et al. Development of a matrix of cost domains in economic evaluation of rheumatoid arthritis. J Rheumatol. 2001;28(3):657–61.
25. Panopalis P, Yazdany J, Gillis JZ, Julian L, Trupin L, Hersh AO, et al. Health care costs and costs associated with changes in work productivity among persons with systemic lupus erythematosus. Arthritis Rheum. 2008;59(12):1788–95.
26. Clarke AE, Petri M, Manzi S, Isenberg DA, Gordon C, Senecal JL, et al. The systemic lupus erythematosus Tri-nation Study: absence of a link between health resource use and health outcome. Rheumatology (Oxford). 2004;43(8):1016–24.
27. Clarke AE, Panopalis P, Petri M, Manzi S, Isenberg DA, Gordon C, et al. SLE patients with renal damage incur higher health care costs. Rheumatology (Oxford). 2008;47(3):329–33.
28. Clarke AE, Esdaile JM, Bloch DA, Lacaille D, Danoff DS, Fries JF. A Canadian study of the total medical costs for patients with systemic lupus erythematosus and the predictors of costs. Arthritis Rheum. 1993;36(11):1548–59.
29. Reilly MC, Zbrozek AS, Dukes EM. The validity and reproducibility of a work productivity and activity impairment instrument. PharmacoEconomics. 1993;4(5):353–65.
30. Zhang W, Bansback N, Kopec JA, Anis AH. Measuring time input loss among patients with rheumatoid arthritis: validity and reliability of the Valuation of Lost Productivity Questionnaire. J Occup Environ Med. 2011;53(5):530–6.
31. McCormick N, Marra CA, Sadatsafavi M, Kopec JA, Avina-Zubieta JA. Excess productivity costs of systemic lupus erythematosus, systemic sclerosis, and Sjogren's syndrome: a general population-based study. Arthritis Care Res (Hoboken). 2019;71(1):142–54.
32. Bojke L, Spackman E, Hinde S, Helliwell P. Capturing all of the costs in NICE appraisals: the impact of inflammatory rheumatic diseases on productivity. Rheumatology (Oxford). 2012;51(2):210–5.
33. Koopmanschap MA, Rutten FF, van Ineveld BM, van Roijen L. The friction cost method for measuring indirect costs of disease. J Health Econ. 1995;14(2):171–89.

34. Targoutzidis A. Some adjustments to the human capital and the friction cost methods. Eur J Health Econ. 2018;19(9):1225–8.
35. Kariburyo F, Xie L, Sah J, Li N, Lofland JH. Real-world medication use and economic outcomes in incident systemic lupus erythematosus patients in the United States. J Med Econ. 2019:1–9.
36. Greco CM, Nakajima C, Manzi S. Updated review of complementary and alternative medicine treatments for systemic lupus erythematosus. Curr Rheumatol Rep. 2013;15(11):378.
37. Turchetti G, Yazdany J, Palla I, Yelin E, Mosca M. Systemic lupus erythematosus and the economic perspective: a systematic literature review and points to consider. Clin Exp Rheumatol. 2012;30(4 Suppl 73):S116.
38. Husereau D, Drummond M, Petrou S, Carswell C, Moher D, Greenberg D, et al. Consolidated health economic evaluation reporting standards (CHEERS) statement. PharmacoEconomics. 2013;31(5):361–7.
39. Gavan S, Bruce I, Payne K. Generating evidence to inform health technology assessment of treatments for SLE: a systematic review of decision-analytic model-based economic evaluations. Lupus Sci Med. 2020;7(1):e000350.
40. Yeo AL, Koelmeyer R, Kandane-Rathnayake R, Golder V, Hoi A, Huq M, et al. Lupus low disease activity state is associated with reduced direct healthcare costs in patients with systemic lupus erythematosus. Arthritis Care Res (Hoboken). 2019;72(9):1289–95.
41. Furie R, Petri M, Zamani O, Cervera R, Wallace DJ, Tegzová D, et al. A phase III, randomized, placebo-controlled study of belimumab, a monoclonal antibody that inhibits B lymphocyte stimulator, in patients with systemic lupus erythematosus. Arthritis Rheum. 2011;63(12):3918–30.
42. Urowitz MB, Ohsfeldt RL, Wielage RC, Kelton KA, Asukai Y, Ramachandran S. Organ damage in patients treated with belimumab versus standard of care: a propensity score-matched comparative analysis. Ann Rheum Dis. 2019;78(3):372–9.
43. Morand EF, Furie R, Tanaka Y, Bruce IN, Askanase AD, Richez C, et al. Trial of anifrolumab in active systemic lupus erythematosus. N Engl J Med. 2020;382(3):211–21.
44. Wallace DJ, Furie RA, Tanaka Y, Kalunian KC, Mosca M, Petri MA, et al. Baricitinib for systemic lupus erythematosus: a double-blind, randomised, placebo-controlled, phase 2 trial. Lancet. 2018;392(10143):222–31.

# Index





Z. Touma (ed.), *Outcome Measures and Metrics in Systemic Lupus Erythematosus*, https://doi.org/10.1007/978-3-030-73303-2

## C